MOSBY'S EMERGENCY DICTIONARY

EMS, Rescue, and Special Operations

SECOND EDITION

Edited by

Bill Garcia, MICP
Paramedic Special Operations Analyst
Trident Operations
Knoxville, TN

MOSBY Inc.
A *Harcourt Health Sciences Company*
St. Louis   Philadelphia   London   Sydney   Toronto

MOSBY Inc.
A *Harcourt Health Sciences Company*

Dedicated to Publishing Excellence

Second Edition

Mosby Inc.
11830 Westline Industrial Drive
St. Louis, Missouri 63146

Library of Congress Cataloging in Publication Data
Mosby's emergency dictionary : EMS, rescue, and special operations /
 edited by Bill Garcia. -- 2nd. ed.
     p.   cm.
  Includes bibliographical references.
  ISBN 0-8016-7941-9
  1. Emergency medicine--dictionaries.   I. Garcia, Bill.
  [DNLM: 1. Emergency Medicine--dictionaries.   W 13 M894 1997]
  RC86.7.M883   1998
  616.02'5'03--dc21
  DNLM/DLC
                        97-34822

00 01 / 9 8 7 6 5 4 3

Dedicated
to my sons,
Anthony and Eric Garcia,
and
to the memory of my grandfather,
William Donald Gibson, M.D.,
author, historian, and
one of the last country doctors

DEDICATION TO THE FIRST EDITION

JAMES G. YVORRA

This first edition of *Mosby's Emergency Dictionary* is dedicated to James G. Yvorra. On January 29, 1988, as this project was nearing completion, Jim was killed while attempting to provide emergency care to victims of an automobile accident on Washington D.C.'s Capitol Beltway. At the time of his death, Jim held the rank of Volunteer Deputy Fire Chief with the Prince George's County, Maryland, Fire Department (Berwyn Heights Station).

Jim Yvorra was born in Elwood City, Pennsylvania, in 1952. After graduating from high school, he attended Indiana University of Pennsylvania, where he received his B.A. in English and journalism. He began his career in 1974 as an EMS education and training coordinator for Pennsylvania's Lycoming, Sullivan, and Tioga counties.

From 1976 to 1978, Jim served as senior instructor with the Maryland Fire and Rescue Institute at the University of Maryland's main campus in College Park. During his tenure, he was responsible for certifying more than 1,000 emergency medical technicians throughout the state.

In 1978, Jim joined the Robert J. Brady Company in Bowie, Maryland, where he was executive editor of emergency medical and fire service publications. While at Brady, he worked on an impressive list of projects, including *Emergency Care, Trench Rescue,* and *Investigating the Fire Ground.*

In 1983, Jim formed his own publishing company. His first book was Alan Brunacini's highly acclaimed text, *Fire Command.* Other works include the recently published *Hazardous Materials: Managing the Incident.*

Jim was dedicated to the emergency response profession. His friends and coworkers will miss him deeply. We hope that the *Emergency Dictionary* continues Jim's work by providing an additional asset to your response program.

FOREWORD

The old saying really is true: If you're not careful, you might get what you wish for. It was 1989 and the first edition of *Mosby's Emergency Dictionary* had just been published. For emergency medical services personnel who were previously frustrated by the lack of EMS terms in traditional medical dictionaries, the new book that represented *their* vocabulary was gladly received.

But *Mosby's Emergency Dictionary* wasn't without its critics. In a review in *Rescue* magazine, technical editor and paramedic Bill Garcia celebrated the book's arrival and recommended it to all EMTs and paramedics, but also pointed out its shortcomings in the way of rescue terminology and "basic concepts of EMS, like telemetry and defensive driving." He wrote that the book was "not bad for a first edition, but not *great* either." We all know where those kinds of comments can get us: "Well, if you're so smart, why don't *you* do it?" And in fact, editor Nancy Peterson challenged Garcia to walk the walk and write the second edition. When he took on the project, Bill Garcia never imagined what an awesome task he had before him.

The second edition has over 7,800 terms, more comprehensive coverage of rescue and special operations, and the EMS basics Garcia desired. Equally important is the comprehensive reference guide in the Appendices, which includes everything from windchill charts to an airway sizing guide. From rookie first-responders to the most seasoned paramedics, readers will find the virtual alphabet soup of EMS vocabulary is made clear and understandable. Garcia went back to the first "Orange EMT Book" and gleaned information from all the latest paramedic, EMT, and rescue texts to update the old words and add new ones. His own curiosity spurred him to find the origins and histories of words: "ambulance," he found, was coined by Napoleon in 1805 when he used the term *Ambulance Volantes* to describe the French "war wagons."

In modern EMS, proper usage of vocabulary and terminology is more important than ever. It can be easily argued that communication is as important a rescue skill as administering oxygen or cutting a "B" post. All emergency services and public safety personnel, from street EMTs to administrators, must be able to write and converse in the unique language of EMS and rescue. When that communication falters, so too does the way we work with each other and the way we treat our patients. Clear and understandable communication is vital to our doing a good job.

This has resonance for me and for the rest of the editorial staff at *JEMS (Journal of Emergency Medical Services)* and *Fire-Rescue Magazine.* Each magazine we produce monthly has close to 40,000 words. Every single one of those words must be correct and understood by our readers. Sometimes the acronyms and jargon can be overwhelming. It's our job to sift through the sea of words to ensure the reader can easily process the writer's thoughts. I have no doubt our editors and our paramedic and EMT authors in the field will have a copy of *Mosby's Emergency Dictionary: EMS, Rescue, and Special Operations* (second edition) close at hand as we create our magazines each month. This new reference is a giant step toward documenting in an easy-to-read style the depth and breadth of our emergency services vocabulary.

While you probably won't be packing this book in your trauma kit and hauling it on calls, you'd do well to keep a copy at the station or at home. Clear written and spoken communication will help get us what we wish for—raising the level of EMS as a profession and providing better care for our patients.

Jeff Berend
Associate Publisher, *JEMS/Fire-Rescue Magazine*

PREFACE

Emergency Medical Services (EMS) as we know them today developed in the late 1960s in Ireland and the United States. Programs in the United States developed sporadically, depending on geography and need. Although many systems developed based on nearby systems, a great deal of isolation existed among EMS providers, and techniques and equipment were developed only as needs were perceived. Procedures of care, and tools and tricks of the trade, were not shared beyond their local areas until after the majority of systems developed, so there was a great deal of "reinventing the wheel." Much of this isolation did not end until around the time our profession placed itself on a more scientific basis during the 1980s. As emergency medical research has grown and contact among providers has been stimulated by new technology and the need to compare ideas, EMS has found itself drawn increasingly to areas of medical care considered nontraditional.

Although the rescue profession has been with us since before system development, the two professions did not grow together. Fire departments and rescue squads assimilated new types of equipment and increasing levels of professionalism, but these organizations generally considered EMS as a separate function, devoted to caring for the patient only after the patient was rescued. Likewise, EMS providers declared that they were "too busy" and that rescue was "not our job."

Research and experience have shown us the need for competent care during rescue. Rapid progression of an evolution is also necessary so that the victims of trauma may be safely, but expeditiously, moved to the surgeons who hold the key for definitive resolution of their injuries.

Across the country today, teams of EMTs and paramedics provide patient care and rescue on land, sea, and air. Helicopter rescue/aeromedical care, wilderness search and rescue (SAR), dive rescue, confined space rescue, vehicle extrication, cave/mine rescue, urban SAR, and technical rescue all have EMS providers as their practitioners. Increases in public awareness of emergency care and of changes in legislative funding for medical care have added mass-gathering EMS and interhospital critical care transport to emergency services' list of challenges.

With the rise of domestic and international terrorism, drug use, and crime in general, law enforcement agencies are better funded and more sophisticated than ever before. Their awareness of both trauma (medical and legal implications) and community relations has led to a demand for the availability of advanced-level care. EMS providers are meeting this challenge with new equipment, advanced patient assessment techniques, demanding physical fitness requirements, weapons qualifications, and training in law enforcement, special weapons and tactics, and antiterrorism.

These capabilities are inevitably fusing into special operations teams within emergency medical/fire services.

Along with this expansion of EMS' arena of operations comes the need for standardization of terminology and access to important information. Understanding disciplines outside the spectrum of medical care has been a necessity that will grow in the future.

English is a rich and living language with the world's largest vocabulary (over a million words). This vocabulary has been published in dictionary or encyclopedic form since the mid-1700s, with the first *American Dictionary of the English Language* published by Noah Webster in 1828. Increasing sophistication of our civilization has given rise to many specialty dictionaries, allowing practitioners to standardize the terminology of their professions. The availability of common, known language is the foundation of all civilization.

A dictionary can also tell a story by relating terminology and biographical information about those responsible for our past, by giving us the information we need to effectively function in the present, and by presenting information that we will use to create the future. Collectively, dictionaries represent what we are and what we have been.

It is hoped that the volume you are holding will provide you a foundation from which to learn and grow within one of the most interesting occupations yet developed by humankind.

Bill Garcia
Knoxville, Tennessee
February, 1997

AUTHOR ACKNOWLEDGMENTS

Some of the contributions to this project were direct and aimed at producing this book, whereas others were, by example, an inspiration that stretched my abilities or brought me greater understanding.

Thom (Dick) Hillson, Richard Land, and Chris Olson—You are among the EMS pioneers; you set the example for those who follow.

Stephen Roberts, Dave Schloss, Linda Sheldone, and Sergeants Sang Moua and Wayne White, USMCR—There are no bonds stronger than those forged on the blackest of nights.

Many thanks to Captain Bill Sorensen (SEAL), USNR, Major Timothy Armstrong, USMC, and HM1 (FMF) Craig Bennett, USN.

To Nancy Peterson, Christi Mangold, Cecilia Reilly, and Claire Merrick at Mosby Lifeline—thank you. Without your encouragement, ideas, and support, this project would not be a reality.

Thanks also to Bonnie Davis of the U.S. Navy Experimental Diving Unit and Sherley Tsagris of the California Emergency Medical Services Authority.

To Anita Masterson goes my love and heartfelt thanks. Problem solving, layout and artwork, manuscript preparation and review, and patience were never beyond your capabilities. Without you, this book would not exist.

Publisher Acknowledgments

The editors wish to acknowledge and thank the many reviewers of this book, who devoted countless hours to intensive review. Their comments were invaluable in helping develop and fine-tune this manuscript.

Randall W. Benner, MEd, NREMT-P
Instructor of Health Professions
Director of Emergency Medical Technology
Youngstown State University
Youngstown, Ohio

Brenda Crawford-Garcia
Paramedic—Hartson Medical Services
San Diego, California

Lafond Davis
Paramedic—Evergreen Medic One
Redmond, Washington

Robert Elling, MPA
Elling & Associates
Quality Educational Endeavors
Niskayuna, New York

Mark Hanshue
Helicopter Rescue Swimmer/EMT—U.S. Navy
Naval Air Test Center
Patuxent River, Maryland

Anita Masterson, RN, CEN, TNCC
Medical Case Manager
Knoxville, Tennessee

Steve McGraw, REMT-P
Assistant Professor, Department of Emergency Medicine
The George Washington University
Washington, DC

Joseph J. Mistovich, MEd, NREMT-P
Chairperson, Department of Health Professions
Associate Professor of Health Professions
Youngstown State University
Youngstown, Ohio

William Raynovich, NREMT-P, MPH, BS
Senior Program Manager
EMS Academy
University of New Mexico
Albuquerque, New Mexico

Norman W. Rooker, EMT-P
City of San Francisco
Department of Public Health
Paramedic Division
San Francisco, California

S. Rutherfoord Rose, Pharm D, FAACT
Director, Carolinas Poison Center
Clinical Associate Professor,
Department of Emergency Medicine
Carolinas Medical Center
Charlotte, North Carolina

Mick J. Sanders, EMT-P, MSA
Training Specialist
St. Charles, Missouri

Consultants to the First Edition

Donna C. Aguilera, PhD, FAAN
Consultant in Clinical Psychology
Beverly Hills, California

Matt Anderson
Training Coordinator
Emergency Medical Services Section
Juneau, Alaska

Kathleen G. Andreoli, DSN, FAAN
Vice President for Educational Services
Interprofessional and International Programs;
Professor of Nursing
University of Texas
Health Science Center at Houston
Houston, Texas

Miriam G. Austrin, RN, BA
Allied Health Care Consultant;
Past Coordinator-Director
Medical Assistant Program
St. Louis Community College
St. Louis, Missouri

Diane M. Billings, RN, MSEd
Associate Professor of Nursing
Indiana University School of Nursing
Indianapolis, Indiana

Violet A. Breckbill, RN, PhD
Dean and Professor, School of Nursing
State University of New York at Binghamton
Binghamton, New York

Carolyn H. Brose, EdD, RN
President, Nu-Vision, Inc.
Liberty, Missouri

Charlene D. Coco, RN, MN
Assistant Professor of Nursing
Louisiana State University Medical Center
School of Nursing, Associate Degree Program
New Orleans, Louisiana

Mary H. Conover, RN, BS
Instructor of ECG and Arrhythmia Workshops
West Hills Hospital
Canoga Park, California
and throughout the western United States

Helen Cox
Principal Nurse Educator, School of Nursing
St. Vincent's Hospital
Ascot Vale, Victoria
Australia

Joyce E. Dains, RN, MSN
Assistant Professor of Nursing
University of Texas
Health Science Center at Houston,
Houston, Texas

Rene A. Day, RN, MSc
Associate Professor, Faculty of Nursing
University of Alberta
Edmonton, Alberta
Canada

Pamela Bakhaus doCarmo, MS, REMT/P
Associate Professor, Program Head
Emergency Medical Services Technology
Northern Virginia Community College
Annandale, Virginia

James J. Dillon, Jr.
Fire/Emergency Ambulance Division
Washington, DC

Gerald M. Dworkin, Consultant
Lifesaving Resources
Springfield, Virginia

Craig Dunham, MS, EMT-P
Tecumseh, Michigan

Claire M. Fagin, PhD, FAAN
Dean and Professor
University of Pennsylvania
School of Nursing
Philadelphia, Pennsylvania

A. Jolayne Farrell, RN, MPH
Gerontological Consultant
Toronto, Ontario
Canada

William F. Finney, MA, RT
School of Allied Medical Professions
Ohio State University
Columbus, Ohio

Richard D. Flinn
Executive Director, Pennsylvania Emergency
Health Services Council
Camp Hill, Pennsylvania

Marilyn E. Flood, RN, PhD
Associate Director of Nursing
University of California Hospitals
San Francisco, California

Catherine Ingram Fogel, RNC, MS
Associate Professor
School of Nursing
Department of Primary Care
University of North Carolina
Chapel Hill, North Carolina

Anne Gray, MEd, BA, DipNEd
Head, Department of Nursing
Kuring-gai College of Advanced Education
Lindfield, New South Wales
Australia

Janet Gray, BSN, MA
Nursing Assistant Program, Wascana Institute
Regina, Saskatchewan
Canada

Susan J. Grobe, RN, PhD
Associate Professor
University of Texas at Austin
Austin, Texas

Maureen W. Groër, RN, PhD
Professor of Nursing
University of Tennessee, Knoxville
College of Nursing
Knoxville, Tennessee

Janet A. Head, RN, REMT-A
Associate Director for Basic Life Support Programs
Emergency Medical Training Department
Kansas University Medical Center
Kansas City, Kansas

Jane Hirsch, RN, MS
Assistant Director of Nursing
Assistant Clinical Professor
Department of Biodysfunction
School of Nursing
University of California
San Francisco, California

Eugene M. Johnson, Jr., PhD
Professor, Department of Pharmacology
Washington University Medical School
St. Louis, Missouri

Virginia Burke Karb, RN, MSN
Assistant Professor
University of North Carolina at Greensboro
School of Nursing
Greensboro, North Carolina

Judith Belliveau Krauss, RN, MSN
Associate Dean and Associate Professor
Psychiatric Mental Health Nursing
Yale University School of Nursing
New Haven, Connecticut

Mavis E. Kyle, RN, MHSA
Assistant Dean, Associate Professor
College of Nursing
University of Saskatchewan
Saskatoon, Saskatchewan
Canada

Linda Armstrong Lazure, RN, MSN
Creighton University
School of Nursing
Omaha, Nebraska

Sgt. Art Long
California Highway Patrol
Emergency Planning Officer

Maxine E. Loomis, RN, PhD, FAAN
Professor and Assistant Dean, Professional
Development
University of South Carolina
College of Nursing
Columbia, South Carolina

Jannetta MacPhail, RN, PhD, FAAN
Dean and Professor, Faculty of Nursing
University of Alberta
Edmonton, Alberta
Canada

Ann Marriner, RN, PhD
Professor, Graduate Department of Nursing
Administration and Teacher Education
Indiana University
School of Nursing
Indianapolis, Indiana

Edwina A. McConnell, RN, MS
Independent Nurse Consultant
Madison, Wisconsin

Janice M. Messick, RN, MS, FAAN
Consultant
Laguna Hills, California

Patricia A. Mickelsen, PhD
Associate Director
Clinical Microbiology Laboratory
Stanford University Hospital
Stanford, California

Susan I. Molde, RN, MSN
Associate Professor
Yale University School of Nursing
New Haven, Connecticut

Mary N. Moore, PhD, RN
School of Nursing
University of Pennsylvania
Philadelphia, Pennsylvania

Helen K. Mussallem, OC, BN, MA, EdD, OStJ, LLD, DSc, FRCN, MRSH
Special Advisor to National and International
Health-Related Agencies;
Former Executive Director, Canadian Nurses Association
Ottawa, Ontario
Canada

Susan Jenkinson Neuman, RN, BA
Nursing Practice Officer
College of Nurses of Ontario
Toronto, Ontario
Canada

Marie L. O'Koren, RN, EdD, FAAN
Dean, School of Nursing
University of Alabama In Birmingham
Birmingham, Alabama

Kathleen Deska Pagana, RN, MSN
Instructor of Nursing
Lycoming College
Williamsport, Pennsylvania

Ann M. Pagliaro, RN, MSN
Associate Professor, Faculty of Nursing
University of Alberta
Edmonton, Alberta
Canada

Anne Griffin Perry, RN, MSN
ANA-Certified Adult Nurse Practitioner;
Associate Professor, Graduate Nursing Program—
Cardiopulmonary Option
School of Nursing
St. Louis University
St. Louis, Missouri

Susan Foley Pierce, RN, MSN
University of North Carolina
Chapel Hill, North Carolina

Patricia A. Potter, RN, MSN
Clinical Director of Surgical Nursing
Barnes Hospital
St. Louis, Missouri

Jack D. Preston, DDS
Harrington Professor of Esthetic Dentistry;
Director, Advanced Education in Prosthodontics
University of Southern California
School of Dentistry
Los Angeles, California

Betti Reiber, RN
Director of Installation and Training, Clinicom
Denver, Colorado

Ginette Rodger, RN, BScN, MNAdm
Executive Director, Canadian Nurses Association
Ottawa, Ontario
Canada

Charlotte Searle, DPhil, RN
Professor and Head, Department of Nursing
Science
University of South Africa
Pretoria, South Africa

Carolyn R. Schmidt
EMS Administrator/Certification
Office of Emergency Medical Services
Arkansas Department of Health
Little Rock, Arkansas

Kay See-Lasley, MS, RPh
Medical Editorial Consultant,
Writer/Consultant in Medicine and Christian
Literature
Board Member, Chairman of Missions
Christian Pharmacy Fellowship International
Lawrence, Kansas

Susan Budassi Sheehy, RN, MSN, CEN
Clinical Nurse Specialist
Emergency and Ambulatory Services
St. Joseph Hospital and Health Care Center
Tacoma, Washington;
Associate Professor of Clinical Nursing
Department of Physiological Nursing
University of Washington School of Nursing
Seattle, Washington

Sandra L. Siehl, RN, MSN
Oncology Clinical Nurse Specialist
The Jewish Hospital of St. Louis
Washington University Medical Center
St. Louis, Missouri

Margretta M. Styles, RN, EdD, FAAN
University of California
San Francisco, California

Mary Ann Talley, BSN, MPA
Program Director of EMS Education
University of South Alabama
Mobile, Alabama

June D. Thompson, RN, MS
Assistant Professor of Nursing
University of Texas
Health Science Center at Houston
Houston, Texas

Freida B. Travis, EMT, MEd
EMS Training Coordinator, State of Florida
Tallahassee, Florida

Diana M. Uhler, RN
Department of Dermatology
Gundersen Clinic, Ltd.
La Crosse, Wisconsin

Lerma Ung
Senior Lecturer, Department of Clinical Nursing
Phillip Institute of Technology
School of Nursing
Bundoora Campus
Bundoora, Victoria
Australia

Mildred Wellbrock, MSc
Instructor Coordinator
EMT Program at Wichita State University
Wichita, Kansas

Pam West, RN, MSN
Director, Emergency Medical Services Division
Texas Department of Health
Austin, Texas

Lucille Whaley, RN, MS
Pediatric Nurse Specialist;
Formerly Professor of Nursing
San Jose State University
San Jose, California

Casie Williams, RN, MEd
Southern Region EMS Council, Inc.
Anchorage, Alaska

Bethany L. Wise, MS, MT(ASCP)CLS
Instructor, Medical Technology Division
School of Allied Medical Professions
Ohio State University
Columbus, Ohio

GUIDE TO THE DICTIONARY

This book is a dictionary, but it is also a reference work in that it defines both words and facts. The information presented is related to Emergency Medical Services, Rescue, and Special Operations.

This information is presented in a single alphabetical listing without regard to the category of information being presented. The body of vocabulary defines current words that relate to many overlapping fields of endeavor. While there is not always agreement on definitions for many terms, there is usually consensus. This consensus is used whenever possible.

Entries are alphabetized in dictionary style rather than telephone-book style. Therefore, hyphens and spaces are disregarded in listing entries. Numbers are positioned as though they were spelled out, but subscript and superscript numbers are disregarded entirely. With few exceptions, compound headwords (any alphabetized and non-indented defined terms that consist of more than one word) are given in their natural order (as amniotic fluid rather than fluid, amniotic; or radiation sickness, not sickness, radiation).

Pronunciation is emphasized using the system found in most English dictionaries today. That is, all symbols for English sounds are ordinary letters of the alphabet with few adaptions. The exception to this rule is the use of the schwa (the neutral vowel), /ə/.

Medical spelling is consistent with current acceptable usage. Where there is more than one form of spelling, common American usage prevails.

Terms that might normally be abbreviated are spelled out (CPR will be found as cardiopulmonary resuscitation). Standard abbreviations are found within the main body of vocabulary only when necessary to improve clarity. A separate comprehensive list of abbreviations is found in the appendices.

Terms involving concepts of the future have been included as they can be anticipated. Likewise, words that may now be obsolete or outdated are not accidental. Many of these terms are from sources decades or centuries old and are included for historical interest.

Drugs incorporated into the vocabulary are those used primarily in emergency care and they are listed by generic name.

Other features include the following:

• Appendices—information is included here that would be confusing or difficult to locate in the main body of terms, such as tables, charts, and drawings.

• Biographical information—people important to the development of emergency medicine and rescue are described with the concepts to which they are connected. Infrequently, some people may be found listed alphabetically by last name when sufficient information about them is available and a separate listing was deemed more appropriate.

• Cross references—terms related to a defined word are listed at the end of an entry to facilitate a greater understanding of the word/topic.

See also terms are related to the defined word and can be found elsewhere in the vocabulary.

Compare terms are those that may be confused with the defined word but are usually related. They are also found within the body of the vocabulary.

Also known as terms are synonyms (additional terms for the same concept) and may be defined elsewhere in the vocabulary.

PRONUNCIATION KEY

Vowels

SYMBOLS	KEY WORDS
/a/	hat
/ä/	father
/ā/	fate
/e/	flesh
/ē/	she
/er/	air, ferry
/i/	sit
/ī/	eye
/ir/	ear
/o/	proper
/ō/	nose
/ô/	saw
/oi/	boy
/ōō/	move
/o͞o/	book
/ou/	out
/u/	cup, love
/ur/	fur, first
/ə/	(the neutral vowel, schwa, always unstressed, as in) ago, focus
/ər/	teacher, doctor

Consonants

SYMBOLS	KEY WORDS
/b/	book
/ch/	chew
/d/	day
/f/	fast
/g/	good
/h/	happy
/j/	gem
/k/	keep
/l/	late
/m/	make
/n/	no
/ng/	sing, drink
/ng•g/	finger
/p/	pair
/r/	ring
/s/	set
/sh/	shoe, lotion
/t/	tone
/th/	thin
/*th*/	than
/v/	very
/w/	work
/y/	yes
/z/	zeal
/zh/	azure, vision

Non-English sounds are represented by the following symbols:

/œ/   as in (French) **feu** /fœ/, **Europe** /œrôp´/; (German) **schön** /shœn/, **Goethe** /gœ´te/

/Y/   as in (French) **tu** /tY/, **déjà vu** /dāzhävY´/; (German) **grün** /grYn/, **Walküre** /vulkY´rə/

/kh/   as in (Scottish) **loch** /lokh/; (German) **Rorschach** /rôr´shokh/, **Bach** /bokh, bäkh/

/*kh*/   as in (German) **ich** /i*kh*/, **Reich** /rī*kh*/ (or, approximated, as in English **fish:** /ish/, /rīsh/)

/N/   This symbol does not represent a sound but indicates that the preceding vowel is a nasal, as in (French) **bon** /bôN/, **en face** /äNfäs´/, or **international** /aNternäsyōnäl´/.

/nyə/   Occurring at the end of French words, this symbol is not truly a separate syllable but an /n/ with a slight /y/ (similar to the sound in "onion") plus a near-silent /ə/, as in **Bois de Boulogne** /bo͞olō´nyə/, **Mal-gaigne** /mälgā´nyə/.

CONTENTS

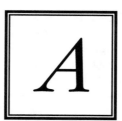

abalienation /abāl´yənā´shən/, a state of physical decline or mental illness.

abandonment, the termination of care by a medical provider without the patient's consent and without providing for continued care at the same treatment level or higher.

abarticulation /ab´ärtik´yəlā´shən/, dislocation of a joint.

abasia /əbā´zhə/, inability to walk.

Abbreviated Injury Scale, a trauma scoring system that categorizes injuries according to their severity. The scale divides the body into six regions, and it assigns a numerical score to each injury. Scores range from 1 to 6, with the higher scores reflecting more serious injury. Although used for blunt and penetrating injuries, the scale is more sensitive for blunt injury.

abdomen /ab´dəmən, abdō´mən/, the part of the body between the chest and the hips. The **abdominal cavity** holds part of the esophagus, stomach, small intestines, liver, gallbladder, pancreas, spleen, kidneys, and tubes (ureters) that deliver urine from the kidneys to the bladder.

abdominal regions, nine parts of the abdomen divided by four imaginary lines. The **epigastric region** is the upper middle abdomen, just below the breastbone. The **hypochondriac region** is the portion of the upper abdomen on both sides and beneath the lower ribs. The **inguinal region** is the part of the groin surrounding the inguinal canal. The **lateral region** is the part of the abdomen on both sides of the navel. The **pubic region** is the inferior portion of the intestinal area and below the umbilicus. The **umbilical region** is the part of the abdomen around the umbilicus.

abdominal thrust, a procedure used to generate high intrathoracic pressure during attempts to relieve complete airway obstruction caused by a foreign body. It involves using the hands to forcefully compress on the abdomen between the xiphoid process and navel. Also known as the **Heimlich maneuver** (named for American surgeon Henry J. Heimlich, 1920-).

abducens nerve /abdoo´sənz/, the sixth cranial nerve or oculomotor nerve.

abduction, movement away from the midline.

abductor, a muscle that moves a body part away from the midline of the body, or to move one part away from another, as the triceps muscle straightens the arm. Compare **adductor.**

aberrant /aber´ənt/, not found in the usual or expected course, such as a blood vessel that appears in an unusual place.

aberration, 1. any change from the normal course or condition. **2.** abnormal growth. **3.** a thought or belief lacking reason. **4.** poor image caused by unequal bending of light rays through a lens.

ability, being able to act because of skill and fitness.

abiotrophy /ab´ē·ot´rəfē/, an early loss of energy or the breakdown of certain parts of the body, usually because of a lack of certain foods. **–abiotrophic,** *adj.*

abirritant /abir´ətənt/, a substance that relieves irritation.

ablation, the act of removing a growth or damaged tissue.

abnormal behavior, acts outside the range of that considered normal. May range from short-term inability to deal with a stress to total withdrawal from the realities of everyday life. *See also behavior disorder.*

abnormal psychology, the study of mental and emotional dysfunctions, such as neuroses and psychoses. It also includes normal states not fully understood, such as dreams and other states of consciousness.

abort, **1.** termination of a pregnancy before the fetus is able to survive. *See also abortion, miscarriage.* **2.** to end anything in the early stages, as to stop the course of a disease.

abortifacient /əbôr´tifā´shənt/, a substance that causes abortion.

abortion, a spontaneous or deliberate ending of pregnancy before the fetus can be expected to survive. The end of a pregnancy before the twentieth week is called an **embryonic abortion.** With a **fetal abortion,** the pregnancy ends after the twentieth week but before the fetus is able to live outside the uterus. The intentional ending of a pregnancy before the fetus has developed enough to live is called an **induced abortion.** A **criminal abortion** is the intentional ending of pregnancy under any condition not allowed by law. An **elective abortion** refers to ending a pregnancy by choice of the woman. A **therapeutic abortion** refers to ending the pregnancy as thought necessary by a physician. A **complete abortion** is one in which the fetus or embryo is entirely removed. **Incomplete abortion** refers to an end of pregnancy in which the products of conception are not entirely expelled or removed. A **tubal abortion** is a condition in which an embryo implants outside the uterus in the fallopian tube. *See also dilation and curettage, miscarriage.*

abortus, a fetus weighing less than 600 g (1⅓ pounds) at time of abortion.

abrasion, a scraping or rubbing away of a surface. It is usually the result of injury. Compare **laceration.**

abreaction, an emotional release from recalling a painful past event. *See also catharsis.*

abruptio placentae, parting of the placenta from the uterus before birth, often resulting in severe bleeding. Compare **placenta previa.**

abscess, a cavity filled with purulent material and surrounded by red, swollen tissue. It forms as a result of a local infection. Healing usually occurs after it drains or is opened. A **cold abscess** is an infection that does not show the usual signs of edema, injection, and warmth.

abscissa /absis´ə/, one of two coordinates used as a point of reference, usually in a graph. This coordinate is in the horizontal plane, which lies at a right angle to the vertical, or y axis. Also known as x **axis.** *See also ordinate.*

abseil /ab´sāl/, a rappel from the top of a structure to a lower level; a roof rappel. It is used primarily for rapid access to a floor below the roof level and involves entering through a window or door.

absolute expansion, the true expansion of a liquid without regard to the expansion of its containing vessel.

absolute humidity, humidity as measured by the number of grams of water vapor present in 1 cubic meter of air.

absolute pressure, total barometric pressure exerted. This pressure value is derived by adding the atmospheric pressure to the gauge pressure. *See also atmospheric pressure, gauge pressure.*

absolute refractory period, **1.** the time during which any cell, capable of responding to a stimulus, is unable to respond. **2.** that period of the cardiac cycle during which the heart cannot respond to electrical stimulation. After each depolarization, the heart must redistribute its electrical charge across the myocardial membranes before it can accept another stimulus. This period corresponds with the time from the beginning of the QRS complex to the peak of the T wave. *See also relative refractory period.*

absolute scale, the Kelvin scale of temperature measurement.

absolute temperature, a temperature scale in which absolute zero corresponds to the absence of any molecular movement; 273 kelvins (K) is the temperature at which water freezes, and 373 K is the temperature at which water boils. The increments are equal. Also known as the **Kelvin temperature scale.**

absolute zero, the temperature at which no molecular movement occurs; the lowest temperature that can be reached on the Kelvin scale. *See also absolute temperature.*

absorbed dose, the energy imparted to matter by ionizing radiation. The unit of absorbed dose is the rad.

absorbifacient /-fā´shənt/, anything that aids absorption.

absorption, taking one substance into another, as dissolving a gas in a liquid or removing a liquid with a sponge.

absorption rate constant, a value that describes how much drug is taken up by the body in a given amount of time.

abstinence, choosing to avoid some activity, such as no food during a religious day.

abuse, inappropriate or harmful treatment or use.

abutment, the supporting structure of a bridge.

acalculia /a´kalko͞o´lyə/, the inability to solve simple mathematic problems.

acampsia /əkamp´sē·ə/, a defect whereby a joint becomes rigid. *See also ankylosis.*

acanthocyte /əkan´thəsīt´/, abnormal red blood cells with spurlike projections. **Acanthocytosis** refers to the presence of acanthocytes in the blood.

acanthoma /ak´ənthō´mə/, any tumor of the skin.

acanthosis /ak´ənthō´sis-/, a thickening of the skin, as in eczema and psoriasis.

acarbia /akär´bē·ə/, a decrease in the bicarbonate level in the blood.

acariasis /ak´ərī´əsis/, any disease caused by an acarid mite. Several types can infect humans. *See also chigger, scabies.*

acathisia /ak´əthizh´ə, ak´əthize·ə/, an inability to remain seated because doing so causes severe anxiety; an urgent restlessness accompanies this anxiety. It is generally seen as a complication of phenothiazine administration. Also spelled as **akathisia, akatizia.**

accelerated A-V conduction, abnormal conduction between the atria and the ventricles that allows electrical impulses to initiate ventricular depolarization earlier than usual. Such rapid conduction occurs due to aberrant conduction pathways that bypass the A-V node and bundle of His. It may be precipitated by certain drugs or by medical conditions, such as myocardial infarction. Also known as **anomalous conduction, preexcitation.** *See also delta wave, Lown-Ganong-Levine syndrome, preexcitation, Wolff-Parkinson-White syndrome.*

accelerated junctional rhythm, EKG rhythm characterized by narrow QRS complexes at a rate between 60 and 100 per minute. P waves are either absent or abnormally formed and are found at locations other than normal. Pulses are usually present.

accelerated ventricular rhythm, EKG rhythm characterized by ventricular complexes at a rate between 40 and 100 per minute. Pulses may or may not be present with this rhythm. Also known as **accelerated idioventricular rhythm.**

acceleration, the rate at which speed, or velocity, increases.

acceleratory forces, those physical forces exerted on aircraft occupants during landing, takeoff, and turning maneuvers. **Centrifugal acceleratory force** is a stress encountered during aircraft turns. **Linear acceleratory force** is encountered during vertical or horizontal flight. Although these stresses are of major concern during flights involving high-performance aircraft and space flight, they also may compromise patients with limited cardiopulmonary function onboard air ambulances.

accessory, a structure that serves one of the main systems of the body. For example, the hair, the nails, and the sweat glands are accessories of the skin.

accessory muscle, any secondary muscle that assists a primary muscle in function.

accessory nerve, either of a pair of nerves needed for speech, swallowing, or movements of the head and shoulders. Also known as **eleventh cranial nerve.**

acclimate /əklī´mit, ak´limāt/, to adjust to a different climate, especially to changes in altitude and weather.

accommodation (A, acc, Acc), the state of adapting to something, such as the ongoing process of a person to adjust to his or her surroundings, both physically and mentally. **Visual accommodation** refers to the way the eye is able to change its focus while seeing things either close up or far away.

accretion /əkrē´shən/, **1.** growth or increase. **2.** the growing together of parts that are normally separated. **3.** the gathering of foreign material, especially within a hole.

Ace bandage, trade name for a woven, cotton-elastic bandage. This bandage is used in prehospital care as a pressure bandage to decrease hemorrhage and to provide support to an injured extremity. The name is commonly used and has often been corrupted to denote any bandage possessing similar qualities. Also known as **ace, ace wrap, elastic bandage.**

acetabulum /as´ətab´yələm/, *pl.* **acetabula,** the large, cup-shaped, hip socket holding the ball-shaped head of the femur.

acetoacetic acid /as´ətō·əsē´tik/, a colorless organic acid found in normal urine in small amounts and large amounts in the urine of patients with diabetes (ketoacidosis).

acetone /as´ətōn/, a colorless, sweet-smelling liquid found in normal urine and in large amounts in the urine of patients with diabetes.

acetylcholine /as´ətilkō´lēn/, a chemical nerve transmission mediator in the body that allows messages to travel from one nerve to another.

acetylcholinesterase /-es´tərās/, an enzyme that blocks acetylcholine. It reduces or prevents the movement of nerve impulses.

acetylsalicylic acid /as´ətilsal´əsil´ik/. See **aspirin.**

achalasia /ak´əlā´zhə/, the inability of a muscle to relax.

ache, a pain that is steady and dull. An ache may be local, such as a stomach ache or headache. It may be systemic, such as the ache of flu. *See also pain.*

Achilles tendon /əkil´ēz/, the tendon of the calf muscles. It is the thickest and strongest tendon in the body. It begins in the midline of the posterior leg and connects to the heel. Also known as **calcaneal tendon.**

Achilles-tendon reflex. See **deep tendon reflex.**

achlorhydria /ā´klôrhī´drē·ə/, a state in which hydrochloric acid is missing from the gastric juice in the stomach.

acholia /əkō´lyə/, **1.** the absence or decrease of bile fluids. **2.** anything that stops the flow of bile from the liver into the small intestine.

achondroplasia /ākon´drōplā´zhə/, a hereditary condition with growth of cartilage in the long bones and skull. The bones fuse prematurely. Growth stops and dwarfism results.

achylia /əkī´lyə/, a lack of hydrochloric acid and pepsinogen needed for digesting food in the stomach.

achylous /əkī´ləs/, **1.** a lack of gastric or other digestive juices. **2.** lack of chyle, a milky fluid made in the intestines during digestion.

acid, 1. a substance that turns blue litmus paper red, has a sour taste, and reacts with bases to form salts. *See also alkali.* **2.** *(slang)* **LSD.** See **lysergide.**

acid-base balance, the phenomenon in which the body makes acids and bases at the same rate they are removed. *See also acid, base.*

acid-base metabolism, biochemical reactions involving changes in hydrogen ion concentration. These reactions maintain a balance of acid and base. Disruption of this metabolism may cause acidosis or alkalosis. Among the numerous causes are cardiac arrest, diarrhea, diabetes, drug use, emesis, and kidney disease. *See also acidosis, alkalosis, metabolism.*

acid dust, highly acidic bits of dust that collect in the air, causing much of the smog over cities. High levels can be dangerous for patients with respiratory problems. *See also acid rain.*

acidophilic adenoma /as´idōfil´ik/, a tumor of the pituitary. These can cause the pituitary to make excess growth hormone, causing abnormal growth.

acidosis, lower than normal pH due to increased hydrogen ion concentration; increased acidity in the body. When this occurs due to inadequate respirations, it is known as **respiratory acidosis. Metabolic acidosis** occurs when the chemical processes of the body are impaired in their function. *See also acid-base metabolism, alkalosis, metabolism.*

acid phosphatase, an enzyme found in the kidneys, blood serum, semen, and prostate. *See also alkaline phosphatase.*

acid rain, rain with high acid content caused by air pollution from industry, motor vehicles, and other sources.

acinus /as´inəs/, *pl.* **acini,** any small saclike structure. Also known as **alveolus.**

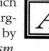

acmesthesia /ak´misthē´zhə/, the feeling of a pinprick or a sharp point touching the skin.

acneform drug eruption, an acnelike skin response to a drug.

acne rosacea. See **rosacea.**

acoria /akôr´ē·ə/, state of always being hungry even when the desire for food is small.

acousma /əkōōz´mə/, hearing sounds which are not there.

acoustic, referring to sound or hearing.

acoustic nerve, a pair of nerves important to hearing. The nerves connect the inner ear with the brain. Also known as **eighth cranial nerve.**

acoustic trauma, a loss of hearing. This can be caused by loud noise over time. A sudden loss of hearing may be caused by an explosion, a blow to the head, or other accident. Hearing loss may be temporary or permanent, partial or total. *See also deafness.*

acquired, a feature, state, or disease that happens after birth. It is not inherited but is a response to the environment. Compare **congenital, familial, hereditary.**

acquired immune deficiency syndrome (AIDS) /ādz/, a disease of the system that fights infection. The cause is a virus called HIV, spread through exchange of body fluids, as in sexual intercourse. Symptoms are extreme fatigue, fever, night sweats, loss of appetite with weight loss, severe diarrhea, and depression. As the disease progresses, the patient is subject to many infections. A form of pneumonia (*Pneumocystis carinii*) often occurs, as does meningitis or encephalitis. The death rate is 90% for patients who have had the disease more than 2 years.

acrid, sharp, bitter, and unpleasant to the smell or taste.

acrocyanosis, cyanosis of the hands or feet due to decreased circulation. The term is particularly used to describe the skin condition of a newborn infant. Also known as **Raynaud's sign.** *See also hypothermia.*

acrodynia, a disease of infants with digestive disturbances, extremity edema, and skin lesions on the hands and feet. Later stages of disease are characterized by arthritis and muscle weakness. Although mercury may be involved in the process, the cause is unknown. Also known as **erythredema, pink disease.**

acromegaly /-meg´əlē/, a disorder in which bones of the face, jaw, arms, and legs grow larger. It occurs in middle-aged patients, caused by excess growth hormone. *See also gigantism, growth hormone.*

acromioclavicular joint /-mī´əkləvik´yələr/, the hinge between the clavicle and scapula.

acromion /əkrō´mē·ən/, the lateral portion of the scapula. It forms the highest point of the shoulder and connects with the clavicle.

acrophobia, a fear of heights. *See also phobia.*

ACTH. See **adrenocorticotropic hormone.**

actin, a protein in muscles that helps them contract and relax.

actinomycosis, an animal fungal disease sometimes transmitted to humans. It causes lesions in the brain, lungs, GI tract, and mandible. The slow-growing lesions discharge purulent drainage in later stages. Also known as **lumpy jaw.**

action potential, a differential in the electrical charge across a cellular membrane.

activated charcoal, a substance that adsorbs toxins from the GI tract and prevents absorption into the circulation. Side effects include nausea and vomiting. If ipecac is to be used in conjunction, charcoal should not be administered prior to ipecac-induced emesis.

activator, a substance, force, or device that stimulates activity.

active transport, the movement of solute across cellular membranes in a process that requires the consumption of energy. This process is utilized by the body to move substances against the concentration differences that exist between the inside and outside of a cell.

activity, the rate at which a particular material decays. It is generally expressed in terms of the average number of nuclear disintegrations per second. Since this number is generally large, it is given in units of curies or fractions thereof. *See also curie.*

acuity, **1.** the clarity of one of the senses, as visual acuity. **2.** seriousness.

acute, **1.** sudden onset, usually within 12 hours. **2.** serious. **3.** intense, sharp. *See also chronic.*

acute abdomen, acute abdominal pain in which emergency surgical intervention must be considered. Diarrhea, nausea, or vomiting may also occur. Pain can be a symptom of most abdominal conditions, including appendicitis, constipation, cholecystitis, and pelvic inflammatory disease.

acute care, treatment for serious illness or trauma. Compare **chronic care.**

acute health hazard, marked by a single dose or exposure generally having a sudden onset, as in acute toxicity or acute exposure.

acute mountain sickness, a syndrome occurring after rapid ascent to altitudes above 2500 m (about 7500 ft) that begins with headache, malaise, and nausea. If progression beyond mild sickness occurs, anorexia, ataxia, and dry cough may be noted. Difficulty with walking is the most useful sign for determining a progression from mild to severe. Alterations in level of consciousness follow, with unconsciousness occurring as soon as 24 hours after onset of ataxia. Oxygen administration and/or descent to lower altitudes terminates symptoms. Also known as **AMS.** *See also high-altitude cerebral edema, high-altitude pulmonary edema.*

acute stress reaction, sudden alteration of behavior and thought process due to a high level of stress for which an individual may be unprepared. Although the stress may be negative or positive, it usually involves negative stressors.

Adam's apple, *(informal)* the bulge on the anterior neck made by the thyroid cartilage of the larynx. Also known as **laryngeal prominence.**

adaptation, a change or response to stress.

addiction, disease characterized by a compulsion to use mind- or mood-altering substances or to be in certain situations to an extent that the patient is unable to maintain normal relationships and lifestyles. Examples include alcohol, drugs, gambling, and sex.

Addison's disease, a life-threatening condition caused by partial or complete adrenal gland failure. Symptoms are weakness, lack of appetite, weight loss, anxiety, and sensitivity to cold. The onset is usually gradual. Causes include autoimmune diseases, infection, tumor, or bleeding in the adrenal gland.

additive effect, the combined effect of two drugs that have similar effects. The combination creates an effect much more pronounced than either drug creates alone. *See also potentiation, synergism.*

adduction, movement of a limb toward the body. Compare **abduction.**

adductor, a muscle that acts to draw a part toward the midline of the body. The **adductor brevis** is a triangular muscle in the thigh. It acts to pull and turn the thigh toward the midline of the body and to bend the leg. The **adductor longus** is the superior of the three adductor muscles of the thigh. It flexes the thigh. The **adductor magnus** is the long, heavy, triangular muscle in the middle of the thigh. Compare **abductor, tensor.**

adenectomy /ad´ənek´təmē/, the removal by surgery of any gland.

adenitis /ad´ənī´tis/, an inflammation of a lymph gland.

adenoid /ad´ənoid/, one of two pharyngeal tonsils on the posterior throat, behind the nasal space. During childhood these masses often swell with infected material and block air passing from the nose to the throat, preventing the child from breathing through the nose.

adenoidal speech, a muted, nasal way of speaking caused by large adenoids.

adenoidectomy /-ek´-/, removal of the adenoids. *See also tonsillectomy.*

adenoma /ad´ənō´mə/, a tumor that develops from glandular tissue.

adenopathy /ad´ənop´əthē/, the enlargement of any gland, especially a lymph gland. –**adeno-pathic,** *adj.*

adenovirus, a virus that infects the respiratory and GI tract.

adhesion, a band of scar tissue that binds two surfaces. This occurs most commonly in the abdomen after surgery, inflammation, or injury.

Adie's syndrome, a disorder of the eyes in which one pupil reacts much more slowly to light or focusing than the other.

adipocele /ad´ipōsel´/, organ or tissue protruding through an opening. Also known as **lipocele.**

adiponecrosis /-nikrō´-/, breaking down of fatty tissue in the body. –**adiponecrotic,** *adj.*

adipose /ad´ipōs/, tissue made of fat cells. *See also fat, fatty acid, lipoma.*

adipsia /ədip´sē·ə/, absence of thirst.

adjustment reaction, a sudden response to great stress in people who have no mental illness. It may occur at any age and can be mild or severe. Symptoms include withdrawal, depression, crying spells, and loss of appetite. *See also neurotic disorder.*

administrative law, regulations and rules established by agencies formed by federal or state legislatures. The legislative statutes establishing these agencies give them their authority. *See also common law, constitutional law, statutory law.*

adnexa, *sing.* **adnexus,** tissue or structures in the body that are next to or near another structure. The ovaries and the uterine tubes are adnexa of the uterus.

adnexitis, an inflammation of the adnexal organs of the uterus, such as the ovaries or the fallopian tubes.

adolescence, the time in growth between the onset of sexual maturity (puberty) and adulthood. This usually begins between 11 and 13 years of age, when breast growth, beard growth, pubic hair growth, and other related changes occur (secondary sex characteristics). It spans the teen years, and ends at 18 to 20 years of age when the person has a fully developed adult body. During this time the adolescent undergoes great physical, psychologic, emotional, and personality changes. *See also puberty.*

adrenal crisis, a life-threatening decrease of glucocorticoid made by the adrenal cortex. There is a drop in fluids, such as blood, urine, and saliva, and hyperkalemia. The patient develops low blood pressure and may have Addison's disease. The cause for the adrenal crisis is not known. Infection is a common cause of crisis in patients who have Addison's disease.

adrenalectomy /-ek´-/, removal of one or both adrenal glands.

adrenal gland, the gland that sits on the superior portion of each kidney. The gland has two parts: the cortex and the medulla. The **adrenal cortex** is the outer part of the gland. It is divided into three parts. The **zona glomerulosa** is the outer portion of the adrenal cortex. The middle portion (**zona fasciculata**) acts together with the innermost segment (**zona reticularis**) in producing male sex hormones (androgens) and some female sex hormones (estrogen and progesterone). They also produce hormones (aldosterone and hydrocortisone) that aid in fluid balance. The inner portion of the gland is the **adrenal medulla.** It produces epinephrine and

norepinephrine to regulate blood pressure and heart rate.

adrenalin, 1. substance manufactured in the adrenal gland and used to stimulate the body during time of heavy work or stress. This hormone acts to speed the heart, constrict blood vessels, and dilate the bronchi. **2.** a natural catecholamine used in the treatment of allergic reactions, anaphylaxis, and cardiac dysrhythmias. Side effects include supraventricular tachycardias and ventricular irritability. There are no contraindications for field use. Also known as **epinephrine.**

adrenaline /ədren´əlin/. See **epinephrine.**

adrenalize /ədrē´nəlīz/, to stimulate or excite.

adrenergic /ad´rinur´jik/, nerves that release epinephrine or epinephrine-like substances. Compare **cholinergic.** *See also sympathomimetic.*

adrenergic blocking agent. See **antiadrenergic.**

adrenergic drug. See **sympathomimetic.**

adrenocorticotropic hormone (ACTH), a hormone made by the pituitary gland that stimulates the growth of the adrenal gland cortex and secretion of corticosteroids. ACTH secretion is controlled by the hypothalamus. ACTH increases when a patient has stress, fever, or low blood sugar. Commercially made ACTH is used to treat rheumatoid arthritis, severe allergy, skin diseases, and many other disorders. Also known as **corticotropin.**

adsorb, to attract and adhere a gas or liquid to a solid.

adulteration, a lowering of quality and purity of any substance, process, or act.

adult respiratory distress syndrome, increased capillary permeability due to illness or injury, which causes pulmonary edema and results in acute respiratory failure. The increased permeability reduces lung compliance and decreases perfusion capacity across alveolar membranes. Also known as **ARDS, Da Nang lung, noncardiogenic pulmonary edema, shock lung.**

advanced life support, an intervention that utilizes cardiac monitoring, advanced airways, and pharmacology for the treatment of life-threatening emergencies. This term refers to care given prehospital or in-hospital. Also known as **ALS.**

adventitia, the outer covering of an organ or structure.

adventitious, a state that is brought on by accident or random action.

adventitious bursa, a defect of the liquid sacs in a joint due to friction or pressure.

adverse drug effect, a harmful side effect of a drug given in normal amounts.

adynamia /ad´īnā´mē·ə/, physical and mental fatigue caused by disease.

AEIOU TIPS, an acronym used to remember the causes of altered levels of consciousness: **A**cidosis/**A**lcohol, **E**pilepsy, **I**nfection, **O**verdose, **U**remia, **T**rauma, **I**nsulin, **P**sychogenic, and **S**troke.

aerate /er´āt/, to mix with air or other gas.

aerial torch, an ignition device suspended under a helicopter, capable of dispensing ignited fuel to the ground for assistance in backfiring or burnout.

aerobe /er´ōb/, a microorganism that needs oxygen to live and grow. Compare **anaerobe.**

aerobic exercise, any physical exercise that makes the heart and lungs work harder to meet the muscles' need for oxygen. Running, bicycling, swimming, and cross-country skiing are types of aerobic exercise. Also known as **aerobics.** See also exercise.

aerobic metabolism, body processes that function most efficiently or can take place only in the presence of oxygen.

aerodontalgia /er´ōdontal´jə/, pain in the teeth caused by air trapped in the teeth when the air pressure changes, as may occur at high altitudes.

aerophagia /er´ōfā´jə/, swallowing air, often leading to stomach upset and gas.

aerosinusitis, inflammation or bleeding of the sinuses, caused when air expands in the sinuses. This occurs when air pressure drops. Also known as **barosinusitis.**

aerosol, 1. small particles in a gas or air. 2. a gas under pressure that contains an inhaled drug.

Aerospace Rescue and Recovery Service, rescue agency of the United States Air Force that operates the Air Force Rescue Coordination Center and the rescue resources of the Air Force. Included in the operations of the Rescue and Recovery Service are long-range rescue resources available around the world. These resources include personnel trained in emergency medical care, parachuting, skiing, survival, and water rescue who are transported from fixed- and rotary-wing aircraft. The parachute jumpers, or PJs, originally known as **paramedics,** are used during combat and peacetime search and rescue. Also known as **ARRS.** See also Air Force Rescue Coordination Center.

aerotitis media, soreness or bleeding in the middle ear, caused by a difference between air pressure inside the middle ear and outside. This occurs with changes in altitude or depth. Symptoms include pain, tinnitus, and vertigo. Also known as **barotitis media.**

Aesculapius /es´kyəlā´pē·əs/, Latin name for the Greek god of medicine. An ancient symbol for healing and medicine was a stick with a snake wound around it, known as the **staff of Aesculapius.**

affect, the way in which a person's feelings are exhibited. –**affective,** adj.

afferent /af´ərənt/, moving toward the center of an organ or system. This usually refers to blood vessels, lymph channels, and nerves. Compare **efferent.**

affinity, an attraction between two substances.

aflatoxins, a group of poisons made by Aspergillus flavus food molds. These poisons cause liver necrosis and cancer in test animals. They are thought to be the cause of the high rate of liver cancer in people in regions of Africa and Asia who may eat moldy grains, peanuts, or other Aspergillus-infected foods. See also aspergillosis.

African sleeping sickness. See **trypanosomiasis.**

aft, toward the rear, or stern, of a ship or aircraft.

afterbirth, the material expelled from the womb after a baby is born.

afterdamp, the toxic gases that remain in a mine after an explosion of methane. See also firedamp.

afterdrop, a continued drop in core temperature following the removal of a hypothermic victim from a cold environment; it is caused by cooler peripheral blood being circulated back to the body core.

afterload, the pressure against which the left ventricle must eject blood during a contraction. The pressure is created by blood flow and the vessel walls themselves.

afterpains, cramps that often occur in the first days after giving birth.

agenesis /ājen´əsis/, **1.** birth without an organ or part. **2.** the state of sterility or impotence. Also known as **agenesia.** Compare **dysgenesis. –agenic,** *adj.*

ageniocephaly /ājen´ē·ōsef´əlē/, faulty skull growth in which the brain, skull, and sense organs are normal but the lower jaw is malformed.

agenitalism /ājen´itəlizm/, the absence of ovaries or testicles or problems of function. It is caused by lack of sex hormones.

Agent Orange, a U.S. military code name for a mixture of two chemicals, 2,4-D and 2,4,5-T, used to kill vegetation in Southeast Asia during the war in Vietnam. The compound contained the highly poisonous chemical dioxin. This chemical causes cancer and birth defects in animals and chloracne and long-term scarring in humans. *See also dioxin.*

agglutinin /əglo͞o´tinin/, an antibody that interacts with antigens by agglutination.

aggression, energetic activity of the body and mind which can be destructive or productive. **Destructive aggression** is an act of hostility that is not needed for self-protection. It is directed toward an object or person. **Inward aggression** is destructive behavior against oneself.

aging, the process of growing old, caused in part by a failure of body cells to function or to make new cells to replace those that are dead or defective. Cells may be lost through infection, poor nutrition, or gene defects. *See also senile.*

agitated, being in a state of physical and mental excitement evidenced by restless actions that have no purpose.

agitophasia /-fā´zhə/, rapid speech in which words, sounds, or parts of words are left out, slurred, or distorted. Also known as **agitolalia.**

agnosia /agnō´zhə/, total or partial loss of the ability to know familiar objects or persons, due to brain damage. The state may affect any of the senses and is noted as auditory, visual, olfactory, gustatory, or tactile agnosia. **Body-image agnosia** is an inability to recognize and identify the parts of one's own body.

agonal respiration, irregular breathing pattern seen immediately prior to respiratory arrest. These shallow, gasping, ineffective respirations are most commonly witnessed immediately after cardiac arrest.

agonal rhythm, EKG rhythm typically seen in the last stages of myocardial hypoxia. Although characterized by an irregular bradycardia, the complexes may vary in amplitude and duration. Also known as **dying heart rhythm.**

agonist /ag´ənist/, **1.** a contracting muscle that is opposed by another muscle (an antagonist). **2.** a drug or other substance that causes a known response.

agoraphobia /ag´ərə-/, fear of being alone in an open, crowded, or public place, such as a field, tunnel, bridge, or store, where escape may be difficult.

agranulocytosis /əgran´yəlōsītō´-/, a decrease in the number of white blood cells (granulocytes).

agraphia /əgraf´ē·ə/, the condition in which a patient can no longer write due to an injury to the language center in the brain.

agrypnotic /ag´ripnot´ik/, a substance that prevents sleep.

air, the atmosphere; the mixture of gases that surrounds the earth. It is made of 78% nitrogen; 21% oxygen; almost 1% argon; small amounts of carbon dioxide, hydrogen, and ozone; and traces of helium, krypton, neon, and xenon.

air bag, **1.** vehicular restraining device that protects occupants during an accident. Inflated bags decrease injury to front seat passengers; they inflate automatically on impact. **2.** extrication device used to lift vehicles for removal or to allow access to victims. These devices use high-pressure compressed air for inflation and come in varying sizes. Also known as **air lifting bag, lift bag.** *See also air cushion.*

airboat, flat-hulled boat propelled by a large fanlike propeller that is located above water on the rear of the vessel. This boat is used in areas of swamp or shallow water, where there is not enough depth to allow safe use of a submerged propeller.

airborne transmission, the movement and spread of disease vectors through air, as by coughing or sneezing.

air chisel, air-powered chisel used as a cutting tool during vehicle extrication. *See also air gun.*

air cushion, extrication device utilizing low-pressure compressed air for lifting thin-skinned vehicles. Even though these bags are constructed of thinner material than air bags and are more susceptible to damage, the low pressure prevents their penetration of the thin skin of an aircraft or truck trailer. *See also air bag.*

air cushion vehicle, vehicle that travels on a cushion of air created by propellers between the vehicle and ground or water surface. Also known as **ACV, hovercraft, skim.** *See also hovercraft.*

air cylinder, any container that can hold a supply of compressed air for breathing or tool operation. Also known as **BA cylinder, SCBA cylinder, scuba tank.**

air embolism. See **embolism.**

Air Force Rescue Coordination Center, the operations center for coordination of all civilian and military search and rescue activities within the contiguous, 48 states. Located at Scott Air Force Base, near St. Louis, Missouri, the Center is operated by Air Force personnel. Also known as **AFRCC.**

airframe, the parts and structure of an aircraft that pertain to flight, such as cowlings, fuselage, landing gear, nacelles.

air gun, pneumatic chisel used as an extrication cutting tool for heavy-gauge metal, particularly on trains and trucks. *See also air chisel.*

air hole, an air pocket encountered during flight.

air purifier, an air-purification system for compressed breathing air.

airspeed, the speed of an aircraft in relation to the air. It is not necessarily the same as ground speed.

air splint, a clear, plastic inflatable splint used to immobilize a suspected extremity fracture and/or control extremity bleeding.

air tanker, any fixed-wing aircraft certified by the FAA as being capable of transporting and delivering fire-retardant solutions.

air traffic control, the agency that exercises control over air traffic by operating major airport control towers; in the United States it is the Federal Aviation Administration.

air trapping, inability of air to escape from portions of the lung owing to bronchospasm, infection, or thickened secretions. The pressure of trapped air may be higher than surrounding pressure, increasing the danger of embolism or pneumothorax.

airway, **1.** the passageway for air movement in and out of the body. The airway consists of the mouth and nose, pharynx, trachea, bronchi, bronchioles, and alveoli. **2.** any device that corrects or prevents an obstruction of the airway, such as an **endotracheal tube, oral airway, or nasal airway. 3.** a ventilation passageway inside a mine.

airway obstruction, complete or partial blockage of a respiratory passageway. *See also airway.*

akathisia. See **acathisia.**

akinesia /āˊkinēˊzhə/, an abnormal state of physical and mental inactivity or inability to move the muscles.

Akja /äˊchä/, a rigid transport litter used for snow evacuation. Constructed of aluminum, it has a rounded bottom to facilitate towing by skiers. *See also rigid transport vehicles.*

ala /āˊlə/, *pl.* **alae,** any winglike structure.

alanine (Ala) /alˊənin/, an amino acid found in many proteins in the body. It is broken down by the liver. *See also amino acid, protein.*

alanine aminotransferase (ALT), an enzyme normally present in blood serum and tissues of the body, especially the tissues of the liver. Also known as **glutamic-pyruvic transaminase.**

alar ligament /āˊlər/, one of a pair of ligaments that joins the cervical vertebra (axis) to the occipital bone at the base of the skull and limits head movement.

alarm reaction, the first stage of adapting. One uses the many defenses of the body or the mind to cope with a stress. *See also stress.*

albinism /alˊbinizm/, a birth defect marked by partial or total lack of pigment in the body. Total albinos have pale skin that does not tan, white hair, and pink eyes. Compare **piebald, vitiligo.**

albumin /albyo͞oˊmin/, a protein found in almost all animal tissues and in many plant tissues.

albumin (human), substance that expands blood volume and is used for treating hypovolemia.

Alcock's canal, a canal formed by the muscles in the pelvis (obturator internus muscle and the obturator fascia). The nerves and vessels affecting the outer sex organs pass through the canal. Also known as **pudendal canal.**

alcohol, 1. (USP) an organic compound that contains between 92.3% and 93.8% ethyl alcohol, used as a sink cleanser and solvent. **2.** a clear, colorless liquid that is made by brewing sugar with yeast, such as beer or whiskey. **3.** a compound derived from a hydrocarbon.

Alcoholics Anonymous (AA), a worldwide nonprofit group founded in 1935, whose members are alcoholics who no longer drink. The purpose of AA is to help others stop drinking and develop sobriety.

alcoholism, an illness characterized by a loss of control over alcohol consumption and chronic alcohol overuse. The etiology is unknown; prolonged alcohol use causes cirrhosis, malnutrition, and neurological disorders. *See also delirium tremens.*

alcohol poisoning, an acute intoxication with (usually) ethyl alcohol, causing unconsciousness, which may progress to respiratory/cardiac arrest. Also known as **acute alcoholism.**

aldolase /al´dəlās/, an enzyme in muscle tissue that is necessary for storing energy in the cells.

aldosterone /al´dōstərōn´, aldos´tərōn/, a steroid hormone made by the adrenal cortex that controls sodium and potassium in the blood. *See also adrenal gland.*

aldosteronism /al´dōstərō´nizm/, a state in which there is an increase in aldosterone. Increased aldosterone causes the body to retain salt and lose potassium. Symptoms include increased blood pressure, weakness, paresthesias, nephropathy, and congestive heart failure. Also known as **hyperaldosteronism.**

aldosteronoma /al´dōstir´ənō´mə/, an aldosterone-secreting tumor (adenoma) of the adrenal cortex that causes the body to retain salt and to increase blood volume and blood pressure.

aleukemic leukemia /ālōōkē´-/, a type of leukemia in which the white blood cell count is normal and few abnormal leukocytes are found in the blood. Also known as **subleukemic leukemia.** *See also leukemia.*

aleukia /ālōō´kē·ə/, a marked decrease or total lack of white blood cells or blood platelets.

alexia /ələk´sē·ə/, a nervous system defect, in which the person cannot understand written words. Compare **dyslexia. –alexic,** *adj.*

algologist /algol´-/, a person who studies or treats pain.

alienation, the act or feeling of being separated from others or isolated. *See also depersonalization disorder.*

alimentary canal. See **digestive system.**

alkali /al´kəlī/, a compound with the chemical qualities of a base. Alkalis join with acids to make salts, turn red litmus paper blue, and enter into chemical reactions. *See also acid, base.* **–alkaline,** *adj.;* **alkalinity,** *n.*

alkaline-ash /al´kəlīn/, substance in the urine that has a pH higher than 7.

alkaline phosphatase, an enzyme in bone, kidneys, intestine, blood, and teeth. It may be present in the blood serum in high levels in some diseases of bone or liver.

alkaloid, any of a large group of organic compounds, both natural and synthetic, such as atropine, caffeine, cocaine, morphine, nicotine, and procaine.

alkalosis, an increase in the body's alkalinity. **Metabolic alkalosis** occurs with heavy vomiting, not enough minerals, or increased adrenal hormones. Symptoms include dyspnea, headache, nausea, vomiting, and tachycardia. **Respiratory alkalosis** occurs with low blood levels of carbon dioxide and large amounts of alkali in the blood. Causes include asthma, pneumonia, aspirin poisoning, anxiety, fever, and liver failure. Symptoms include lightheadedness, numbness of the hands and feet, muscle weakness, and tachypnea. Compare **acidosis.**

alkaptonuria /alkap´tənur´ē·ə/, a genetic disorder that causes incomplete metabolism of the amino acids phenylalanine and tyrosine. This causes a darkening of the urine and may lead to a condition of dark pigmentation known as **ochronosis.**

alkylating agent /al´kilā´ting/, substance that causes a disruption of cell division, especially in fast-growing tissue. Such drugs are useful in the treatment of cancer. Types of alkylating agents include the alkyl sulfonates, the ethylenimines, the nitrogen mustards, the nitrosoureas, and the triagenes. The most widely used agent is cyclophosphamide.

allergen /alˊərjən/, a foreign substance that can cause an allergic response in the body. Some common allergens (antigens) are pollen, dust, feathers, and various foods. Some people are immune to allergens, but in others the immune system may be sensitive to foreign substances and even substances made by the body. –**allergenic,** *adj. See also allergy, antigen.*

allergic reaction, a reaction of the body (antibody response) to any substance (antigen) to which it has developed a hypersensitivity. It is characterized by erythema, pruritus, and urticaria with no corresponding decrease in blood pressure. *See also anaphylactic shock.*

allergy, a reaction to generally harmless substances. Allergies are classified according to how the body's cells react to the allergen. Allergies are also divided into acute and chronic. *See also allergy testing.*

allergy testing, any one of the many tests used to find the allergens that cause allergy. Skin tests are used most often for allergy testing.

allocated resources, resources dispatched to an incident that have not yet checked in with the incident communications center.

allogenic, **1.** a being or cell that is from the same species but looks distinct due to different genes. **2.** referring to tissues that are transplanted from the same species but have distinct genes.

allopathic physician, a doctor who treats disease and injury with active treatments, as medicine and surgery. Almost all doctors in the United States are allopathic. Compare **chiropractic, homeopathy.**

allopathy /əlopˊəthē/, a system of treatment in which a disease is treated by creating a state in which it cannot thrive. For example, an antibiotic that kills a certain germ is given for an infection.

all-or-none principle, a rule that states that when a cell is stimulated it either responds completely or not at all.

alloxan /alˊoksən/, a substance found in the intestine in diarrhea. Because it can kill the cells of the pancreas that secrete insulin, alloxan may cause diabetes.

aloe /alˊō/, the juice of the varied species of *Aloe* plants.

alopecia /alˊəpēˊshə/, partial or complete loss of hair that results from aging, hormone defects, drug allergy, anticancer treatment, or skin disease. *See also baldness.*

alpha (α), the first letter of the Greek alphabet, often used in chemistry to denote one type of a chemical compound from others.

alpha adrenergic receptor, any of the adrenergic chemical receptor tissues that respond to norepinephrine and various blocking agents.

alpha particle or alpha radiation, alpha particles are ejected spontaneously from the nuclei of some radioactive elements. The alpha particle is identical to a helium-4 nucleus ($^4_2$He), which has an atomic mass number of 4 and an electrostatic charge of +2. It has low penetrating power and short range. The most energetic alpha particle will generally fail to penetrate the skin. The major hazard occurs when matter containing alpha-emitting nuclides is introduced into the body. Symbol: α.

alpha receptor, the nerve cells to which norepinephrine and certain drugs attach. When attached, the receptors cause the blood vessels to get smaller, the pupils of the eyes to get bigger, and some skin muscles to contract. Compare **beta receptor.**

alpha-tocopherol. See **vitamin E.**

alphavirus, any of a group of very small viruses made of a single molecule. Many alphaviruses live in the cells of insects and are given to humans through insect bites.

altered state of consciousness, any state of awareness that differs from normal consciousness.

alternobaric vertigo, transient vertigo, nausea, and tinnitus occurring due to increased pressure in the inner ear. The symptoms can occur before or after equilibration of pressure on the ears and can be seen during pressure changes. The vertigo can last from a few seconds to 15 minutes and may cause vomiting or disorientation.

altitude sickness. See **acute mountain sickness, polycythemia.**

alum, a substance that causes the skin cells to contract (astringent). It is used mainly in lotions and douches.

aluminum (Al), a widely used metal and the third most abundant of all the elements. It is found in many antacids, antiseptics, astringents, and styptics. Aluminum salts, such as aluminum hydroxychloride, can cause allergies in some people. Aluminum hydroxychloride is the most often used agent in antiperspirants.

alveolar ventilation, the exchange of oxygen for carbon dioxide and other waste products between the alveoli and pulmonary capillaries.

alveolectomy /-ek´-/, removal of part of the mandible to take out a tooth, change the line of the mandible after tooth removal, or prepare the mouth for false teeth.

alveolitis /al´vē·əlī´-/, an inflammation of the tiny air sacs in the lungs. *See also hypersensitivity pneumonitis.*

alveolus /alvē´ələs/, *pl.* **alveoli,** a small saclike structure, such as one of the tiny air sacs in the lungs.

alymphocytosis /əlim´fəsītō´-/, an abnormal decrease in the number of white cells (lymphocytes) in the blood.

Alzheimer's disease /älts´hīmərz, ôls´-/, a form of brain disease that can lead to confusion, memory loss, restlessness, and hallucinations. The patient may refuse food and lose bowel or bladder control. The disease often starts in late middle life with slight defects in memory and behavior. The exact cause is not known, but breakdown of the cells of the brain occurs. Also known as **senile dementia-Alzheimer type (SDAT).**

Amanita /-ī´tə/, a genus of mushrooms. Some species, such as *Amanita phalloides,* are poisonous if eaten, causing hallucinations, stomach upset, and pain. Liver, kidney, and nervous system damage can result.

amasesis /am´əsē´-/, a defect in which the person is not able to chew food. This may be caused by failure of the chewing muscles to function, crowded teeth, poorly fitted false teeth, or a mental problem.

amaurosis /am´ôrō´-/, blindness caused by something outside the eye, as by a disease of the optic nerve or brain, diabetes, kidney disease, or poisoning from alcoholism.

amaurosis fugax /am´ôrō´sis foo´gäks/, temporary, unilateral vision loss due to diminished blood flow to the eye. Amaurosis is due to arterial spasm, glaucoma, hypertension, or trauma. Also known as **transient blindness.**

ambient air standard /am´bē·ənt/, the highest amount allowed of any air pollutant, such as lead, nitrogen dioxide, sodium hydroxide, or sulfur dioxide.

ambient pressure, the pressure of the environment that exists at a particular altitude or depth; the pressure surrounding a person at any particular moment.

ambivalence /ambiv´ələns/, **1.** a state in which a person has conflicting feelings, attitudes, drives, or desires, such as love and hate, tenderness and cruelty, pleasure and pain. To some degree, ambivalence is normal. **2.** the state of being uncertain or unable to choose between opposites.

amblyopia /am´blē·ō´pē·ə/, reduced vision in an eye that appears to be normal.

ambu-bag. See **bag-valve mask.**

ambulance, transportation and treatment vehicle for the sick or wounded. The U.S. Department of Transportation categorizes ground vehicles into Type I (truck chassis with modular ambulance body), Type II (van type), and Type III (van chassis with modular ambulance body).

ambulance volantes, *(historical)* horse-drawn carriages designed during the Napoleonic Wars (1805) to transport the ill and injured. This invention was adopted in the United States in 1835 when the U.S. Army implemented ambulance transport during the Seminole War.

ambulatory, able to walk; referring to a patient who is not confined to bed.

ambulatory care, health services given to those who come to a hospital or other health care center and who leave after treatment on the same day.

ambulatory surgery center, a health care center that deals with relatively minor surgeries, which do not need overnight hospitalization.

ameba, any of a genus of microscopic, single-celled protozoa, which reproduce by binary fission. One species, *Entamoeba histolytica,* is found in the human colon and can cause amebic dysentery. Also known as **amoeba.**

amebiasis /am´ēbī´əsis/, an infection of the intestine or liver by an ameba, often *Entamoeba histolytica.*

amebic dysentery. See **dysentery.**

amelogenesis imperfecta, an inherited defect in which the teeth are yellow or brown in color where the dentin under the enamel is showing. Also known as **hereditary brown enamel.**

amenorrhea /ā´menôrē´ə/, the absence of the monthly flow of blood and discharge of mucous tissues from the uterus through the vagina (menstruation).

American Medical Association (AMA), a society composed of licensed physicians in the United States, which publishes journals and medical standards.

American Red Cross (ARC), a national organization that seeks to help people with many health, safety, and disaster relief programs. It is connected with the International Committee of the Red Cross. The Red Cross was begun at the Geneva Convention of 1864 and has more than 130 million members in about 3100 chapters. It depends largely on volunteers. The symbol for the American Red Cross is a red cross on a field of white.

Ameslan /am´islan/, abbreviation for American Sign Language, a way of communicating with the deaf. Words and letters are made with the hands and fingers.

ametropia /am´itrō´pē·ə/, an image seen incorrectly by the eye because of the way light is bent when it enters the eye. Astigmatism, farsightedness (hyperopia), and nearsightedness (myopia) are types of ametropia. –**ametropic,** *adj.*

amide-compound local anesthetic, a compound that causes a loss of feeling in an area. Some types are **bupivacaine, dibucaine, etiodocaine, lidocaine, mepivacaine, prilocaine.**

amino acid /am´inō, əmē´nō/, an organic compound necessary for forming peptides, a piece of protein, and proteins. Digestion releases the individual amino acids from food. Over 100 are found in nature, but only 22 occur in animals.

aminoaciduria /-as´ido͞or´ē·ə/, the abnormal presence of amino acids in the urine. It usually indicates an inborn chemical defect, as in cystinuria.

aminophylline /-fil´in/, a drug used in treating asthma, emphysema, and bronchitis. It is used with caution in patients in whom cardiac stimulation would be harmful. Side effects include stomach and intestinal upsets, tachycardia or irregular heart beat, and anxiety.

aminotransferase, an enzyme that helps move an amino group from one chemical compound to another. Aspartate amino transferase (AST) is present in blood and many tissues, especially the heart and liver. It is given off by cells that have been damaged. Also known as **transaminase.**

ammonia, a pungent colorless gas composed of nitrogen and hydrogen. It is used as a stimulant, a detergent, and an emulsifier.

amnesia, a loss of memory due to brain damage or severe emotional stress. **Anterograde amnesia** is the loss of memory of the events that occur after an injury. **Retrograde amnesia** is the loss of memory for events occurring before a set time in a patient's life, often before the event that caused the amnesia. The condition may result from disease, or injury.

amniocentesis /am´nē·ōsentē´-/, removing a small amount of the fluid (amniotic) in the womb during pregnancy. It is usually done between the sixteenth and twentieth weeks. Testing the fluid can reveal fetal abnormalities, such as Down's syndrome, spina bifida, and Tay-Sachs disease, as well as sex and age of the fetus.

amnion. See **amniotic sac.**

amniotic fluid /am´nē·ot´ik/, a liquid made by the amnion and the fetus. It usually totals about 1500 ml (a little over 1½ quarts) at 9 months. It surrounds the fetus during pregnancy, providing it with protection. It is swallowed, processed, and excreted as fetal urine at a rate of 50 ml (more than 2 ounces) every hour. Amniotic fluid is clear, though cells and fat give it a cloudy look.

amniotic sac, a thin-walled bag that contains the fetus and fluid during pregnancy. The wall of the sac extends from the edge of the placenta and surrounds the fetus. There are two layers of membranes forming the sac. The **amnion** is the inner layer. It contains the amniotic fluid. The **chorion** is the outermost of the two layers of membrane. This membrane at first contains fluid and loose pieces of tissue. As pregnancy proceeds, the amnion grows into the chorionic space. The chorion continues to expand around the fetus as it grows. In this way the amniotic sac protects the fetus and separates it from the wall of the uterus. Also known as **bag of waters.**

amperage, strength of electrical current flowing between two points; expressed in units of amperes or milliamperes.

AMPLE, a patient evaluation acronym that stands for **A**llergies, **M**edications, **P**ast medical history, **L**ast meal (or other oral intake), and **E**vents causing an emergency.

amplitude, amount; extent; size; the peak positive or negative value of a wave or signal. The height and depth, or waveform size, of an EKG complex is a reflection of its amplitude.

amplitude modulation, **1.** modulation of the amplitude of a carrier wave of constant frequency by varying the signal's strength. **2.** referring to a broadcasting system between 118 and 136 mHz that utilizes amplitude modulation. Also known as **AM.** *See also frequency modulation.*

ampule /am´pyo͞ol/, a small, sterile glass or plastic container.

ampulla /ampul´ə, -po͞ol´ə/, a rounded, saclike opening of a duct, canal, or tube, such as the tear duct, fallopian tube, or rectum.

amputation, the removal of a part of the body, often a leg, arm, finger, or toe.

amputee, a patient who has had one or more arms or legs amputated.

amygdalin /əmig´dəlin/, a chemical that is found in bitter almonds and apricot pits. Thought by some to be a cure for cancer, it is sold under the trademark of Laetrile. Also known as **vitamin B₁₇.**

amyl nitrate, a nitrate agent used in the treatment of cyanide poisoning. Although there are no contraindications for field use, this agent is most effective when used in conjunction with sodium thiosulfate.

amylo-, amyl-, a combining form referring to starch.

amyotonia /ā´mī·ətō´nē·ə/, a defect of the muscles, whereby the muscles lose tone and become weak. It is usually due to disease of the motor neurons.

amyotrophic lateral sclerosis (ALS) /-trof´ik/, a nervous system disease of the nerves that supply the muscle (motor neurons). It usually occurs in middle age and can cause death within 2 to 5 years. There is no known treatment. Also known as **Lou Gehrig's disease.**

anabolism /ənab´əlizm/, any process that produces energy in which simple substances are converted into more complex matter. It is a process that occurs in living matter. Compare **catabolism. –anabolic,** *adj.*

anadipsia /-dip´sē·ə/, extreme thirst. It often occurs in the manic phase of manic-depressive psychosis.

anaerobe /aner´ōb/, a microorganism that grows and lives without oxygen.

anaerobic infection, an infection caused by an anaerobic organism. It usually occurs in deep puncture wounds or any tissue that has decreased oxygen due to injury, cell death, or increased bacteria.

anal canal, the end of the intestinal tract, about 4 cm (about 1½ inches) long, that ends at the anus.

anal crypt, the area in the wall of the rectum that holds networks of veins. These veins can become enlarged (hemorrhoids). An **anal fistula** is an open sore on the skin surface near the anus, usually as a result of an infection of the anal crypt.

analeptic. See **central nervous system stimulant.**

analgesia, relief of pain.

analgesic /an´əljē´zik/, a drug that relieves pain. There are two kinds, narcotic and nonnarcotic.

analog /an´əlog/, **1.** something that is similar in appearance or function to another object. However, the source or final product differ, as in the eye of a fly and the eye of a human. **2.** a drug or other compound that acts like another substance but has different effects. Compare **homolog.**

analog signal, a waveform that communicates information by varying the signal's magnitude of strength.

analysis, **1.** the act of breaking down substances into their parts. It is done so that the nature and qualities of these parts may be understood. **Qualitative analysis** is naming the elements in a substance; **quantitative analysis** is the measurement of the amount of each element in a substance. **2.** *(informal)* psychoanalysis.

anaphase, a stage of mitosis that involves duplicate chromosomes migrating to two sides of a dividing cell. *See also prophase, metaphase, telophase.*

anaphylactic shock, decreased tissue perfusion occurring when the body is exposed to a substance (antigen) that causes a severe allergic reaction (antibody response). Symptoms include hives, pale and clammy skin, and urticaria, with a corresponding decrease in blood pressure. As with other low-resistance-types of shock, patients with anaphylaxis exhibit normal or bradycardic heart rates. *See also allergic reaction.*

anaplasia /-plā´zhə/, a breakdown in the structure of cells and in their relation to each other. Anaplasia occurs in cancer. Compare **metastasis. –anaplastic,** *adj.*

anasarca, general edema. Anasarca is often seen in kidney disease when fluid retention is a chronic problem. *See also edema.*

anastomosis /ənas´tōmō-/, joining two parts, such as blood vessels, to allow flow from one to the other. *See also aneurysm, bypass.*

anatomic curve, a normal curve of the segments of the spinal column. When looking at the spine from the side, the cervical curve is seen to go inward, as does the lumbar curve. The thoracic spine shows an outward curve.

anatomic dead space, that portion of the airway that conducts air from the external environment to the alveoli. The term "dead space" refers to the fact that blood oxygenation cannot occur in this portion of the airway—only in the alveoli.

anatomical position, standing erect with feet and palms facing forward.

anatomy, **1.** the study of structures and organs of the body. In **applied anatomy,** body structures in relation to disease are studied. **Comparative anatomy** relates the various stages of growth in different animals. **Cross-sectional anatomy** studies the relation of the structures of the body to each other. This involves examining cross sections of the tissue or organ. **Descriptive anatomy** is the study of the form and structure of various systems of the body, as the digestive system and the nervous system. **Gross anatomy** is the study of organs of parts of the body large enough to be seen with the naked eye. **2.** the structure of an organism. Compare **physiology.**

anchor, **1.** device that holds a boat or ship in a fixed position by weight and/or resistance due to its construction. Types include the Danforth, mushroom, Northill, and stockless. **2.** solid holding point used to attach carabiners, rope, or webbing for use during climbing or rappelling. Natural anchors include rocks and trees. Artificial anchors include bolts and hangers, chocks, and pitons. *See also anchor point, anchor system.*

anchor point, the place at which an anchor is attached. *See also anchor, anchor system.*

anchor system, two or more anchor points joined together to form a stable anchor for belaying, climbing, or rappelling. *See also anchor, anchor point.*

Andersen's disease. See **glycogen storage disease.**

andro-, andr-, a combining form referring to man or to the male.

androgen /an´drəjen/, any steroid hormone that increases growth of male physical qualities.

androgynous /androj´ənəs/, having some qualities of both sexes. Social role, behavior, personality, and appearance are not due to the physical sex of the person. **–androgyny,** *n.*

androsterone /andros´tərōn/, one of the male sex hormones (androgens). *See also testosterone.*

anecdotal, knowledge based on observations and not yet confirmed by scientific studies.

anemia, a decrease in red cells in the blood. The ability to carry oxygen is reduced. Anemia is noted by the hemoglobin content of the red cells and by red cell size. Depending on its severity, anemia may cause respiratory difficulty, fatigue, headache, and insomnia. With **aplastic anemia,** the bone marrow can no longer make blood cells. **Hemolytic anemia** is a disorder involving the premature destruction of red blood cells. **Hypochromic anemia** refers to any of a large group of anemias marked by decreased hemoglobin in the red blood cells. **Hypoplastic anemia** refers to a broad class of anemias marked by decreased production of red blood cells. **Microcytic anemia** has small red blood cells, linked to long-term blood loss or a disease of poor nutrition, such as iron deficiency anemia. **Anemia of pregnancy** results from a problem in the manufacture of erythrocytes, a loss of red blood cells through bleeding, or a lack of iron, folic acid, or vitamin B_{12}. *See also nutritional anemia, sickle cell anemia, antianemic.*

anencephaly /an´ənsef´əlē/, a birth defect in which there is no brain or spinal cord, the skull does not close, and the spinal canal remains a groove.

anergy, **1.** lack of activity. **2.** an immune defect in which the body fights off foreign substances inadequately. This state may be seen in advance tuberculosis, in AIDS, and in some cancers. **–anergic,** *adj.*

anesthesia, the lack of sensation, especially awareness of pain. It may occur due to an anesthetic drug or damage to nerve tissue. *See also general anesthesia, local anesthesia, regional anesthesia, topical anesthesia.*

anesthesiologist /an´əsthē´zē·ol´-/, a physician trained to administer anesthetics and to support the cardiovascular system during surgery. Also known as **anesthetist.**

anesthesiology, the branch of medicine that deals with the control of sensations of pain during surgery.

aneurysm /an´yo͞orizm/, a bulging of the wall of a blood vessel, usually caused by atherosclerosis and hypertension. It may be caused by injury, infection, or a congenital weakness in the vessel wall. Sign of an arterial aneurysm is a pulsating mass. An **aortic aneurysm** is a bulging of a portion of the thoracic or abdominal aorta. In many cases the first sign is rupture of the lesion. A **dissecting aneurysm** is one with a tear in one of the layers of the arterial wall, occurring most often in the aorta. Symptoms include severe pain and unequal pulses in the extremities. A **ventricular aneurysm** is one that occurs in the wall of the ventricle of the heart. Scar tissue may be formed as a result of inflammation caused by myocardial infarction. This tissue weakens the myocardium, allowing it to bulge outward when the ventricle contracts.

Intracranial aneurysm refers to any aneurysm of the cerebral arteries in the brain. Rupture results in mortality approaching 50%. There is high risk of recurrence in survivors. **Cerebral aneurysm** refers to one in the cerebrum. It is the result of congenital defect, infection, tumors, or injury. Depending on the size and location, symptoms may include headache, dizziness, weakness, and altered levels of consciousness. About half of all cerebral aneurysms rupture.

angiitis /an´jē·ī´-/, an inflamed state of a blood or lymph vessel.

angina /anjī´nə, an´jinə/, a symptom of some diseases that creates a feeling of choking, suffocation, or crushing pressure and pain. **Angina dyspeptica** is a painful state caused by gas swelling of the stomach. It has the same symptoms as angina pectoris. **Angina epiglottidea** refers to pain caused when the epiglottis becomes inflamed. **Angina pectoris** is a pain in the chest caused by oxygen deprivation to the heart. It is often linked to atherosclerosis of the heart. The pain may occur in the chest, arms, or jaw. It often occurs with a feeling of suffocation. Attacks are often related to exertion, emotional stress, and contact with intense cold. **Angina decubitus** is a type of angina pectoris that occurs when the patient is lying down. **Prinzmetal's angina** is a form that occurs during rest rather than from activity. With **streptococcal angina,** pain occurs as the result of a streptococcal infection. *See also Ludwig's angina.*

angiocardiogram /-kär´dē·ōgram/, an x-ray of the heart and its vessels. Dye that is visible on x-ray is injected into a vein that goes directly to the heart. X-rays are taken as the fluid passes through the heart and its vessels.

angiography /an´jē·og´rəfē/, x-ray study done with dye to locate myocardial infarction, vascular occlusion, tumors, and lung emboli. **Cerebral angiography** refers to dye studies of the brain.

angioneurotic, paralysis or spasm of blood vessels.

angioplasty, repair of damaged blood vessels.

angiospasm /an´jē·ōspazm´/, a sudden spasm of a blood vessel. Also known as **vasospasm.** *See also vasoconstriction.*

angiotensin /-ten´-/, a substance in the blood that causes blood vessels to constrict, raising blood pressure. It causes the hormone aldosterone to be released from the adrenal cortex.

angle,   the geometric relationships between surfaces.

angle of Louis,   the anatomical point where the manubrium joins the body of the sternum. The angle can usually be palpated as a protrusion on the superior portion of the sternum. Also known as **sternal angle.**

angle of repose,   the largest angle above a horizontal plane where loose material will rest, without sliding (trench rescue).

angular movement,   one of the four basic kinds of movement by the joints of the body. For example, the angle between the forearm and upper arm gets smaller when the arm is flexed and gets larger when the arm is extended. Compare **circumduction, gliding, rotation.**

angulated fracture,   a break in which the fragments of bone are angled.

anima /an´imə/,   **1.** the soul or life. **2.** the active substance in a drug. **3.** a person's true, inner being, as distinct from outward personality (persona). **4.** the female part of the male persona.

animus /an´iməs/,   **1.** the active or rational soul; the active agent of life. **2.** the male part of the female persona. **3.** a deep resentment that is under control but may assert itself under stress.

anion,   a negatively charged ion. *See also anode.*

aniseikonia /an´īsīkō´nē·ə/,   a defect in which each eye sees the same image differently in size or shape.

ankle,   **1.** the junction of the tibia, talus, and fibula. **2.** the part of the leg where it joins the foot.

ankle hitch,   an improvised attachment, usually made from a cravat (a folded triangular bandage) that is tied around the ankle and attached to a traction splinting device, as a means of applying traction to a fractured femur. Also known as a **Collins hitch, improvised Collins hitch.**

ankylosing   spondylitis /ang´kilō´sing/,   a chronic disease with inflammation of the spine and nearby structures. It often progresses to a fusing (ankylosis) of the bones of the spinal column.

ankylosis /ang´kilō´-/,   fusing of a joint, due to destruction of cartilage and bone, as occurs in rheumatoid arthritis.

anode,   any positively charged electrical source. In the body, anions are attracted to anodes. *See also anion.*

anomalous conduction.   See **accelerated A-V conduction.**

anomaly /ənom´əlē/,   **1.** change from what is regarded as normal. **2.** inherited problem with growth of a structure, as the lack of a limb or the presence of an extra finger. **–anomalous,** *adj.*

anorexia /an´ôrek´sē·ə/,   a loss of appetite that results in the patient not eating. **Anorexia nervosa** is a disorder in which there is refusal to eat. It is often linked with mental stress or conflict, as worry, anger, or fear. **–anorexic,** *adj.*

anosmia /anoz´mē·ə/,   loss or damage of the sense of smell. Also known as **olfactory anesthesia.** Compare **hyperosmia.**

anoxia /anok´sē·ə/,   a lack of oxygen. Anoxia may occur locally or affect the whole body. It can occur when the blood is not able to carry oxygen to the tissues or the tissues are not able to absorb oxygen from the blood. A condition in which little oxygen reaches the brain is called **cerebral anoxia.** This state, caused by failure of circulation or respiration, can exist for no more than 4 to 6 minutes before permanent brain damage occurs.

antacid /antas´id/,   **1.** opposing acidity. **2.** a drug or substance in the diet that buffers, makes neutral, or absorbs hydrochloric acid in the stomach.

antagonist,   **1.** a chemical or pharmacological agent that inhibits the effects of another substance. **2.** a muscle that counteracts the action of another. *See also synergist.*

antecubital /an´təkyōō´bitəl/,   at the bend of the elbow on the anterior of the arm.

antecubital fossa.   See **antecubital space.**

antecubital space,   the anterior portion of the elbow; the bend of the elbow. Also known as **AC space, antecubital fossa.**

antecubital veins,   the portions of the basilic and cephalic veins located in the antecubital space, which are frequently accessed sites for venipuncture.

antepartal care,   care of a pregnant woman throughout maternity. *See also intrapartal care, postpartal care.*

anterior (A),   the front of a structure or a part facing toward the front. *See also ventral.* Compare **posterior.**

anterior chamber of the eye,   the chamber located between the cornea and the iris. *See also posterior chamber of eye.*

anterior communicating artery, the artery that connects with the anterior cerebral arteries and completes the circle of Willis.

anterior cord syndrome, injury to the spinal cord caused by pressure on the anterior cord due to a ruptured disc or fractured vertebral body. This injury is usually seen with flexion injuries of the spinal cord.

anterior cutaneous nerve, one of a pair of branches of the network of nerves near the cervical plexus. It arises from the second and the third nerves in the neck and branches to the neck and upper chest.

anterior longitudinal ligament, the broad, strong ligament attached to the anterior surfaces of the vertebrae; from the skull to the lower back.

anterior superior iliac spine, one of the two bony segments forming the iliac crest.

anterior tibial artery, one of the two branches of the popliteal artery which starts posterior to the knee, splits into six branches, and supplies the muscles of the leg and foot.

anteroposterior /an´tərō-/, from the front to the back of the body. Also known as **AP.**

Anthozoa, the class of sea life that includes the sea anemones, soft corals, and true (stony) corals. These creatures generally exist in fixed locations and exhibit great beauty. They are a danger to swimmers and scuba divers because of their capability to envenomate via stinging cells. In addition, true corals maintain a rigid structure, which can cause deep cuts when brushed against.

anthracosis /an´thrəkō´-/, a chronic lung disease of coal miners caused by coal dust in the lungs. It forms lumps on the bronchioles that lead to emphysema. Also known as **black lung.**

anthrax /an´thraks/, a disease that affects primarily farm animals. Humans most often contract it through a break in the skin when in direct contact with infected animals and their hides. Symptoms include internal bleeding, pain, weeping sores, fever, nausea, and vomiting. Anthrax of the lungs (**woolsorter's disease**) occurs after bacterial inhalation. Early symptoms are similar to influenza. However, the patient soon develops fever, dyapnea, and cyanosis.

anthropometry /an´thrəpom´ətrē/, the science of measuring the human body for height, weight, and size of different parts. Also known as **anthropometric measurement.**

antiadrenergic /an´ti·ad´rənur´jik/, **1.** impulses sent by nerves that release the chemical norepinephrine. These nerves (adrenergic nerves) have two types of receivers, alpha and beta. **2.** drugs that block the response to norepinephrine by alpha-adrenergic receptors. They cause blood flow to increase and blood pressure to decrease. Drugs that block beta-adrenergic receptors slow the heart rate. Also known as **sympatholytic.** Compare **andrenergic.**

antiantibody, an antibody formed by the blood to fight off a foreign antibody that can cause an allergic response. *See also antibody, immune gamma globulin.*

antiarrhythmic. See **antidysrhythmic.**

antibacterial, a substance or drug that kills bacteria or prevents their growth.

antibiotic, the ability to kill or prevent the growth of a living organism. Therapeutic substances which have this ability are known as antibiotic, antibacterial, or anitimicrobial drugs.

antibody (Ab), a molecule produced by lymph tissue. It defends the body against bacteria, viruses, or other antigens. Each antibody reacts to a particular foreign body. Also known as immunoglobulins.

anticholinergic, **1.** interfering with the action or impulses of parasympathetic nerve fibers. **2.** any substance that causes parasympathetic blocking activity. Also known as **parasympatholytic.**

anticholinesterase, a substance which halts the action of acetylcholine. Anticholinesterase drugs are used to treat myasthenia gravis.

anticoagulant, a substance or drug that prevents or delays coagulation.

anticonvulsant, a drug or a treatment that prevents seizures, such as in epilepsy, or makes them less severe.

antidepressant, a drug or a treatment that prevents or relieves depression. *See also antipsychotic.*

antidiuretic, a drug or substance that prevents the body from making urine. **–antidiuresis,** *n.*

antidiuretic hormone (ADH), a hormone produced in the hypothalamus of the brain and stored in the pituitary gland. It decreases the production of urine by causing water to be absorbed in the kidneys. ADH is released when blood volume falls, when a large amount of sodium occurs in blood, or when stress is present. Also known as **vasopressin.**

antidote /an´tidōt/, a substance which counteracts the action of another substance. **Chemical antidote** refers to any substance that reacts to form a compound that is harmless or less harmful. There are few true antidotes. Treatment of poisoning depends largely on destroying the toxic agent before it can be absorbed by the body.

antidysrhythmic, any drug or treatment that corrects or prevents abnormal cardiac rhythms.

antiemetic, a substance that prevents or relieves nausea and vomiting.

antifogging chemical, a chemical that keeps condensation from forming on the inside of a facepiece lens.

antifungal, a substance that kills or controls fungi.

antigen /an´tijən/, a substance foreign to the body, often a protein. It causes the body to form an antibody that responds only to that antigen. Antigens can cause allergic reactions in some people. *See also allergen.*

antigen-antibody reaction, a process of the immune system in which certain lymphocytes respond to an antigen by making antibodies. The antigens are made harmless when they are bound to these antibodies.

antigenic site, a site capable of binding and reacting with an antibody.

antihistamine /-his´təmin/, a substance that reduces the effects of histamine, a chemical released by cells of the body. Although histamine has a role in the body, it also causes the symptoms of allergic reactions.

antihypertensive, a drug or treatment that reduces high blood pressure. Some diuretics lower the blood pressure by decreasing blood volume.

antiinflammatory, a drug or treatment that reduces heat, redness, swelling, and pain (inflammation).

antilipidemic /-lip´idem´-ik/, a diet or drug that reduces the amount of fats (lipids) in the blood. *See also hyperlipidemia.*

antilymphocyte serum (ALS). See **antiserum.**

antimalarial /-məler´ē·əl/, **1.** a drug that kills or stops the growth of malarial organisms (plasmodia). **2.** a method to kill mosquitos that carry the disease, as spraying insecticides or draining swamps. *See also malaria.*

antimicrobial, a substance that kills microorganisms, as bacteria, or stops their growth.

antimony /an´təmōnē/, a natural chemical element used to treat parasitic infections. Antimony is common in many substances used in medicine and industry.

antiparasitic, a drug or treatment that kills parasites or stops their growth.

antiparkinsonian, a drug or treatment used to treat a nervous system defect (parkinsonism). The drugs are of two types. One replaces the lack of dopamine in the brain. Another balances the effects of increased acetylcholine in the brain.

antipruritic, a drug or treatment that helps relieve or prevent itching.

antipsychotic, a drug or treatment that lessens the symptoms of severe mental illness (psychosis).

antipyretic, a drug or treatment that reduces fever. The most widely used drugs are acetaminophen, aspirin, and other salicylates.

antiseptic, a substance, technique, or treatment used to stop the growth of microorganisms.

antisocial personality disorder, repeated behavior patterns that lack morals and ethics. These patterns bring a person into conflict with society. A person with this deficit may be aggressive, impulsive, irresponsible, hostile, immature, and show poor judgment.

antitoxin. See **antiserum.**

antitussive /-tus´iv/, any of a large group of drugs that act on the nervous system to reduce the action of the cough reflex. These drugs should not be used with a cough that produces sputum because the cough is needed to clear fluids. Antitussives may be either habit-forming (narcotic) or not habit-forming (nonnarcotic).

antivenin. See **antiserum.**

antiviral, destructive to viruses.

antivitamin, a substance that stops the action of a vitamin.

anuria /əno͞or´ē·ə/, unable to urinate. Anuria may be caused by kidney failure, a severe decline in blood pressure or blockage of the urinary tract. Also known as **anuresis** /an´yo͞orē´-/.

anus /ā´nəs/, the opening at the end of the anal canal.

anxiety, a feeling of worry, uncertainty, and fear that comes from thinking about threat or danger. Anxiety is often mental, rather than a response to real events.

anxiety attack, a sudden response of intense anxiety and panic. Symptoms often include tachycardia, shortness of breath, dizziness, stomach upset, and a vague feeling of doom. Attacks occur suddenly, and last from a few seconds to 1 hour or longer. They may occur many times a month.

anxiety neurosis, a mental conflict or problem in which anxiety lasts for a long time. The person may feel tense, worried, afraid, unable to make a decision, and restless. There may be hostility toward others. In extreme cases, the condition may lead to physical problems.

aorta /ā·ôrtə/, the largest artery in the body, arising from the left ventricle of the heart. The **abdominal aorta,** one of the four segments of the aorta, is approximately 1 inch in diameter as it passes through the abdomen. It supplies blood to many different parts of the body, such as the testicles, ovaries, kidneys, stomach, and lower extremities. The **ascending aorta** branches into the right and left coronary arteries. It continues as the **arch of the aorta.** From the aortic arch, the **descending aorta** leads into the inferior portion of the body and supplies blood to many areas, including the throat, ribs, chest muscles, and stomach.

aortic arch syndrome, a blockage of the section of the aorta that forms the arch. Conditions such as atherosclerosis, arteritis, and syphilis may precipitate the syndrome. Symptoms include syncope, blindness, loss of use of an extremity, and memory loss.

aortic regurgitation, the reverse flow of blood from the aorta back into the left ventrical. Also known as **aortic insufficiency.**

aortic stenosis. See **stenosis.**

aortitis /ā´ôrtī´-/, inflammation of the aorta.

aortopulmonary fenestration, a birth defect in which there is an opening between the ascending aorta and the pulmonary artery. This allows oxygenated blood to mix with deoxygenated blood, decreasing oxygen to the tissues.

apathy /ap´əthē/, a lack of emotion; a lack of care for things that are normally exciting or moving.

aperture /ap´ərchər/, an opening in an object or structure, as the **aperture of larynx,** the opening between the pharynx and larynx.

apex /ā´peks/, *pl.* **apices** /ā´picēz/, the top end or tip of a structure, as the **apex pulmonis,** the rounded superior border of each lung.

apex beat. See **point of maximum impulse.**

apex of the heart, the left-sided protrusion on the inferior portion of the heart, opposite the base. *See also base of the heart.*

Apgar score /ap´gär/ (Virginia Apgar, U.S. anesthesiologist, 1909-1974), an assessment to determine a newborn's physical health. It is done 1 minute and 5 minutes after birth. Scoring is based on rating heart rate, breathing, muscle tone, reflexes, and color from a low value of 0 to a normal value of 2. The five scores are combined, and the totals at 1 minute and 5 minutes are assessed. For example, Apgar 9/10 is a score of 9 at 1 minute and 10 at 5 minutes. A score of 0 to 3 is given to infants with severe distress, a score of 4 to 7 means moderate distress, and a score of 7 to 10 is normal. About 50% of infants with 5-minute scores of 0 to 1 die, and infants that survive have three times as many defects at 1 year of age as at birth. See Appendix 1-10.

aphagia /əfā´jə/, loss of the ability to swallow. *See also dysphagia.*

aphakia /əfā´kē·ə/, a state in which part or all of the lens of the eye is missing, usually from removal, as in the treatment of cataracts.

aphasia /əfā´zhə/, a nerve deficit in which there are difficulties with speaking or speech is lost. There are many forms and aphasia may result from a head injury, lack of oxygen, or CVA. **Anomia** is a form of aphasia in which the patient cannot name objects. It is caused by an injury to the brain. With **conduction aphasia,** the patient has problems in self-expression. Words can be understood, but the patient may mix words similar in sound or meaning. The patient is alert and aware of the problem. **Motor aphasia** is the inability to say words because of a lesion in the brain. Most commonly, the cause is a

CVA. The patient knows what to say but cannot make the mouth movements for words. With **receptive aphasia,** the patient may see or hear words but does not understand what they mean.

aphonia /əfō´nē·ə/, loss of voice as a result of laryngeal disease or injury.

-aphrodisia, a combining form meaning a state of sexual arousal.

apical odontoid ligament, a ligament that connects the spine to the skull.

aplasia /əplā´zhə/, failure of normal development of an organ or tissue.

apnea, absence of respiration.

apneustic breathing /apnoo´stik/, a pattern of breathing in which the person breathes in for a prolonged time and then fails to breathe out. The rate of apneustic breathing is usually around 2 cycles per minute. *See also respiratory rate.*

aponeurosis /ap´ōnoorō´-/, *pl.* **aponeuroses,** a strong sheet of fiberlike tissue that attaches muscles to bone (tendon) or holds muscles together (fascia).

apophysis /əpof´i·sis/, a projection or outgrowth, especially from a bone.

A-post, first roof pillar from the windshield of a vehicle.

apothecaries' measure /əpoth´əker´ēz/, a system of liquid measurements. It was first based on the minim, equal to one drop of water. It is now 0.06 ml. 60 minims equal 1 fluid dram, 8 fluid drams equal 1 fluid ounce, 16 fluid ounces equal 1 pint, 2 pints equal 1 quart, 4 quarts equal 1 gallon. *See also metric system.*

apothecaries' weight, a system of weights. The system was based on the weight of a plump grain of wheat. It is now 65 mg. Weights are 20 grains equal 1 scruple, 3 scruples equal 1 dram, 8 drams equal 1 ounce, 12 ounces equal 1 pound. Compare **avoirdupois weight.**

apparatus, a vehicle with a purpose; usually used to denote a fire department vehicle, as an engine, truck.

appendage, an extra piece that is attached to a part or organ. Also known as **appendix.**

appendectomy /-dek´-/, removal of the appendix. *See also peritonitis.*

appendicitis, inflammation of the appendix. The most common symptom, known as **Aaron's sign,** is constant pain in the right quad-rant of the abdomen. Symptoms include vomiting, fever, tenderness, a rigid abdomen, and few or no bowel sounds. The condition is caused by a blockage at the opening of the appendix, disease of the bowel wall, an adhesion or a parasite. Treatment delay usually results in rupture and infection. *See also peritonitis.*

appendicular skeleton, the bones of the upper and lower extremities. *See also axial skeleton.*

appendix, *pl.* **appendices,** a closed sac extending from the large intestine. Its length varies from 3 to 6 inches, and its diameter is about ⅓ inch. Also known as **vermiform appendix.**

appliance, apparatus made for a purpose, such as a lifting appliance.

apraxia /əprak´-sē·ə/, loss of the ability to do simple or routine acts.

apron, paved area designed to accommodate parked aircraft.

aprosody /āpros´ədē/, absence in speech of pitch, sound, and rhythm.

aptitude, a natural talent to learn or know a skill.

aqueous /ā´kwē·əs, ak´-/, **1.** watery or water-like, as the **aqueous humor,** the clear fluid that moves in the eyeball. **2.** a drug manufactured with water.

aqueous film forming foam, fire-fighting liquid that forms a film over volatile liquids, thus minimizing vapor escape and ignition. Also known as **AFFF.**

aqueous humor, clear fluid produced by the ciliary body, cornea, and iris that fills the anterior and posterior chambers of the eye. *See also vitreous humor.*

arachnoid /ərak´noid/, a weblike structure, as the **arachnoid membrane,** one of the three thin membranes covering the brain and the spinal cord.

arbovirus, any one of more than 300 viruses carried by insects. These viruses may cause infections. The infections have symptoms of two or more of the following: fever, rash, brain inflammation, and bleeding into the internal organs or skin. There are vaccines that prevent infection from some arboviruses.

arc, completing an electrical pathway or current, usually through a medium, such as air or other electrically conductive materials.

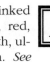

archetype /är´kətīp/, **1.** an original model or pattern from which something is made. **2.** (in Jungian psychology) an idea or way of thinking that is inherited from the experiences of the human race. It is believed present in the unconscious of a person in the form of drives or moods.

arcing, visible light produced by the flow of electricity between two points.

area, a space that contains a specific structure of the body or within which certain functions take place, as the aortic area is the space around the artery.

area navigation, an aircraft computer navigation system that uses ground radio signals to determine flight position. Also known as **RNAV.**

areflexia /ā´rēflek´sē·ə/, absence of reflexes.

areola /erē´ōlə/, *pl.* **areolae, 1.** a small area **2.** a circular area of an altered color surrounding a lesion. **3.** one of the spaces in areolar tissue.

arginine (Arg) /är´jinin/, an amino acid made by digestion of proteins or synthetically. Some compounds made from arginine are used to treat excess ammonia caused by liver disease.

argininemia /-ē´mē·ə/, an inherited disorder with an increased amount of arginine in the blood from a lack of an enzyme (arginase).

ariboflavinosis /ārī´bōflā´vinō´-/, a condition caused by lack of vitamin B2 in the diet. Symptoms include sores on the mouth, lips, nose, and eyes. *See also riboflavin.*

arm, 1. the part of the upper limb of the body between shoulder and elbow. The bone of the arm is the humerus. The muscles of the arm are the coracobrachialis, biceps brachii, brachialis, and triceps brachii. **2.** *(nontechnical)* the arm and the forearm.

arrest, to inhibit, restrain, or stop, as to arrest the course of a disease. **Developmental arrest** is when fetal growth stops. *See also cardiac arrest.*

arrhythmia, 1. *(literal)* absence of cardiac electrical activity. **2.** a term often used to refer to dysrhythmias. *See also dysrhythmia.*

arsenic (As) /är´sənik/, an element that occurs throughout the earth's crust. This element continues to have limited use in drugs used to treat trypanosomiasis. The introduction of drugs without arsenic that have fewer dangerous side effects have greatly reduced its use. **–arsenic** /är´senik/, **arsenical,** *adj.*

arsenical stomatitis, an oral condition linked to arsenic poisoning. Symptoms are dry, red, and painful mucous membrane in the mouth, ulcers, bleeding gums, and loosened teeth. *See also stomatitis.*

arterial gas embolism, gas bubbles in the arterial circulation, usually introduced into the pulmonary capillaries as air, which can obstruct cerebral or myocardial circulation. Overpressurization of the lungs or air introduced during vascular catheterization are the primary precipitating causes of this disorder. Also known as **AGE.** *See also cerebral arterial gas embolism, embolism, pulmonary overpressurization syndrome.*

arterial insufficiency. See **vascular insufficiency.**

arteriogram /ärtir´ē·ə gram´/, a radiological study of an artery that has been injected with a dye. *See also angiography.*

arteriole /ärtir´ē·ōl/, any of the smaller vessels of the arterial circulation. Blood from the heart is pumped through the arteries to the arterioles, which form part of the capillaries. The blood flows from the capillaries into the veins and returns to the heart. The wall of the arterioles constrict and dilate in response to chemicals regulated by nerves. *See also artery.*

arteriosclerosis /ärtir´ē·əsklerō´-/, thickening, loss of elasticity, and hardening of the arterial walls. The condition often develops with aging, high blood pressure, kidney disease, diabetes, and excess lipids in the blood. Symptoms include leg cramps when walking (intermittent claudication), changes in skin temperature and color, altered pulses, headache, dizziness, and memory defects. *See also atherosclerosis.*

arteriovenous fistula, 1. abnormal connection between arteries and veins that results from congenital defects, inflammation, and penetrating injuries. **2.** a surgically created connection between an artery and a vein (in an extremity) used for cannulation to connect a patient to a hemodialysis machine. Due to the arterial connection, field providers should access the fistula only in life-threatening situations. Also known as **AV shunt.**

arteritis /är´tərī´-/, inflammation of the walls of arteries. It may occur as a disease in itself.

artery, vessel that carries blood away from the heart. This hollow tube is composed of the three layers: tunica intima (inner), tunica media (middle), and tunica adventitia (outer). Most arteries are approximately 3⁄16 inch (4 mm) in diameter.

arthralgia /ärthral´jə/, any pain that affects a joint. **–arthralgic,** *adj.*

arthritis, any inflammation of the joints. **Acute pyogenic arthritis** is a bacterial infection of one or more joints. It occurs most often in children and is caused by injury. Symptoms include pain and swelling in the joint, muscle spasm, chills, fever, and sweating. **Septic arthritis** may be caused by the spread of bacteria through the bloodstream from an infection elsewhere in the body or by infection of a joint. *See also osteoarthritis, rheumatoid arthritis.*

arthrocentesis /är´thrōsentē´-/, aspirating a joint with a needle and withdrawing synovial fluid from the joint.

arthrodesis /ärthrod´əsis/, repairing a joint by uniting the bones through surgery to relieve pain or give support.

arthropathy /ärthrop´əthē/, any disease or abnormal condition affecting a joint.

arthroplasty /är´thrəplas´tē/, surgery for a painful deteriorating joint. Arthroplasty gives movement to a joint in osteoarthritis and rheumatoid arthritis. It can correct a congenital defect.

arthropod /-pod/, a member of *Arthropoda,* the largest major group (phylum) of animal life that includes crabs and lobsters, mites, ticks, spiders, and insects. Arthropods generally have a jointed shell (exoskeleton) and paired, jointed legs.

arthroscopy /ärthros´kəpē/, examination of the interior of a joint. A specially designed microscope-like device (endoscope) is inserted through a small incision. Arthroscopy permits removal of cartilage or fluid (synovial) from the joint, and the diagnosis of a torn meniscus.

articular capsule, an envelope of tissue that surrounds a joint. *See also fibrous capsule.*

articular cartilage, fibrous or soft tissue that lines the opposing surfaces of joints.

articular disk, the platelike end of some bones in movable joints. It can be closely linked to surrounding muscles or with cartilage.

artifact, anything irrelevant or unwanted, as a substance, structure, or piece of information.

artificial limb. See **prosthesis.**

artificial pacemaker. See **pacemaker.**

artificial respiration, continuation of respiratory movement by artificial means. The methods are manual or mechanical. Manual methods include mouth-to-mouth breathing and several relatively ineffective techniques utilizing compression of the chest. Mechanical methods include resuscitators and ventilators. *See also back-pressure arm-lift, Byrd-Dew method, chest-pressure arm-lift, resuscitator, ventilator.*

asbestosis, a lung disease caused by breathing asbestos fibers. It results in lung disorders, such as pleural fibrosis, with shortness of breath. The disease can occur in people who have been exposed to asbestos building materials. *See also pulmonary disease.*

ascariasis /as´kərī´əsis/, an infection caused by a parasitic worm, *Ascaris lumbricoides.* The eggs are passed in human feces. The infection is transmitted to others through hands, water, or food.

ascend, to go up; to move toward a source. *See also descend.*

ascender, devices used for climbing up rope, classified as soft or hard. **Soft ascenders** are generally simple knots formed from small sling rope and attached to climbing rope. Popular knots include the Prusik, the Bachmann, and the Kreuzklem. **Hard ascenders** include any mechanical device designed as a rope clamp. Common mechanical ascenders include the Clog, the Gibbs, and the Jumar.

ascending pharyngeal artery, one of the smallest arteries to branch from the outer carotid artery. It provides blood to the head.

ascites /əsī´tēz/, an abnormal pooling of fluid in the abdominal cavity containing large amounts of protein and other cells. *See also paracentesis.* **–ascitic,** *adj.*

ascorbemia /as´kôrbē´mē·ə/, the presence of vitamin C (ascorbic acid) in the blood in larger than normal amounts.

ascorbic acid. See **vitamin C.**

ascorburia /-o͞or´ē·ə/, ascorbic acid in the urine in larger amounts than normal.

asepsis /āsep´-/, the absence of germs. **Medical asepsis** is the removal of disease organisms or infected material. **Surgical asepsis** is protection against infection before, during, or after surgery by use of sterile technique. **–aseptic,** *adj.*

aseptic bone necrosis, changes in bone seen after repeated exposure to increased barometric pressure. Whereas both divers and compressed air workers are affected, pressures equivalent to and greater than 50 meters (about 150 feet) of depth are generally necessary for the condition to occur. Radiographic changes in the shoulder, hip, and knee may be the only evidence of change, but arthritis and pain may eventually occur.

asexual /āsek´sho͞o·əl/, **1.** an organism that has no sexual organs. **2.** a process that is not sexual. **–asexuality,** *n.*

asparagine (Asn) /asper´əjin/, an amino acid found in many proteins in the body. It acts as a drug that promotes the release of urine. *See also amino acid.*

aspartame, a white, almost odorless crystalline powder with an intensely sweet taste. It is used as an artificial sweetener. It is about 180 times as sweet as the same amount of sugar. Aspartame tends to lose its sweetness in the presence of heat and moisture.

aspartate aminotransferase (AST) /aspär´tāt/, an enzyme normally present in blood serum and in the heart and liver. AST is released into the blood after injury or heart and liver damage.

aspartic acid (Asp), an amino acid in sugar cane, beet molasses, and the breakdown products of many proteins. Aspartic acid is used in dietary supplements and in drugs that kill funguses and germs. *See also amino acid.*

aspergillosis /as´pərjilō´-/, an infection caused by the fungus *Aspergillus.* It usually affects the ear but is capable of infecting any organ. Relatively uncommon, it typically occurs in a patient already weakened by another disorder.

asphyxia /asfik´sē·ə/, severe oxygen deprivation. It leads to loss of consciousness and, if not corrected, death. Some of the more common causes of asphyxia are drowning, electric shock, cardiac arrest, aspiration, and airway obstruction. *See also artificial respiration.* **–asphyxiate,** *v.,* **asphyxiated,** *adj.*

asphyxiant, any gas capable of causing death due to oxygen displacement.

aspiration, 1. the act of withdrawing fluid, such as mucus or blood, from the body by a suction device. **2.** The act of taking foreign material or emesis into the lungs. **–aspirate,** *n.*

aspiration pneumonia. See **pneumonia.**

aspirator, any instrument that removes a substance from body cavities by suction, as a bulb syringe, pump, or hypodermic needle.

aspirin, a drug used to reduce fever, increase blood clotting time, and relieve pain and inflammation. Side effects include ulcers, bleeding, and ringing in the ears. Use of large doses can cause blood clotting defects and liver and kidney damage. Reye's syndrome in children may be caused by aspirin. There are no contraindications for field use.

assault, 1. creating apprehension or fear of injury. **2.** unauthorized handling and/or treatment of a patient.

assessment, evaluation of patient condition. Field assessment is conducted as the primary survey (ABCs) and secondary survey (chief complaint, history of present illness, past medical history, physical examination, diagnosis, and differential diagnosis). Although patient assessment will vary, depending on the situation, the above information is critical to proper diagnosis and treatment.

assigned resources, resources checked in and assigned work tasks on an incident.

assimilation, 1. the process of incorporating nutrition into living tissue. **2.** the incorporation of new experiences into a person's consciousness.

assisting agency, an agency directly contributing suppression, rescue, support, or service resources to another agency.

association, 1. a connection, union, joining, or combination of things. **2.** connecting feelings, emotions, sensations, or thoughts with particular persons, things, or ideas.

assured crew return vehicle, rescue craft designed for use in the event of an emergency onboard NASA space station *Freedom.* This vehicle will be capable of isolating the crew from the emergency, separating from the space station, and reentering Earth's atmosphere. Also known as **ACRV.**

astereognosis /əstir´ē·ognō´-/, a nervous system disorder marked by an inability to recognize objects by touch.

asthenia /asthē´nē·ə/, the lack or loss of strength or energy; weakness.

asthenic personality, a personality with low energy, lack of enthusiasm, and oversensitivity to physical and emotional strain.

asthenopia /as´thənō´pe·ə/, a condition in which the eyes tire easily because of weakness of the eye muscles. Symptoms include pain in or around the eyes, headache, dimness of vision, dizziness, and slight nausea.

asthma /az´mə/, a lung disorder with periods of dyspnea which range from occasional periods of wheezing, mild coughing, and slight breathlessness to airway obstruction and apnea. Asthmatic attacks are caused by a narrowing of the airways due to smooth muscle spasm, inflammation, and swelling of the bronchi or excess mucus. **Allergic asthma** occurs from breathing in an allergen. Antibodies form in the cells of the alucoli to fight the allergen. The histamine released causes bronchial smooth muscles to contract, which leads to the coughing and wheezing of asthma. **Intrinsic asthma** is a nonseasonal, nonallergic form of asthma that tends to be chronic and long-lasting rather than episodic. Trigger factors include pollutants, as dust particles, smoke, aerosols, paint fumes, and other volatile substances. Persons who work with soaps, Western red cedar, cotton, flax, hemp, grain, flour, and stone are subject to **occupational asthma.** Bronchospasm may also occur in cold, damp weather, after sudden breathing of cold, dry air and after exercise or violent coughing. A severe asthma episode is known as **status asthmaticus.** Cyanosis and unconsciousness may follow.

astigmatism /əstig´mətizəm/, a condition of the eye in which the curve of the cornea is unequal. As a result, light rays cannot be focused clearly. Vision is blurred.

astringent /əstrin´jənt/, a substance that causes tissues to contract. It is usually used on the skin. Alum and tannic acid are common astringents.

astroblastoma /as´trōblastō´mə/, a cancerous tumor of the brain and spinal cord. Cells of an astroblastoma lie around blood vessels or connective tissue.

asymmetrical, referring to parts that are unequal in size or shape, or that are different in arrangement. Compare **symmetrical.**

asynclitism /āsing´klitizm/, during labor, a presentation of the top of the baby's head that is not in proper alignment with the mother's pelvis for birth.

asynergy /āsin´ərjē/, faulty coordination among groups of organs or muscles that normally function together.

asyntaxia /ā´sintak´sē·ə/, any interference with the proper order of growth of the fetus during development.

asystole, absence of cardiac electrical activity; an absence of upward or downward deflections on the isoelectric line of the EKG. Also known as **flat line, straight line.**

atavism /at´əvizm/, traits or characteristics in a person that are more like those of a grandparent or earlier ancestor than like the parents.

ataxia /ətak´sē·ə/, inability to coordinate movements, due to damage to the spinal cord or brain.

atelectasis /at´ilek´təsis/, collapse of alveoli, which prevents the exchange of carbon dioxide and oxygen by the blood. Symptoms include dyspnea and fever. The condition may be caused by pressure on the lung from fluid or air in the area around the lungs (pleural space) or by pressure from a tumor outside the lung.

atheroma /ath´ərō´mə/, an abnormal mass of fat, as in a sebaceous cyst.

atherosclerosis /ath´ərōsklərō´-/, a disorder in which plaques of cholesterol and fats are deposited in the walls of arteries. The vessel walls become thick and hardened, which lessens circulation to areas normally supplied by the artery. These plaques (atheromas) are major causes of heart disease and other disorders of the circulation. *See also arteriosclerosis.*

athetosis /ath´ətō´-/, a condition in which there is a writhing, slow, continuous, and involuntary movement of the hands and feet.

athiaminosis /əthī´əminō´-/, a condition resulting from the lack of thiamine (vitamin B_1) in the diet.

athlete's foot, a chronic fungal infection of the foot. Also known as **tinea pedis.**

athletic habitus. See **somatotype.**

atlantooccipital joint /-oksip´itəl/, one of a pair of joints formed where the atlas of the vertebral column meets the occipital bone of the skull.

atlas. See **vertebra.**

atmosphere, **1.** the combination of gases that exists above the Earth's surface. **2.** measure of barometric pressure with 1 atmosphere equaling 14.7 psi (760 mmHg). **3.** any envelope of gas.

atmospheric pressure, the pressure exerted by atmospheric air upon the Earth's surface or an object above it. The pressure varies with altitude or elevation from 0 psi (0 mmHg) at the edge of the ionosphere to 14.7 psi (760 mmHg) at sea level. Also known as **barometric pressure.**

atom, the smallest particle of an element that retains all the chemical characteristics of the element. It consists of a central core called the nucleus, which contains protons and neutrons and orbiting electrons.

atomic energy, energy released in nuclear reactions. Of particular interest is the energy released when a neutron initiates the splitting of an atom's nucleus into smaller pieces (fission) or when two nuclei are joined together under millions of degrees of heat (fusion). Also known as **nuclear energy.**

atomizer, a device for spraying a liquid as a fine mist or vapor.

atonic /əton´ik/, **1.** weak; lacking normal tone, as a muscle that is soft. **2.** lacking vigor, as an atonic ulcer, which heals slowly.

atopic /ātop´ik/, a congenital tendency to develop immediate allergic reactions, as asthma, allergic skin disease, or hay fever.

atopic dermatitis, an intensely pruritic inflammation of the skin on the face, knees, and elbows, most common in infants.

atopy /at´əpē´/, a state of allergic hypersensitivity to numerous environmental substances. A skin-sensitizing antibody creates edema of the cutaneous tissues. This edema can be seen as bronchospasm, eczema, rhinitis, and urticaria.

atresia /ətrē´zhə/, the absence of a normal body opening, duct, or canal.

atrial fibrillation, cardiac dysrhythmia characterized by ineffective atrial contractions and irregular ventricular response. The atria are unable to contract effectively because of numerous electrical signals occurring simultaneously. EKG rhythm shows an irregular rhythm with normal QRS complexes and no discernible P waves. Fine fibrillatory waves may

be seen between QRS complexes. Ventricular response rates of 100 per minute and below are known as **controlled atrial fibrillation** and are usually considered a benign, chronic condition in older patients. Ventricular response rates above 100 are known as **uncontrolled atrial fibrillation** and may require treatment if symptoms occur. Also known as **AF, A fib, atrial fib.**

atrial flutter, cardiac dysrhythmia with rhythmic atrial depolarizations occurring at 250 to 350 beats per minute and a variable ventricular response. An irritable area (or focus) in the atria causes the rapid atrial rate. Ventricular depolarizations are usually limited to one half or one third of the atrial rate due to the control exerted by the AV node. The EKG rhythm has normal QRS complexes at regular or irregular intervals. The baseline is characterized by a sawtooth pattern of waves known as **F** (or **flutter**) **waves.** Although the rate of the rhythm determines cardiac effectiveness, the patient is almost always symptomatic. Symptomatic patients will deteriorate without intervention. Also known as **A flutter.**

atrial natriuretic factor, a peptide that decreases blood pressure by increasing urine production. When atrial blood pressure increases, this substance is released from the atria to reduce blood volume.

atrial synchronous ventricular pacemaker, an electrical device implanted in the chest that synchronizes with the patient's atrial rhythm so that the ventricles are paced if an AV block occurs. Also known as a **pacemaker.**

atrial tachycardia, a dysrhythmia of the heart in which an atrial irritable focus produces cardiac rates of 150 to 250 impulses per minute with normal, regularly occurring QRS complexes. If discernable, P waves are generally altered in shape but occur before every QRS. When this dysrhythmia begins and ends suddenly, it is known as **paroxysmal atrial tachycardia.** Also known as **AT, A tach, atrial tach, PAT.**

atrial-ventricular demand pacemaker, an implanted electrical device that monitors the rates of both the atria and ventricles and paces either if the rates drop below preset levels. Also known as **pacemaker.**

atrioventricular block, interference with cardiac nerve conduction through the atrioventricular node. Also known as **AV block, heart block.**

atrioventricular dissociation, cardiac phenomenon in which rhythmically occurring P waves and QRS complexes have no relationship to each other. The dysrhythmia in which this occurs most frequently is complete, or third-degree, heart block. This is a life-threatening situation that, if untreated, will lead to death. Also known as **AV dissociation.**

atrioventricular node, an area of specialized cardiac tissue that receives and slows the electrical impulse of the heart from the sinoatrial (SA) node. The impulse then travels to the bundle of His, which carries it to the ventricles. The AV node is located in the septum of the right atrium.

atrioventricular septum, a wall that separates the atria from the ventricles of the heart.

atrioventricular valve, a valve in the heart through which blood flows from the atria to the ventricles. The valve between the left atrium and the left ventricle is called the mitral valve. The valve on the right side is known as the tricuspid valve.

at risk, susceptible to a particular disease or injury. The risk may be environmental or physical.

atrium /ā´trē·əm/, *pl.* **atria,** a chamber or cavity, such as the nasal cavity. The **atrium of the heart** is one of the two upper chambers of the heart. Blood returns from the body to the right atrium. The left atrium receives blood from the veins in the lungs. Blood is emptied into the ventricles from the atria.

atrophy /at´rəfē/, a wasting or loss of size of a part of the body because of disease or non-use. A muscle may atrophy due to lack of physical exercise. Cells of the brain and nervous system may atrophy in old age because of restricted blood flow to those areas.

atropine sulfate, an anticholinergic agent used in the treatment of asystole, unstable bradycardia, pulseless electrical activity, and organophosphate poisoning. Although there are no contraindications for field use, it should be used with caution in the presence of acute myocardial infarction and glaucoma.

attachment, 1. the state or quality of being attached. **2.** a mode of behavior in which one person relates in a dependent manner to another; a feeling of affection or loyalty that binds one person to another.

attending physician, the physician who is responsible for a particular patient.

attention deficit disorder, learning and behavioral problems affecting children, adolescents, and rarely, adults. It may result from genetic factors, chemical imbalance, or injury or disease. Also known as **hyperactivity, minimal brain dysfunction.**

attenuation, the process of reduction, as the weakening of a disease organism.

attraction, the passive mode of search and rescue, when it can be expected that the subject of the search will show up or walk out. The primary focus of these procedures should be to allow the subject to walk out or provide points to guide and encourage mobile subjects to move to particular locations. Techniques—such as balloons, fires, flares, lights, and skywriting—can be used for visual attraction. Sound attraction would use public address systems, sirens, and voice. *See also confinement, detection.*

attrition, the process of wearing away or wearing down by friction.

audiometer /ô´dē·om´ətər/, an electrical device for testing hearing and for measuring the conduction of sound through bone and air. The results are noted on a chart (**audiogram**).

audiometry /ô´dē·om´ətrē/, testing the sense of hearing. **Pure tone** audiometry determines the patient's ability to hear frequencies, usually ranging from 125 to 8000 hertz.

auditory ossicles /ô´ditôr´ē/, the small bones in the middle ear (incus, malleus, and stapes) that connect with each other and the tympanic membrane. Sound waves are carried though these bones as the tympanic membrane vibrates.

auditory tube. See **eustachian tube.**

aura /ôr´ə/, *pl.* **aurae** /ôr´ē/, a sensation of light or warmth that may be noted before a migraine or seizure.

aural /ôr´əl/, referring to the ear or hearing. **–aurally,** *adv.*

auricle /ôr´ikəl/, **1.** the external ear. Also known as **pinna. 2.** the left or right cardiac atrium, so named because of its earlike shape.

auricularis /ôr´ikyələr´is/, referring to the ear, as one of three muscles of the ear.

auriculin /ôrik´yəlin/, a hormonelike substance produced in the atria of the heart. It promotes the release of urine.

auscultation /ôs´kəltā´shən/, the act of listening for sounds within the body to evaluate the condition of the heart, lungs, bowel, or fetal heart beat. This is usually performed with a stethoscope.

autism /ô´tizm/, tending toward self absorption while ignoring reality.

autoantibody, an antibody that reacts against the patient's own body. Normally antibodies attack foreign antigens. Several processes may lead to the manufacture of autoantibodies. For example, antibodies produced against some streptococcal bacteria during infection may react with cardiac tissue and cause rheumatic heart disease.

autoantigen /-an´tijən/, any tissue component that causes a reaction of the body against tissues in the body. *See also autoantibody.*

autodiploid /-dip´loid/, referring to a person, organism, or cell containing two genetically identical or nearly identical chromosome sets.

autoeroticism /-irot´isizm/, sensual, usually sexual, satisfaction of the self, usually done through stimulation of one's own body.

autoerythrocyte sensitization /-ərith´rəsīt/, painful bleeding under the skin on the anterior areas of the arms and legs due to allergy to red blood cells.

autogenous /ôtoj´ənəs/, **1.** self-creating. **2.** originating from within the organism, as a poison or vaccine.

autograft. See **transplant.**

autoimmune disease, one of the large group of diseases marked by a change of the immune system of the body. Normally, the immune system controls the body's defenses against infection. Sometimes these defenses are turned against the body itself.

automated external defibrillator, a cardiac defibrillator, designed for field use, that analyzes dysrhythmias internally and shocks lethal rhythms automatically. Also known as **AED.**

Automated Merchant Vessel Report, an aircraft and vessel location tracking service of the U.S. Coast Guard that is used in an aircraft or vessel emergency. When a distress signal is received, the aircraft or vessels closest to the emergency scene are notified and asked to assist. Also known as **AMVER.**

automatic implanted cardiac defibrillator, an implanted device designed to perform cardiac defibrillation in the presence of life-threatening dysrhythmias. Also known as **AICD.** *See also implantable cardioverter defibrillator.*

automatic transport ventilator, portable respiratory ventilation device for patients requiring respiratory assistance during transport. Requires minimal adjustment to provide appropriate pressure and time parameters for ventilation. Also known as **ATV.**

automatic vehicle locator, a radio subsystem that periodically determines the position of a vehicle and relays that information to a communications center. These locators are equally effective for air, land, or water vehicles. Also known as **AVL.**

automaticity, the ability of cardiac pacemaker cells to initiate spontaneous electrical impulses.

automatism /ôtom´ətizm/, **1.** involuntary function of an organ system. It can be independent of central stimulation, such as beating of the heart, or dependent on central stimulation but not consciously controlled, such as the dilation of the pupil of the eye. **2.** mechanical, repetitive, and undirected behavior that is not consciously controlled as in psychomotor epilepsy, hysteric states, and sleepwalking.

autonomic, **1.** having the ability to function independently without outside influence. **2.** referring to the autonomic nervous system.

autonomic drug, any of a large group of drugs that copy or change the function of the autonomic nervous system.

autonomic nervous system, the involuntary portion of the peripheral nervous system that regulates vital body functions. Separated into parasympathetic and sympathetic divisions, this system controls cardiac and smooth muscle and glandular activity. Also known as **ANS.** *See also central nervous system, parasympathetic nervous system, peripheral nervous system, sympathetic nervous system.*

autonomic reflex, any of a large number of reflexes that regulate the functions of the autonomic nervous system, such as blood pressure, heart rate, intestinal activity, and urination.

autonomy /ôton´əmē/, the ability to function or live independently. –**autonomous,** *adj.*

autoplastic maneuver, a process that is part of adaptation, involving an adjustment within the self. The opposite, **alloplastic maneuver,** involves a change in the external environment.

autopsy /ô´topsē/, an examination after death that is done to determine the cause of death.

autoregulation, the process that regulates body systems independently by various biochemical and pressure parameters, as cerebral blood flow is maintained by vasoconstriction/dilation in response to blood pressure changes.

autosomal /-sō´məl/, **1.** referring to or characteristic of a non-sex-determining chromosome (autosome). **2.** referring to any condition carried by an autosome.

autosome /ô´təsōm/, any chromosome that is not a sex chromosome and appears as an identical (homologous) pair.

autosuggestion, an idea, thought, attitude, or belief suggested to oneself, as a means of controlling one's behavior.

autotoxin, a poison produced within the body.

auxanology /ôks´ənol´-/, the scientific study of growth and development.

available resources, resources assigned to an incident and available for an assignment.

avalanche, a snow mass that slides down a mountainside.

avalanche beacon. See **avalanche transceiver.**

avalanche cord, brightly colored nylon line, attached to a skier, that is used to determine location and depth in the event of being covered in an avalanche. This line, up to 20 meters (about 60 feet) long, is marked in increments, so that depth can be determined.

avalanche fracture zone. See **avalanche path.**

avalanche guard, a rescuer posted near the top of an avalanche path to warn rescuers below of an impending secondary avalanche.

avalanche path, the route an avalanche travels. The initial slide area is known as the **avalanche zone,** or **fracture zone.** This zone is between 25 and 55 degrees of inclination and is the area of initial snow mass fracture. Snow sliding down

from the fracture zone follows what is known as the **avalanche track.** The slope of this track is between 0 and 90 degrees of inclination. The end of the avalanche track, where the snow stops, is known as the **runout zone.**

avalanche search, looking for victims of an avalanche. Search tactics include using avalanche dogs, avalanche transceivers, and probing. Probing can be either hasty (Type I), coarse (Type II), or fine (Type III).

avalanche track. See **avalanche path.**

avalanche transceiver, a transmitter worn by a skier that emits a signal detectable up to 100 feet after being buried in a snow mass. The transmitter signal is emitted at 457 kilohertz and is detected on a receiver carried by a rescuer. Also known as **avalanche beacon, avalanche rescue beacon.**

avascular /āvas´kyələr/, without blood or lymphatic vessels.

avitaminosis /āvī´-/, a lack of one or more essential vitamins. It may result from lack of vitamins in the diet or inability to use the vitamins because of disease. Also known as **hypovitaminosis.**

AV nicking, a blood vessel abnormality on the retina of the eye. The vein appears "nicked" because of narrowing or spasm. It is a sign of hypertension, arteriosclerosis, and other disorders of the blood vessels.

Avogadro's law (Amedeo Avogadro, Italian physicist, 1776-1856), as long as gas pressure and temperature are the same, equal volumes of gases contain equal numbers of molecules.

Avogadro's number, the number of molecules in 1 gram-molecule; 6.0225×10^{23}. Also known as **Avogadro's constant.**

avoidance, a conscious or unconscious defense mechanism, physical or psychologic in nature, in which a person tries to escape from something unpleasant. *See also conflict.*

avoirdupois weight /av´ərdəpoiz´/, the English system of weights in which there are 7000 grains, 256 drams, or 16 ounces to 1 pound. One ounce in this system equals 28.35 grams. 1 pound equals 453.59 grams. *See also metric system.*

AVPU, an acronym used to describe different levels of patient consciousness: **A**lert; responsive to **V**erbal commands; responsive to **P**ain; or **U**nresponsive.

avulsion /əvul´zhən/, the partial or complete separation, by tearing, of any part of a structure.

axial, referring to or situated on the center (axis) of a structure or part of the body.

axial gradient, the variation of the metabolic rate in different parts of the body.

axial loading, traumatic compression force, placed along the axis of the spine, which may result in compression fractures.

axilla /aksil´ə/, *pl.* **axillae,** a pyramid-shaped space forming the underside of the shoulder between the superior portion of the arm and lateral chest.

axillary artery /ak´sələr´ē/, the artery that supplies each arm. Called the subclavian artery at the scapula, it becomes the axillary at the shoulder and the brachial at the bicep.

axillary nerve, the nerve that runs through the axilla, winds around the humerus, and supplies a portion of the deltoid and shoulder joint.

axillary node, one of the lymph glands of the axilla that drains lymph from the chest, neck, and arm. *See also lymphatic system, lymph node.*

axillary vein, one of a pair of veins of the arm that begins near the bicep and becomes the subclavian vein near the clavicle.

axis, **1.** a line around which an object rotates. **2.** one of the reference lines in a coordinate system. **3.** the second cervical vertebra. This is the pivot point around which the first cervical vertebra, the **atlas,** rotates, allowing head movement.

axis artery, one of a pair of extensions of the subclavian artery that supplies the upper arm and continues into the forearm as the palmar interosseous artery.

axon, the cylinderlike extension of a neuron that conducts impulses away from the neuron. Compare **dendrite.**

axon flare, vasodilatation, erythema and increased sensitivity of skin surrounding an injured area due to nerve damage.

azimuth, **1.** bearing; course; direction. **2.** the clockwise angle between a fixed point and the vertical plane through the object of interest; a horizontal arc.

azimuth compass, magnetic compass equipped with sights for measuring azimuth angle or bearing.

azoospermia /āzō´əspur´mē·ə/, lack of sperm in the semen.

azotemia /āz´ōtē´mē·ə/, excess amounts of nitrogen compounds in the blood due to a failure of the kidneys to remove urea from the blood. *See also uremia.* **–azotemic,** *adj.*

azygous /az´igəs/, occurring as a single being or part, as the mouth.

azygous vein, one of the seven veins of the chest.

B

babesiosis /bəbē´sē·ō´-/, an infection caused by the protozoa *Babesia,* which enters the body through the bite of ticks. Symptoms include headache, fever, nausea and vomiting, aching, and blood disorders.

Babinski's reflex (Joseph Babinski, French neurologist, 1857-1932), a reflex movement in which the great toe dorsiflexes and the other toes spread out in response to stroking the plantar aspect of the foot. This response is referred to as a **positive Babinski** and is seen in certain upper-motor neuron diseases, such as amyotrophic lateral sclerosis (Lou Gehrig's disease), or with intracranial bleeding or head injury. It can be a normal finding in children under twelve years of age. Also known as **Babinski's sign.**

baby, **1.** an infant or young child, especially one who is not yet able to walk or talk. **2.** to treat gently or with special care.

Baby Jane Doe regulations, rules established in 1984 by the United States Health and Human Services Department. States governments are required to investigate complaints about parental decisions involving the treatment of handicapped infants. The rules also allow the federal government to have access to children's medical records. Hospitals are required to post notices urging doctors and nurses to report any suspected cases of infants denied proper medical care. Also known as **Baby Doe rules.**

Bacillaceae /-lā´si·ē/, a family of *Schizomycetes* bacteria of the order *Eubacteriales,* consisting of rod-shaped cells. These bacteria commonly appear in soil. Some are parasitic on insects and animals and can cause disease. The family includes the genus *Bacillus,* which requires air (aerobic), and the genus *Clostridium,* which can live without air (anaerobic).

bacille Calmette-Guérin (BCG) /kälmet´gāraN´/, a weakened strain of tubercle bacilli, used in many countries as a vaccine against tuberculosis.

back, the back portion of the trunk between the neck and the pelvis. The back is divided by the spine. The skeletal portion of the back includes the thoracic and lumbar vertebrae and both scapulas.

backache, pain in the spine or muscles of the back. Causes may include muscle strain or other muscular disorders, pressure on the root of a nerve, or a ruptured vertebral disk.

backboard. See **spineboard**.

backdraft, an "explosion" or rapid burning of heated gases resulting from the introduction of oxygen when air is admitted to a building that is heavily charged with smoke from a fire that has depleted the oxygen content of the building.

backfill, **1.** the material used to refill an open trench. **2.** the refilling of an open trench.

background radiation, naturally occurring radiation given off by materials in the soil, ground water, and building material. Radioactive substances in the body, especially potassium 40 (^{40}K), and cosmic radiation also give off background radiation. The average person is exposed each year to 44 millirad (mrad) of cosmic radiation, 44 mrad from the environment, and 18 mrad from naturally occurring internal radioactive sources.

back pressure, pressure that builds in a vessel or a cavity as fluid accumulates. The pressure increases and extends backward if the normal passageway for the fluid is not opened.

back-pressure arm-lift, *(historical)* a manual method of artificial respiration, used in the first half of the twentieth century for victims of respiratory arrest. The technique consisted of kneeling at the patient's head, compressing the back of a prone patient (to cause exhalation), and providing lung expansion by pulling the upper arms toward the rescuer in a rhythmic fashion, twelve times per minute. This technique has since been replaced by mouth-to-mouth ventilation. Also known as **Holger-Nielsen method.** *See also chest-pressure arm-lift, Schäfer prone pressure method.*

backwash, **1.** backward-flowing water, caused by a rapid drop over an obstruction, which creates a hole in the surface water directly below the obstruction. **2.** the drag of a receding wave. **3.** water thrown backward by the passage of a ship.

bacteremia /-tirē´mē·ə/, the presence of bacteria in the blood. Bacteremia is diagnosed by growing organisms from a blood sample. Compare **blood poisoning.**

bacteria /baktir´ē·ə/, *(sing)* **bacterium,** the one-celled microorganisms of the class Schizomycetes. Some are round (cocci), rod-shaped (bacilli), spiral (spirochetes), or comma-shaped (vibrios). The nature, of any infection caused by a bacterium depend on the species.

bactericidal /-sī´dəl/, destructive to bacteria. Compare **bacteriostatic.**

bacteriology, the scientific study of bacteria.

bacteriophage /baktir´ē·əfāj´/, any virus that destroys bacteria. **Bacteriophage typing** is the process of identifying a species of bacteria according to the type of virus that attacks it.

bacteriostatic, tending to restrain the development of bacteria. Compare **bacteriocidal.**

bacteriuria /-ēyoŏr´ē·ə/, the presence of bacteria in the urine. More than 100,000 bacteria per ml of urine usually means a urinary tract infection is present. *See also urinary tract infection.*

Bacteroides /-oi´dēz/, a genus of bacilli that can live without air (anaerobic). They are normally found in the large intestine, mouth, genital tract, and upper respiratory system. Infection may result if the integrity of the mucous membrane is compromised and the bacillus enters the circulation.

bagging, *(informal)* ventilating a patient with a bag-valve unit.

bag of waters. See **amniotic sac.**

baguio. See **tropical cyclone.**

bag-valve mask, a manual breathing device consisting of an oxygen reservoir, a self-refilling bag, a nonreturn valve, and an assortment of masks. The device is squeezed by hand to generate airflow to the nonbreathing or respiratorially compromised patient. Oxygen is added via the reservoir or connecting tubing. It can be used with a face mask, esophageal obturator airway, or endotracheal tube. Also known as **ambu bag, bag-valve, BVM.**

Bainbridge reflex, an increased pulse rate, resulting from stimulation of the wall of the left (cardiac) atrium. It may be produced by large amounts of intravenous fluids.

balaclava /bal´əklä´və/, *(special operations)* a head covering that is worn as protection and/or camouflage during covert or night law enforcement operations. It is a dark-colored, knitted hood that covers the entire head and face, leaving only the eye area exposed.

balance, **1.** an instrument for weighing. **2.** a normal state of physical equilibrium. **3.** a state of mental or emotional equilibrium.

balanic /bəlan´ik/, referring to the penis or the clitoris.

balanitis, inflammation of the penis.

balanoposthitis /-posthī´-/, a generalized inflammation of the penis and foreskin. The symptoms are soreness, irritation, and discharge, occurring as a complication of bacterial or fungal infection. The cause is often a venereal disease.

balisage /bal´isäzh´/, *(special operations)* nighttime route marking, using dim or infrared beacon lights, that allows vehicles to drive without lights at daytime speed.

ball-and-socket joint, a synovial joint in which the round head of one bone is held in the cuplike cavity of another bone. This allows a limb to move in many directions. The hip and shoulder joints are ball-and-socket joints. *See also joint.*

ballistic helmet, protective helmet made of several layers of metal and woven fabric, which absorbs and spreads the impact of bullets or shrapnel across a greater surface area. It is used primarily during high-risk law enforcement and military operations to decrease the danger of head injury.

ballistics, the study of projectiles, their movement and impact. Although this term applies to any projectile, it is most often used to refer to bullets and their damage.

ballistocardiogram /-kär´-/, a recording of the vibrations of the body that are caused by the beating of the heart. When blood is pumped into the aorta and the pulmonary arteries, it causes a vibration beginning at the head and traveling to the feet. The patient is placed on a special table, a ballistocardiograph, that is so delicately balanced that vibrations of the body can be recorded by a machine attached to the table. It is used to determine how elastic the aorta is and the amount of blood the heart is able to handle.

ball mill, a mill containing material to be pulverized in a drum with numerous heavy balls. As the drum is rotated, the balls smash the material. Typically, this is used to crush ore to facilitate its separation.

ballottement /bä´lôtmäN´, bəlot´mənt/, a technique of palpating an organ or structure by bouncing it gently and feeling it rebound. In late pregnancy, a fetal head that can be ballotted is said to be **floating** or **unengaged.** This is in contrast to a fixed or an engaged head which cannot be easily dislodged from the pelvis.

ball-valve action, the opening and closing of a hole by a buoyant, ball-shaped mass that acts as a valve. Some kinds of objects that may act in this manner are kidney stones, gallstones, and blood clots.

bamboo spine, the typically rigid spine of advanced ankylosing spondylitis. Also known as **poker spine.**

band, a bundle of fibers that encircles a structure or binds one part of the body to another.

bandage, 1. (verb) covering a body part by bandage application. 2. (noun) gauze or other material, applied to a portion of the body to apply pressure, hold dressing, provide support, and/or immobilize. Types include **adhesive** (absorbent gauze with a fabric or plastic covering that is covered with adhesive), **elastic** (a stretchable material that provides pressure), **roller** (variable-width material, formed into a roll, so as to aid application), **stockinet** (a variable length of elastic material that can be applied to an extremity to hold a dressing), and **triangular** (cloth cut in a triangular shape and folded or tied into various configurations). Various methods of application have particular names, such as **Barton's** (bandaging around the head, so as to support the mandible), **butterfly** (strips of adhesive applied across a small laceration to approximate the wound edges together), **capeline** (covering an amputation or head like a cap), **chest, cravat** (a triangular bandage folded lengthwise after bringing the point of the triangle down to the middle of its base), **figure-of-eight** (a bandage applied to two separate areas so that its turns resemble a figure 8), **oblique** (progressive turns of the bandage proceed obliquely around an extremity), **pressure, sling, Velpeau** /velpō´/ (material that immobilizes an arm to the chest wall with the hand pointing upward toward the opposite clavicle). *See also Ace bandage, dressing, pressure bandage, rubber bandage.*

bandage shears, angled scissors with a rounded, blunt tip, used to cut bandaging material. The blunt tip prevents damage to the skin when the point is inserted under the bandage. When equipped with a serrated edge and used to cut material, such as clothes, they are also known as **trauma shears, trauma scissors.**

bank blood, preserved blood collected from donors in pints (500 ml) and refrigerated for future use. Bank blood is used after it is matched to the recipient's blood. *See also blood bank.*

Banti's syndrome /ban´tēz/, blockage of the blood vessels that lie between the intestine and liver, causing an enlarged spleen, abdominal bleeding, cirrhosis of the liver, and destruction of red and white blood cells. Early symptoms are weakness, fatigue, and anemia.

barbiturates, organic derivatives of barbituric acid, which act as central nervous system depressants.

barbiturism /bärbich´ər-/, **1.** sudden or long-term poisoning by any of the barbiturates. Excessive amounts of these drugs may be fatal or may produce physical and psychologic changes, as depressed respiration, hypoxia, disorientation, and coma. **2.** addiction to a barbiturate.

Bard-Pic syndrome, a condition of jaundice and enlarged gallbladder. Syndrome worsens with advanced pancreatic cancer.

Bard's sign, nystagmus when the patient tries to follow a target moved from side to side.

bariatrics /ber´ē·at´riks/, the field of medicine that focuses on the treatment and control of obesity and diseases associated with obesity.

barium (Ba) /ber´-/, a pale yellow, metallic element classified with the alkaline earths. Fine, milky barium sulfate is given to patients before x-rays films are taken of the digestive tract.

Barlow's syndrome, an abnormal heart condition with the sound of a murmur and a click. These symptoms are associated with back flow of blood caused by prolapse of the mitral valve located between the left atrium and ventricle.

barodontalgia /ber´ōdontal´jə/, tooth pain associated with pressure changes. Most commonly, this pain occurs during scuba diving when a faulty dental filling traps air during descent or ascent.

baroreceptor /-risep´-/, one of the pressure-sensitive nerve endings in the walls of the atria of the heart and in some larger blood vessels. Baroreceptors stimulate reflex mechanisms that allow the body to adapt to changes in blood pressure by dilating or constricting blood vessels.

barosinusitis, sinus pain and/or damage during exposure to pressure changes. This pain or damage to a sinus is due to an inability to equalize internal air pressure, within the sinus cavity, with higher or lower surrounding external pressure. Scuba diving is the usual provoking activity. Also known as **sinus squeeze, squeeze.**

barotitis, ear pain and/or trauma during exposure to pressure changes. The pain is due to an inability to equalize internal ear pressure with surrounding external pressure. Also known as **ear squeeze, squeeze.**

barotrauma, injury due to exposure to increased ambient pressure, such as a pneumothorax that occurs to a scuba diver while submerged.

barrel chest, a large, rounded chest, considered normal in some stocky people and others who live in high-altitude areas. They develop larger lung capacities. Barrel chest, however, may also be a sign of emphysema.

Barrett's syndrome, an ulcerlike area in the esophagus. It is caused most often by long-term irritation of the esophagus from digestive juices flowing back into the esophagus. Treatment is similar to that for heartburn.

barrier, **1.** a wall or other obstacle that can block the passage of substances. Barrier methods of contraception, as the condom or diaphragm, prevent sperm from entering the uterus. Membranes of the body act as screenlike barriers to permit water or certain other molecules to move from one side to the other, while preventing the passage of other substances. **2.** something nonphysical that obstructs, as barriers to communication.

Bartholin's gland, small glands located on the wall near the opening of the vagina. These glands help lubricate the vagina. **Bartholinitis** is an inflammation of one or both Bartholin's glands, caused by bacterial infection.

Barton's fracture, a fracture of the forearm involving the bone on the thumb side of the arm (radius) near the wrist. A dislocated wrist may also be present.

Bartter's syndrome, a rare hereditary disorder with kidney enlargement and overactive adrenal glands.

basal /bā´səl/, referring to the fundamental or the basic. For example, "basal metabolic rate" means the lowest rate at which chemical activity (metabolism) occurs in the body.

basal bone, **1.** the bone of the upper and lower jaw, which provides support for artificial dentures. **2.** the fixed bone structure that limits the movement of teeth.

basal cell, any one of the cells in the base layer of the epithelium. The epithelium is the lining of the internal and external surfaces of the body, including organs, blood vessels, and skin (epidermis).

basal cell carcinoma, a slow-growing cancer on the face that begins as a small bump and enlarges to the side. It develops a central crater that erodes, crusts, and bleeds.

basal ganglia, the islands of gray matter within the lobes of the brain (cerebrum). They are involved in posture and coordination.

basal membrane, a sheet of tissue that lies just under the pigmented layer of the retina in the eye.

basal metabolism, the amount of energy needed to maintain essential body functions, such as respiration, circulation, temperature, intestinal activity, and muscle tone.

basaloid carcinoma, a rare, malignant tumor of the anal canal. These tumors contain areas that resemble basal cell carcinoma of the skin. The tumor may spread to the skin of the genital area.

base, 1. a chemical compound that combines with an acid to form a salt. Compare **alkali. 2.** the major ingredient of a compounded material, particularly one that is used as a drug. Petroleum jelly is frequently used as a base for ointments.

base hospital, 1. the emergency department to which a paramedic unit is assigned and from which it receives its on-line medical direction. **2.** the hospital where a paramedic unit is stationed.

base leg, that position in an aircraft landing pattern where the aircraft is at a 90° angle to the runway. *See also final approach.*

baseline fetal heart rate, the fetal heart rate during labor between contractions of the uterus. Very fast or slow rates (less than 120 or more than 160 per minute) can mean the baby's oxygen supply has been interrupted.

base of the heart, the right-side inferior portion of the heart; the opposite of the apex. *See also apex of the heart.*

base station, 1. the nonmobile transceiver and antenna used at a communications center that connects that facility with mobile units. **2.** the building or room containing a fixed radio system, telephones, and intercoms.

bas-fond /bäfôN´/, the bottom or base of any structure, especially the urinary bladder.

basilar artery, the artery at the base of the skull that is formed by the junction of the two vertebral arteries. It supplies blood to the internal ear and parts of the brain.

basilar artery insufficiency syndrome, a lack of blood flow through the basilar artery. The cause can be a blockage. Symptoms include dizziness, blindness, numbness, depression, speech problems, and weakness on one side of the body.

basilic vein /bəsil´ik/, one of the four veins of the arm near the surface. It runs along the inside of the forearm.

basin, a low, bowl-shaped landform surrounded by elevated land.

basioccipital /-oksip´-/, referring to the occipital bone.

basophilic adenoma, a tumor of the pituitary gland. Cushing's syndrome is often caused by a basophilic adenoma. *See also adenoma.*

basophilic leukemia, a cancer of blood-forming tissues, characterized by larger numbers of immature basophils. *See also leukemia.*

basophilic stippling, the presence of spotted basophils in the red blood cells. Stippling is characteristic of lead poisoning.

basosquamous cell carcinoma /-skwā´-/, a malignant skin tumor composed of basal and squamous cells.

bathesthesia /bath´əsthē´zhə/, a sensitivity of internal parts of the body. It is associated with organs or structures beneath the surface, as muscles and joints.

bathycardia /bath´ə-/, an unusually low position of the heart in the chest. It usually does not affect function.

batter boards, horizontal boards that span a trench.

battered woman syndrome, repeated episodes of physical assault on a woman by the man with whom she lives, often resulting in serious physical and emotional damage to the woman. Such violence tends to follow a pattern, such as verbal abuse on almost any subject—housekeeping, money, or childrearing. Often the violent episodes become more frequent and severe over time. Studies show that the longer the woman stays in the relationship the more likely she is to be seriously injured.

battery, **1.** a group of cells or condensers used for making electricity. **2.** the striking or touching of person against their will or without their consent.

Battey bacillus, any of a group of mycobacteria that cause a long-term lung disease resembling tuberculosis.

Battle's sign, an area of ecchymosis behind the ear. It may indicate a fracture of the basilar skull.

Baudelocque's method /bôdloks´/, turning the baby from a face-first position to a crown-first position just before delivery.

bay, **1.** part of a lake, ocean, or sea that extends into the land. It is usually smaller than a gulf. **2.** a section of an enclosed parking area, usually related to a fire station, that will accommodate one or more vehicles.

B cell, a type of white blood cell (lymphocyte) that comes from the bone marrow. It is one of the two lymphocytes that play a major role in the body's immune response. Compare **T cell.** *See also plasma cell.*

B complex vitamins, a large group of water-soluble substances that includes **vitamin B$_1$ (thiamine), vitamin B$_2$ (riboflavin), vitamin B$_3$ (niacin), vitamin B$_6$ (pyridoxine), vitamin B$_{12}$ (cyanocobalamin), biotin, choline, carnitine, folic acid, inositol,** and **para-aminobenzoic acid.** The B complex vitamins are essential in breaking down carbohydrates into glucose to provide energy, and for breaking down fats and proteins. They are also needed for normal functioning of the nervous system, for maintenance of muscle tone in the stomach and intestinal tract, and for the health of skin, hair, eyes, mouth, and liver. They are found in brewer's yeast, liver, whole-grain cereals, nuts, eggs, meats, fish, and vegetables and are produced by the intestinal bacteria. Symptoms of vitamin B deficiency include nervousness, depression, insomnia, anemia, hair loss, acne or other skin disorders, and excessive cholesterol in the blood. *See also specific vitamins.*

Beck's triad, a combination of three symptoms that show compression of the heart: high pressure in the veins, low pressure in the arteries, and a small heart.

Beckwith's syndrome, a hereditary disorder in infants of hypoglycemia and overproduction of insulin.

bed, a supporting tissue, as the nail beds of specialized skin over which the fingernails and the toenails move as they grow.

bedbug, a bloodsucking arthropod of the species *Cimex* that feeds on humans and other animals. The bite causes itching, pain, and redness.

bedding, material placed in the bottom of a trench as a foundation for pipe. This material is usually fine or crushed stone. Also known as **bedding stone.**

bedsore, an ulcer (decubitus) on the skin over a bony projection of the body. It results from prolonged pressure.

bee sting, an injury caused by the venom of bees, usually accompanied by pain and swelling.

behavior, **1.** the manner in which a person acts or performs. **2.** any or all of the activities of a person, including physical and mental activity.

behavioral crisis, an incapacitating manner of behavior that occurs suddenly in an otherwise functional person.

behavior disorder, any of a group of antisocial behavior patterns occurring mainly in children and adolescents. The behavior disorder include overaggressiveness, overactivity, destructiveness, cruelty, truancy, lying, disobedience, perverse sexual activity, criminality, alcoholism, and drug addiction. The most common reason for such behavior is hostility. It is provoked by a disturbed relationship between the child and the parents, an unstable home situation, and, in some cases, organic brain dysfunction. *See also antisocial personality disorder.*

bel, a unit that expresses intensity of sound. An increase of 1 bel approximately doubles the intensity or loudness of most sounds.

belay, **1.** a sturdy projection around which a rope can be passed in order to secure it. The rope is then used to secure a climber who will act as a safeguard to prevent another climber from falling. **2.** the act of assuming a secure position and protecting another climber from significant falls.

3. *(verb, transitive)* to secure or make fast. **4.** *(interjection)* disregard; stop.

belayed boat rescue, river rescue technique using a boat that is tethered to both banks and that can be moved between them. Used primarily on wide rivers or those devoid of suitable anchorage.

belladonna, the dried leaves, roots, and flowering or fruiting tops of *Atropa belladonna,* a common perennial called deadly nightshade. It contains hyoscyamine, which is a source of atropine.

Bell's law, an axiom stating that the nerves at the internal part of the spinal cord control the muscles and those at the outer part control the senses.

Bell's palsy, paralysis of the facial nerve, caused by injury to the nerve, compression of the nerve by a tumor, or an infection.

belonephobia /bel´ənə-/, fear of sharp-pointed objects, especially needles and pins.

benching, mining procedure in which horizontal slices of the floor of a mine are removed in order to extract the ore it contains. *See also heading, shrinkage.*

bending fracture, a fracture indirectly caused by bending an extremity, such as the foot or the big toe.

bends. See **decompression sickness.**

benign /bənīn´/, not harmful; describing a condition or disorder that is not a threat to health. Compare **malignant.**

benign prostatic hypertrophy, enlargement of the prostate gland, common among men after 50 years of age. The condition is not malignant or inflammatory. It may lead to blockage of the urethra and interfere with the flow of urine. This can increase frequency of urination, the need to urinate during the night, pain, and urinary tract infections. Compare **prostatitis.**

bent fracture, a fracture caused by the bone being forcibly bent. The actual fracture may be some distance from the area that was bent.

benzene poisoning, poisoning caused by swallowing benzene, inhaling benzene fumes, or exposure to benzene-related products, such as toluene or xylene. Symptoms include nausea, headache, dizziness, and incoordination. In severe cases, respiratory failure or extremely rapid heart beat may cause death. Long-term exposure may result in aplastic anemia or a form of leukemia. Benzene poisoning by inhalation is treated with breathing assistance and oxygen. Poisoning from swallowing benzene is treated by flushing the stomach with water. *See also nitrobenzene poisoning.*

benzodiazepine derivative /ben´zōdī·az´əpin/, one of a group of drugs used to relieve anxiety or insomnia, including tranquilizers and hypnotics. Tolerance and physical dependence occur with prolonged high doses. Withdrawal symptoms, including seizures and serious psychosis, may occur if the drug is abruptly stopped. Side effects include drowsiness, muscle incoordination, and increased aggression and hostility. However, these reactions are not commonly seen in patients who take only the usual recommended dose.

benzyl alcohol, a clear, colorless, oily liquid, derived from certain balsams. It is used as an anesthetic on the skin and to prevent bacteria from growing in solutions for injection.

benzyl benzoate, a clear, oily liquid with a pleasant, aromatic odor. It is used to destroy lice and scabies, as a solvent, and as a flavor for gum.

bergschrund /burk´shrōōnt/, the giant crevasse created when the leading edge of a glacier encounters rocky terrain and breaks off.

beriberi, a nervous system disease affecting the arms and legs caused by a deficiency of thiamine. It is usually caused by a diet limited to polished white rice and is common in eastern and southern Asia. Rare cases in the United States are linked with stressful conditions, such as underactive thyroid gland, infections, pregnancy, breast feeding, and alcoholism. Symptoms include fatigue, diarrhea, appetite and weight loss, disturbed nerve function causing paralysis and wasting of limbs, water retention, and heart failure. *See also thiamine.*

Berlock dermatitis, a skin disorder caused by a reaction to oil of bergamot (psoralens), which is commonly used in perfumes, colognes, and pomades. Dark patches and sores appear on the skin. This condition affects primarily women and children and may result from using products that contain psoralens and exposure to ultraviolet light. The level of ultraviolet radiation reaching the earth on a sunny day is enough to cause the condition to appear.

Bert, Paul (19th century French physiologist), first scientist to demonstrate that the symptoms of decompression sickness are caused by bubbles of nitrogen that form in the blood during rapid decompression. His book *Barometric Pressure* began the scientific approach to the study of decompression sickness in 1878. He also discovered that oxygen is toxic when breathed under pressure and that symptoms we now know as belonging to hypoxia are due to a lack of oxygen. *See also Paul Bert effect.*

berylliosis /bəril´ē·o´-/, poisoning that results from inhaling dusts or vapors that contain beryllium, a steel-gray light-weight metallic element.

bestiality, **1.** sexual relations between a human being and an animal. **2.** sodomy.

beta (β), the second letter of Greek alphabet, used as a combining form with chemical names to distinguish one of two or more forms or to show the position of substituted atoms in certain compounds. Compare **alpha.**

beta-adrenergic blocking agent. See **antiadrenergic.**

beta-adrenergic receptor, adrenergic receptor tissues that respond to beta agonists, such as epinephrine and the beta-blocking substances atenolol, labetalol, or propranolol.

beta-adrenergic stimulating agent. See **adrenergic.**

beta-carotene, an ultraviolet screening agent used to reduce sensitivity to the sun.

beta cells, **1.** cells in the pancreas that produce insulin. The insulin production by the beta cells tends to speed up the movement of glucose, amino acids, and fatty acids out of the blood and into the cells. **2.** cells in the pituitary gland.

beta-hydroxybutyric acid, a ketone body produced in large amounts during the fatty acid oxidation that occurs in diabetic ketoacidosis.

beta particle or **beta ray,** a small particle ejected spontaneously from a nucleus of a radioactive element. It has the mass of the electron and a charge of minus 1 or plus 1. It has a medium or intermediate penetrating power; its range in air

is from a few inches to several feet. The most energetic beta particles will penetrate the skin and a fraction of an inch of tissue. The damage is manifested primarily as skin burns. Symbol: β^- or β^+.

beta receptor, any one of the adrenergic receptors of the nervous system that responds to adrenaline (epinephrine). Activation causes relaxation of the smooth muscles and an increase in cardiac rate and contractility.

bicarbonate buffer system, one of the three compensatory mechanisms of the body that uses bicarbonate, carbon dioxide, and carbonic acid to maintain pH within a normal range. This system, acting with the kidneys and lungs, provides a balance between the acids and bases produced during normal body metabolism.

biceps brachii, the long muscle that stretches over the humerus. It flexes the arm and the forearm. Also known as **biceps.**

biconcave, concave on both sides, usually applied to a lens.

biconvex, bulging out (convex) on both sides, usually applied to a lens.

bicuspid /bīkus´pid/, **1.** having two cusps or points. **2.** one of two teeth between the molars and canines of the upper and lower jaw.

bidactyly /bīdak´tilē/, condition in which the second, third, and fourth fingers on the same hand are missing.

bifocal, referring to an eyeglass lens that has two areas, one for near vision and the other for distant vision.

bifurcation, a splitting into two branches, as the trachea, which branches into the two bronchi of the lungs.

bigeminy /bījem´ənē/, cardiac electrical activity characterized by a pattern of one ectopic beat followed by one normal beat. These ectopic beats can be atrial or ventricular in origin and are indicative of cardiac irritability. *See also trigeminy, quadrigeminy.*

bight, **1.** a portion of slack rope; a loop or coil. **2.** a bend in a coast or river.

bilateral, **1.** having two sides, or layers. **2.** occurring or appearing on two sides. A patient with bilateral hearing loss may have partial or total deafness in both ears.

bile, a bitter, yellow-green secretion of the liver. Bile is stored in the gallbladder and is released when fat enters the duodenum. Bile emulsifies these fats, preparing them for further digestion and absorption in the small intestine. Also known as **gall.**

bile ducts, any of several passageways that convey bile from the liver to the small intestine. Also known as **biliary ducts.**

bilge, the portion of a ship from the keel to where the sides begin to rise; the lowest part of a boat or ship.

Bilgeri method, a crevasse rescue technique that utilizes two ropes to which a climber is secured by foot loops or prusiks. The victim is then raised to the top of the crevasse by alternating rope movements from above.

biliary /bil´ē·er´ē/, referring to bile or to the gallbladder and its ducts, which transport bile to the duodenum. These are often called the **biliary tract** or the **biliary system.**

biliary atresia, an inborn absence or poor development of one or more of the biliary structures. It causes jaundice and early liver damage. *See also biliary cirrhosis.*

biliary calculus. See **gallstone.**

biliary cirrhosis, an inflammatory condition in which the flow of bile through the liver is obstructed. With **primary biliary cirrhosis,** there is abdominal pain, jaundice, and enlargement of the liver and spleen. Other symptoms include weight loss and diarrhea with pale, bulky stools. Blood coagulation defects may also occur with petechia and epistaxis. Fractures may occur from a lack of absorbed vitamin D and calcium. *See also cirrhoses.*

biliary duct. See **bile ducts.**

biliary fistula, an abnormal passage from the gallbladder, a bile duct, or the liver to an internal organ or to the surface of the body. A biliary fistula may open into the large intestine, duodenum, liver duct, or abdominal cavity.

biliary obstruction, blockage of the common or cystic bile duct, usually caused by one or more gallstones. Stones, consisting chiefly of cholesterol, bile pigment, and calcium, may form in the gallbladder and liver duct in persons of either sex at any age but are more common in middle-aged women. This obstruction interferes with bile drainage and produces an inflammatory reaction. Symptoms of biliary obstruction include severe pain near the sternum that may radiate to the back/shoulder, nausea, vomiting and diaphoresis.

biliary tract cancer, an uncommon malignant tumor in a bile duct, occurring slightly more often in men than in women. Symptoms include progressive jaundice, itching, weight loss, and, in the later stages, severe pain.

bilious /bil´yəs/, referring to bile, such as an excessive secretion of bile, or a disorder affecting the bile.

bilirubin /-roo´-/, the orange-yellow pigment in bile, formed mainly by the breakdown of hemoglobin in red blood cells. Bilirubin normally travels in the bloodstream to the liver, where it is changed to a water-soluble form and excreted into the bile. In a healthy person, most of the bilirubin produced daily is excreted from the body in the stool. The yellow skin of jaundice is caused by bilirubin in the blood and in the tissues of the skin. *See also jaundice.*

biliuria /-yoor´ē·ə/, the presence of bile in the urine.

bimaxillary /bīmak´siler´ē/, referring to the right and left maxilla.

bilobate /bīlō´bāt/, having two lobes.

bimanual, the use of both hands.

binary fission, direct division of a cell or nucleus into two equal parts. It is the common form of asexual reproduction of bacteria, protozoa, and other lower forms of life.

bind, **1.** to bandage or wrap. **2.** to join together with a band. **3.** to combine or unite molecules.

binocular, **1.** referring to both eyes, especially regarding vision. **2.** a microscope, telescope, or field glass that can accommodate viewing by both eyes.

binocular fixation, the process of having both eyes directed at the same object at the same time. This is essential to having good depth perception.

binocular vision, the use of both eyes together so that the images seen by each eye are combined to appear as a single image. Compare **diplopia.**

bioavailability, the amount of drug or other substance that is active in the tissues.

biochemistry, the chemistry of living organisms and life processes.

bioelectricity, electric current that is produced by living tissues, as nerves, brain, heart, and muscles. The electric impulses of human tissues are recorded by electrocardiograph, electroencephalograph, and similar sensitive devices.

bioequivalent, referring to a drug that has the same effect on the body as another drug, usually one nearly identical in its chemical structure.

bioethics, the application of morals and values to solve dilemmas in biology and medicine.

biofeedback, a method used in learning to alter certain functions of the body, such as blood pressure, muscle tension, and brain wave activity, through relaxation. A device may be used to allow the patient to monitor this information. Some conditions, such as high blood pressure, insomnia, and migraine headache, may be treated this way.

bioflavonoid /-flā´-/, any of a group of substances found in many fruits and essential for the absorption and processing of vitamin C (ascorbic acid). Also known as **vitamin P.** *See also vitamin C.*

biogenic /-jen´ik/, **1.** produced by the action of a living organism, as fermentation. **2.** essential to life and the maintenance of health, such as food, water, proper rest.

biologic, any substance made from living organisms or the products of living organisms that is used in the diagnosis, prevention, or treatment of disease. Kinds of biologics include **antigens, antitoxins, serums, vaccines.**

biological death, the beginning of organ death due to hypoxia. The brain is the body's most hypoxia-sensitive organ, with cell death beginning 4-6 minutes after oxygen deprivation. *See also clinical death.*

biological half-life, the time required for the body to eliminate one half of an internally deposited substance by normal processes of elimination. This time is also the same for stable and radioactive isotopes of a particular element.

biology, the scientific study of plants and animals.

biomechanics, the study of mechanical laws and their application to living organisms, especially the human body and its movement.

biomedical engineering, a system of techniques in which knowledge of biologic processes is applied to solve practical medical problems.

bionics /bī·on´iks/, the science of applying electronic principles and devices, such as computers and solid-state miniaturized circuitry, to medical problems, such as artificial pacemakers. **–bionic,** *adj.*

biopsy /bī´əpsē/, removing a small piece of living tissue from an organ or other part of the body for microscopic examination to establish a diagnosis or follow the course of a disease.

biorhythm, any cyclic, biologic event, such as the sleep cycle, the menstrual cycle, or the respiratory cycle. **–biorhythmic,** *adj.*

biostatistics. See **vital statistics.**

biosynthesis /-sin´thəsis/, any of thousands of chemical reactions continually occurring throughout the body. In biosynthesis, molecules form more complex biomolecules, especially carbohydrates, fats, proteins, nucleotides, and nucleic acids.

biotechnology, the study of the relationships between humans or other living organisms and machinery.

biotelemetry. See **telemetry.**

biotin /bī´ətin/, a colorless, crystalline, water-soluble B complex vitamin that helps produce fatty acids. It also helps the body use protein, folic acid, pantothenic acid, and vitamin B_{12}. Rich sources are egg yolk, beef liver, kidney, unpolished rice, brewer's yeast, peanuts, cauliflower, and mushrooms.

biotoxicology, the science of poisons, divided into animal and plant poisons. *See also phytotoxicology, zootoxicology.*

biotransformation, the chemical changes a substance undergoes in the body, as by the action of enzymes. *See also metabolism.*

Biot's respirations /bēōz´/ (Camille Biot, 19th-century French physician), abrupt, irregular, alternating periods of apnea and breathing of a constant rate and depth, as a result of increased intracranial pressure. Also known as **ataxic breathing, ataxic respirations, Biot's breathing, respiratory ataxia.**

bipolar /bīpō´lər/, **1.** having two poles, as in certain types of electrotherapy using opposite poles (positive and negative). **2.** referring to a nerve cell that has electric signals traveling both to and away from the center (afferent and efferent).

bipolar disorder, a mental disorder with periods of mania and depression. The manic phase shows excess emotional displays, excitement, overactivity, excess joy, a high degree of energy, inability to concentrate, and reduced need for sleep, often coupled with unrealistic ideas about one's worth. In the depressive phase, apathy and underactivity are seen along with feelings of excess sadness, loneliness, guilt, and lowered sense of one's worth.

bipolar lead, two electrodes of opposite polarity forming a single lead.

birth, event of being born, the coming of a new person out of its mother into the world. Kinds of birth are **breech birth, live birth, stillbirth.**

birth canal, *(informal)* the passage that extends from the opening in the pelvis to the vaginal opening, through which an infant passes during birth.

birth defect, any abnormality present at birth, primarily a structural one. Also known as a **congenital anomaly,** it may be inherited, obtained during pregnancy, or inflicted during childbirth. A **developmental anomaly** refers to any birth defect that results when the normal growth of the fetus is disturbed.

birth injury, damage to a baby while being born. Also known as **birth trauma.**

birthmark. See **nevus.**

birth rate, the number of births during a given period in relation to the total population of a certain area. The birth rate is usually counted as the number of births per 1000 of population.

birth weight, the weight of a baby when born, usually about 3500 g (7.5 lbs). In the United States, 97% of newborns weigh between 2500 g (5.5 lbs) and 4500 g (10 lbs). Babies who are full term but weigh less that 2500 g are termed **small for gestational age.** This is smaller than 90% of all babies born. Babies who weigh more than 4500 g are called **large for gestational age,** whether delivered prematurely, at term, or later than term. Diabetes mellitus in the mother is a cause of rapid fetal growth. These infants are generally obese, listless, limp, feed poorly, and have hypoglycemia within the first few hours.

bisect, to cross; to intersect; to divide into two equal parts.

bisexual, 1. having sex organs of both sexes (hermaphroditic). **2.** engaging in both heterosexual and homosexual activity.

bismuth (Bi) /biz´məth/, a reddish metal element. It is combined with other elements, such as oxygen, to make salts used in pharmaceutical production.

bite, 1. the act of cutting, tearing, holding, or gripping with the teeth. **2.** relationship of the teeth to each other. An **open bite** is a condition in which the lower front teeth do not touch the upper front teeth when the jaws are closed. **Overbite** refers to the vertical overlapping of lower teeth by upper teeth. A **closed bite** is an abnormal overbite.

biteblock, device inserted into the mouth to prevent trauma to the teeth or tongue during seizures or with orally intubated patients. Its use with orally intubated patients also prevents obstruction of the endotracheal tube if the patient bites down on it.

bitter end, the end of any line or rope.

bivalent, a chemical element or molecule having the ability to accept or donate two electrons in a chemical reaction.

black, 1. without color; reflecting no light. **2.** covert; having a classified or unknown nature.

black box, 1. any removable electronic unit in an aircraft, particularly voice or data recorders. **2.** a portable electronic device that utilizes unknown principles of operation.

blackdamp, air with carbon dioxide replacing oxygen due to combustion or explosion. Protective, self-contained breathing equipment is required in these atmospheres because of inadequate oxygen concentrations.

black ice, ice containing a large amount of debris and dirt. The term is generally used when referring to ice encountered on mountains and in gullies.

black lung. See **anthracosis.**

blackout, *(informal)* a temporary loss of vision or consciousness resulting from lack of oxygen to the brain.

blackwater fever. See **malaria.**

black widow spider, a poisonous spider (arachnid) found in many parts of the world.

The poison injected with its bite causes sweating, abdominal cramps, nausea, headaches, and dizziness. Small children, the elderly, and those with heart conditions are most severely affected.

bladder, **1.** a sac that holds fluids. **2.** the urinary bladder.

blanch, **1.** causing to become white or pale. **2.** becoming white or pale, as from narrowing of the blood vessels that happens with fear or anger.

bland, mild or having a soothing effect.

blast cell, any immature cell, as a red blood cell (erythroblast), a white blood cell (lymphoblast), or a nerve cell (neuroblast).

blast injury, trauma resulting from the energy released when pressure waves, generated by an explosion, strike body surfaces. These injuries can occur without obvious external injury after exposure to an air blast, an immersion (underwater) blast, or a solid (pressure wave transmission through solid objects) blast. *See also primary injury, secondary injury, tertiary injury.*

blastid, the site in the fertilized egg (ovum) where the nucleus forms.

blastin, any substance that gives food to or helps the growth or reproduction of cells.

blastocyte /blas´təsīt/, a very early embryonic cell before any cell layer has formed.

blastogenesis /-jen´əsis/, **1.** nonsexual reproduction by budding. **2.** the theory that hereditary traits are carried by the first cell of an organism (germ plasm). **3.** the development of the embryo during the separation and formation of the germ layers. –**blastogenetic,** *adj.*

blastomycosis /-mīkō´sis/, an infectious disease caused by a fungus, *Blastomyces dermatitidis.* It usually affects the skin but may invade the lungs, kidneys, nervous system, and bones. The disease is most common in young men living in the southeastern United States. Skin infections often begin as small lumps on exposed areas where there has been an injury. When the lungs are involved, symptoms include cough, shortness of breath, chest pain, chills, and a fever with heavy sweating.

blastula /blas´tyələ/, an early stage of the process in which a fertilized egg develops into an embryo. The blastula is the form in which the embryo becomes planted in the wall of the uterus. Also known as **blastosphere.**

bleb, a gathering of fluid under the skin, forming bumps that a smaller than normal blisters.

bleed, **1.** to lose blood from blood vessels. The blood may flow out through a natural opening, a break in the skin, or into the interstitial spaces. **2.** to cause blood to flow from a vein or an artery.

bleeder, **1.** *(informal)* a patient who has a blood clotting disease (hemophilia) or any other vessel or blood condition linked to a tendency to bleed. **2.** *(informal)* a bleeding blood vessel.

blepharitis /blef´ərī´tis/, an inflammatory, often contagious condition of the eyelash and oil glands of the eyelids. Swelling, redness, and crusts of dried mucus on the lids are the primary symptoms.

blepharoplegia /-plē´jə/, paralysis of the eyelid.

blepharospasm /blef´ərospazm´/, spasm of the eyelid.

blighted ovum, a fertilized egg (ovum) that fails to develop.

blind loop, a part of the intestine that is blocked from the rest of the intestine so that nothing can pass through it. Blind loops are sometimes created surgically during bowel operations.

blindness, loss of eyesight.

blind spot, **1.** a small, normal gap in sight caused when an image is focused on the optic disc of the retina. **2.** an abnormal gap in sight caused by an injury of the retina or other part of the eye. It is often sensed as light spots or flashes.

blister, **1.** a bleb or swelling containing serum, caused by burns or irritation. Also known as **bulla, vesicle. 2.** transparent housing protruding from an aircraft fuselage.

bloat, swelling or filling with a gas, as when the stomach is distended from swallowing air.

blockade, **1.** the inability of a body system to function due to chemical intervention or trauma, such as neuromuscular blockade. **2.** barriers used to divert, halt, or slow pedestrian or vehicular traffic.

blocking, **1.** preventing the sending of an impulse of the nervous system. For example, spinal anesthesia blocks the nerve signals to part of the body. **2.** interrupting body processes, as with some drugs. **3.** being unable to remember an event.

blood, the liquid pumped by the heart through all arteries, veins, and capillaries. It is composed of a clear yellow fluid, called plasma, and many cells called the formed elements. The formed elements include red blood cells (erythrocytes), white blood cells (leukocytes), and platelets. The erythrocytes move oxygen and food to the cells and remove carbon dioxide and other wastes from the cells. The leukocytes defend the body against foreign invaders. The platelets function in blood clotting. Hormones and proteins are also contained in the blood. The normal adult has about 1 ounce of blood per pound of body weight (70 ml/kg for men and 65 ml/kg for women).

blood agent, chemical compound, used in chemical warfare, that interferes with enzyme production and oxygen-carrying capability of the blood. Cyanogen chloride (CK) and hydrocyanic acid (AC) are the most common agents. These cyanide gases are systemic poisons that act rapidly but persist in the air for only short periods of time.

blood bank, an organization that collects, processes, and stores blood to be used for transfusions and other purposes.

blood-brain barrier, capillary walls within the central nervous system that function to slow or prevent chemical passage from the circulatory system into central nervous system tissue.

blood buffers. See **buffer.**

blood cell, any one of the many cells (formed elements) of the blood, including red cells (erythrocytes), white cells (leukocytes), and platelets. Together they normally make up about 50% of the total volume of the blood. *See also erythrocyte, leukocyte, platelet.*

blood clot, a semisolid, gelatin-like mass that results from the clotting process of blood. It is made up of red cells, white cells, and platelets mixed in a protein (fibrin) grouping. Compare **embolus, thrombus.**

blood clotting, changing blood from a liquid to a semisolid gel. The process usually begins with tissue damage and exposure of the blood to air. Within seconds of injury to the vessel wall, platelets clump at the site. A chain reaction of clotting factors (prothrombin, thrombin, and fibrinogen) produces a substance called fibrin. Fibrin forms a mesh over the wound. Clotting can also occur in abnormal conditions within the blood vessel, forming an embolus or thrombus. Also known as **blood coagulation.**

blood colloid osmotic pressure, osmotic pressure generated by the presence of plasma protein. The protein, consisting primarily of albumin, remains in the circulation because its size precludes passage through the capillary walls. Also known as **oncotic pressure.**

blood count, a measure of the number of cells found in the blood. A **complete blood count (CBC)** is the number of red and white blood cells per cubic millimeter of blood. It is one of the most valuable diagnostic tests, performed by staining a smear of blood on a slide and counting the types of cells under a microscope. Most laboratories use an electronic counter. In a **red blood cell count (RBC),** only the red blood cells (erythrocytes) are measured in a sample of whole blood. In a **differential white blood cell count,** the number of different types of white blood cells (leukocytes) are measured in a small blood sample. The different kinds of white cells are reported as percentages of the total examined. A **hematocrit** is a measure of the number of red cells found in the blood, stated as a percentage of the total blood volume. The normal range is between 43% and 49% in men, and between 37% and 43% in women.

blood donor, anyone who donates blood to a blood bank or to another person. A **universal donor** is a person with blood of type O, Rh factor negative. Such blood may be used for emergency transfusion with little risk of incompatibility.

blood dyscrasia, a condition in which any of the blood elements are abnormal, such as leukemia or hemophilia.

blood gas, a diagnostic test used to determine the adequacy of oxygenation and ventilation by assessing acid-base status and the partial pressures of oxygen and carbon dioxide from a blood sample (usually arterial).

blood group, the labeling of blood based on the presence or lack of specific chemical substances on the surface of the red cell. There are several different grouping systems. **ABO blood groups** refers to the primary system for labeling blood based on properties of the red blood cell. The four blood types in this group are A, B, AB, and O.

blood plasma. See **plasma.**

blood poisoning, *(informal).* See **septicemia.**

blood pressure, 1. the pressure exerted by blood on any vessel wall. **2.** the vital sign, usually obtained with a blood pressure cuff (sphygmomanometer) and stethoscope, that indirectly measures the existing arterial pressure within the large arteries. This pressure can also be obtained with doppler devices or venous/arterial lines (transducers). *See also pulse pressure.*

blood serum. See **serum.**

blood substitute, a substance used to replace circulating blood or to increase its volume, such as plasma, human serum albumin, or leukocytes. *See also transfusion.*

blood sugar, 1. one of a group of closely related substances, such as glucose, fructose, and galactose, that are normally in the blood and are necessary for metabolism. **2.** the amount of glucose in the blood. Also known as **blood glucose.** *See also hyperglycemia, hypoglycemia.*

blood transfusion, giving whole blood or part, such as red cells, to replace blood lost through injury, surgery, or disease. Whole blood may be given to a patient by transfusion directly from a donor, but more often the donor's blood is collected and stored by a blood bank. Blood must be checked, typed, and cross matched. A healthy donor's blood group and specific chemical substances must match those of the patient.

blood typing, noting the specific chemical substances (antigens) on the surface of the red blood cell. This process is used to determine a person's blood group. It is the first step in testing donor's and patient's blood to be used in transfusion and is followed by cross matching. *See also blood group, crossmatching of blood.*

blood urea nitrogen, the amount of nitrogen in the blood in the form of urea. As a waste product of normal body functions, it is a rough gauge of kidney function. It is high in kidney failure, shock, bleeding, diabetes mellitus, and some tumors. Levels are lowered in liver disease, poor diet, and normal pregnancy.

blood vessel, any one of the group of vessels that carries blood, such as **arteries, arterioles, capillaries, veins, venules.**

bloody show. See **vaginal bleeding.**

blow-out fracture, a fracture of the orbit of the eye.

blue baby, an infant born with cyanosis caused by a congenital heart problem or incomplete expansion of the lungs. **Tetralogy of Fallot** is the most common congenital cyanotic heart defect. These defects are corrected surgically, usually in early childhood. *See also congenital heart disease.*

blue nevus, a steel-blue nodule with a diameter between 2 and 7 mm (less than 1/3 inch). It is found on the face or arms, grows very slowly, and lasts throughout life. Those on the buttocks occasionally become cancerous. Compare **melanoma.**

blue spot, 1. any of the small grayish-blue spots (macula cerulea) that may appear near the axilla or groin of individuals infested with body or pubic lice. **2.** any of the dark blue or mulberry-colored round or oval spots (Mongolian spots) that may appear as a temporary defect on the buttocks.

blunt trauma, trauma induced by sudden changes of speed and compression of body surface areas. *See also penetrating trauma.*

blush, a brief reddening of the face and neck, commonly the result of the widening of small blood vessels. Blushing may be a response to heat or emotion.

board and care facility, a group residential home for people (generally the elderly) who require supervision without medical care.

boatswain's chair. See **breeches buoy.**

body, 1. the whole structure of an individual including the organs. **2.** the largest or the main part of any organ.

body armor, protective vests made of hard ceramic plate and/or synthetic fabrics that reduce the chances of injury from projectiles. Vests made with ceramic plates are helpful in protecting from blast injuries, whereas those of synthetic fabric (Kevlar™) are useful in protection from the low-velocity projectiles of most handguns. Also known as **bulletproof vest** *(inaccurate),* **ballistic vest.** *See also ballistic helmet.*

body fluid, a liquid contained in the three fluid spaces of the body: the blood plasma, the fluid between the cells (interstitial), and the cell fluid within the cells. Blood plasma and interstitial fluid make up the extracellular fluid. The cell fluid is the intracellular fluid.

body image, a person's own concept of physical appearance. The mental picture, which may be realistic or unrealistic, is created from self-observation, the reactions of others, and the interaction of attitudes, emotions, memories, fantasies, and experiences.

body language, a set of nonspeaking signals that can express many physical, mental, and emotional states. These include body movements, postures, gestures, expressions, and what one wears.

body mechanics, the movement and positioning required to perform physical activity. Using proper positioning with an awareness of the body's musculature can prevent injuries by avoiding those positions that provide inadequate support.

body movement, motion of all or part of the body, especially at a joint. Some kinds of body movements are **abduction, adduction, extension, flexion, rotation.**

body odor, a smell linked to stale sweat. Fresh sweat is odorless, but after exposure to the air and bacteria on the surface of the skin, chemical changes occur to make the odor. Body odors also can be the result of discharges from many conditions, including cancer, fungus, hemorrhoids, leukemia, and ulcers.

body-righting reflex, any one of the nerve and muscle responses to restore the body to its normal upright position when it has been displaced. The righting reflexes involve complex mechanisms linked to the structures of the internal ear. Also involved in the righting mechanism are the many nerves to the inner ear, to muscles and tendons, and to the eyes. Interruption of the nerve signals linked to body-righting reflexes may disturb the sense of balance and cause nausea and vomiting.

body temperature, the level of heat manufactured by the body. Variations in body temperature may be signs of disease or illness. Heat is created in the body through metabolism of food. Heat is lost from the body surface through radiation, convection, and evaporation of sweat. Heat production and loss are regulated by the hypothalamus and brain stem. Fever is usually caused by increased heat production. Diseases of the hypothalamus may cause below-normal body temperatures. **Basal body temperature** is the temperature of the body taken in the morning, after at least 8 hours of sleep. Normal adult body temperature, as measured by mouth, is 98.6° F. Mouth temperatures ranging from 96.5° F to 99° F are consistent with good health, depending on the physical activity and the normal body temperature for that person. When the axillary temperature is taken, it is usually 1° F lower than the oral temperature. Rectal temperatures may be 0.5° to 1.0° F higher than oral readings. Body temperature appears to vary 1° to 2° F throughout the day, with lows recorded early in the morning and peaks between 6 PM and 10 PM. *See also fever.*

Boerhaave's syndrome, ruptured esophagus resulting from forceful vomiting. The inferior esophagus is the usual rupture site with immediate contamination of the mediastinum with gastric contents. Signs/symptoms include pleuritic pain in the back, epigastrium, or substernal chest; change in voice quality to a nasal tone; and mediastinal-subcutaneous emphysema. Also known as **postemetic rupture, spontaneous esophageal rupture.** *See also Hamman's sign.*

boil, **1.** an acute, localized inflammation of the subcutaneous layers of the skin, gland, or hair follicle. The inflammation's severity obstructs blood flow to the area, causing necrosis of tissue and pain. Also known as **furuncle. 2.** the point in a hydraulic backwash where the current separates and flows downstream and upstream.

boiling liquid expanding vapor explosion, explosions that occur when the vapors from rapidly heated flammable liquids exceed the venting capabilities of the container, causing structural failure of the container. Also known as **BLEVE.**

boiling point, the temperature at which a substance passes from a liquid to a gas at a particular air pressure, such as when water boils at 212° F (100° C) at sea level.

bollard. See **snow anchor.**

bolo, a line with a small padded weight on the end that serves to carry the line across a distance when thrown.

bolt, a type of anchor in rock that utilizes a bolt that is drilled or screwed into a rock face. This bolt or stud incorporates a hanger that will then support a carabiner and the weight of a fall. *See also anchor, nut.*

bolus /bō´ləs/, **1.** a chewed, round lump of food ready to be swallowed. **2.** a large round mass of a drug for swallowing that is usually soft and not prepackaged. **3.** a dose of a drug or a drug injected all at once into the vein.

bonding, the attachment process that occurs between an infant and the parents. These ties of affection later influence the physical and mental growth of the child. Mothers are usually more concerned with touching and holding the infant. Fathers are more intent on eye contact with the child.

bone, 1. the dense, hard, and slightly elastic connective tissue that makes up the 206 bones of the human skeleton. It is made up of dense bone tissue (osseous) surrounding spongy tissue that contains many blood vessels and nerves. Covering the bone is a membrane called the periosteum. Long bones contain yellow marrow in the long spaces and red marrow in the ends near the joints. Red marrow also fills the spaces of the flat and the short bones, the vertebrae, the skull, the sternum, and the ribs. Blood cells are made in active red marrow. **2.** any single element of the skeleton, such as a rib, the sternum, or the femur. *See also connective tissue.*

bone marrow, soft tissue filling the spaces in the spongy part of bone shafts. Its main function is to make the blood cells. Fatty, **yellow marrow** is found in the compact bone of most adult long bones, such as in the arms and legs. **Red marrow** is found in many bones of infants and children and in the smaller bones, such as the sternum, ribs, and vertebrae of adults. Red blood cells are made in red marrow.

booster injection, giving an antigen, such as a vaccine or toxoid, usually in a smaller amount than the original vaccination. A booster is given to keep the immune response at an active level.

booster pump, a pump used to continue or increase pressure.

borborygmus /bôr´bərig´məs/, *pl.* **borborygmi,** an abdominal and bowel sound caused by overactive intestine movement (peristalsis). Borborygmi are rumbling and gurgling noises. Although increased intestinal movement may be noted in cases of gastroenteritis and diarrhea, true borborygmi are more intense and periodic. Borborygmi along with vomiting and cramps may mean blockage of the small intestine.

boron (B), a nonmetal element, similar to aluminum. It is the principal component of boric acid.

Boston exanthem, a viral disease with a scattered, pale red rash on the face, chest, and back, sometimes with small ulcers on the tonsils and soft palate. The lymph glands usually do not swell, and the rash disappears by itself in 2 or 3 weeks. It requires no treatment.

botulism /boch´əlizm/, an often fatal form of food poisoning caused by a poison (endotoxin) made by rod-shaped germs *(Clostridium botulinum)*. Most botulism occurs after eating improperly canned or cooked foods. In rare cases, the toxin may enter the human body through a wound infected by the organism. Botulism differs from most other types of food poisoning in that it develops without stomach upset. Nausea and vomiting occur in less than one half of the cases. Symptoms may not occur from 18 hours up to 1 week after the infected food has been eaten. Muscles become weak, and the patient often develops difficulty in swallowing. About two-thirds of the cases of botulism are fatal, usually as a result of late diagnosis and pulmonary difficulty.

boutonneuse fever /boo´tənooz´/, an infectious disease carried to humans through the bite of a tick. The disease begins with a sore at the site of the bite. A fever lasting from a few days to 2 weeks and a red rash that spreads over the body including the palms and soles develop. It is common in parts of Europe, Asia, Africa, and the Middle East. *See also Rocky Mountain spotted fever.*

bow, the forward, or front, section of a boat or ship.

bowel. See **intestine.**

bowleg, a deformity in which one or both legs are bent out at the knee. Also known as **genu varum.**

Boyle's law (Robert Boyle, English scientist, 1627-1691), at a constant temperature the volume of a given mass of gas is inversely proportional to its pressure. Also known as the **general gas law.**

B-post, second roof pillar from a vehicle's windshield.

brace, 1. material, usually wood or metal, that provides additional support for a structure. **2.** a device, sometimes jointed, that supports a moveable part of the body in a position that allows function, as a leg brace allows standing and walking. Compare **splint.**

brachial /brā´kē·əl/, referring to the arm.

brachial artery, the main artery of the upper arm. It ends just below the inside bend of the elbow where it branches into the radial artery and the ulnar artery.

brachialis /brā´kē·ā´lis/, a muscle of the upper arm that extends from the shoulder to the medial elbow. It lies under the biceps and flexes the forearm.

brachial plexus, a group of nerves that branch from the upper spine and neck. The brachial plexus supplies the muscles and skin of the chest, shoulders, and arms.

brachial pulse, arterial pulsation felt on the medial upper arm. It is used for palpation of pulse if the radial pulse is absent and as a pressure point for bleeding of the distal arm.

brachiocephalic /brāk´ē·ōsəfal´ik/, relating to the arm and head.

brachioradialis /-rā´dē·ā´lis/, the muscle on the thumb (radial) side of the forearm. It flexes the forearm.

brachycephaly /brak´ēsef´əlē/, a birth defect of the skull in which premature closing of the coronal suture results in excess growth of the head from side to side, giving it a short, broad appearance.

Bradley method, a method of preparing for childbirth developed by Robert Bradley, MD. It includes education about the physical nature of childbirth, exercise and diet during pregnancy, and ways of breathing for control and comfort during labor and birth. The father is involved in the classes and is the mother's "coach" during labor. Also known as **husband-coached childbirth.** Compare **Lamaze method.** *See also natural childbirth.*

bradycardia, 1. a heart rate below 60 beats per minute, when related to atrial or sinus rhythms. **2.** *(informal)* a slow heart rate.

bradycardia-tachycardia syndrome, a heart rate that shifts from very slow to very fast rhythms.

bradykinesia /-kinē´zhə/, slowness of all voluntary movement and speech. This may be caused by nerve disorders and some tranquilizers.

bradykinin, a chemical made by the body that dilates blood vessels.

bradypnea, a consistent respiratory rate below 12 breaths per minute.

Braille /brāl/, a system of printing for the blind. It consists of patterns of raised dots or points that can be read by touch.

brain, the portion of the brain and spinal cord (central nervous system) contained within the skull. It is composed of the cerebrum, cerebellum, and brainstem (pons, medulla, and mesencephalon). The **cerebrum** is the largest and uppermost section of the brain, divided by a deep groove at the top into the left and the right halves of the brain. **Cerebral hemisphere** refers to one of the halves of the cerebrum. The two cerebral hemispheres are connected at the bottom by the corpus callosum. Each cerebral hemisphere is made up of the large outer **cerebral cortex** layer (the "gray matter" of the brain), the underlying white substance, the internal basal ganglia, and certain other structures. The internal structures of the hemispheres join with the brainstem through the cerebral stalks. Prominent grooves further subdivide each hemisphere into four major lobes. The **frontal lobe** is the largest of the brain. The **occipital lobe** lies under the occipital bone of the skull. The **parietal lobe** rests on the side of the skull next to the parietal bone. The **temporal lobe** is the outer lower region of the brain. The **cerebellum** is the part of the brain located at the base of the skull behind the brainstem. It consists of two cerebellar lobes, one on each side, and a middle section called the vermis. Three pairs of stalks link it with the brainstem. **Cerebellar cortex** refers to the outer layer of gray matter of the cerebellum. It covers the white substance in the core. The **brainstem** is the part of the brain that includes the medulla oblongata, the pons, and the mesencephalon. It has motor, sense, and reflex functions and contains the spinal tracts. The 12 pairs of nerves from the brain to the rest of the body branch off the brainstem. The **medulla oblongata** continues as the bulblike part of the spinal cord just above the opening into the skull (foramen magnum). It contains mostly white substance with some gray substance. The medulla contains the heart, blood vessel, and breathing centers of the brain. Thus, any injury or disease in this area is often fatal. The **mesencephalon,** also called midbrain, is mostly composed of white matter with some gray matter. A red nucleus is in the mesencephalon. It contains the ends of nerve fibers from the other parts of the brain. Deep inside the mesencephalon are nuclei of several skull nerves. The mesencephalon also contains nerve nuclei for certain hearing and seeing reflexes. The **pons** is a mass of nerve cells on the surface of the brainstem. It has nuclei of various nerves, including the facial and the trigeminal nerves.

Special cells in the brain's mass of complex, soft, gray or white tissue bring together and control the functions of the central nervous system. The cerebrum has sensory and motor functions, and functions linked to integration of many mental activities. The cerebral cortex has cells that integrate higher mental functions, general movement, stomach functions, and behavioral reactions. Research has described more than 200 different areas and 47 separate functions of the cerebral cortex. The left cerebral hemisphere is dominant in right-handed people, and those who are left-handed have dominant right hemispheres. The motor speech area is better developed in the left hemisphere of right-handed persons, for example. Its destruction causes aphasia or other speech defects. Stimulation of the frontal area affects circulation, breathing, widening of the pupils, and other activity. Some of the other processes that are controlled by the cerebrum are memory, speech, writing, and emotional response. The frontal lobe influences personality and is linked to the higher mental activities, such as planning and judgment. Damage to the parietal lobe causes disorders of speech and sight. The parietal lobe also help to tell the sizes, shapes, and textures of objects.

The center for smell is located within the temporal lobe of the brain. It also has some association areas for memory and learning, and a region where thoughts are selected. **Association area** refers to any part of the cerebrum involved in integrating sensory information, such as vision. The cerebellum is concerned with coordinating voluntary muscular activity, such as walking and maintaining equilibrium.

brain death, loss of cerebral function due to tissue death, usually from hypoxia. Although cerebral tissue death begins 4 to 6 minutes after the onset of hypoxia, this process takes much longer to complete. Absence of reflexes, respirations, and brain wave activity (as indicated by a flat-line electroencephalogram) are indicative of brain death.

brain fever, *(informal)* any inflammation of the brain or lining of the brain (meninges). *See also encephalitis.*

brainstem. See **brain.**

brake bar, a solid aluminum bar added to a carabiner, over which a rappel rope is run to create friction and control a descent.

brake bar rack. See **rappel rack.**

brake block, a hardwood block used as a belaying device when cable is being used instead of rope to lower a climber or rescuer.

braking distance, the distance required for a vehicle to come to a complete stop. This distance is different for every vehicle and is modified by mechanical, terrain, and weather factors. Also known as **stopping distance.** *See also following distance, 3-second rule.*

branch, that organizational level having functional/geographic responsibility for major segments of incident operations. The branch level is organizationally between section and division/group.

branchial fistula /brang´kē·əl/, an inborn, abnormal passage from the throat to the outside surface of the neck. Also known as **cervical fistula.**

brand name. See **trade name.**

brattice, a wall that controls ventilation in the shaft or gallery of a mine.

Braxton Hicks contraction. See **false labor.**

breakdown, a canvas or nylon stretcher that folds in the middle for storage. A **minor breakdown** also has folding pegs that can be used to elevate the stretcher off the ground. A **major break-down** incorporates folding wheels at one end and pegs at the other end, which afford the above-noted capability and allow single-person transport of a victim for short distances. Also known as **emergency stretcher, folding stretcher.** *See also rigid transport vehicle.*

breaking,   a controversial technique of gastric or pulmonary drainage in which the rescuer grasps the prone patient around the abdomen and lifts. This technique is used with drowning victims in the belief that it will clear the lungs and stomach of debris and/or water. Its use during cardiac arrest facilitates emptying of the stomach in patients at risk for aspiration, as in those who have recently eaten or have ingested alcohol.

breaking strength over an edge,   the amount of weight a rope will bear, when bent over an edge, before breaking.

breakthrough bleeding.   See **vaginal bleeding.**

breast,   the anterior portion of the surface of the chest. *See also mammary gland.*

breast cancer,   a malignant tumor of breast tissue, the most common cancer in women in the United States. The rate increases between 30 to 50 years of age and reaches a second peak at 65 years of age. Risk factors include a family history of breast cancer, no children, exposure to radiation, young age when menstruation began, late menopause, being overweight, diabetes, high blood pressure, long-term cystic disease of the breast, and, possibly, hormone therapy after menopause. Women who are over 40 years of age when they bear their first child or with cancer in other areas also have a greater risk of getting breast cancer. First symptoms include a small painless lump, thick or dimpled skin, or nipple withdrawal. As the tumor grows, there may be a nipple discharge, pain, ulcers, and swollen lymph glands under the arms. *See also mastectomy.*

breast feeding,   **1.** suckling or nursing, giving a baby milk from the breast. Breast feeding causes the uterus to return to its nonpregnant size. **2.** taking milk from the breast.

breathing.   See **respiration.**

breathing air,   compressed air that contains no more contaminants than are suitable for breathing in toxic atmospheres.

breathlessness.   See **dyspnea.**

breath sound,   the auscultated sound of air movement within the respiratory system. **Tracheal** sounds are those heard while listening over the normal trachea and/or bronchi. Absent tracheal sounds mean a complete airway obstruction. **Absent** lung sounds may mean a bilateral pneumothorax, a complete airway obstruction from a foreign body, or an obstructive condition, such as asthma. **Diminished** breath sounds are due to partial airway obstruction or chronic respiratory disease, such as emphysema. Diminished sounds on one side of the chest are indicative of pneumothorax. **Wheezing** occurs when the smooth muscle of the lungs is constricted, as during asthma or an anaphylactic reaction. Fine, crepitus-like sounds during respirations are the result of fluid in the small airways. Known as **crackles** (formerly **rales**), these sounds are indicative of early pulmonary edema. **Rhonchi** (loud, bubbling lung sounds) signify fluid in the larger airways. Advanced pulmonary edema filling the bronchi will generate this sound. **Vesicular** sounds are the normal rustling, swishing noises heard during respirations.

breech birth,   birth in which the baby comes out feet, knees, or buttocks first. Breech birth is often dangerous. The body may come out easily, but the head may become trapped by an incompletely widened cervix because babies' heads are usually larger in diameter than their bodies. A **complete breech** is a position of the fetus in the womb in which the buttocks and feet are toward the birth canal. The posture of the fetus is the same as in a normal head-first position, but upside down. A **footling breech** refers to a position in which one or both feet are folded under the buttocks. One folded foot coming out is a single footling breech, both feet a double footling breech. **Frank breech** means the buttocks of the baby are at the mother's pelvic opening. The legs are straight up in front of the body, and the feet are at the shoulders. Babies born in this position tend to hold their feet near their heads for some days after birth.

breeches buoy,   a transfer device used to move passengers between ships or ship-to-shore, consisting of a transfer chair with flotation that is suspended on a rope. This device can be used during an emergency when the water or weather does not allow other means of transport. Also known as **boatswain's chair.**

bregma /breg´mə/, the joining of the frontal and parietal bones on the superior portion of the skull.

bretylium tosylate, an antidysrhythmic agent used in some cases of malignant ventricular ectopic beats, ventricular fibrillation, and pulseless ventricular tachycardia. It is contraindicated for use in children under 12 years of age. Generally, this drug is used only after defibrillation, epinephrine, and lidocaine have been unsuccessful during cardiac arrest.

BRIM, Breathing (airway/respiratory rate), **R**esponse to stimulus (level of consciousness), eyes (pupils), **M**ovement (type of extremity movement). This acronym is used to remember high-priority information needed about a patient with an altered level of consciousness. It is also useful with trauma patients if chest/abdomen and capillary refill categories are added. *See also PQRST.*

British thermal unit, the amount of heat necessary to raise the temperature of 1 pound of water from 39° F to 40° F. This is equal to 0.2522 calorie, or 1055 joules. Also known as **BTU.**

broach, the turning of a boat or ship so that its side is facing current, wind, or waves. This frequently precedes the capsizing of the vessel.

broad beta disease, a hereditary disorder (a type of hyperlipoproteinemia) in which lipoprotein gathers in the blood. The condition causes yellowish lumps (xanthomas) on the elbows and knees, disease of the blood vessels, and high blood cholesterol levels. Patients with this disease are at risk of developing early heart disease. *See also hyperlipoproteinemia.*

broad ligament, peritoneum that is draped over the uterine tubes, the uterus, and the ovaries.

Broca's area /brō´kəz/, the part of the brain that is involved in speech. It is located on the anterior portion of the brain.

bromhidrosis /brō´midrō´sis/, a condition in which the sweat has an unpleasant odor. The odor is usually caused by the breakdown of sweat by bacteria on the skin.

bronchial hyperreactivity /brong´kē·əl/, an abnormal respiratory problem with spasms of the bronchus. It is a reflex response to histamine or a cholinergic drug. This is a feature of asthma that is used to differentiate between asthma and heart disease.

bronchial sounds. See **breath sounds—tracheal.**

bronchial tree, a complex of the bronchi and the bronchial tubes. The bronchi branch from the trachea, and the bronchial tubes branch from the bronchi. The right bronchus is wider and shorter than the left bronchus. The right bronchus branches into three bronchi, one passing to each of the lobes that make up the right lung. The left bronchus is smaller in diameter but about twice as long as the right bronchus and branches into the bronchi for the upper and the lower lobes of the left lung.

bronchiectasis /brong´kē·ek´təsis/, widening and destruction of the bronchial walls. It usually results from bronchial infection or blockage by a tumor or a foreign body, but sometimes occurs as a birth defect. Symptoms include a constant cough with excess, blood-stained sputum, chronic sinus infection, clubbing of the fingers, and continual moist breath sounds.

bronchiole /brong´kē·ōl/, a small airway of the respiratory system from the bronchi to the lobes of the lung. The bronchioles allow the exchange of air and waste gases between the alveolar ducts and the bronchi. **–bronchiolar,** *adj.*

bronchiolitis, a viral infection of the lower respiratory tract that occurs mainly in infants under 18 months of age. The condition typically begins with watery nasal discharge and, often, mild fever. Rapid breathing and tachycardia, cough, wheezing, and fever develop. The chest may appear barrel-shaped, and breathing becomes more shallow. The infection typically runs its course in 7 to 10 days, with good recovery.

bronchitis /brong·kī´tis/, inflammation of the mucous membranes of the bronchi with a productive cough. **Acute bronchitis** causes cough, fever, and back pain. Caused by the spread of viral infections to the bronchi, it often occurs with childhood infections, such as measles, whooping cough, diphtheria, and typhoid fever. With **chronic bronchitis** there is an excess release of mucus in the bronchi with a productive cough for at least 3 months in at least 2 years.

Dyspnea results from bronchospasm with cyanosis. Cor pulmonale or heart failure is common in end-stage disease. Factors that may cause chronic bronchitis include cigarette smoking, air pollution, chronic infections, and abnormal growth of the bronchi.

bronchodilator /-dī´lātər/, a drug that relaxes the smooth muscle of the lungs to improve breathing.

bronchopneumonia, an inflammation of the lungs and bronchioles. Symptoms include chills, fever, cough with bloody sputum, and severe chest pain. The disease usually results from the spread of bacterial infection from the upper to the lower respiratory tract. *See also pneumonia.*

bronchopulmonary /-pul´mənər´ē/, referring to the bronchi and the lungs.

bronchoscopy /brongkos´kəpē/, an examination of the bronchial tree, using a bronchoscope. It contains fibers that carry light down the tube and project a large image up the tube to the viewer. Used to suction, obtain a tissue or fluid sample for examination, to remove foreign bodies, and to diagnose disease.

bronchospasm, spasm of the smooth muscle of the bronchi due to allergy, aspiration, exertion, infection, or other irritation. Partial obstruction of the airway occurs, with severity dependent on degree of spasm.

bronchovesicular sounds, the sounds that are intermediate in quality between bronchial/tracheal and vesicular. *See also breath sounds.*

bronchus /brong´kəs/, pl. **bronchi,** either of the two large branches of the trachea, beginning at the carina. Each bronchus has a wall composed of three layers. The outer layer is made of dense fiber strengthened with cartilage. The middle layer is smooth muscle. The inner layer is composed of mucous membrane with hairlike structures (cilia). The right bronchus is a more direct continuation of the trachea than the left. As a result, foreign bodies in the trachea usually lodge in the right bronchus.

Brooke formula, estimation of the amount of fluid to be replaced in a burn patient. This formula, now modified, requires 2 milliliters of fluid times the patient's body weight in kilograms times the percentage of body surface area burned (2 ml × kg × %BSA = ml (of fluid to be administered)). One-half of the total should be given in the first 8 hours from time of injury and the remainder given in the next 16 hours. Also known as the **Modified Brooke formula.** *See also consensus formula, Parkland formula, Shrine burn formula.*

Broselow resuscitation tape, system for evaluating pediatric drug dosages and equipment needs during resuscitation by measuring height and weight via a measuring tape. The tape is marked in increments indicating desirable dosages and equipment for a patient of that height and weight.

brown fat, a type of fat in newborn infants that is rarely found in adults. Brown fat is a unique source of heat energy for the infant because it creates more heat than ordinary fat.

brownout, 1. diminished visibility from loose dirt or sand that is blown into the air by a helicopter's rotor wash and/or prevailing winds. *See also whiteout.* **2.** dimming of light caused by loss of power in local area.

Brown-Séquard syndrome /-sākär´/, nerve dysfunction resulting from pressure on one side of the spinal cord at about the level of the inferior scapula. The disorder includes paralysis on the injured side of the body and loss of pain and heat sensation on the other side of the body.

brown spider, a poisonous spider, also known as the brown recluse or violin spider, found in both North and South America. The poison from its bite usually creates a bleb surrounded by white and red circles. This so-called "bull's eye" appearance is helpful in telling it apart from other spider bites. The wound usually ulcerates and can become infected. Pain, nausea, fever, and chills are common.

brucellosis /broo͞´səlō´sis/, a disease caused by any of several species of *Brucella* bacteria. Primarily a disease of livestock, humans contract it by drinking infected milk or milk products or through a break in the skin. Fever often comes in waves, rising in the evening and decreasing during the day, occurring at times separated by periods of no symptoms. Although brucellosis itself is rarely fatal, pneumonia, meningitis, and encephalitis can develop. **Abortus fever** is a form of brucellosis with similar routes of infection and of symptoms.

Brudzinski's sign /brōōdzin´skēz/, an involuntary flexing of the legs when the neck is flexed. This is seen in patients with meningitis.

bruise. See **contusion.**

bruit /brōōē´, brōōt/, an auscultated murmur or sound, usually referring to that produced by turbulence in blood vessels (or other abnormal sounds).

bruxism /bruk´sizm/, the continuous, unconscious grinding of the teeth. This occurs especially during sleep, or during waking hours to release tension in periods of high stress.

bubo /byōō´bō/, *pl.* **buboes,** a swollen lymph node in the axilla or groin. Buboes are linked to diseases such as chancroid, bubonic plague, and syphilis.

bubonic plague /byōōbon´ik/. See **plague.**

buccal /buk´əl/, referring to the inside of the cheek, or the gum or side of a tooth next to the cheek.

buccinator /buk´sinā´tər/, the main muscle of the cheek, one of the 12 muscles of the mouth. It puts pressure on the cheek, acting as an important muscle of chewing by holding food under the teeth.

buccopharyngeal /buk´ōfərin´jē·əl/, referring to the cheek and the throat (pharynx) or to the mouth and the pharynx.

bucket-handle tear, a tear in the meniscus that occurs lengthwise. It is a common injury in athletes and active young people. The usual cause is twisting of the knee. Symptoms are pain when squatting or twisting, some swelling, and tenderness.

bucking, *(informal)* resisting assisted ventilations. Confused or unconscious patients who require airway management may not breathe at the same time as a manual or cycled ventilator. This may manifest as exhaling against a forced ventilation, thrashing movements, or biting on tubing placed in the oropharynx.

Budd-Chiari syndrome /-kē·är´ē/, a disorder of liver circulation. Blockage of the portal veins leads to hepatomegaly and ascites. There is severe elevation of blood pressure within the portal vessels.

buddy system, utilization of two-person teams when undertaking hazardous operations. The second person provides a resource for communications, equipment, or rescue in the event of injury or unforeseen circumstances.

Buerger's disease, a condition in which the veins close, usually in a leg or a foot. The small and medium-sized arteries become inflamed and clotted. Early signs of the condition are burning, numbness, and tingling of the foot or leg. Gangrene may develop as the disease progresses. Pulses in the affected extremity may be absent. Also known as **thromboangiitis obliterans.**

buffer, a substance or group of substances that controls hydrogen ion levels in a solution. Buffer systems in the body balance the acid-base levels of the blood. **Blood buffers** are composed primarily of dissolved carbon dioxide and bicarbonate.

bulbar paralysis /bul´bər/, a wasting nerve condition with continually worsening paralysis of the lips, tongue, mouth, throat, and vocal cords.

bulimia /byōōlē´mē·ə/, an eating disorder with unsatisfied desire for food, often resulting in periods of continuous eating. This is followed by periods of depression and, in some cases, forced vomiting. –**bulemic,** *n., adj.*

bulkhead, the wall of an aircraft or ship.

bulk packaging, bulk packaging has an internal volume greater than 119 gallons (450 L) for liquids, a capacity greater than 882 pounds (400 kg) for solids, or a water capacity greater than 1000 pounds (453.6 kg) for gases. They can be an integral part of a transport vehicle (e.g., tank cars and barges), packaging placed on or in a transport vehicle (e.g., portable tanks, intermodal portable tanks, ton containers), or fixed or processing containers.

bulla /bul´ə/, *pl.* **bullae,** a thin-walled blister, generally 5 mm or larger, of the skin or mucous membranes containing clear fluid. Compare **vesicle.** –**bullous,** *adj.*

bullet tumble, forward rotation of a projectile around its center of mass. *See also bullet yaw, nutation, precession.*

bullet yaw, horizontal and vertical oscillation of a projectile around its axis. This deviation from its longitudinal axis increases the projectile's surface area, increasing tissue damage. *See also bullet tumble, nutation, precession.*

bullous myringitis /bul´əs/, inflammation in the ear with fluid-filled sores on the tympanic membrane. The condition often occurs with otitis media. *See also otitis media.*

bumper, an energy-absorbing bar across the front and back of cars and trucks, designed to reduce the damage and shock of vehicular impact. These bars are joined to the vehicle frame with energy-absorbing pistons, which retract when struck. *See also bumper strike zone.*

bumper strike zone, the area around the front and rear of a damaged vehicle, particularly when burning, that presents the greatest hazard from injury by a compressed bumper or energy-absorbing piston. The compressed (loaded) bumper and piston may eject and be launched distances up to 300 feet. Avoiding these zones during evolutions around burning or wrecked vehicles is necessary for safety.

bundle branch block, a disruption of the cardiac electrical conduction system in the ventricles. Electrical impulses between the bundle of His and the Purkinje fibers are slowed or blocked, causing notching or widening of the QRS complex or dropped beats. This phenomenon will affect the right and/or left common bundle branches. Also known as **BBB.**

bundle of Kent, fibers that connect atrial muscle to ventricular muscle, creating an accessory pathway that bypasses the AV node. These fibers may allow the rapid electrical impulses and EKG changes seen in preexcitation to occur. Also known as **Kent fibers.**

bunion /bun´yən/, swelling of the joint at the base of the great toe. It is caused by inflammation of the bursa, usually as a result of long-term irritation and pressure from poorly fitted shoes.

bunker coat, *(informal)* jacket worn during extrication and firefighting that protects from injury due to flame or debris. Also known as **turnout coat.**

burette, intravenous measuring device that allows for the delivery of specific volumes of drugs and fluids.

burn, tissue injury that is due to excessive exposure to chemical, electrical, thermal, or radioactive agents. Injury varies depending on the agent, the duration and intensity of exposure, and the part of the body affected. Burns are categorized according to the degree of injury. **First-degree** burns cause superficial injury, primarily to the outer layer of epidermis (skin redness). **Second-degree** burns damage tissue into the dermal layer but no so much that it prevents regeneration of epidermis (skin vesicles). **Third-degree** injury destroys dermis and epidermis and damages tissue below the dermal layer (skin charring). **Fourth-degree** burns destroy muscle tissue. **Fifth-degree** destroys bone tissue, and **sixth-degree** vaporizes areas of the body.

burn center, a health care center that is set up to care for patients who have been severely burned.

burnout, job dissatisfaction that occurs when mental and physical coping mechanisms fail to provide protection from the stresses of the job. Inadequate fitness and health, inappropriate education and training, poor personnel management, and unrealistic job expectations are all contributing factors.

bursa /bur´sə/, *pl.* **bursae,** one of the many closed sacs in the connecting tissue between the muscles, tendons, ligaments, and bones. Lined with a membrane that releases fluid (synovial), the bursa acts as a cushion. This makes the gliding of muscles and tendons over bones easier, as does the **bursa of Achilles** that separates the tendon of Achilles and the heel.

bursitis /bərsī´tis/, an inflammation of the bursa, the connective tissue structure surrounding a joint. Bursitis may be caused by arthritis, infection, injury, or excess activity. The primary symptom is severe pain in the joint, particularly on movement.

bursting fracture, any broken bone that scatters bone fragments, usually at or near the end of a bone.

bus conductor, a metal bar, used in place of cable or wire, to transfer electrical power. Also known as **bar(s), bus bar.**

butte, a small flat-topped hill.

butterfly fracture, a fracture in which two cracks form a triangle.

butterfly rash, a scaling erythema of both cheeks joined by a narrow band across the nose. It is seen in lupus erythematosus, rosacea, and seborrheic dermatitis.

buttocks, the external prominences posterior to the hips, formed by the gluteal muscles. Also known as **clunes, nates.**

butyl alcohol /byo͞o´til/, a clear, poisonous liquid used as a solvent. Also known as **butanol.**

bypass, **1.** circumvention; an alternate route. **2.** surgical procedure that reroutes blood flow around an obstruction, usually related to the coronary arteries.

Byrd-Dew method (Harvey Byrd, American physician, 1820-1884; James Dew, American physician, 1843-1914), *(historical)* procedure for artificial respiration in the apneic newborn. The infant was held face up, allowing the head to fall backward. The forearms were straightened and pulled toward the feet, flexing the body, causing expiration. The forearms were then flexed toward the upper arms, causing extension of the body and inspiration.

byssinosis /bis´ino͞´sis/, a job-related respiratory disease that is an allergic reaction to dust or fungus in cotton, flax, and hemp fibers. Symptoms are dyspnea, cough, and wheezing. The disease is curable in the early stages. Exposure for several years results in bronchitis and emphysema.

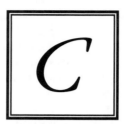

C

cabin, cargo or passenger compartments onboard aircraft or ships.

cable, **1.** a strong length of chain, rope, or wire. **2.** wire rope used for rescue in Canada, Europe, and New Zealand. Although it is desirable in that cable has minimal elasticity, its stiffness makes kinking a significant problem. Its use requires more training and mechanical aptitude than similar evolutions (maneuvers) with rope.

cable cutter, aircraft rescue tool used to sever cables, hoses, and tubing to disarm aircraft ejection systems. Also known as **disarming tool**.

cachet /käshā/, any wafer-shaped, flat capsule that holds a dose of a bitter-tasting drug. It is swallowed whole.

cachexia /kəkek´sē·ə/, general ill health and poor diet. It is usually linked to a wasting disease, such as tuberculosis or cancer.

cachinnation /kak´ənā´shən/, excess laughter for no reason, often part of the behavior in schizophrenia.

cacodemonomania /kak´ədē´mənō-/, a confused state in which a person claims to be possessed by the devil or an evil spirit.

cadaver, a dead body used for study.

cadmium, a bluish-white metal element. It is used in engraving, printing, and photography. Breathing the fumes during metal-plating processes can cause poisoning. A lung disease (**cadmiosis**) is caused by breathing in cadmium dust. Acid foods (such as tomatoes and lemonade) that are prepared and stored in cad-

mium-lined containers can also cause poisoning.

cadmium poisoning, the effects of swallowing cadmium, eating foods stored in cadmium cans, or breathing cadmium fumes from welding, smelting, or other industrial processes. Symptoms from breathing fumes include vomiting, difficulty in breathing, headache, and fatigue. Cadmium causes severe stomach and bowel symptoms 30 minutes to 3 hours after swallowing.

caduceus /kədoo´sē·əs/, medical insignia consisting of a staff entwined with two serpents and surmounted by two wings. Although it is the official symbol of the U.S. Army Medical Corps, it otherwise has limited medical significance. In mythology, it is the wand of the god Hermes, or Mercury; and it is often confused with the staff of Aesculapius, the Greco-Roman god of medicine. *See also staff of Aesculapius.*

café-au-lait spot /kaf´ā·ōlā´/, a pale tan patch of skin. It occurs in a type of bone disease (Albright's syndrome), but these spots can also occur normally. Many café-au-lait spots may develop with a tumorlike growth all over the body (neurofibromatosis).

cafe coronary, *(informal)* complete airway obstruction from a foreign body, particularly food.

caffeine /kafēn´, kaf´ē·in/, a substance found in coffee, tea, cola, and other plant products. It is used as a stimulant and given to treat migraine headaches. Patients with heart disease and peptic ulcer must use it with caution. Side effects include tachycardia, excess urination, stomach and bowel distress, restlessness, and lack of sleep.

caffeinism, poisoning condition caused by the chronic use of excess amounts of caffeine in beverages or other products. Symptoms include restlessness, anxiety, general depression, rapid heart beat, tremors, nausea, high urine output, and lack of sleep. A fatal dose is estimated to be 10 g (equal to 100 cups of coffee) for a healthy adult. *See also xanthine derivative.*

caisson disease. See **decompression sickness**.

calcaneal spur /kal´kā´nē·əl/, a painful, bony growth on the lower surface of the heel (calcaneus). The spur is usually caused by chronic pressure on the heel.

calcaneus /kal´kā´nē·əs/, the heel bone. The largest of several bones that form the ankle.

calcar /kal´kär/, *pl.* **calcaria,** a spur or spurlike structure that occurs normally on many bones of the human skeleton.

calcemia, an excess level of calcium in the blood.

calcific aortic disease, abnormal deposits of calcium in the aorta.

calcification, abnormal calcium deposits in body tissues. Normally, about 99% of all the calcium in the human body is deposited in the bones and teeth. The remaining 1% is dissolved in body fluids, such as the blood. Disorders that cause deposits in arteries, kidneys, lungs, and other soft tissues usually are related to parathyroid hormone activity and vitamin D levels.

calcinosis /kal´sənō´-/, an abnormal condition with deposits of calcium in the skin and muscles. The disease usually occurs in children.

calcitonin /-tō´nin/, a hormone produced in the thyroid gland. It controls the levels of calcium and phosphorus in the blood and acts to prevent the loss of calcium from the bones.

calcium, an alkaline earth metal element. It is the most common mineral and the fifth most common element in the human body, found mainly in the bones and teeth. The body needs calcium to conduct nerve impulses, contract muscles, clot blood, and enable cardiac and enzyme functions. Calcium is absorbed primarily by the small intestine. The adult human body contains about 2.5 pounds of calcium. Only about one-third of the calcium taken in by humans is absorbed. Excess calcium in the body can cause calculi in the kidney. Inadequate calcium can cause rickets in children and osteoporosis, especially in older women.

calcium channel blocker, chemicals that antagonize calcium, thereby allowing arterial vessel dilation and decreasing the myocardial cells' ability to respond to electrical stimulation. This decrease in electrical activity reduces both myocardial oxygen demand and consumption. Patients with angina at rest and/or occasional rapid heart rates are often prescribed these medications.

calcium chloride, an electrolyte used in cases of calcium channel blocker toxicity, suspected hyperkalemia in hemodialysis patients, and in transfusion-induced hypocalcemia. Although there are no contraindications for field use, this agent is a potent local irritant that can precipitate with sodium bicarbonate.

calculus /kal´kyələs/, *pl.* **calculi,** a stone formed in tissues from mineral salts. Calculi may form anywhere in the body, with the most common locations being the kidneys, the gallbladder, and the joints.

calefacient /kal´əfā´shənt/, making or tending to make anything warm or hot.

calenture /kal´əncho͞or´/, tropical fever, caused by exposure to excessive heat. The fever may cause hallucination.

calf, *pl.* **calves,** the fleshy mass at the back of the leg below the knee. It is composed primarily of the gastrocnemius and soleus muscles.

calibration, **1.** conforming an EKG monitor or printer to a known standard voltage (1 millivolt) for purposes of equality in interpretation. The amplitude of the waveform is adjusted to the height of the standardization waveform. **2.** sending a signal to a base station, which sets off a tone that alerts radio personnel to incoming radio traffic. **3.** adjusting electronic or mechanical parameters of a device to allow proper function, as with a gas or radiation detector.

caligo /kəlī´gō/, dim sight, usually caused by cataracts, a cloudy cornea, or failure of the pupil to widen properly.

calipers, instrument for measuring diameter or distance, such as EKG calipers, or pelvic calipers.

calisthenics /kal´isthen´-/, exercising the many muscles of the body according to certain routines. They may be done with or without equipment. The goal of calisthenics is to keep physical health while increasing muscle strength.

callbox, a publicly located phone, used for calling for emergency services. This is a direct-dial, no-cost phone, located on streets and interstates, in public buildings, and along long sections of deserted highway. It may be used for EMS, fire, police, or towing service.

callout, response of rescuers when the need arises. This response is composed of the primary and secondary responses. **Primary callout** involves mobilizing those agencies likely to become involved in an operation. When a high-profile or long-term operation is expected, secondary callout would be initiated and includes additional personnel for search, preparing public information links to the media, and establishing liaison with administrators removed from field operations.

callus, 1. a common, usually painless thickening of the skin at locations of pressure or friction. 2. a bony deposit formed around the broken ends of a broken bone during healing. The bone callus is replaced by normal hard bone as the bone heals.

calor /kā´lər/, heat in the body. Examples are heat caused by inflammation or from the normal processes of the body.

caloric /kəlôr´ik/, referring to heat or calories.

caloric balance, the proportion of the number of calories taken in in food and beverages to the number of calories used during work and exercise.

calorie, the amount of heat needed to raise 1 g of water 1° C at 1 atmosphere pressure.

calorimetry /kal´ərim´ətrē/, the method of measuring heat loss or energy loss. Human body heat can be measured by putting a subject in a tank of water and noting the temperature change in the water, caused by body heat. Human calorie use can also by measured in terms of the amount of oxygen breathed in and the amount of carbon dioxide breathed out during a given time.

calyx /kā´liks/, a cup-shaped structure of the body. An example is the kidney (renal) calyx,

which collects urine and directs it into a tube (ureter) that carries the urine to the bladder.

camel, a machine for lifting sunken objects out of water.

camp, a geographical site, used during incident command operations, that is equipped and staffed to provide food, sanitary services, and water to incident personnel.

camphor, a clear or white crystal-like substance with a strong odor and taste. It is used as a mild irritant and antiseptic in lotions and soaps.

camptomelia /-mē´lyə/, a congenital defect in which one or more limbs are curved.

canal, 1. any narrow tube or channel through an organ or between structures. An example is the **adductor canal,** a channel for vessels and nerves in the thigh muscle. The **canal of Schlemm** is a tiny vein at the corner of the eye that drains the fluid in the eye (aqueous humor) and funnels it into the bloodstream. A blockage of the canal can result in glaucoma. 2. waterway built to carry water for irrigation or navigation.

cancellous /kan´sələs/, referring to the spongy, inner portion of many bones, primarily bones that have marrow.

cancer, a general term for a malignant tumor or for forms of new tissue cells that lack a controlled growth pattern. Cancer cells usually invade and destroy normal tissue cells. A cancer tends to spread to other parts of the body by releasing cells into the lymph or bloodstream. The most common sites for the growth of cancers are the lung, breast, colon, uterus, mouth, and bone marrow. Many cancers are curable if found in the early stage.

cancroid, 1. resembling a cancer. 2. a mild skin cancer.

cancrum oris, a cankerlike sore of the mouth. It can begin as a small sore of the gum and spread to the mouth and face.

Candida albicans /kan´didə al´bəkanz/, a yeastlike fungus normally found in the mouth, digestive tract, vagina, and on the skin of healthy persons. In some situations, it may cause chronic infections of the skin, nails, scalp, mucous membranes, genitals, or internal organs. *See also candidiasis.*

candidiasis /kan´didī´əsis/, any infection caused by a species of the *Candida* genus of yeastlike fungi. Many common diseases, such as diaper rash, thrush, vaginitis, and dermatitis, are caused by *Candida* infestations.

canine tooth, any one of the four teeth, two in each jaw, found on either side of the four front teeth (incisors) in humans. Canine teeth are larger and stronger than the front teeth and have deeper roots. Canines in the upper jaw are also called **eyeteeth**.

canker, a sore, found generally in the mouth. Causes include food allergy, herpes infection, and emotional stress. *See also gingivitis, stomatitis.*

cannabis /kan´əbis/, American or Indian hemp *(Cannibus sativa)* used as a source of marijuana, hashish, and other mind-altering drugs. The dried flower tops contain the chemical tetrahydrocannabinol (THC). Cannabis and its products are classified as controlled substances by the U.S. government.

cannula, **1.** a sheath enclosing a trochar, such as an intravenous cannula. **2.** *(informal)* a nasal cannula, an oxygen delivery device.

canopy, the transparent enclosure over an aircraft cockpit.

canopy jettison, the blowing away of an aircraft canopy by explosive or mechanical action during aircraft emergencies. It can be done when an aircraft is in the air or on the ground. Ground emergencies dictate a canopy jettison only when fire is involved or when the canopy cannot be opened normally or manually.

cantharis /kan´thəris/, *pl.* **cantharides** /kanther´idēz/, the dried insects *Cantharis vesicatoria,* which contain an irritating chemical once thought to stimulate sex. Also known as **Spanish fly.**

canthus /kan´thəs/, *pl.* **canthi,** each corner of the eye; the angle at which the upper and lower eyelid meet on either side of the eye.

capacitor, a device that stores electrical energy. Designed with conducting plates separated by layers of nonconducting material, the electrical charge is separated, creating a difference of potential, thereby storing electrical energy.

cape, a projecting part of coastline that extends into a bay, gulf, lake, ocean, or sea.

capillary /kap´iler´ē/, any of the tiny blood vessels in the system that link the arteries and the veins. The size of a capillary may be 0.008 mm, so tiny that red blood cells must pass through one at a time. Through their walls, blood and tissue cells exchange various substances. The blood gives oxygen and nutrients to the cells and collects waste from the cells.

capillary refill, the flow of blood back into a capillary bed, as into a cuticle after pressure has been applied. The refill time of the capillaries is judged as the time that it takes for the area involved to change from blanched to pink. Normal refill time is 2 seconds or less. Prolonged refill is due to decreased circulation caused by cold, diminished cardiac output, hypovolemia, or other obstruction of blood flow.

capitate bone, a large bone in the midline of the wrist.

capitulum /kəpich´ələm/, *pl.* **capitula,** a small, rounded protuberance on a bone where it joins another bone. The capitula of the wrist and ankle can be seen as bulges under the skin.

capnometry, noninvasive measurement of carbon dioxide levels. Used primarily in intubated patients, this measurement is used as a determinant for proper endotracheal tube placement and as an indication of ventilatory status. **Analog/digital capnometers** measure levels using scales of analog or digital numbers, via a probe placed in or near the patient's endotracheal tube or oropharynx. **Color capnometers** measure the presence or absence of carbon dioxide via a carbon dioxide–sensitive filter paper that changes color in its presence.

capsule, **1.** a small, oval-shaped, gelatin container that holds a powdered or liquid drug. It is taken by mouth. Liquid drugs are usually packaged in soft gelatin capsules that are sealed to prevent leakage. Powdered drugs may be packaged in hard capsules. A capsule is coated with a substance to keep it from dissolving in the stomach when the drug must be absorbed in the small intestine. Compare **tablet**. **2.** a membrane or other body structure that covers an organ or part, such as the capsule of the adrenal gland or a joint.

caput /kā´pət, kap´ət/, the head or the enlarged portion of an organ or part, such as **caput costae,** for the head of a rib.

carabiner /ker´əbē´nər/, a ring of highly tensile aluminum alloy or steel with a moveable gate that is used to attach equipment or a harness to other anchor points, such as a cargo ring, piton, or rope. Designed in either oval or D-ring styles, their openings (gates) are either locking or non-locking. Also known as **biner, D-ring, oval**.

carbide lamp, a device used underground that generates acetylene to create light. Water is dripped over crystals of calcium carbide to produce acetylene gas. The gas is ignited as it escapes through a burner tip and the flame is focused by a metal reflector into useable light.

carbohydrate, a large group of sugars, starches, celluloses, and gums that all contain carbon, hydrogen, and oxygen in similar proportions. Carbohydrates are the main source of energy for all body functions and are needed to process other nutrients. They are formed by all green plants, which use the sun to combine carbon dioxide and water into simple sugar molecules. They can also be made in the body. Lack of carbohydrates can result in fatigue, depression, breakdown of body protein, and mineral imbalance.

carbolic acid, a germ-preventing and germ-killing compound made from coal tar. While fairly safe in very weak solutions of about 1% for cleaning small wounds or to relieve itching, carbolic acid is a strong poison. It can be absorbed through the skin and destroy the tissue. If swallowed, it depresses the nervous system and causes respiratory and cardiac arrest. Because carbolic acid has no color, it often contains a dye to warn against mistaken use. Also known as **phenol.**

carbon, a nonmetallic chemical element. Carbon occurs throughout nature as a part of all living tissue and is essential to the chemistry of the body. It occurs in all organic compounds. Carbon dioxide is important in the acid-base balance of the body and in controlling respiration. Dusts with carbon in them can cause many pulmonary diseases, such as coal worker's pneumoconiosis, black lung disease, and byssinosis. Also known as **C.**

carbon dioxide, a clear, odorless gas, found in nature. Plants and animals produce carbon dioxide during respiration. The acid-base balance of the body is affected by the level of carbon dioxide in the blood and other tissues. Also known as **CO_2.**

carbon monoxide, a clear, odorless, poisonous gas produced when fuel is burned in an oxygen-poor mixture. **Carboxyhemoglobin** is a compound produced when carbon monoxide links with red blood cells. It blocks the sites on the cells that carry oxygen, limiting the ability of the blood to transport oxygen. Oxygen in the blood decreases and suffocation and death result. A late sign of carbon monoxide poisoning is a cherry-red skin color. In a small enclosed space, death can occur within minutes.

carbon tetrachloride, a clear, poisonous liquid that quickly vaporizes. It is used as a solvent in dry-cleaning fluids. Accidentally swallowing the liquid or breathing the fumes results in headaches, nausea, abdominal pain, and seizures.

carbuncle /kär´bungkəl/, a group of staphylococcal sores in which purulent material is present in deep, connected pockets under the skin. Common sites for carbuncles are the back of the neck and the buttocks. **Carbunculosis** refers to the presence of a group of carbuncles. The infecting bacteria invade the skin through hair follicles.

carcinectomy /kär´sinek´-/, the removal of a cancerous tumor.

carcinogen /kärsin´əjən, kär´sinəjən/, a substance that can cause the growth of cancer. An **environmental carcinogen** is any of many natural or manufactured substances that can cause cancer. These substances may be chemical agents, physical agents, or certain hormones and viruses. They include arsenic, asbestos, uranium, vinyl chloride, radiation, ultraviolet rays, x-rays, and various things derived from coal tar. **Carcinogenic** refers to the ability to cause cancer.

carcinolysis /kär´sinol´isis/, the killing of cancer cells, as by chemotherapy.

carcinoma /kär´sinō´mə/, any cancerous tumor that starts with the cells (epithelial) that cover inner and outer body surfaces. Carcinomas invade nearby tissue and spread to far regions of the body. It occurs most often in the skin, large intestine, lungs, stomach, prostate gland, cervix, and breast. The tumor is usually a firm, uneven, knotty mass, with a well-defined edge in some places.

carcinosarcoma /-särkō´mə/, a cancerous tumor composed of two kinds of cancer cells that are called carcinoma and sarcoma. Tumors of this type may occur in the throat, thyroid gland, and uterus.

carcinosis /kär′sinō′-/, the growth of many cancers throughout the body.

cardiac, 1. the heart **2.** (informal) a person with heart disease. **3.** the portion of the stomach where it is joined by the esophagus.

cardiac arrest, cessation of functional circulation and respiration. Effective resuscitation is necessary to prevent death. *See also biological death, brain death, cardiopulmonary resuscitation, clinical death.*

cardiac asthma, wheezing in the presence of pulmonary edema. This bronchospasm is due to smooth muscle irritation caused by the fluid of pulmonary edema. Also known as **cardiasthma.**

cardiac atrophy, a breaking down of the heart muscle.

cardiac catheterization, a diagnostic procedure in which a catheter is passed into the heart through a large blood vessel in an arm or a leg. The blood pressures in the atria and ventricles and nearby blood vessels are measured during catheterization. Many conditions may be identified, including narrowing of vessels or cardiac valves.

cardiac conduction defect, any impairment in conduction of electrical impulses within the heart. The cardiac conduction system is composed of the **sinoatrial node, intranodal pathways, atrioventricular node, bundle of His, and Purkinje fibers.** Medications, myocardial infarction, hypoxia, or trauma may disrupt a portion of the conduction system, prolonging conduction time and causing reciprocal changes in the electrocardiogram. *See also heart block.*

cardiac contusion, bruising of the heart muscle due to trauma. This injury may lead to dysrhythmias or cardiac tissue death in extreme cases.

cardiac hypertrophy, enlargement of the heart.

cardiac massage, artificial internal or external rhythmic compression of the heart performed as an immediate method of circulatory support when effective circulation is absent. Using the hands, the heart is compressed externally via the sternum or internally by direct compression. This technique is ineffective unless combined with respiratory support when respirations are absent.

cardiac monitoring, observation of the cardiac electrical cycle via oscilloscope. Even though changes in the cardiac electrical pattern may indicate cardiac dysfunction, actual cardiac output and effectiveness are not measured by this technique. Also known as **EKG monitoring.** *See also electrocardiograph.*

cardiac murmur. See **heart murmur.**

cardiac muscle, striated muscle of the myocardium, responsible for the movement of blood throughout the body, by the force of its contraction.

cardiac output, the volume of blood pumped by the heart, usually measured in milliliters per minute. It is a product of the heart rate multiplied by the left ventricular stroke volume. The normal adult resting output varies from 2.5 to 4 quarts (2.3-3.8 liters) per minute.

cardiac pacemaker. See **pacemaker.**

cardiac plexus, one of several nerve complexes located near the arch of the aorta. These complexes contain both parasympathetic and sympathetic nerve fibers that innervate the heart.

cardiac reserve, the potential of the heart to increase output and blood pressure above its normal level in response to needs of the body.

cardiac sphincter, a ring of muscle fibers where the esophagus joins the stomach. Its function is to keep the stomach contents from backing into the esophagus. **Cardiochalasia** is a state in which the muscle is relaxed. This allows the stomach contents to back up.

cardiac tamponade, compression of the heart resulting from excess fluid in the pericardial sac. This fluid may be blood resulting from trauma to the heart or major blood vessels or serous fluid from infection or inflammation. Also known as **pericardial tamponade.**

cardiac valve. See **heart valve.**

cardialgia /kär′dē·al′jə/, any pain in the region of the heart. The term is used even if the heart is not directly involved. Also known as **cardiodynia.**

cardiectomy /-ek′-/, removing the portion of the stomach where it joins the esophagus.

cardinal, the main feature of an organ or its function.

cardinal point, one of the main points of the compass, i.e., North, East, South, West.

cardinal position of gaze, one of the positions to which the normal eye may be turned. Each position depends on certain eye muscles and nerve fibers. The positions include to the left, to the right, up, up and to the right, up and to the left, down, down and to the right, and down and to the left.

cardiocele /kär´dē·əsēl/, an event in which the heart pushes through the muscle that holds it in place above the stomach (diaphragm), or through a nearby wound.

cardiogenic shock. See **shock.**

cardiogram. See **electrocardiogram.**

cardiology, the study of the heart. A physician who specializes in this area is called a **cardiologist**.

cardiolysis /-ol´isis/, a procedure to separate scar tissue (adhesions) that constrict the heart.

cardiomegaly /-meg´əlē/, enlargement of the heart caused most often by high blood pressure within the heart. It can also occur with various cardiac defects. In athletes an enlarged heart may be normal.

cardiomyopathy /-mī·op´əthē/, any disease that affects the heart muscle. **Secondary cardiomyopathy** refers to a problem that is linked to another form of heart disease or illness, such as high blood pressure.

cardiopericarditis /-per´ikärdī´-/, inflammation of the heart and the pericardium.

cardioplegia /-plē´jə/, paralysis of the heart, which may be caused by drugs, hypothermia, or electric shock.

cardiopulmonary /-pul´məner´ē/, the heart and the lungs.

cardiopulmonary resuscitation, 1. maintenance of cerebral perfusion during cardiac arrest, by the performance of closed chest cardiac massage in conjunction with mouth-to-mouth (or similar variation) ventilation. This procedure can be performed with one or two persons. Also known as **CPR. 2.** generally referring to basic or advanced variations of the maintenance of cerebral perfusion via artificial circulation and ventilation techniques.

cardiospasm, dysfunction of distal esophageal muscle and the esophageal orifice to the stomach (cardiac sphincter), creating an inability for food substances to reach the stomach. The name is misleading because it does not pertain to the heart muscle.

cardiotachometer /-təkom´ətər/, a device that monitors and records heartrate.

cardiotomy /-ot´-/, an operation in which an opening is made into the heart.

cardiotonic, increasing the tone (tonicity) of the heart, as by medication.

cardiotoxic, a substance that has a poisonous or harmful effect on the heart.

cardiovascular /-vas´kyələr/, the heart and blood vessels

cardiovascular disease, any one of many disorders that may cause conditions of the heart and blood vessels. In the United States cardiovascular disease is the leading cause of death. It accounts for more than 50% of all deaths from disease every year. More than a quarter of a million persons under 65 years of age in the United States die each year from this disease.

cardiovascular system, the network of structures, which include the heart and the blood vessels, that pump and carry blood through the body. The system has thousands of miles of arteries, veins, and capillaries. The arteries deliver nutrients to the cells, and the veins take away waste products from the cells. The cardiovascular system works closely with the respiratory system to transport oxygen from the lungs to the tissues and carry carbon dioxide to the lungs to be exhaled. Many conditions, such as diet, exercise, and stress, affect the cardiovascular system.

cardioversion, 1. conversion of a pathological cardiac dysrhythmia, such as ventricular fibrillation or symptomatic atrial fibrillation, to a stable rhythm. It can be done electrically (defibrillation, synchronized cardioversion), mechanically (carotid sinus massage), or pharmacologically. **2.** commonly applied to mean synchronized cardioversion, wherein an organized, perfusing (but deteriorating) cardiac rhythm is electrically converted to a stable rhythm. This technique requires a device known as a **cardioverter**, which synchronizes the electrical shock so that it lands on the nonvulnerable portion of the cardiac rhythm. Rhythms that may require this technique include ventricular tachycardia with pulses, supraventricular tachycardia, atrial flutter, and atrial tachycardia. *See also cardioverter.*

cardioverter, device that synchronizes a defibrillator's electrical output so that the delivered energy is timed to land approximately 10 milliseconds after the peak of the R wave of the cardiac cycle. By sensing and avoiding the relative refractory period of the cardiac cycle, dysrhythmias may be halted and allowed to convert to a stable rhythm without as much danger of creating a lethal, disorganized rhythm. *See also cardioversion.*

carditis /kärdī´-/, an inflammation of the muscles of the heart. It usually results from infection. Chest pain and damage to the heart may occur.

caries /ker´ēz/, decay, breaking down, and destruction of a bone or tooth.

carina, the portion of the airway where the trachea separates into the right and left bronchi; the end of the trachea.

carotene /ker´ətin/, a red or orange compound found in carrots, sweet potatoes, milk fat, egg yolk, and leafy vegetables. Carotene is changed to vitamin A in the body. A body that cannot make use of carotene may become deficient in vitamin A. *See also vitamin A.*

carotenemia /-ē´mē·ə/, the presence of too much carotene in the blood. This results in yellow appearance of the blood and skin.

carotenoid /kərot´ənoid/, any of a group of red, yellow, or orange pigments that are found in such foods as carrots, sweet potatoes, and leafy green vegetables. They can also be found in some animal tissue. Many of these substances, such as carotene, are needed to make vitamin A in the body.

carotid artery /kərot´id/, one of the major blood vessels supplying blood to the head and neck. The **common carotid artery** begins at the aorta on the left side and at the innominate artery on the right side. About an inch above the scapula it forms two branches. The **external carotid** supplies the face, scalp and most of the neck and throat tissues. The **internal carotid** supplies the brain, ears, and eyes. The carotid artery pulse can be felt anteriorly on the neck on either side of the larynx.

carotid body, the structure at the bifurcation of the common carotid artery, which contains the chemoreceptor cells that respond to changes in blood pressure and oxygen concentration.

carotid body reflex, the reflex that exists in the chemoreceptors located at the branch of the carotid arteries. It controls the oxygen content of the blood by sending nerve impulses to the medulla of the brain, which in turn increases the breathing rate.

carotid plexus, a network of nerves around the carotid artery and its branches.

carotid sinus, the area at the bifurcation of the common carotid artery with a large number of sensory nerve endings supplying the vagus nerve. This nerve, when stimulated, causes reflex slowing of heart rate along with vasodilation. The sinus is the object of stimulation when performing carotid sinus massage.

carotid sinus massage, technique of applying pressure over the carotid sinus to slow a rapid heart rate. The technique stimulates the vagus nerve, which innervates the carotid sinus. Caution should be used with this technique as it can induce bradycardia, cerebral embolism, or syncope. Also known as **CSM.**

carotid sinus reflex, the decrease in the heart rate as a reflex response to pressure on the carotid sinus.

carotodynia /kərot´ōdin´ē·ə/, soreness along the length of the common carotid artery.

carpal /kär´pəl/, referring to the wrist (carpus).

carpal tunnel syndrome, a common, painful defect of the carpal tunnel, a channel in the wrist for the median nerve and the tendons of the hand. The middle nerve serves the palm and the thumb side of the hand. Pressure on the nerve causes weakness, pain when the thumb is bent toward the palm, and burning, tingling, or aching that may spread to the forearm and the shoulder. The disorder is seen more often in women, especially pregnant and menopausal women. Symptoms may result from edema, rheumatoid arthritis, or a small carpal tunnel that squeezes the nerve.

carpopedal spasm, contractures of the fingers and rigidity of the toes due to blood chemistry abnormalities resulting from tachypnea of psychological origin. Although painful, the condition is otherwise harmless and will terminate shortly after respirations return to the normal range.

carpus.   See **wrist.**

carrier, 1. a person or animal who carries and spreads disease, such as typhoid fever, to others but who does not become ill. **2.** one who carries a gene that has no effect unless it is combined with the gene of another person (recessive gene).

carrier signal, an analog signal with known amplitude, frequency, and phase characteristics. When the original characteristics are known, a receiver can interpret any changes as modulations and recover information so encoded.

carry, 1. to move a victim to another location while supporting his/her weight. **2.** one of several methods used to move victims by hand, as in **blanket carry, chair carry, fore-and-aft carry, hammock carry, three- or four-man carry, seat carry**. *See also lift.*

cartilage, a tissue that connects and supports. It is composed of cells and fibers, found primarily in the joints, the chest, and stiffened tubes of all types, such as the larynx, trachea, nose, and ear.

caruncle, a small fleshy growth.

cascade system, a series of compressed gas bottles, linked together to provide a means for filling smaller, portable bottles. This system utilizes bottles of varying pressures, with the portable bottles being filled in a cascade from lowest to highest pressure.

cascade toboggan, a rescue litter generally used to move victims across snow or ice. This rigid transport vehicle is made of fiberglass, with detachable handles used by a skier or attached to a snowmobile. *See also rigid transport vehicle.*

caseation /kā´sē·ā´shən/, a form of tissue death in which the area looks like crumbly cheese. It is common in tuberculosis.

cast, a solid dressing applied to a body part for temporary immobilization. Made of fiberglass or plaster, the dressing is applied while wet and allowed to harden until rigid.

castration, the removal of one or both testicles or ovaries. It is usually done to reduce hormone production that may cause the growth of cancer cells in women with breast cancer or in men with cancer of the prostate. The removal of both ovaries or testicles causes the person to become sterile.

catabasis /kətab´əsis/, the phase in which a disease declines and health begins to return.

catabiosis /kat´əbī·ō´sis/, the normal aging of cells.

catabolism /kətab´əlizm/, a complex, chemical process of the body in which energy is released for use in work, energy storage, or heat production. The energy is released in the cells by breaking down complex substances into simple compounds. Compare **anabolism. –catabolic,** *adj.*

catalase /kat´əlās/, an enzyme, found in most living cells. It speeds up (catalyzes) the breakdown of hydrogen peroxide to water and oxygen.

catalepsy /kat´əlep´sē/, a trancelike level of awareness and muscle rigidity. It occurs in hypnosis and in some physical and mental conditions, such as schizophrenia, epilepsy, and hysteria.

catalyst /kat´əlist/, a substance that speeds up the rate of a chemical reaction without being changed by the process. *See also enzyme.*

catalytic converter, a metallic pollution-control device located in vehicle exhaust systems. The interior of the converter consists of a glass element coated with platinum. As the vehicle exhaust passes over the platinum, it is changed into carbon dioxide and water vapor. Converter temperatures are generally around 1200° F, but a stationary vehicle with engine running may approach 2000° F.

cataplexy /kat´əplek´sē/, a state in which sudden muscle weakness and loss of muscle tone occurs. It is caused by emotions, such as anger, fear, or surprise. It is linked with narcolepsy, a desire to sleep that cannot be controlled. **–cataplectic,** *adj.*

cataract, a condition in which the eye lens loses its transparency. Most cataracts are caused by a loss of function in the lens tissue, most often after 50 years of age.

catastrophe, a sudden, negative event; a disaster.

catastrophic reaction, the confused response to a sudden threatening state. This reaction occurs in victims of accidents and disasters.

catch basin, a concrete box found in storm sewers.

catchment area, a geographic area, defined on the basis of population, natural geography, or need, that serves as the responsibility or target area for a health program or institution.

catharsis /kəthär´-/, **1.** cleaning out. **2.** the process of bringing memories of events that were not pleasant to the surface of thought.

cathartic /kəthär´-/, a substance that aids bowel movement by increasing peristalsis. The term *cathartic* implies a fluid bowel movement; this is in contrast to *laxative*, which implies a soft, formed stool. *See also laxative.*

catecholamine, organic compounds that have a sympathomimetic effect on the body. These compounds, derived from the amino acid tyrosine, include dopamine, epinephrine, and norepinephrine.

catheter, a metal, plastic, or rubber tube used for injecting or removing fluids, such as **Foley catheter, intravenous catheter.**

catheterization, placing a catheter into a body cavity or organ to inject or remove fluid. The most common practice is putting a catheter into the bladder through the urethra to empty it when a sterile urine sample is needed or if voluntary urination is not possible. *See also cardiac catheterization.*

catheter shear, the tearing off of the plastic portion of an intravenous catheter by the needle within. This shearing occurs when the needle has been partially withdrawn from the catheter and is then reinserted. This may cause a portion of the torn catheter to be introduced into the circulation as an embolus.

cathexis /kəthek´sis/, to attach importance and feeling to a set idea, person, or object.

cation, a positively charged ion, which is attracted to a negatively charged cathode or pole. *See also anion.*

cat's-paw, 1. a slight movement on the surface of water, caused by a light breeze. **2.** a hitch or loop in rope to which tackle is attached.

CAT scan. See **computerized tomography.**

cat-scratch fever, a disease that may be caused by a virus. It results from the scratch or bite of a cat that looks healthy. Lymph nodes in the neck, head, groin, or axilla enlarge. The symptoms

can last for months. Also known as benign inoculation reticulosis, cat scratch disease.

catwalk, a narrow, usually high, walkway with a safety chain or rail spanning its length.

cauda equina /kô´də/, the nerve roots that come out from the end of the spinal cord and go down the spinal canal through the lower part of the spine and coccyx.

caudal, 1. inferior in position; at or near the foot end of the body. **2.** pertaining to any tail-like structure.

caudate, having a tail.

caudate process, a small, raised tissue that arises from the inferior portion of the liver.

caul, the intact bag of waters (amniotic sac) that surrounds a baby at birth. The sac usually breaks open during the course of labor or birth. If it remains whole it must be torn or cut to allow the baby to breathe. In the past, pieces of the caul were sold to sailors as a good luck charm that would protect from death by drowning.

cauliflower ear, a thick, deformed ear caused by being hit many times, as suffered by boxers.

caumesthesia /kô´məsthē´zhə/, low body heat while having a sensation of intense heat.

causalgia /kôzal´jə/, a feeling of severe burning pain, sometimes with local irritation of the skin. It is caused by damage to a sensory nerve.

causation, that which brings about a particular condition or result; the relation of cause and effect.

cause, anything that has an effect.

causeway, a raised roadway across water or low-lying ground.

caustic, any substance that destroys living tissue or causes burning or scarring, such as silver nitrate, nitric acid, or sulfuric acid.

cave-in, 1. yielding to pressure and collapsing inward. **2.** the collapse of unsupported dirt or rock walls.

cavernous sinus /kav´ərnəs/, one of a pair of unevenly shaped channels for blood vessels between the bone of the skull and the dura mater. It is one of five sinuses in the inferior portion of the skull that drain the blood into the jugular vein.

cavernous sinus syndrome, a condition with swelling of the membrane that lines the conjunctiva, the upper eyelid, and the base of the nose. It is caused by a thrombus in a blood vessel of the cavernous sinus.

cavitation,   **1.** the formation of a cavity, such as from a high-velocity projectile striking the body or from tuberculosis in the lung. **2.** the inability of a boat's propeller to develop thrust due to slipping.

cavity,   a hollow space in a larger structure, such as the peritoneal cavity or the oral cavity. A space in a tooth formed by decay of the tooth (caries) is also called a cavity.

cay,   a bank or reef of sand.

cecal /sē´kəl/,   **1.** referring to the top part of the large intestine (cecum). **2.** referring to a blind spot in the field of vision.

cecum /sē´kəm/,   the first portion of the large intestine.

ceiling,   **1.** the cloud level above clear air. **2.** the maximum altitude at which an aircraft can continue to climb at a rate of 100 feet per minute. Also known as **service ceiling. 3.** the upper limit of ability or capacity.

celiac artery /sē´lē·ak/,   a branch of the blood vessel that serves the abdomen (abdominal aorta). It begins below the diaphragm and divides into three arteries that serve the stomach, the liver, and the spleen.

celiac disease,   a defect in the chemistry of food breakdown that is present from birth. A person with this defect cannot digest the gluten of some grain foods. The disease affects adults and young children, who may suffer from an enlarged abdomen, vomiting, diarrhea, muscle wasting, and extreme fatigue. *See also malabsorption syndrome, sprue.*

cell,   the basic unit of all living tissue. The **cell body** is the part of a cell that contains the nucleus and cytoplasm around it. Within the **nucleus,** the controlling part of the cell, are the nucleolus (containing RNA) and chromatin granules (containing protein and DNA) that grow into chromosomes, which determine hereditary traits. Some cells lack a nucleus when they are mature, as do red blood cells. The **cytoplasm** (also called protoplasm) is all of the substance of a cell other than the nucleus. Bits of substance in the cytoplasm, the organelles, are a network of membrane-enclosed tiny tubes (endoplasmic reticulum), ribosomes, the Golgi complex, mito-

chondria, lysosomes, and the centrosome. The thin and fragile outer wall of a cell is called the **cell membrane,** which controls the exchange of materials between the cell's cytoplasm and the area around it.

cell death,   the point in the process of dying at which cells no longer perform their work.

cell division.   See **meiosis, mitosis.**

cellular phone,   a radio communications system (800-900 MHz) that gains access to telephone circuits, allowing telephone communication in remote locations.

cellulitis,   an infection of the skin in one area, as in the lower leg. Symptoms include heat over the area, redness, pain, and swelling. Abscess and tissue destruction may follow.

cellulose /sel´yəlōs/,   a colorless, transparent solid carbohydrate that is the major component of the cell walls of plants. It is nondigestible by humans. However, it provides the bulk needed for proper functioning of the stomach and intestines.

cell wall,   the structure that covers and protects the cell membrane of some kinds of cells, as in certain bacteria and all plant cells.

Celsius /sel´sē·əs/,   a temperature scale in which 0° is the freezing point of water and 100° is the boiling point of water at sea level. Also known as **centigrade.** Compare **Fahrenheit.**

cement,   **1.** a sticky, gluelike substance that helps neighboring tissue cells stay together. **2.** a material used to position an artificial joint in adjacent bone.

cementum,   the bonelike connective tissue that covers the roots of the teeth and helps to support them.

cenesthesia /sē´nəsthē´zhə/,   the general sense of existing, based on all the various stimuli and reactions throughout the body at any specific moment.

censor,   a form of holding back thoughts and only letting them rise to consciousness if they are heavily masked.

center,   **1.** the midline of the body. **2.** a group of cells with a common function.

Centers for Disease Control and Prevention, an agency of the United States government that offers facilities and services for the investigation, identification, prevention, and control of disease. Interests include environmental health, smoking, hunger, poisoning, and problems of health in the workplace. Also known as **CDC.**

centigrade. See **Celsius.**

centimeter /sen´timē´tər/, a metric unit of measurement. It is equal to 1 hundredth of a meter, or 0.3937 inch.

centimeter-gram-second system, an internationally accepted scientific system of expressing length, mass, and time in basic units of centimeters, grams, and seconds. This system is slowly being replaced by the International System of Units based on the meter, kilogram, and second.

central cord syndrome, spinal cord injury usually seen with flexion or hyperextension types of cervical trauma, which causes greater impairment of the upper extremities than the lower extremities.

central nervous system, one of the two main divisions of the nervous system of the body. It is made up of the brain and the spinal cord. The central nervous system carries impulses to and from the peripheral nervous system. It is the main network of coordination and control for the entire body. The brain controls many functions and sensations, such as sleep, sexual activity, muscle movement, hunger, thirst, memory, and the emotions. The spinal cord contains various types of nerve fibers from the brain and acts as a switching and relay terminal for the peripheral nervous system. The 12 pairs of cranial nerves emerge directly from the brain. The nerves of the peripheral system leave the spinal cord separately between the vertebrae of the backbone. However, they unite to form 31 pairs of spinal nerves containing sensory fibers and motor fibers. Sensory nerves carry impulses to the spinal cord and brain. Motor nerves carry impulses from the central nervous system to the muscles and glands. The brain contains more than 10 billion nerve cells. Billions of other cells help form the soft, jellylike substance of the brain. Flowing through many cavities of the central nervous system is the fluid of the brain and spine. This fluid helps to protect the central nervous system from injury. It affects the rate of breathing through cells that measure its content of carbon dioxide. The brain and the spinal cord are made up of gray matter and white matter.

The gray matter primarily consists of nerve cells and linked filaments. The white matter is made up of bundles of insulated (myelinated) nerve fibers. Also known as **CNS.** Compare **peripheral nervous system.** *See also autonomic nervous system, brain, parasympathetic nervous system, spinal cord, sympathetic nervous system.*

central nervous system oxygen toxicity, oxygen poisoning sustained while breathing pure oxygen under pressure. This syndrome may be seen when breathing 100% oxygen in a recompression chamber or with divers using closed-circuit oxygen rebreathers below 30 feet of depth. Symptoms include auditory changes, nausea, seizures, and tunnel vision. Also known as **oxygen toxicity.**

central processing unit, the portion of a computer that does computing. Composed of the arithmetic logic unit and the control unit, this piece of equipment, along with the clock and main memory, make up a computer. Also known as **CPU.**

central scotoma, an area of blindness or lowered vision involving the central area of the retina.

central thermoreceptors, nerve endings sensitive to heat, which are located near the hypothalamus.

central venous return, the blood from the body's veins that flows into the right upper chamber (atrium) of the heart through the major vein in the trunk (vena cava).

central vision, vision that results from images falling on the center of the retina.

centrifugal /sentrif´yəgəl/, referring to a force that is directed outward, away from a central point or axis. *See also centripetal.*

centrifugal force, an inertial force that pushes an object, moving along a curved path, to the outside of the curve. The tighter a turn radius, the more centrifugal force exerted. *See also centripetal force.*

centriole /sen´trē·ōl´/, an organ within a cell usually as a part of the center of a cell (centrosome). Often occurring in pairs, centrioles are linked to cell division. The precise function of centrioles is still unclear.

centripetal /sentrip´ətəl/, **1.** referring to a direction, as a sensory nerve impulse traveling toward the brain. **2.** the direction of a force pulling an object toward the center or an axis of rotation, as opposed to a centrifugal force.

centripetal force,   the inertial force that pushes an object, moving along a curved path, to the inside of the curve. The opposite of centrifugal force. *See also centrifugal force.*

centromere /sen´trəmir/,   a specialized region of the chromosome. It joins 2 chromosome halves (chromatids) to each other and attaches to the spindle fiber in cell reproduction. During cell division the centromeres split lengthwise, half going to each of the new daughter chromosomes.

centrosome /-sōm/,   a region present in animal cells and in some plants. It is located near the nucleus and is involved in cell division.

centrosphere /-sfir/,   a condensed area of cytoplasm surrounding the centrioles in the centrosome of a cell.

cephalalgia /sef´əlal´jēə/,   headache, often combined with another word to describe the type of headache, such as histamine cephalalgia. *See also headache.*

cephalhematoma /sef´əlhē´mətō´mə/,   swelling caused by the pooling of blood under the scalp. It may begin to form in the scalp of a baby during labor and slowly become larger in the first few days after birth. It is usually a result of injury, often from forceps. Compare **molding.**

cephalic /səfal´ik/,   referring to the head.

cephalic presentation,   a baby's position during labor in which the head is at the narrow lower end of the uterus (cervix). Cephalic presentation is usually further qualified by the part of the head presenting, as the back (occiput) or front (bregma).

cephalic vein,   one of the four superficial veins of the arm. It begins in the network of veins in the hand and ends near the shoulder.

cephalopelvic disproportion /sef´əlōpel´vik/,   a condition in which a baby's head is too large or a mother's birth canal too small to allow normal labor or birth.

cephalothorax,   the united head and thorax of spiders, ticks, and mites.

cercaria /sərker´ē·ə/, *pl.* **cercariae,**   a tiny worm of the class Trematoda. Cercariae enter the body through the skin and form cysts in many organs of the body. Each species tends to go to a particular organ, such as *Fasciola hepatica,* which becomes a liver fluke. *See also fluke, schistosomiasis.*

cerebellar /ser´əbel´ər/,   referring to a part of the brain (cerebellum).

cerebellum /ser´əbel´əm/.   See **brain.**

cerebral /ser´əbrəl, sərē´brəl/,   referring to the cerebrum.

cerebral cortex.   See **brain.**

cerebral dominance,   the role of each of the two halves of the cerebrum (cerebral hemispheres) in the integration and control of different functions. The left hemisphere houses the logical, reasoning activities and controls reading, writing, speech, and analytic activities. The right hemisphere concerns imagination, intuitions, creativity, spatial skills, art, and left-hand control. In 90% of the population, the left cerebral hemisphere dominates the ability to speak, write, and understand spoken and written words. In the other 10% of the population, either the right hemisphere or both hemispheres dominate. The right cerebral hemisphere also dominates the integration of certain sounds other than speaking, such as the sounds of laughter, crying, and melodies. The right cerebral hemisphere perceives touch stimuli and visual relationships better than the left cerebral hemisphere.

cerebral hemisphere.   See **brain.**

cerebral hemorrhage,   bleeding from a blood vessel in the brain. Cerebral hemorrhages are classified by location, the kind of vessel involved, and the cause. Each type has its own symptoms, some of which include headache, partial paralysis, loss of consciousness, nausea, vomiting, and seizures. They are caused by the rupture of an artery as a result of high blood pressure. Other causes of rupture include congenital ballooning of brain arteries (aneurysm) and head injury. Bleeding may lead to destruction of brain tissue. Extensive bleeding leads usually to death. Blood may be found in the spinal fluid. Depending on the extent and the location of the damaged tissue, effects may include aphasia, diminished mental function, or loss of the function of one of the special senses.

cerebral herniation, brain tissue forced into the inferior cranial orifice (foramen magnum) due to increased intracranial pressure. This commonly occurs after serious head injury and precipitates altered levels of consciousness, pupillary changes, decerebrate or decorticate posturing, and respiratory arrest.

cerebral palsy, a motor nerve disorder caused by a permanent brain defect or an injury at birth or soon after. Symptoms depend on the area of the brain involved and the extent of damage. Milder cases have spastic paralysis of the legs or both limbs on one side and normal intelligence. More severe cases have widespread loss of normal muscle control, seizures, numbness, mental retardation, and blocked speech, vision, and hearing. The disorder is usually linked to premature or abnormal birth and lack of oxygen during birth, causing damage to the nervous system.

cerebrocerebellar atrophy /ser´əbrōser´əbel´- ər/, a breakdown of the cerebellum caused by nutritional diseases.

cerebroma /ser´əbrō´mə/, any unusual mass of brain tissue.

cerebroretinal angiomatosis /-ret´ənəl/, a hereditary disease of small tumorlike growths in the retina of the eye and part of the brain (cerebellum). Similar growths on the spinal cord, pancreas, kidneys, and other organs are also common. Seizures and mental retardation may be present.

cerebrospinal /-spī´nəl/, the brain and the spinal cord.

cerebrospinal fluid (CSF), the fluid that flows through and protects the brain and the spinal canal. It has small amounts of proteins, glucose, and electrolytes. Changes in the carbon dioxide content of CSF affect the respiratory center in the brain, helping to control breathing. A brain tumor may obstruct the flow of fluid. This results in hydrocephalus. Other blockages of the flow of cerebrospinal fluid may occur, such as those caused by blood clots. Examination of CSF is important in diagnosing diseases of the central nervous system.

cerebrovascular /-vas´kyələr/, referring to the blood vessels and blood supply of the brain.

cerebrovascular accident, sudden alteration in level of consciousness, sensation, and/or voluntary movement due to obstruction or rupture of an artery in the brain. These effects may be temporary or permanent. Also known as **CVA, stroke.** *See also transient ischemic attack.*

cerebrum /ser´əbrəm, səre´brəm/. See **brain.**

cerium, a gray rare earth element. A compound of cerium (cerium oxalate) is used as a sedative, to relieve nausea, and to control coughing.

ceroid /sir´oid/, a golden, waxy pigment appearing in the stomach and intestines, the nervous system, and the muscles. It is sometimes found in the livers of people with cirrhosis.

certification, 1. the process by which a person or program is evaluated, based on certain recognized standards. **2.** the recognition that a person or program meets a predetermined standard. This standard attempts to ensure quality performance.

certify, to guarantee that certain requirements have been met based on expert knowledge.

cerumen /sirōō´mən/, a yellowish or brownish waxy substance, made by glands in the ear canal. Also known as **earwax.**

cervical /sur´vikəl/, referring to the neck or a necklike structure, such as the narrow inferior end of the uterus (cervix).

cervical collar, a soft, adjustable collar, used during and after hospitalization, to remind the patient with neck injury to restrict movement of the head. This device is not suitable for field use as it does not provide the stabilization necessary for cervical immobilization. Also known as **C-collar, collar.** *See also extrication collar.*

cervical disk syndrome, a spinal disorder in which the cervical nerves (neck) are compressed or irritated. The cause may be herniated disks, degenerative disk disease, or neck injuries, especially those that overextend the vertebrae. Fluid usually pools around the injured area. Pain, the most common symptom, usually centers around the neck. It may also radiate down the arm to the fingers. *See also herniated disk.*

cervical erosion, a condition in which the lining (epithelium) of the narrow lower end of the uterus (cervix) is eroded as a result of infection or injury, as during childbirth.

cervical fistula, an abnormal passage from the cervix to the vagina or bladder. The cause may be cancer, x-ray therapy, surgical injury, or injury during childbirth. A cervical fistula connecting with the bladder permits leakage of urine.

cervical immobilization device, foam or nylon pads, placed on either side of the head, that serve to diminish lateral movement in a patient with suspected spinal injury. This device replaces sandbags previously used for lateral immobilization. Also known as **CID.**

cervical plexus, the network of nerves formed by divisions of the first four cervical nerves in the neck.

cervical polyp, an outgrowth of tissue on the wall of the cervical canal through the uterine cervix. It is usually attached to the wall by a slender skin flap. Often there are no symptoms. However, polyps may cause bleeding, especially from contact during intercourse. Polyps are most common in women over 40 years of age. The cause is not known.

cervical vertebra. See **vertebra.**

cervicitis /sur´visī´-/, sudden or chronic inflammation of the inferior uterus (cervix). **Acute cervicitis** is an infection with edema and bleeding of the cervix. The primary causes are *Trichomonas vaginalis, Candida albicans,* and *Haemophilus vaginalis.* **Chronic cervicitis** is a persistent inflammation of the cervix that occurs among women in their reproductive years. Symptoms are like those of the acute form. The cervix is congested and swollen. Cysts are often present. *See also Candida albicans, cautery, cervical cancer, cervical polyp.*

cervix /sur´viks/, the part of the uterus that protrudes into the cavity of the vagina. The cervix is divided into two parts: the portion above the vagina (supravaginal) and the vaginal portion. They are separated by a band of tissue. The vaginal portion of the cervix has the **cervical canal,** the opening within the cervix. The canal is a passageway through which the menstrual flow escapes. It is completely widened during labor. The infant passes through this canal when childbirth occurs vaginally.

cesarean section /səser´ē·ən/, childbirth performed surgically through an incision in the abdomen and uterus. It is done when conditions exist that are judged likely to make vaginal birth dangerous for mother or child, as in placenta previa, abruptio placenta, preeclampsia, and fetal distress.

Chaddock reflex, an abnormal reflex induced by firmly stroking the skin of the forearm on the side opposite the thumb. This causes the wrist to flex and the fingers to spread like a fan. This reflex occurs on the affected side in partial paralysis.

Chaddock's sign, a variation of the Babinski reflex. It is induced by firmly stroking the side of the foot. This causes the great toe to extend and the other toes to fan. It is seen in disease of the pyramidal tract of the brain.

chafe, an irritation of the skin by friction, as when rough material rubs against an unprotected area of the body.

Chagres fever /chag´ris/, an arbovirus infection carried to humans through the bite of a sandfly. Symptoms include fever, headache, and muscle pains of the chest or stomach. Also known as **Panama fever.**

chain, **1.** a length of units linked together, such as a polypeptide chain of amino acids. **2.** a group of individual bacteria linked together, such as streptococci formed by a chain of cocci. **3.** the relationship of some body structures, such as the chain of small bones in the middle ear.

chain reaction, **1.** a chemical reaction that makes a compound needed for the reaction to continue. **2.** an atomic reaction that continues itself by continuing the splitting of nuclei and the release of atomic particles, which causes more nuclear splitting.

chain saw, electric or gas-powered saw that cuts by means of a rotating chain of teeth, used to cut holes in roofs and obstructing vegetation.

chalasia /kəlā´zhə/, the abnormal relaxation of the muscle (cardiac sphincter) at the junction of the esophagus with the stomach. This results in the stomach contents backing up into the esophagus. Infants with this disorder vomit after every feeding. Most grow out of it by about 6 months of age. *See also reflux.*

chalazion /kəlā´zē·on/, a small swelling of the eyelid. It results from obstruction of the glands in the eyelid. *See also sty.*

chalkitis /kalkī´-/, an inflammation of the eyes, caused by rubbing the eyes with the hands after touching or handling brass. Also known as **brassy eye.**

chamber, a hollow but not always empty space or cavity in an organ, such as the atrial and ventricular chambers of the heart.

chancre /shang´kər/, **1.** a skin sore, usually from syphilis (venereal sore). It begins as a small lump and grows into a bloodless, painless ulcer. It heals without treatment, but is highly contagious. It leaves no scar. **2.** an ulcerated area of the skin that marks the point of infection of a nonsyphilitic disease, such as tuberculosis.

chancroid /shang´kroid/, a highly contagious, sexually transmitted disease caused by infection with *Haemophilus ducreyi*. It usually begins on the skin of the external genitals as an ulceration.

channel, 1. a passageway that passes fluid, such as the central channels that connect arterioles with venules. **2.** single or dual frequencies used to carry data or voice communications. **3.** a short waterway used by vessels to transit between bodies of water.

channel guard. See **continuous tone-controlled subaudible squelch.**

chapped, skin that is roughened, cracked, or reddened by exposure to cold or excess evaporation of sweat. Stinging or burning sensations are often felt.

character, the group of traits and behavioral tendencies that enable a person to react in a relatively consistent way. Character, as contrasted with personality, implies choice and morality.

character disorder, a persistent, habitual, badly adaptive, and socially unacceptable pattern of behavior and emotional response. *See also antisocial personality disorder.*

Charcot's fever /shärkōz´/, a disorder with fever, jaundice, and stomach pain in the right upper quadrant linked to inflammation of the bile ducts. It is caused by a gallstone becoming lodged in the bile ducts.

charging station, a filling device for the refill of portable compressed gas (usually air) bottles. An air compressor is usually used to fill a fixed reservoir from which the bottles are then filled. *See also cascade system.*

Charles's Law (Jacques Alexandre César Charles, French physicist, 1746-1823), at a constant pressure, the volume of a given mass of gas is proportional to its absolute temperature.

CHART, 1. (*informal*) a patient record. *See also patient record.* **2.** acronym for an emergency medical services documentation method that stands for: **C**hief complaint, **H**istory (subjective information), **A**ssessment (objective information), **R**x, or treatment (on scene), **T**ransport (events and treatment en route to hospital). An **E** is sometimes added to stand for **E**xceptions, which occurred during the call, such as a prolonged on-scene time.

chauffeur's fracture, any fracture of the wrist, caused by a twisting or a snapping type injury.

check-up, a study of the health of an individual.

cheek, a fleshy rise, especially the fleshy parts on the lateral face between the eye and jaw. Also known as **bucca.**

cheilitis /kīlī´-/, inflammation and cracking of the lips. There are several forms including those caused by excessive exposure to sunlight, allergic sensitivity to cosmetics, and vitamin lack.

cheiromegaly /kī´rōmeg´əlē/, extremely large hands.

chelation /kēlā´shən/, a chemical reaction in which a metal combines with another chemical to form a ring-shaped molecular complex. The process is used in treatment for metal poisoning.

chemical, a substance composed of elements that can react with other substances; a substance produced by or used in chemical processes.

chemical abstract service number, used by state and local right-to-know regulations for tracking chemicals in the workplace and the community.

chemical action, any process in which natural elements and compounds react with each other to produce a chemical change or a different compound. For example, hydrogen and oxygen combine to produce water.

chemical agent, toxic chemical compounds used for crowd control or incapacitation. Classified by effect, they are either casualty producing, harassing, or incapacitating. Harassing chemicals (riot control agents) include oleoresin capsicum (pepper spray), tear gas, and vomiting agents, and are most commonly used by civilian law enforcement. They are short-duration gases, which are nonlethal in their effect. *See also blood agents, choking agents, lacrimator, nerve agents, sternutator, vesicants.*

chemical burn. See **burn.**

chemical equivalent, a drug with similar amounts of the same ingredients as another drug.

chemical gastritis, inflammation of the stomach, caused by swallowing a chemical compound. **Corrosive gastritis** is caused by swallowing an acid, alkali, or other substance that eats away the lining of the stomach. **Erosive gastritis** is a wearing away of portions of the mucous membrane lining the stomach. Symptoms include nausea, loss of appetite, pain, and hematemesis. *See also acid poisoning, alkali poisoning, gastritis.*

chemical name, the name of a drug based on its chemical structure.

chemical restraint, the pharmacological sedation of a combative patient. Also known as **rapid sequence induction.**

chemistry, the science of the structure and interactions of matter. **Applied chemistry** refers to the practical use of the study of chemical elements and compounds.

chemonucleolysis /kē´mōnoo͞´klēol´isis, kem´ō-/, a method of dissolving the cartilage between the vertebrae of the spine (intervertebral disk) by injecting a substance, such as chymopapain. It is done mainly to treat a herniated disk.

chemoreceptor, a sensory nerve cell that is activated by chemicals. An example is the chemoreceptor in the main artery (carotid) in the neck. It is sensitive to carbon dioxide in the blood, which signals the breathing center in the brain to increase or decrease breathing. The activity or reflex triggered by the stimulation of chemoreceptors is called **chemoreflex.**

chemosis /kimō´-/, an abnormal swelling of the mucous membrane covering the eye and lining the eyelids. It is usually the result of injury or infection. A blockage of normal lymph flow may be the cause of chemosis. Also known as **conjunctival edema.**

chemosurgery, the destruction of cancerous, infected, or dead (gangrenous) tissue by applying chemicals. This technique is used to remove skin cancers.

chemotherapy, the treatment of disease with chemicals or drugs, most often in treating cancer.

cherry-red spot, an abnormal red area with white tissue on the retina of the eye. It is linked to retinal artery disorders. It sometimes appears with Tay-Sachs disease. Also known as **Tay's spot.**

chest. See **thorax.**

chest harness, nylon webbing, made into a strapping system, that fits around the chest. This device is used during climbing activities and various types of rescue when an equipment platform or a secure tie-off location around the chest is needed. Various types include baudrier, cross-shoulder, and swimmers.

chest-pressure arm-lift, *(historical)* manual method of artificial respiration used in the first half of the twentieth century for victims of respiratory arrest. The technique involves pressing the wrists (arms) of a supine patient onto their lower chest (as a means of causing exhalation) and then pulling the arms above the head as far as possible (as a means of causing inhalation). With the rescuer positioned at the patient's head, this technique was rhythmically repeated 12 times per minute. Also known as **Silvester method.** *See also back-pressure arm-lift, Schäfer prone pressure method.*

Cheyne-Stokes respiration (Cheyne, John, Scottish physician, 1777-1836; Stokes, William, Irish physician, 1804-1878), periods of apnea, followed by tachypnea. The tachypnea manifests as a gradual increase in depth and, occasionally, rate, followed by a gradual decrease in rate and depth. This will persist for 30 seconds to 2 minutes, to be followed by 5 to 30 seconds of apnea. This pattern is usually due to a head injury with an alteration in the respiratory center, a toxic drug ingestion, or a metabolic encephalopathy.

chickenpox, a highly contagious disease caused by a herpes virus, varicella zoster. It occurs primarily in children and causes blisterlike eruptions on the skin. The fluid and blebs are infectious until entirely dry. The disease may also be spread by droplets from the breathing tract of infected persons, usually in the early stages of the disease. The rash begins as flat red spots and develops in a day or two to become blisters surrounding a reddened base and containing clear fluid. Within 24 to 48 hours the blisters turn cloudy. They are easily broken and become encrusted. They erupt in groups so that all three stages are present at the same time. They appear first on the back and chest, and then spread to the face, neck, and limbs. In severe cases, blisters in the throat may cause breathing difficulty and pain with swallowing. Fever, swollen lymph glands, and extreme irritability from itching are other symptoms. The symptoms last from a few days to 2 weeks. One attack of the disease gives permanent immunity. However, herpes zoster virus (HZV), like all herpes viruses, lies dormant in certain sensory nerve roots following a main infection. The virus is sometimes reactivated later in life (usually after age 50), with the eruption following the path of a nerve on the trunk, face, or limbs. Common complications are secondary bacterial infections, such as abscesses, pneumonia, and blood poisoning. Also known as **varicella.**

chief complaint, a patient's primary presenting sign or symptom.

chigger, the larva of *Trombicula* mites found in tall grass and weeds. They stick to the skin, causing irritation and severe itching.

chilblain, inflammation and cyanosis of the ears, hands, lower legs, and feet caused by cold. In severe cases, it may be accompanied by skin lesions (ulcerations, vesicles). Although there is no actual tissue freezing, as in frostbite, rewarming does cause intense pruritus and burning paresthesias. Also known as **pernio.** *See also frostbite, immersion foot.*

child, **1.** a person between the time of birth and adolescence. **2.** a descendant or offspring. **3.** for medical treatment purposes, a person between 1 and 8 years or 7 and 25 kilograms (15 and 55 pounds).

child abuse, the physical, sexual, or emotional mistreatment of a child. It may result in permanent physical or mental injury, or, sometimes, death. Factors that contribute to child abuse include a stressful environment, such as poor economic conditions, lack of physical and emotional

support within the family, and any major life change or crisis, especially those arising from marital strife. Marks on a child's body, such as burns, welts, or bruises, and signs of emotional distress, including symptoms of failure to thrive, are common signs of neglect or abuse.

childbirth. See **birth.**

child development, the various stages of physical, social, and psychological growth that occur from birth to adulthood.

childhood, the period in human development that extends from birth until the beginning of puberty.

child neglect, failure of guardians or parents to provide the essentials necessary for survival, such as clothing, food, or shelter. Neglect may be medical (deprivation of medical care), nutritional (inadequate food), and/or physical (inadequate clothing, shelter).

chill, **1.** the sensation of cold from exposure to a cold environment. **2.** an attack of shivering with a feeling of coldness.

Chinese restaurant syndrome, a reaction that may occur after eating food with the flavor additive monosodium glutamate. Symptoms include tingling and burning sensations of the skin, headache, and chest pain.

chin lift, a technique for opening the airway by hyperextending the head, using the chin as a lift point for hyperextension. This procedure is usually combined with pressure on the forehead (head tilt). It is then known as head-tilt chin-lift.

chip, a relatively small piece of a bone or tooth.

chiropodist /kirop´ədist, shir-/, a health professional trained to diagnose and treat diseases and disorders of the foot. Also known as **podiatrist.**

chiropody /kirop´ədē, shir-/, the study of disorders of the feet and the practice of treating these disorders.

chiropractic /kī´rōprak´-/, a system of treatment that involves manipulation of the spinal column. It is based on the theory that the state of a person's health is determined by the condition of the musculoskeletal and nervous systems.

Chlamydia /kləmid´ē·ə/, a genus of microorganisms that live as parasites within the cell. Two species of *Chlamydia* cause diseases in humans. *Chlamydia trachomatis* are organisms that live in the eye, urethra, and cervix. They cause inflammation of the conjunctiva (inclusion conjunctivitis), venereal disease (lymphogranuloma venereum), and eye disease (trachoma). *Chlamydia psittaci* cause a type of pneumonia in humans. *See also psittacosis.*

chloasma /klō·az´mə/, tan or brown coloring, particularly of the forehead, cheeks, and nose. The condition is commonly linked to pregnancy and the use of birth control pills.

chloride /klôr´īd/, a chemical compound with chlorine.

chlorine /klôr´ēn/, a yellowish-green, gaseous element of the halogen group. It has a strong, distinctive odor. It is irritating to the breathing tract. It is poisonous if swallowed or inhaled. It occurs in nature chiefly as a component of sodium chloride in sea water and in salt deposits.

chloroform /klôr´əfôrm/, a nonflammable liquid. It was the first gas anesthetic to be discovered. Chloroform is a dangerous anesthetic drug, however. Delayed poisoning, even weeks after apparently complete recovery, can occur.

chloroformism /klôr´-/, the habit of inhaling chloroform for its narcotic effect.

chloroleukemia /klôr´əlōōkē´mē·ə/, a kind of myelocytic leukemia in which body fluids and organs get a green color. *See also leukemia.*

chloroma /klôrō´mə/, a cancerous, greenish tumor. It occurs anywhere in the body in patients with myelocytic leukemia. The green pigment has no definite function. Also known as **granulocytic sarcoma, green cancer.**

chlorophyll /klôr´əfil/, a plant pigment that absorbs light and changes it to energy. Chlorophylls a and b are found in green plants. Chlorophyll c occurs in brown algae. Chlorophyll d occurs in red algae. *See also photosynthesis.*

chock, 1. a block of metal or wood, placed under a wheel, to prevent aircraft or vehicle movement. **2.** device resembling a nut that provides an anchor point to guard against falls while climbing. *See also nut.*

choke, 1. constrict; tighten. **2.** disruption of respirations due to compression or obstruction of the trachea. **3.** passing the end of a cable or rope sling through the eye formed at the opposite end and tightening until secure around an object to be lifted.

choke damp. See **black damp.**

chokes, decompression sickness with respiratory distress caused by nitrogen bubbles mechanically obstructing pulmonary blood vessels. Symptoms include chest pain, cyanosis, dyspnea, and nonproductive cough. Although similar to gas embolism, the mechanism of injury is due to inadequate decompression time and not due to holding the breath. Also known as **pulmonary decompression sickness.** *See also decompression sickness.*

choking agent, casualty-producing chemical agent that irritates the bronchi and causes pulmonary edema. These chemicals, such as chlorine or phosgene, can cause extensive destruction of alveoli, precipitating pulmonary edema. Signs and symptoms may not occur for 2–6 hours after exposure and include chest tightness, painful cough, cyanosis, and hypotension. Treatment is symptomatic. Also known as **lung agents.**

cholangioma /kōlan´jē·ō´mə/, a cancer of the bile ducts.

cholangitis /kō´lanjī´-/, inflammation of the bile ducts. Causes include bacterial infection and blocking of the ducts by stones or a tumor. Symptoms include severe pain in the right upper quadrant of the abdomen, jaundice, and fever.

cholecalciferol. See **vitamin D₃.**

cholecystectomy /kō´lisistek´-/, the surgical removal of the gallbladder. A tube is placed in the incision temporarily to drain bile to the outside of the body.

cholecystitis /-sistī´/, inflammation of the gallbladder, usually caused by a gallstone that cannot pass through the bile duct.

cholecystokinin /kō´ləsis´təkī´nən/, hormone that stimulates the secretion of pancreatic enzyme and contraction of the gallbladder. It is secreted by mucosa of the small intestine.

cholelithiasis /-lithī´əsis/, the presence of gallstones in the gallbladder. The condition affects about 20% of the population over age 40. It is more common in women. Many patients complain of general stomach discomfort and intolerance to certain foods. *See also gallstone.*

cholelithotomy /-lithot´-/, a surgical operation to remove gallstones through an incision in the gallbladder.

cholera /kol´ərə/, a serious bacterial infection of the small intestine. Symptoms include severe diarrhea and vomiting, muscular cramps, and dehydration. The disease is spread by water and food that have been contaminated by feces of infected persons. The symptoms are caused by toxic substances made by the bacterium *Vibrio cholerae*. Mortality is as high as 50% if untreated. A vaccine is available.

cholestasis /-stā´-/, interruption in the flow of bile through any part of the biliary system, from liver to intestine. Causes include hepatitis, drug and alcohol use, and an obstruction in the common bile duct. Symptoms of both types of cholestasis include jaundice, dark urine, and intense itching of the skin.

cholesterase /koles´tərās/, an enzyme in the body that forms cholesterol and fatty acids.

cholesterol /koles´trôl/, substance found in animal fats and oils, egg yolk, and the human body. It is most common in the blood, brain tissue, liver, kidneys, adrenal glands, and around nerve fibers. It helps to absorb and move fatty acids. Cholesterol is necessary for the production of vitamin D on the surface of the skin. Cholesterol is found in foods from animals and is constantly produced in the body, mainly in the liver and the kidneys. High amounts of cholesterol in the blood may be linked to the development of cholesterol deposits in the blood vessels (atherosclerosis).

cholesterolemia /-ē´mē·ə/, the presence of increased cholesterol in the blood.

choline /kō´lēn/, one of the B-complex vitamins, essential for the use of fats in the body. The richest sources of choline are liver, kidneys, brains, wheat germ, brewer's yeast, and egg yolk. Lack of choline leads to cirrhosis of the liver, resulting in stomach ulcers, damage to the kidney, high blood pressure, high blood levels of cholesterol, atherosclerosis, and arteriosclerosis. *See also inositol, lecithin.*

cholinergic, nerve fibers that liberate acetylcholine at the myoneural junctions.

cholinergic blocking agent, any drug that blocks the action of acetylcholine and similar substances.

cholinesterase /-es´tərās/, enzyme that causes the breakdown of acetylcholine.

chondrectomy /kondrek´-/, surgical removal of cartilage.

chondrocostal /-kos´təl/, the ribs and the cartilages of the ribs.

chondromalacia /-məlā´shə/, a softening or stretching of cartilage with accompanying pain and stiffness.

chondroplasty /kon´drəplas´tē/, the surgical repair of cartilage.

chordae tendineae /kôr´dē tendin´i·ē/, *sing.* **chorda tendinea,** strong fibrous bands in the heart that attach the corners of the heart valves to the muscles of the ventricles. They prevent the valves from protruding into the atria as the heart beats.

chordencephalon /kôrd´ənsef´əlon/, the part of the central nervous system that develops in the early weeks of pregnancy from the nerve tube. It later becomes the nerves of the spinal cord that control sensation and movement.

chorditis /kôrdī´-/, inflammation of a spermatic cord or of the vocal cords.

chordotomy /kôrdot´-/, an operation in which parts of the spinal cord are surgically divided to relieve pain.

chorea /kôrē·ə/, a condition of uncontrolled, purposeless, rapid motions. Typical movements are bending and extending the fingers, raising and lowering the shoulders, or grimacing.

chorioamnionitis /-am´nē·onī´-/, inflammation in the amniotic sac caused by organisms in the fluid surrounding the fetus.

choriocele /kôr´ē·əsēl´/, a hernia or bulging of tissue in the back (choroid layer) of the eye.

chorion /kôr´ē·on/. See **amniotic sac.**

chorioretinitis /-ret´ənī´-/, inflammation of the outer membrane and retina of the eye, usually as a result of infection. Symptoms are blur-red vision, sensitivity to light, and distorted images.

chorioretinopathy /-ret´inop´əthē/, a disease of the eye that involves the outer membrane of the eye (choroid) and the retina. Inflammation does not occur.

choroid /kôr´oid/, a thin membrane richly supplied with blood that covers the white of the eyeball. It begins near the iris and wraps around the back of the eye. The choroid supplies blood to the retina. It conducts nerves and arteries to the front of the eye.

choroiditis, inflammation of the outer membrane of the eye (choroid). *See also chorioretinitis.*

choroidocyclitis /-siklī´-/, an inflammation of the eye that affects the outer membrane and the process that controls focusing of the lens.

choroid plexus, any one of the tangled masses of tiny blood vessels found in several parts of the brain.

chromaffin cell /krō´məfin/, any of the cells linked to sympathetic nerves, which produce the "flight or fight" response. Chromaffin cells in the adrenal glands secrete epinephrine and norepinephrine, which increase heart rate, raise blood pressure, increase respiration, and slow digestion. They are highly responsive to stress.

chromatic, 1. referring to color. **2.** able to be stained by a dye. **3.** referring to chromatin, **chromatinic.**

chromatic dispersion, the splitting of light into its wavelengths or frequencies. A prism is often used to separate and study the different colors.

chromatid /krō´mətid/, one of the two identical threadlike fibers of a chromosome. It results when the chromosome reproduces itself. The two chromatid fibers making up each chromosome are joined in the center. During cell division, it divides lengthwise to form identical chromosomes.

chromatin /krō´mətin/, the material in the nucleus that forms the chromosomes. It is made up of fine, threadlike strands of DNA attached to protein. During cell division, parts of the chromatin condense and coil to form the chromosomes. **Chromatin-negative** refers to nuclei that lack sex chromatin. This is distinctive of the normal male. **Chromatin-positive** refers to the nuclei that contain sex chromatin. This is distinctive of the normal female.

chromatism, 1. condition in which a patient has hallucinations and sees colored lights. **2.** abnormal pigmentation.

chromatopsia /-top´sē·ə/, **1.** a visual defect that makes colorless objects appear touched with color. **2.** a form of color blindness in which the patient may not see various colors correctly. It may be caused by a lack of one or more of the cells in the retina or from incorrect color messages being carried. *See also color blindness.*

chromesthesia /krō´məsthē´zhə/, a condition in which the person confuses other senses, such as hearing, taste, or smell, to be sensations of color.

chromhidrosis /krō´midrō´-/, a rare disorder in which the sweat glands secrete perspiration that may be yellow, blue, green, or black and often also glows (fluoresces). A cause is regular exposure to copper, catechols, or ferrous oxide.

-chromic, -chromatic, 1. a combining form meaning the number of colors seen by the eye. **2.** a combining form meaning a specific color of the blood indicating the hemoglobin content. **3.** a combining form meaning the ability of bacteria and tissues to be stained. **4.** a combining form meaning a specified skin color as a symptom of disease.

chromium, a hard, brittle, metallic element. It does not occur naturally in pure form but exists with iron and oxygen in chromite. Traces of chromium occur in plants and animals. This element may be important in human nutrition, especially in digestion of carbohydrates. Workers in chromite mines are susceptible to a long-term lung disorder (pneumoconiosis) caused by breathing chromite dust.

chromobacteriosis /krō´məbaktir´ē·ō´-/, a rare, usually fatal infection caused by bacteria found in fresh water in tropic and subtropic regions. They enter the body through an opening in the skin. Symptoms are fever, liver abscesses, and severe fatigue.

chromoblastomycosis /-blas´təmīkō´-/, an infectious skin disease caused by a fungus. Symptoms include itching and growths that develop in a cut or other break in the skin. These first appear as a small dull-red papule, slowly becoming a large ulcerlike growth. Over weeks or months, more growths may appear on the skin.

chromosomal aberration /-sō´məl/, any change in the normal structure or number of any of the chromosomes. This can result in birth defects and a number of physical disabilities. Some of these include Down's syndrome, Turner's syndrome, and Kleinfelter's syndrome.

chromosome /krō´məsōm/, any one of the threadlike structures in the nucleus that carry genetic information. Each is made up of a double strand of twisted DNA (deoxyribonucleic acid). Along the length of each strand of DNA lie the genes, which contain the genetic material that controls the inheritance of traits. In cell division, chromosomes reproduce themselves. Each species has a certain number of chromosomes, called a **chromosome complement**. Humans have 46 chromosomes. These include 22 pairs of nonsex chromosomes (autosomes) and one pair of sex chromosomes. Each parent contributes one sex chromosome. **–chromosomal,** *adj.*

chronic, disease or disorder that persists for long periods of time. *See also acute.*

chronic brain syndrome, a condition that is due to damage to brain tissue, causing loss of memory and disorientation. It may occur in dementia paralytica, cerebral arteriosclerosis, cerebral injury, and Huntington's chorea.

chronic care, a type of medical care that concentrates on lasting care of people with long-term disorders. This care may be given either at home or in a medical facility.

chronic health hazard, marked by a long or permanent duration, consistent or continuous. Often occurs from repeated exposures over a period of time.

chronic lymphocytic leukemia. See **leukemia.**

chronic mountain polycythemia, abnormally high red blood cell production due to high-altitude hypoxia. Symptoms include headache, insomnia, and lethargy. This chronic condition is noted in both natives of high altitude and those who relocate there. Susceptibility of males is much greater than females. Also known as **chronic mountain sickness, Monge's disease.** *See also acute mountain sickness.*

chronic myelocytic leukemia. See **leukemia.**

chronic obstructive pulmonary disease, any disease process that decreases the pulmonary system's ability to perform ventilation. Those chronic diseases responsible for this condition include asthma, bronchitis, and emphysema. Symptoms include persistent dyspnea on exertion (with or without chronic cough) and less than one-half normal maximum breathing capacity. Increased chest diameter and pursed-lip breathing are often seen in patients with more advanced forms of this condition. Also known as **chronic obstructive lung disease, COLD, COPD.** *See also specific condition.*

chronologic age, the age of a person stated as the amount of time that has passed since birth. For example, the age of an infant is stated in hours, days, or months, and the age of children and adults is stated in years.

chronotropic, a substance that affects heart rate. When the heart rate increases, the agent used has a positive chronotropic effect. *See also dromotropic, inotropic.*

chronotropism /krənot´rəpizm/, anything that affects the rhythm of a function of the body, such as interfering with the rate of heartbeat.

chute, **1.** a clear passage through white water. **2.** a quick descent of water over a slope. **3.** *(informal)* parachute.

Chvostek's sign /khvosh´teks/, an abnormal spasm of the face muscles when the facial nerve is lightly tapped. This spasm occurs in patients who have low blood calcium. It is a sign of tetany.

chyle /kīl/, the cloudy liquid that results from digestion in the small intestine. Consisting mainly of fats, chyle passes through tiny fingerlike bulges (lacteals) in the small intestine. It then goes into the lymph system for transport to the veins.

chylothorax /kī´lōthôr´aks/, a condition in which fluid caused by digestion in the intestine (chyle) makes its way through the thoracic duct in the chest to the space around the lungs. The cause is usually trauma or a tumor of the thoracic duct. Treatment is surgical repair of the duct.

chyluria /kīloor´ē·ə/, milky-appearing urine caused by the presence of digestive juices (chyle) from the intestine.

chyme /kīm/, the contents of the stomach during digestion of food. Chyme then passes to the small intestine (duodenum), where further digestion takes place.

chymotrypsinogen /-tripsin´əjən/, a substance that is produced in the pancreas. It is turned into the digestive enzyme chymotrypsin by trypsin.

cibophobia /sē´bō-/, an aversion to food or to eating.

cicatrix /sik´ətriks, sikā´-/, scar tissue that is pale, tight, and firm. As the skin begins to heal, it becomes red and soft.

cicutism /sik´yətizm/, poisoning caused by water hemlock. Symptoms include hypoxia, which results in cyanosis, seizures, and coma.

ciguatera poisoning /sē´gwəter´ə/, food poisoning that results from eating fish infected with the ciguatera poison. The poison comes from tiny creatures that the fish eat. Over 400 types of fish from the Caribbean and South Pacific are thought to carry this poison. Symptoms include vomiting, diarrhea, tingling or numbness, muscle weakness, and pain. Symptoms last 6 to 18 hours. Abnormal nerve sensations may last for months.

cilia /sil´e·ə/, *sing.* **cilium, 1.** the eyelashes. **2.** small, hairlike projections on the outer layer of some cells, promoting processing by creating motion in a fluid. **–ciliary,** *adj.*

ciliary body /sil´ē·er´ē/, the part of the eye that joins the iris with the blood vessel layer (choroid). Continuous with the ciliary body is the **ciliary margin,** the outer border of the iris of the eye.

ciliary gland, one of the many sweat glands found on the eyelids. These glands lie near the lashes. Bacterial infection of one or more of the ciliary glands causes sties.

ciliary muscle, a band of smooth muscle fibers of the eye. These help adjust the eye to view near objects.

ciliary reflex.   See **accommodation reflex.**

Ciliata /sil´ē·ā´tə/, a type of tiny primitive creature (protozoa) that has cilia through its whole life. The only important ciliate in humans is the intestinal parasite *Balantidium coli,* which causes dysentery.

ciliated tissue, any tissue with hairlike projections from its surface. This type of tissue is present in the fallopian tubes and respiratory tract. Also known as **ciliated epithelium.**

ciliospinal reflex /sil´ē·ōspī´nəl/, a normal reflex caused by scratching or pinching the skin of the posterior neck. This results in dilation of the pupils. Also known as **pupillary-skin reflex.**

circadian rhythm /sərkā´dē·ən, sur´kədē´ən/, the biological clock in humans based on a 24-hour cycle. At regular intervals each day, the body becomes active or tired. Body temperature is highest in the afternoon or evening. It drops to its lowest point from 2 AM to 5 AM. Heart beat, blood pressure, breathing, urine flow, hormones, and enzymes rise and fall in a rhythmic pattern. Interference with this rhythm can cause impatience, decreased mental alertness, problems with sleep, and tachycardia. Jet lag and some sleeping disorders are common causes of circadian disturbance. Some drugs affect the body more at certain times during the day than at others.

circle of Willis, a group of arteries at the base of the brain. The circle is formed by the connections between branches of the arteries that supply the brain.

circular bandage, a bandage wrapped around an injured part, usually an arm or leg.

circular fold, one of the many ring-shaped folds in the small intestine formed by mucous tissue.

circulation, 1. the movement of blood through the blood vessels by pumping action of the heart. This flow distributes nutrients and oxygen to the cells and removes carbon dioxide and wastes. **2.** any movement in a circuit that generally returns to a starting point.

circulation time, the time it takes for blood to flow from one part of the body to another. A dye or radioactive substance is injected into a vein and timed to find how long it takes to return to the same point in the body.

circulatory failure, cardiovascular system inability to provide body tissues with the necessary amount of blood for proper functioning.

circulatory system, the network consisting of the heart, blood vessels, and lymph vessels through which the blood and lymph circulate. *See also cardiovascular system, lymphatic system.*

circumcision, a surgical removal of the foreskin of the penis or, rarely, the hood of the clitoris.

circumduction, movement in a circular motion.

circumoral /sur´kəmôr´əl/, the part of the face around the mouth.

circum-speech, the behaviors that are linked to conversation. They include body language, keeping of personal space between persons, handsweeps, head nods, and activity, such as walking while carrying on a conversation.

circumstantiality, a disorder in which a person is unable to separate important from unimportant facts while describing an event. The person may include every detail, losing the train of thought. Very often the person may need to have questions repeated. It may be a sign of chronic brain dysfunction. Compare **flight of ideas.**

circus movement, the abnormal circular movement of cardiac electrical impulses via intranodal pathways, so that these impulses continually excite the sinoatrial node, atrial tissue, and atrioventricular node. The tachydysrhythmias that result may cause a drop in cardiac output, thus altering blood pressure and patient level of consciousness. Also known as **circus reentry.**

cirrhosis /sirō´-/, a chronic disease of the liver in which the liver becomes covered with fiber-like tissue. This causes the liver tissue to break down and fill with fat. All functions of the liver then decrease, such as production of glucose and vitamin absorption. Stomach and bowel function and making of hormones are also affected. Blood flow through the liver is blocked. Symptoms include nausea, anorexia, weight loss, light-colored stools, weakness, abdominal pain, and noticeable veins (often on the face). Unless the cause of the disease is removed, coma, bleeding in the stomach and bowels, and kidney failure occur. Cirrhosis is most often the result of long-term alcohol abuse. It can also result from malnutrition, hepatitis, or other infection. The liver may be able to repair itself, but recovery may be very slow. *See also biliary cirrhosis.* –**cirrhotic,** *adj.*

cisterna /sistur´nə/, *pl.* **cisternae,** a cavity that holds lymph or other body fluids. An example is a **cisterna subarachnoidea,** any one of many spaces in the brain that hold cerebrospinal fluid.

cisvestitism /sisves´titizm/, wearing clothing correct for the sex, but not the age, occupation, or status of the wearer.

citric acid, a white, crystal-like organic acid which dissolves in water and alcohol. It is taken from citrus fruits, especially lemons and limes. Citric acid is used to flavor foods, carbonated drinks, and medicinal products such as laxatives. It is also used to prevent scurvy.

civil disturbance, the loss of control and order in a civilian population, such as a riot.

civil law, a system of laws combined into a code, with decisions about law based on the principles of that code. This system is the most widely distributed of the three systems of law. The other two are the common law system and the socialist system.

clairvoyance /klervoi´əns/, the alleged ability to be aware of objects or events without the use of the physical senses such as sight or hearing.

clamp, any instrument that holds things together to compress, grasp, join, or give support, such as a hemostat.

clampstick, a tool of nonconducting material, used to safely move energized electrical wires. Also known as **hot stick, shotgun.**

clang association, the mental connection between unrelated ideas that is made because the two words sound similar. This happens often during manic depression (bipolar disorder).

clasp-knife reflex, an abnormal reflex in which a spastic arm or leg cannot be moved and then suddenly jerks, like the blade of a jackknife. It indicates damage to the brain's involuntary control system.

class A fire, fire in ordinary combustible materials, as in canvas, mattresses, paper, or wood. Extinguishing agents include carbon dioxide, dry chemical, foam, and water.

class B fire, petroleum-based fires, as in gasoline, oils, paints, or solvents. Extinguishing materials include carbon dioxide, dry chemical, and foam.

class C fire, electrical equipment fires. Methods of extinguishing include turning off power to equipment, carbon dioxide, foam, and dry chemical.

class D fire, metal fires, such as powdered aluminum, magnesium, potassium, sodium, titanium, or zinc. Use high-velocity water fog, dry sand, sodium chloride, or talc to extinguish.

classic second-degree heart block. See **Mobitz II.**

claudication, pain of the legs with cramps caused by poor circulation of blood in the legs. The condition is often linked to atherosclerosis and may include lameness or limping. **Intermittent claudication** is a form of the disorder that occurs only at certain times, often after a period of walking. It is relieved by rest.

claustrophobia /klôs´trə-/, a great fear of being trapped in closed or narrow places. This fear is seen more often in women than in men. Sometimes it can be traced to some very frightening event involving closed spaces, usually occurring in childhood.

claustrum /klôs´trəm/, *pl.* **claustra,** **1.** a barrier, such as a membrane that partly closes an opening. **2.** a thin sheet of gray matter in the brain.

clavicle /klav´ikəl/, the collarbone. It is a long, curved, horizontal bone just above the first rib, forming the front portion of the shoulder. It is shorter, thinner, and smoother in women than in men. In persons who perform regular heavy manual labor, it becomes thicker, more curved, and more ridged for muscle attachment.

clawhand, a hand seriously bent into a fixed position. Also known as **main en griffe** /menäNgrēf´/.

clearance, the removal of a substance from the blood by the kidneys. Kidney function can be tested by measuring how much of a specific substance appears in the urine in a given length of time.

clear text, the use of plain English in radio communications. No codes are used when using clear text.

cleavage, the series of repeated cell divisions of the egg (ovum) immediately after fertilization. A mass of cells is formed into an embryo capable of growth.

cleavage line, any of a number of lines in the skin that mark the basic structural pattern and tension of the skin tissue. They are present in all areas of the body but are visible only in certain sites, such as the palms of the hands and soles of the feet. In general, the lines run in the direction in which the skin is most loose.

cleft, **1.** divided. **2.** a crack, most often one that begins in the embryo.

cleft foot, an abnormal condition in which the division between the third and fourth toes extends into the foot.

cleft lip, a birth defect consisting of one or more fissures in the upper lip. This results from the failure of the maxilla and nasal area to close in the embryo.

cleft palate, a birth defect in which there is a hole in the middle of the roof of the mouth (palate). This results from the failure of the two sides to join during the development of the embryo.

cleft uvula, birth defect in which the uvula is split into two halves.

click. See **heart sound.**

cliff evolution, rescue procedure, utilizing a rope suspended from a helicopter, by which a rescuer rappels to a victim on a cliff face. The victim is placed in a stretcher or attached to the rescuer and lifted from the cliff. The rescuer and victim are flown to a safe landing site while suspended from the aircraft. *See also long line haul, short haul.*

climate, the average conditions of the weather in any place. Climate may be considered in the diagnosis and treatment of some illnesses, especially those affecting breathing –**climatic,** *adj.*

climbing nut. See **nut.**

clinic, **1.** an outpatient facility where persons not needing to stay in the hospital receive medical care. Formerly known as a dispensary. **2.** a group practice of doctors, such as the Mayo Clinic. **3.** a meeting place for doctors and medical students where lessons can be given at the bedside of a patient or in a similar place.

clinical, information or practice based on actual observation and treatment of patients.

clinical death, cessation of breathing and circulation; cardiopulmonary arrest. *See also biological death.*

clinical horizon, a point in a disease at which detectable symptoms first begin to appear.

clinical laboratory, a laboratory in which tests are done to help diagnose a patient's illness.

clinical research center, an organization that studies and describes medical cases. Such centers are often linked to a medical school or teaching hospital. Clinical research centers often offer free or low-cost care for patients taking part in research programs.

clinical specialist, a physician or other health care professional who has advanced training in a certain field of medicine. These include nurse-midwife, pediatrician, or radiologist.

clinical trials, organized studies to provide clinical data for assessment of a treatment.

clinocephaly /klī´nōsef´əlē/, a birth defect in which the upper surface of the skull dips in the middle, making it saddle-shaped.

clinodactyly /-dak´tilē/, a birth defect in which one or more fingers are bent to either side.

clitoris /klit´əris/, the female structure that corresponds to the penis. It is a pea-shaped projection made up of nerves, blood vessels, and erect tissue. It is partially hidden by the labia minora.

clo, a unit of measurement for the thermal insulation capability of clothing. It is calculated as the amount of insulation necessary to maintain comfort in a resting subject at a temperature of 70° F (21° C) and relative humidity of less than 50% in a normally ventilated room.

clone, a group of cells or organisms that have identical genes. They are a result of cell division.

clonus /klō´nəs/, abnormal activity of the nerves sending signals to the muscles. In this state the person cannot control rapid tensing and relaxing of muscles. Compare **tonus, -clonic,** *adj.*

closed injury, internal injury, sustained without obvious penetration of the body's surface.

clostridial /klostrid´ē·əl/, referring to bacteria that form spores and need no oxygen to live. They are of the genus *Clostridium*. Gangrene, botulism, and tetanus are examples of disease caused by this kind of bacteria.

closure /klō´zhər/, the surgical closing of a wound by sutures.

clotting time, the time required for blood to form a clot. It is tested by putting a small amount of blood in a glass tube. The first clot is noted and timed. It is primarily used to evaluate treatment with anticlotting drugs. Also known as **coagulation time.**

clubbing, enlargement of the distal portion of the fingers and toes. This condition is usually due to chronic or congenital cardiovascular or respiratory disease.

clubfoot, a birth deformity of the foot, sometimes resulting from crowding in the uterus. In a clubfoot the bones in the front part of the foot are misaligned. In 95% of clubfoot deformities the front half of the foot turns in and down **(equinovarus).** In the rest of the defects the front part of the foot turns out and up **(calcaneovalgus** or **calcaneovarus).**

cluster breathing, respiratory pattern of tachypnea interspersed with periods of apnea. *See also Cheyne-Stokes respirations.*

cluster headache. See **headache.**

cluttering, a speech defect in which words are rapid, confused, nervous, and uneven. Letters or syllables may be reversed or left out. The condition is often linked to other language disorders, such as problems in learning to speak, read, and spell. It also seen in some personality and behavioral problems.

coagulase /kō·ag´yəlās/, an enzyme produced by bacteria, particularly *Staphylococcus aureus*. It helps to form blood clots.

coagulation /kō·ag´yəlā´shən/, clotting; the process of turning a liquid into a solid, especially the blood. *See also blood clotting.*

coagulation factor, one of 13 elements in the blood that help to form blood clots. *See also blood clotting, factor.*

coagulopathy /-lop´əthē/, any disorder of the blood that makes it difficult for blood to coagulate.

coarctation /kō·ärktā´shən/, a narrowing or contraction of the walls of a blood vessel, as in the aorta.

coarctation of the aorta, a birth defect of the heart in which the aorta is narrowed. This results in higher blood pressure on one side of the defect and lower pressure on the other side. In its most common form it causes high blood pressure in the arms and head and low blood pressure in the legs. Symptoms include dizziness, headaches, epistaxis, and muscle cramps in the legs during exercise.

coarse, gross movement, generally absent fine movement, as in coarse fibrillation.

coastal flooding, the flooding of low-lying coastal areas due to earthquake **(tsunami),** hurricane, or other tropical storm.

coat, **1.** a membrane that covers the outside of an organ or part. **2.** one of the layers of a wall of an organ or part, especially a canal or a vessel.

cobalt, a metallic element that is found in certain minerals. Cobalt is a part of vitamin B_{12}, and is found in most foods. It is easily absorbed by the stomach and intestines. The amount the body needs is not known. A radioactive form, **cobalt 60,** is the source often used in treatment for cancer.

coca, a species of South American shrub that is native to Bolivia and Peru. It is also grown in Indonesia. It is a natural source of cocaine.

cocarcinogen /kō´kärsin´əjən/, a substance that becomes cancerous only when combined with another substance.

coccidioidomycosis /koksid´ē·oi´dōmīkō´-/, an infectious disease caused by breathing in spores of the fungus *Coccidioides immitis*. These spores are carried on dust particles in the wind. The disease occurs in hot, dry regions of the southwest United States. Early symptoms resemble the common cold or influenza. Later symptoms include low fever, weight loss, breathing difficulty, and pain in the bones and joints. Also known as **valley fever.**

coccidiosis /kok´sidē·ō´-/, a parasitic disease found in tropical and subtropical regions. It is caused by swallowing eggs of a tiny organism (*Isospora belli* or *I. hominis*). Symptoms include fever, malaise, abdominal pain, and diarrhea. The infection usually lasts 1 to 2 weeks.

coccus /kok´əs/, *pl.* **cocci** /kok´sī/, a bacterium that is round, spherical, or oval. **–coccal,** *adj.*

coccygeus /koksij´ē·əs/, one of the muscles in the floor of the pelvis, which stretches across the pelvic cavity like a hammock.

coccygodynia /kok´sigōdin´ē·ə/, a pain in the coccygeal area of the body.

coccyx /kok´siks/. See **vertebra.**

cochlea /kok´lē·ə/, a small bone of the inner ear that is the organ of hearing. It is coiled 2½ times into the shape of a snail shell. This bone has many small holes through which passes the acoustic nerve. The cochlea connects with the organs of the acoustic nerve. **–cochlear** /kok´lē·ər/, *adj.*

code, **1.** a system of signals used for passing on information, such as genetic code or Morse code. **2.** (*informal*) cardiac arrest.

code of ethics, written and unwritten rules and moral principles on which the behavior of an individual or group is based.

coelenterates /səlen´tərāts´/, a group of marine invertebrates, comprising approximately 9000 species, including anemones, jellyfish, and soft corals. These organisms are divided into the cnidaria (those with venom-charged stinging cells) and acnidaria (without stinging cells). The cnidaria are dangerous to humans and are divided into three main groups: anthozoans (anemones, corals), hydrozoans (Portugese man-of-war), and scyphozoans (true jellyfish).

coenzyme /kō·en´zīm/, a substance that combines with other substances to form a complex enzyme. Coenzymes include some vitamins, such as B_1 and B_2.

coffee-ground emesis, dark brown vomitus, with a composition like that of coffee grounds. This symptom of bleeding in the upper gastrointestinal tract is caused by the breakdown of blood by the gastric secretions. *See also hematemesis.*

cofferdam, **1.** a watertight structure, placed next to a ship, from which repairs below the ship's waterline are made. **2.** a temporary structure, enclosing a portion of a body of water, from which the water is pumped, to enable construction on the bottom.

coffin, a container, used to transport radioactive materials, that is resistant to penetration by radiation.

cognition, the mental process of knowing, thinking, learning, and judging.

cognitive development, the process by which an infant gains knowledge and the ability to think, learn, and reason.

cognitive dissonance, a state of mental stress. This comes from learning new information that conflicts with old ideas or knowledge.

cogwheel rigidity, an abnormal stiffness in muscle tissue. There are jerky movements when the muscle is made to stretch.

coherence, **1.** the property of sticking together, such as the molecules of a substance. **2.** the logical pattern of speech and thought of a normal, stable person.

cohesive, firmly holding together.

cohort, a group of people born in the same year.

coign of vantage /koin/, the better, usually higher, position for observation or action. Also known as **high ground.**

coining, an Asian folk medicine practice of rubbing an affected body part with a heated coin, as a means of drawing out illness. The practice may leave the area with burns, contusions, or welts.

coitus /kō´itəs/, the sexual union of two people of opposite sex. Also known as **sexual intercourse. –coital,** *adj.*

cold, **1.** the absence of heat. **2.** a contagious viral infection **(common cold)** of the upper respiratory tract.

cold-blooded, referring to animals not able to control body heat, such as fishes, reptiles, and amphibians. Compare **warm-blooded.**

cold damp, gas that is primarily carbon dioxide and unable to support respirations, such as might be found in an underground mine. The gas is usually formed as a result of a natural process and not combustion or explosion. *See also damp.*

cold injury, any of several abnormal conditions caused by exposure to cold temperatures. *See also chilblain, frostbite, hypothermia, immersion foot.*

cold sore. See **herpes simplex.**

cold urticaria, local or generalized wheals sustained after continuous cold exposure or rewarming of areas previously exposed to cold. In addition to wheals, local symptoms may include edema and pruritus. Systemic manifestations may cause dyspnea, fatigue, headache, and tachycardia.

cold zone, safe haven for those agencies directly involved in a hazardous materials operation. Includes the incident commander, command post, representatives from appropriate agencies, and usually the media.

colectomy /kəlek´-/, surgical removal of part or all of the large intestine (colon).

colic /kol´ik/, sharp pain resulting from twisting, blockage, or muscle spasm of a hollow or tubelike organ. These can include a ureter or the intestines. A **baby's colic** is a painful condition common in infants under the age of three months. Causes include swallowed air and allergy to the baby's formula.

coliform /kol´ifôrm/, referring to the bacteria that live in the intestines of humans and other animals.

colitis /kōlī´-/, a general term for inflammation of the large intestine. This can refer to the disorder called **irritable bowel syndrome.** It can also mean one of the inflammatory bowel diseases **(Crohn's disease, ulcerative colitis).** *See also Crohn's disease, irritable bowel syndrome, ulcerative colitis.* **–colitic,** *adj.*

collagen /kol´əjən/, protein consisting of bundle fibers. Collagen forms connective tissue. These include the white inelastic fibers of the tendons, the ligaments, the bones, and the cartilage. **–collagenous,** /kəlaj´ənəs/, *adj.*

collagen disease, any one of many disorders marked by inflammation and breakdown of fiber in connective tissue. Some collagen diseases are rheumatic fever, arteritis, and ankylosing spondylitis.

collagenoblast /kəlaj´ənōblast´/, a cell that forms collagen. It can also change into cartilage and bone tissue.

collagenous fiber /kəlaj´ənəs/, the tough, white fibers that make up much of the connective tissue of the body. These fibers contain collagen. They are often arranged in bundles that strengthen the tissues in which they are found.

collagen vascular disease, any of a group of disorders in which inflammation occurs in small blood vessels and connective tissue. The cause of most of these diseases is unknown. Heredity, deficiencies, environment, infections, and allergies may be involved. Common complications of most of these diseases include arthritis, skin sores, eye inflammations, pleuritis, myocarditis, and nephritis. Diseases included in this category are rheumatic fever, rheumatoid arthritis, scleroderma, and systemic lupus erythematosus.

collapse, **1.** *(informal)* a state of extreme depression or of total exhaustion caused by physical or emotional distress. **2.** an abnormal condition marked by shock. **3.** the abnormal sagging of an organ. **4.** The falling of any structure.

collar, **1.** a structure used to hold something in place or to limit motion. **2.** *(informal)* cervical or extrication collar.

collarbone. See **clavicle.**

collar drag. See **drag.**

collateral, **1.** secondary or accessory. **2.** a small branch, such as any one of the arterioles in the body.

collateral circulation, accessory circulation from a branch of a major blood vessel. Regular exercise causes the body to expand small blood vessels to accommodate the increased oxygenation necessary during exertional states. This allows the body to compensate for diminished blood flow in the major vessels, as seen in atherosclerosis.

collective, one of the major helicopter control devices, consisting of a combination hand throttle, which is used to vary engine speed, and control lever, which varies the angle of the main rotor and determines amount of aircraft vertical movement. *See also cyclic, foot pedals.*

Colles' fascia /kol´ēz/, a strong, smooth sheet of tissue with stretchy fibers that fills a groove between the scrotum and the thigh in a man or between the labia and the thigh in a woman.

Colles' fracture, a fracture of the radius. It occurs 1 inch above the wrist and creates a hand position bent posteriolaterally.

Collin's hitch. See **ankle hitch.**

colliquation /kol´ikwā´shən/, the breakdown of a tissue of the body into liquid. It is normally linked to dead tissue.

colloid, large molecules, such as protein or starch, that, when mixed in a solvent, do not dissolve.

colloid osmotic pressure, the pressure generated by the presence of colloids in interstitial spaces and the vascular system. Also known as **oncotic pressure.**

colon /kō´lən/, the part of the large intestine that extends to the rectum. The **ascending colon** extends upward from the first part of the colon (cecum) in the lower right side of the stomach to where the colon turns. The **transverse colon** goes from the end of the ascending colon at the liver on the right side across the middle intestinal area to the beginning of the **descending colon** at the spleen on the left side. From there the colon descends to the **sigmoid colon,** which extends to the beginning of the rectum. The colon takes the contents of the small intestine, moving them to the rectum by contracting. Water is added to the foodstuff by the stomach and small intestine during digestion. The colon absorbs most of this water through the walls. This firms the feces as they move into the rectum.

colonic fistula /kōlon´ik/, an abnormal passage from the colon to the surface of the body or to another organ or structure. Chronic inflammation of the intestines may cause a fistula between two loops of bowel. An opening from the colon to the surface of the skin may be made

surgically after part of the bowel is removed. *See also colostomy.*

colony, **1.** a mass of microorganisms that grows from a single cell. This mass is grown in a special substance called a culture. **2.** a mass of cells in a culture.

Colorado tick fever, a virus infection that is carried to humans by the bite of a tick. It is most common in the spring and summer months throughout the Rocky Mountains, especially in Colorado. Symptoms occur in two phases between which there are no symptoms. They include chills, fever, headache, pain in the eyes, legs, and back, and sensitivity to light. Compare **Rocky Mountain spotted fever.**

color blindness, the inability to distinguish color. In most cases it is a weakness in discerning colors distinctly.

colorimetry /kol´ərim´ətrē/, **1.** measurement of the intensity of color in a fluid or substance. **2.** measurement of color in the blood to determine the content of hemoglobin.

color index, the ratio between the amount of hemoglobin and the number of red blood cells in a sample of blood.

color vision, the perception of color. Color is seen as the cones in the retina react to changing intensities of red, green, and blue light. *See also color blindness.*

colostomy /kəlos´-/, an opening made by surgery for feces to pass through the abdominal wall.

colostrum /kəlos´trəm/, the fluid released by the breast during pregnancy before lactation begins. Colostrum is a thin, yellow fluid that contains white blood cells, water, protein, fat, and carbohydrate.

colpotomy /kolpot´-/, any surgical incision into the wall of the vagina.

coma, *(informal)* a nonspecific description of an altered level of consciousness where the patient is not awake and cannot be aroused by external stimuli.

combat austerity, the concept and practice of functioning in life-endangering situations with less than optimal equipment and space. As related to military and special operations, necessity prohibits the availability of equipment that would otherwise be utilized. In these situations, equipment for control of airway, hemorrhage, fluid replacement, and splinting take priority over cardiac monitors, drugs, and sophisticated immobilization devices. The degree of austerity practiced is dependent on skill level, location and transportation, number of patients anticipated, operational situation, and threat level. *See also special operations.*

combat fatigue.   See **stress reaction.**

come-along,   a pulling tool utilizing chain, cable, or nylon strapping/rope to lift or pull a moveable object toward a stationary one. Having many applications, this winch is commonly used during vehicular extrication and vertical rescue. Also known as **hand winch, rope puller.**

command,   the act of directing, ordering, and/or controlling resources by virtue of explicit legal, agency, or delegated authority.

command post,   a fixed area from which incident operations are directed.

command staff,   those individuals assigned to assist the incident commander and his or her section officers by gathering and managing information and coordinating communications. They may be fire fighters, EMTs, line officers, or any other knowledgeable individuals on scene.

comminuted fracture,   disruption of a bone into several segments.

commissurotomy /kom´ishoŏrot´-/,   surgically dividing a fiberlike band or ring connecting parts of a body structure. This is often done to separate the thickened flaps of a narrowed mitral valve in the heart.

commitment,   **1.** the placement of a patient in a hospital or other facility designed to deal with the patient's special needs. **2.** the legal act of admitting a mentally ill patient to an institution for psychiatric treatment. The process usually involves court action. This act is based on medical evidence that the person is mentally ill.

common bile duct,   the duct formed by the joining of the cystic duct and hepatic duct.

common carotid artery.   See **carotid artery.**

common cold.   See **cold.**

common hepatic artery,   an artery that branches off the aorta as it goes through the area of the stomach. Its five branches supply blood to the stomach, small intestines, and liver.

common iliac artery,   a division of the abdominal aorta that divides into external and internal iliac arteries. These supply blood to the pelvis and legs.

common law,   a body of legal principles derived from case decisions of the past, but applied to current law in an attempt to fairly judge similar situations.

communicable disease,   any disease carried from one person or animal to another by direct or indirect contact. Direct contact includes touching any discharge from the body, such as saliva. Indirect contact might include contact through something else, such as drinking glasses, toys, water, or insects. To control a communicable disease, it is important to identify the organism causing the disease and prevent its spread. Many communicable diseases, by law, must be reported to the local health department. Also known as **contagious disease.**

communication,   the transmission and reception of information, resulting in mutual understanding. This may be done directly or indirectly, nonverbally or verbally, electronically or visually.

communications center,   a facility that coordinates communication between field units, fixed locations, and personnel.

community medicine,   a branch of medicine concerned with the health of the members of a community or region.

compact soil,   soil that can be indented by a thumb but penetrated only with great difficulty; hard and stable in appearance.

company,   any piece of equipment having a full complement of personnel.

compartment syndrome,   obstruction of extremity blood flow, following an injury (crush, fracture) to a closed muscular compartment. This state of muscular and neurovascular compromise is a surgical emergency.

compatibility,   **1.** the orderly, efficient mixing of elements from one system with those of another. **2.** the ability of several drugs to work together without harming the patient. **3.** the degree to which the body's defense system will accept foreign matter, such as blood or organs. Usually, perfect compatibility exists only between identical twins.

compensated shock,　early hypoperfusion, during which time the body is attempting to maintain homeostasis by shunting blood from the periphery to the brain, heart, and lungs. Symptoms include anxiety, mildly elevated pulse, normal blood pressure, and normal or borderline capillary refill.

compensation,　**1.** correction of a defect or loss of the body by the increased output of another part. **2.** the process of keeping enough blood flow in spite of heart or circulatory problems. **3.** a complex defense mechanism to avoid a feeling of inferiority.

compensation neurosis,　an unconscious process by which one retains the symptoms of an injury or disease. This is usually done to receive other secondary gain. Compare **malingering.**

competence,　**1.** sufficient ability. **2.** legal capacity.

competitive antagonist,　substance with a preference for the same receptor site as an agonist. The antagonistic agent occupies the receptor site without stimulating it, thereby inhibiting the action of the agonist.

complaint,　any illness, problem, or symptom identified by the patient. A **chief complaint** is a statement made by a patient describing his or her most important symptoms of illness or dysfunction. It is often the reason that the person seeks health care.

complement,　complex proteins in the blood that bind with substances that defend the body (antibodies) against foreign invaders (antigens). Complement is involved in reactions such as severe allergic reaction (anaphylaxis). A deficiency or defect of any of the parts of a complement can occur. Patients with complement abnormalities are more likely to get infections and collagen vascular diseases. It is difficult to diagnose.

complete blood count.　See **blood count.**

complete heart block.　See **third-degree heart block.**

complex,　**1.** a group of chemical molecules that are related in structure or function. **2.** a combination of symptoms of disease that forms a syn-

drome. **3.** a group of linked ideas with strong emotional overtones. These ideas affect a patient's attitudes.

compliance,　a measure of the amount of resistance and pressure required to change lung volume.

component therapy,　transfusion in which only certain components of blood are given. In this way it is possible to transfer more of the blood component than would be found in whole blood.

compound,　**1.** a substance composed of two or more elements. **2.** any substance made up of two or more ingredients. **3.** to make a substance by combining ingredients, such as a drug. **4.** referring to an injury marked by several factors.

Comprehensive Emergency Management,　a U.S. federal management system for planning and coordinating multiagency responses to an emergency. Also known as **CEM.**

Comprehensive Environment Response, Compensation, and Liability,　U.S. legislation which addresses hazardous substance releases into the environment and the clean-up of inactive hazardous waste disposal sites. It requires that those individuals responsible for the release of hazardous materials above certain levels (reportable quantities) notify the National Response Center. Also known as **CERCL superfund.**

compress,　a soft pad used to apply pressure over a wound to help stop bleeding. Compare **dressing.**

compression,　the act of applying pressure to an area of the body. A tumor or bleeding may cause compression of brain tissue, for example.

compression fracture,　disruption of bone that occurs when a compressing force causes the bone to collapse into itself. Most frequently seen with injuries of the spinal column. Also known as **burst fracture.**

compromised host,　a patient who is not able to resist infection. This may be due to defective immune system or severe anemia. A severe disease or condition, as cancer or general poor health may also be involved.

compulsion,　an irresistible impulse to perform an act. The impulse is usually the result of an obsession. *See also obsession.* **–compulsive,** *adj.*

compulsive personality disorder, a condition in which a compulsive need interferes with everyday work and normal behavior. The disorder features excessive devotion to order, rules, and detail and clinging to a system of behavior. The person cannot make decisions when faced with unexpected situations.

compulsive ritual, a series of acts a person feels must be carried out. This is done even though the behavior is known to be useless and inappropriate. Failure to complete the acts results in extreme anxiety. *See also obsessive-compulsive neurosis.*

computer-aided dispatch, a computerized communications enhancement, which provides communications personnel with information that is used in the selection and routing of resources. Also known as **CAD.**

computerized tomography, a method for examining structures inside the body. It produces picture that shows relationships of structures in thin slices, which provide a 3D view. The examination is painless and requires no special preparation. Tumors, blood clots, bone displacement, and fluid can be detected. Also known as **CAT, computerized axial tomography, CT.**

conation, the mental process marked by desire, impulse, voluntary action, and striving. Compare **cognition, conative,** *adj.*

concave, having a depressed or hollow surface.

concealment, camouflage that provides hiding but cannot provide protection from projectiles. *See also cover.*

concentration gradient, the difference in concentration of molecules in a solution as related to areas of higher and lower concentration. The molecules tend to move toward an area of lower concentration in an attempt to equilibrate the solution.

concept, an abstract idea or thought that begins and is held in the mind. **–conceptual,** *adj.*

conception, **1.** the beginning of pregnancy. This usually taken to be the instant that a sperm enters an egg (ovum). **2.** the act or process of fertilization. **3.** the process of creating an idea. **4.** the idea created.

conceptional age, the number of weeks since conception of an embryo. Because the exact time of conception is difficult to know, concep-tional age is said to be two weeks less than the pregnancy (gestational) age.

concussion, a transient period of altered level of consciousness, which is usually followed by a complete return of function.

condition, **1.** a state of being. It refers to physical and mental health or well-being. **2.** to train the body or mind, through certain exercises and repeated exposure to an object state.

conditioned reflex. See **reflex action.**

conditioned response, an automatic reaction to a stimulus that has been learned through training. Such responses can be physical or psychological, conscious or unconscious. They are caused by exposure to the stimulus or event. This is done over and over until the response is automatic. Compare **unconditioned response.**

conditioning, a form of learning in which a response to a stimulus is developed. **Avoidance conditioning** establishes certain patterns of behavior to avoid unpleasant or painful stimulation. With **classical conditioning,** an object or event that used to hold no special meaning now causes a predictable response. **Operant conditioning** refers to a way of learning used to change the way a person thinks or does things. The person is rewarded for the right response and punished for the wrong response.

conduction, moving electrons, heat, or sound waves through a conductor or conducting medium.

conductivity, the ability of a substance to conduct electrons, heat, or sound.

condyle, a rounded bone projection that usually interfaces with another bone.

condyloid joint, a joint in which a condyle fits into an oval cavity, such as the wrist joint. *See also joint.*

cone, a cell that receives light in the retina of the eye and causes a person to see colors. There are three kinds of retinal cones, one for each of the colors blue, green, and red. Other colors are seen by combining these three colors. *See also rod.*

cone shell, tropical, cone-shaped mollusks with a highly developed venom apparatus, which cause infrequent fatalities in humans. Of approximately 300 species (class Gastropoda), about 20 have been identified as dangerous to humans, living primarily in shallow waters of the Indo-Pacific regions.

confabulation, the invention of events, often told in a detailed and convincing way. This is done in order to fill in and cover gaps in the memory. It occurs mainly as a way of defense. It is quite common in alcoholics and persons with head injuries or lead poisoning. Also known as **fabrication.**

confidentiality, the presumption that information given to an individual will not be revealed without the explicit consent of the confiding party.

confined area, any space that lacks ventilation.

confinement, 1. the state of being restricted to a specific area, in order to obstruct or reduce activity. **2.** a search technique that attempts to establish a search perimeter, beyond which the subject of the search is unlikely to pass without being detected. Methods that can be used include lookouts, physical barriers (string lines), roadblocks, and track traps. *See also attraction.*

conflict, a painful mental state caused by opposing thoughts, ideas, goals, or desires. This state is worsened by not being able to resolve the conflicts. This kind of stress is found to some degree in every person.

confluence, 1. the flowing together of two or more roads or streams. **2.** the place where roads or streams come together.

confusion, a mental state in which a patient is unsure of time, place, or person. This causes a lack of orderly thought. The person is also not able to make decisions. It often indicates an organic mental disorder. It may, however, appear with severe emotional stress. **—confusional,** *adj.*

congener /kon´jənər/, one of two or more things that are similar in structure, function, or origin, such as muscles that function the same way, or drugs that are similar in effect.

congenital /kənjen´ətəl/, present at birth, such as a congenital defect.

congenital pulmonary arteriovenous fistula, a congenital fistula between the arteries and veins of the lung, that permits deoxygenated blood to enter the circulation.

congestion, abnormal collection of fluid in an organ or body area. The fluid is often blood, but it may be bile or mucus.

congestive heart failure. See **heart failure.**

conjugate gaze, the ability of the eyes to move and focus together. *See also disconjugate gaze.*

conjunctiva /kon´jungktī´və/, two membranes in the eye. The **palpebral conjunctiva** lines the inner surface of the eyelids. The **bulbar conjunctiva** covers the front part of the sclera. It is thin and transparent.

conjunctival reflex, closure of the eyes in response to irritation of the conjunctiva. This response may be diminished during seizures, unconsciousness, or when wearing contact lenses. *See also corneal reflex.*

conjunctivitis /kənjungk´tivī´tis/, inflammation of the lining (conjunctiva) of the eye and eyelids, caused by infection, allergy, or other factors. Symptoms include itching and discharge.

connecting fibrocartilage, a disk of fiberlike cartilage between many joints. It is common between joints with little movement, as the spinal vertebrae. Each disk is made of rings of fiberlike tissue separated by cartilage. The disk swells outward if it is pressed by the vertebrae on either side. *See also intervertebral disk.*

consanguinity /kon´sang·gwin´itē/, a hereditary or "blood" relationship between persons. These persons share a common parent or ancestor.

conscience, the moral sense of what is right and wrong. This includes the ability to judge one's own actions.

conscious, awake.

consensus formula, a formula for calculating the fluid needs of a burn patient, which is 2 to 4 milliliters per kilogram of patient weight for each percent of body surface area burned (2-4 ml × kg × %BSA burned = ml). One-half of the resulting amount is given in the first 8 hours after the burn, and the remainder is given over the following 16 hours. This calculation is the result of combining the modified Brooke and Parkland burn formulas. *See also Brooke formula, Parkland formula, Shrine Burn formula.*

consent, 1. the giving of permission by a patient or guardian that allows care to be administered. **2.** that permission necessary to care for a patient. The two general types of consent are implied (or presumed) and informed (or expressed). Implied consent occurs when a patient requires care and is unable to give consent, as during an emergency, or replies nonverbally, as by holding out their arm. Informed consent presumes that the patient is able to make a decision and is informed of the risks and the benefits of their decision prior to giving consent.

conservation of energy law, energy can be neither created nor destroyed; it can only be changed from one form to another, such as chemical, electrical, mechanical, thermal.

consolidation, 1. combining of separate parts into a single whole. **2.** the process of solidification, as is seen in pneumonia when the lungs become stiff due to fluid engorgement and do not stretch normally.

constipation, difficulty in passing feces. Stomach and bowel pain, loss of appetite, back pain, and headache may occur.

constitutional law, the derivation of power based on enabling constitutions. Federal and state governments represent the rights transferred from individual citizens to the government, but are also limited by the power granted by constitution.

constriction, the binding or contraction of a part.

contact, 1. the merging or touching of two surfaces. **2.** the transfer of an infectious organism from one source to another. **3.** the source of infection.

contact dermatitis, skin rash resulting from exposure to either an irritating or allergic substance. An irritant causes a sore much like a burn. With an allergic substance, the reaction is delayed. Symptoms include inflammation and large amounts of fluid in the body tissues. Poison ivy is a common example of this type. *See also dermatitis.*

contact lens, a small, curved plastic lens shaped to fit the eye and used to correct poor vision. Contact lenses float on the film of tears over the cornea. They must be handled with great care to avoid damage to the eyes. Various types of contact lenses include hard lenses, soft lenses, extended-wear lenses, and tinted lenses.

contagious, communicable, as a disease that is carried by direct or indirect contact. **–contagion,** *n.*

contagious disease. See **communicable disease.**

container, the portion of a shipping package that physically houses the radioactive material.

contamination, deposition of material in any place where it is not desired, particularly where its presence may be harmful.

continuing education, formal adult education after the completion of training.

continuous positive airway pressure, maintaining spontaneous ventilation airway pressures above atmospheric at the end of exhalation. This creates a positive airway pressure throughout the ventilatory cycle and serves to increase the amount of air left in the lungs at the end of expiration (functional residual capacity) in patients who have conditions preventing adequate levels of tissue oxygenation. The technique is only indicated when a patient is able to maintain an adequate tidal volume spontaneously. Also known as **CPAP.** Compare **positive end-expiratory pressure.**

continuous tone-controlled subaudible squelch, a radio filter that screens out extraneous noise in order to improve the quality of reception. Only radios with the same tone-control frequency setting will normally receive these transmissions. If the operator needs to monitor the entire frequency or if a transmitting radio tone is unknown, this filter can be disabled. Also known as **Channel Guard, CTCSS, Private Line.**

contraception, a technique for preventing pregnancy. This may be done with a drug, device, or by blocking a process of reproduction. Also known as **birth control, conception control, family planning.**

contractility, ability of the cardiac muscle to contract in response to electrical stimulation. *See also automaticity, excitability.*

contraction, a shortening or tightening, particularly when referring to muscle fibers.

contracture, a condition of joint rigidity in a contracted position. This is usually a permanent condition. Contractures are caused by shortening and wasting away of muscle fibers or by loss of the normal stretchiness of the skin. Extensive scar tissue over a joint can cause contracture.

contraindication, a medical or physiologic circumstance that makes it harmful to administer a medication or treatment that is otherwise therapeutic.

contralateral, affecting the opposite side of the body.

contrastimulant, any factor that delays or prevents stimulation.

contrecoup /kän´trəko͞o´, kōN´trəko͞o´/, an injury that occurs at a site opposite the side of impact, as that seen in head injuries after trauma.

controlled area, an area in which entry and activities are controlled to ensure radiation protection and prevent the spread of contamination.

contusion, a tissue injury with diffuse bleeding into subcutaneous tissue, causing discoloration under unbroken skin. Also known as **bruise.**

convalescence, the period of recovery after an illness, injury, or surgery.

convalescent home. See **extended care facility.**

convection, the transfer of heat through a liquid or gas.

convergence, the act or state of two or more things having a direction toward the same point in space; coming together.

conversion, 1. changing from one form to another. 2. correcting the position of a fetus during labor.

conversion reaction, a kind of hysterical neurosis. Emotional conflicts are repressed and changed into symptoms of illness without physical cause. Common symptoms are blindness, involuntary muscle movements, as tics or tremors, paralysis, loss of voice, and breathing difficulties. The person who has conversion reaction believes the physical condition exists.

convex, an evenly curved surface or one bulging outward.

convulsion. See **seizure.**

Cooley's anemia. See **thalassemia.**

cooling, reducing temperature.

coordination, the process of systematically analyzing a situation, developing relevant information, and informing appropriate authority of viable alternatives for the most effective combination of available resources to meet specific objectives.

cooperating agency, an agency supplying assistance other than direct suppression, rescue, support, or service functions to the incident control effort (e.g., Red Cross, law enforcement agency, telephone company).

coping, a process by which a person deals with stress, solves problems, and makes decisions. The stress can be either physical or mental. Coping is done through the use of both conscious and unconscious tools.

copper, a metallic element essential to good health. Copper deficiency in the body is rare. Little is needed daily, and it is easily obtained from a number of foods. Increased copper in the body can result from some diseases.

coprolalia /kop´rəlā´lyə/, the excessive use of obscene words.

cor, 1. the heart. 2. relating to the heart.

coracoid process /kôr´əkoid/, the thick, curved part of the upper edge of the scapula. The pectoralis minor muscle stretches between this process and the ribs.

coral, 1. a marine organism of the class Anthozoa; polyps grow in large colonies. Contact with their hard, rough skeletons can result in injury. A few types secrete poison. *See also coelenterates.* 2. the hard substance secreted by these creatures as protection and support. When the animal dies, this substance remains and, over time, builds into the structures known as **coral reefs.**

cord, any long, rounded, flexible structure. The body contains many cords, as the vocal, spinal, nerve, and umbilical cords.

corditis, inflammation of the spermatic cord. Also known as **funiculitis.**

cordonazo. See **tropical cyclone.**

core temperature, body temperature within the central structure of the body. This temperature is maintained at a constant level with little variation under normal circumstances. Normal core body temperature is approximately 99.2° F (37.1° C).

Cori's disease. See **glycogen storage disease.**

corium /kôr´ē·əm/, the layer of skin, just below the outer layer (epidermis). It contains blood and lymph vessels, nerves and nerve endings, glands, and hair follicles.

corn, a cone-shaped mass of thickened skin on the toes.

cornea /kôr´nē·ə/, the transparent front of the eye. It is dense and even in thickness. It projects like a dome beyond the sclera. The amount of curve varies in different persons. It can also change since the cornea tends to flatten with age.

corneal grafting /kôr´nē·əl/, transplanting corneal tissue from one human eye to another. It is done to improve vision in persons with scars or warps of the cornea or when an ulcer in the cornea is removed. *See also transplant.*

corneal reflex, 1. contraction of the eyelids when the cornea is touched. *See also conjunctival reflex.* **2.** the reflection of light from the corneal surface.

corniche /kōrnēsh´/, accumulated snow on the leeward side of a ridge crest. The snow accumulation can collapse due to the weight of a climber, causing the climber to fall or an avalanche to occur.

cornification, thickening of the skin by a build-up of dead cells.

corona /kərō´nə/, **1.** a crown. **2.** a crownlike bulge, such as a place on a bone that protrudes.

coronal plane, a lengthwise plane running from side to side; it divides the body into anterior and posterior portions.

coronal suture, suture between the bones of the skull that crosses the top of the skull from temple to temple.

coronary /kôr´əner´ē/, **1.** referring to circling structures, such as the coronary arteries; referring to the heart. **2.** *(informal)* myocardial infarction.

coronary arteriovenous fistula, a congenital defect with a passageway between a coronary artery and the right heart or the vena cava.

coronary artery, one of a pair of arteries that branch from the ascending aorta. The **right coronary artery** passes along the right side of the heart and divides into branches that supply both ventricles and the right atrium. The **left coronary artery** supplies both ventricles and the left atrium of the heart.

coronary artery disease, any abnormal condition that may affect the arteries of the heart. This refers especially to those that reduce the flow of oxygen and nutrients to the heart muscle. The most common kind of coronary artery disease is coronary atherosclerosis. This is a form of arteriosclerosis in which cholesterol is deposited in the artery walls. The disease affects more men than women. It also occurs more often in whites and the middle-aged or elderly. The disease occurs most often in people with regular diets high in calories, fat (especially saturated fat), cholesterol, and refined carbohydrates. Cigarette smokers are two to six times more likely to develop this disease than nonsmokers. High blood pressure is also a common related cause in atherosclerosis. Other risk factors include heavy alcohol use, obesity, lack of exercise, shortage of vitamins C and E, living in large urban areas, heredity, climate, and viruses. Angina pectoris is the classic symptom of coronary artery disease. *See also angina pectoris, myocardial infarction.*

coronary autoregulation, the widening of an artery of the heart. This happens in response to lack of oxygen to the heart muscle.

coronary bypass, a surgical shunt that allows blood to travel from a major artery to a coronary artery around an obstruction. Also known as **CABG.**

coronary occlusion, blockage of a coronary artery. Also known as **coronary thrombosis.**

coronary sinus, a cavity, which opens into the right atrium, that drains blood from the coronary veins.

coronary thrombosis. See **thrombosis.**

coronary vein, one of the veins of the heart. It takes blood from the capillaries of the heart to the right atrium.

coronaviruses, a group of viruses that cause most common colds.

coroner /kôr´ənər/, a public authority who investigates into the causes and events of a death, especially one resulting from unnatural causes. Also known as **medical examiner.**

corpsman /kōr´mən/, an enlisted military medical practitioner (U.S. Navy), often assigned as the only medical caregiver in a field unit or on a small ship.

cor pulmonale /kôr pŏŏl´mənā´lē/, an increase in size of the right ventricle, resulting from pulmonary hyertension. Long-term cor pulmonale enlarges the right ventricle because it cannot adjust to a rise in pressure as easily as the left ventricle. In some patients, however, the disease also increases the size of the left ventricle. Some diseases linked to cor pulmonale are cystic fibrosis, myasthenia gravis heart disease, and pulmonary arteritis. Chronic obstructive pulmonary disease and emphysema are others. Cor pulmonale accounts for about 25% of all types of heart failure. The disease affects middle-aged and elderly men more than women. It may occur in children. Some of the early signs of cor pulmonale include constant cough, difficulty breathing, fatigue, and weakness. As the disease progresses, breathing difficulty becomes severe.

corpus cavernosum, a type of spongy tissue in the penis or clitoris. The tissue becomes filled with blood during sexual excitement.

corpuscle /kôr´pəsəl/, **1.** any cell of the body. **2.** a red or white blood cell.

corpus luteum, yellow tissue that forms in the ovary. It occurs in the wall of the ovary where an ovum has just been released. Its purpose is to release hormones to help prepare the body for pregnancy. If the egg is impregnated, it grows larger and lasts for several months. If the egg is not impregnated, it shrinks and is shed during menstruation.

corrosive, 1. chemical destruction of a substance or tissue. **2.** a substance that corrodes a substance or tissue. **–corrode,** v., **corrosion,** n.

corrugator supercilii, one of the three muscles of the eyelid. It draws the eyebrow downward and inward, as in a frown.

cortex /kôr´teks/, pl. **cortices** /kôr´tisēz/, the ocouter layer of an organ or other structure.

corticosteroid /kôr´tikōstir´oid/, any one of the hormones made in the adrenal cortex. They influence or control key functions of the body, as by making carbohydrates and proteins. The release of these hormones increases during stress, especially in anxiety and injury. Too much of these hormones in the body is linked with various disorders, as Cushing's syndrome.

corticotropin. See **adrenocorticotropic hormone.**

cortisol /kôr´-/, a steroid hormone produced in the body. Also known as **hydrocortisone.**

cortisone /kôr´-/, a steroid hormone produced in the liver.

Corti's organ, a small, spiral structure inside the cochlea in the inner ear. It contains hair cells that touch the acoustic nerve, sending sound waves to the brain.

Corynebacterium /kôr´inē-/, a group of rod-shaped organisms. The most common disease-causing types are *Corynebacterium acnes,* found in acne, and *C. diptheriae,* the cause of diphtheria.

coseismal, points of simultaneous shock from the pressure wave of an earthquake.

costal, 1. referring to a rib. **2.** located near a rib or on a side close to a rib.

costochondral /kos´təkon´drəl/, a rib and its cartilage.

costovertebral, a rib and the spinal column.

cot, 1. a small, narrow bed, particularly a gurney. **2.** a cover or sheath, such as a finger cot.

cough, a sudden, forceful release of air from the lungs, which clears the lungs and throat of irritants and fluid. It is a common symptom of diseases of the chest and throat. Tuberculosis, lung cancer, and bronchitis can cause chronic coughing. Congestive heart failure and valve disease may be linked with severe coughing. A **productive cough** usually forces sputum from the respiratory tract, clearing the air passages and allowing oxygen to reach the alveoli. Coughing is precipitated by irritation of the respiratory tract.

coulee, 1. a solidified, steep lava flow that is formed in a cooling lava dome volcano. **2.** a steep ravine.

couloir /ko͞olwär´/, a steep gulley on a mountainside.

countershock, electrical stimulation of the heart to effect a change in rhythm.

countertraction, a force that pulls against traction, such as the force of body weight.

coup /ko͞o/, a sudden blow or stroke. **Coup de sabre** is a wound similar to a laceration made by a sword. **Coup de soleil** is sunstroke (heat stroke). **Contrecoup** is an injury to the opposite side from which a blow is struck, as in contrecoup damage in a head injury.

Courvoisier's law /ko͞orvō·äzē·āz´/, the rule that the gallbladder is smaller than usual if a gallstone blocks the common bile duct. However, the gallbladder is enlarged if the common bile duct is blocked by something else, as in cancer of the pancreas.

Cousteau-Gagnon process (Jacques-Yves Cousteau, French naval officer; Emile Gagnon, French engineer), the demand valve apparatus for scuba, developed in 1943. Also known as **Cousteau-Gagnon patent.**

Couvelaire uterus /ko͞ovəler´/, a bleeding condition of the uterus. It may occur after abruptio placenta. *See also abruptio placenta.*

cover, an object that will conceal a person from danger and stop a projectile. *See also concealment.*

cowling, removeable covering around an aircraft engine.

Cowper's gland /kou´pərz/, either of two pea-sized glands found near the urethral sphincter of the male. They consist of several lobes with ducts that join and form a single duct.

cowpox, a mild infectious disease marked by a rash with pus-filled blisters. It is a viral disease of cattle that may be transmitted to humans by direct contact. It may also be administered by deliberate injection as cowpox infection usually makes a person immune to smallpox. Also known as **vaccinia.** *See also smallpox.*

coxa magna, widening of the head and neck of the femur.

coxa valga, a hip defect in which the femur angles out to the side of the body.

coxa vara, a hip defect in which the femur angles toward the center of the body. Also known as **coxa adducta, coxa flexa.**

coxsackievirus /koksak´ē-/, any of 30 different viruses that infect the intestines (enterovirus). These cause a number of symptoms and affect primarily children during warm weather. These infections are linked to many diseases. *See also viral infection.*

C-post, the third roof support post from the front of a motor vehicle. This is the thickest and most rearward post on a sedan. It is the third of four supports on a station wagon.

crab louse, a type of body louse. It infests the hairs of the genital area and is often transmitted between persons by sexual contact. Also known as *Pediculus pubis (informal)* **crab.** *See also pediculosis.*

crackles. See **breath sounds.**

cramp, **1.** a spastic and often painful contraction of one or more muscles. **2.** a pain similar to a muscle cramp, such as a **charley horse, heat cramp, writer's cramp.**

CRAMS, acronym for **C**irculation, **R**espiration, **A**bdomen/chest, **M**otor and **S**peech. This trauma assessment tool gives a score from 0 to 2 in each assessed category, with the highest total score as 10. A score of 7 or less indicates a major trauma patient.

cranial, relating to the cranium.

cranial nerves /krā´nē·əl/, the 12 pairs of nerves emerging from the cranial cavity through openings in the skull. They are referred to by Roman numerals and named as follows: (I) olfactory, sense of smell; (II) optic, sight; (III) oculomotor, eye muscles; (IV) trochlear, eye muscles; (V) trigeminal, jaws, chewing; (VI) abducens, eye muscles; (VII) facial, taste; (VIII) acoustic, hearing; (IX) glossopharyngeal, throat, swallowing; (X) vagal, heart, lungs, digestion; (XI) accessory, upper spine; (XII) hypoglossal, tongue, speaking. See Appendix 1-2.

craniopharyngeal /-fərin´jē·əl/, the skull and the throat.

craniotomy /krā´nē·ot´-/, any surgical opening into the skull. It may be done to relieve pressure, control bleeding, or to remove a tumor.

cranium /krā´nē·əm/, the bony skull that holds the brain. It is made up of eight bones: frontal, occipital, sphenoid and ethmoid bones, and paired temporal and parietal bones. –**cranial,** *adj.*

cravat, triangular bandage folded to form a narrow band. Generally used as a bandage, limb restraint, and traction accessory.

creatine /krē´ətēn/, an important nitrogen compound produced in the body. It combines with phosphorus to form high-energy phosphate.

creatinine /krē·at´inēn/, a substance formed from the making of creatine. It is common in blood, urine, and muscle tissue.

creeping eruption, a skin disorder with irregular, wandering red lines. These are made by burrowing larvae of hookworms and some roundworms that invade the skin when people walk barefoot where these parasites exist. Also known as **larva migrans.**

crepitus, **1.** a grating sensation, that may be palpated, in conditions involving fractures or pathological bone changes. **2.** a crackling sensation noted in the presence of subcutaneous air (subcutaneous emphysema), caused by pneumothorax. **3.** a crackling sound in the lungs, auscultated in the presence of fluid in the small airways (crackles).

cresol /krē´sol/, a liquid obtained from coal tar. It is used as an antiseptic and disinfectant and is poisonous.

cretinism /krē´tənizm/, a condition marked by severe lack of thyroid function during infancy. Signs include dwarfism, mental deficiency, and lack of muscle coordination.

crevasse, **1.** a deep crevice, especially in a glacier. **2.** a breach in a river bank.

crib, technique of supporting an unstable object for the purposes of allowing extrication of victims with relative safety. *See also cribbing.*

cribbing, wedges, usually made of wood, used to shore up a vehicle or part of a structure that must be jacked or lifted. These wedges prevent the item being lifted from falling, if the equipment being used in the lifting process were to fail or slip.

crib death. See **sudden infant death syndrome.**

cricoid /krī´koid/, **1.** having a ring shape. **2.** a ringshaped cartilage in the larynx. It moves as the pitch of the voice changes.

cricopharyngeal /krī´kōfərin´jē·əl/, the cricoid cartilage and the pharynx.

cricothyrotomy, an incision into the larynx to create an airway in cases of complete upper-airway obstruction.

crisis, **1.** a turning point for better or worse. **2.** events that strongly affect the emotional state of a person, such as death or divorce.

crisis intervention, problem-solving used to correct or prevent a crisis.

crisis theory, a way of defining and explaining the events that occur when a person faces a problem that appears to have no solution.

crista supraventricularis /kris´təsoo´prəventrik´yələr´is/, the muscle ridge on the inside wall of the right ventricle of the heart.

critical care. See **intensive care.**

critical constant, the critical temperature, pressure, or density of a substance.

critical density, density of a substance in its critical state.

critical incident stress, a stress reaction often experienced after a stressful emergency response.

critical incident stress debriefing, review of a stressful event to allow a discussion of emotions and feelings. Also known as **CISD.**

critical mass, **1.** the point of accumulation of any substance at which that substance can become explosive. **2.** the point in an accumulation of plutonium at which a nuclear weapon could be exploded.

critical organs, tissues that are the most reactive to radiation, as the sex glands, lymph organs, and intestine. The skin, cornea and lens of the eye, mouth, esophagus, vagina, and cervix are the next most reactive organs to radiation.

critical pressure, vapor pressure of a liquid at its critical temperature.

critical state, condition of a substance when its liquid and vapor phases have the same density.

critical temperature, the temperature beyond which a gas cannot be liquefied by the application of pressure alone.

Crohn's disease, a long-term bowel disease with inflammation. The cause is unknown. It most often affects the ileum or colon.

crossed reflex, any nerve reflex in which stimulating one side of the body causes a response on the other side.

cross-eye. See **strabismus.**

crossmatching of blood, a means used by blood banks to determine whether donated blood can be used by a particular patient. This is done after the samples have been matched for major blood type, as A, B, AB, and O. Serum from the donor's blood is mixed with red cells from the patient's blood, and cells from the donor are mixed with serum from the patient. If agglutination occurs, a foreign substance is present and the blood is not usable. *See also blood group, blood typing.*

croup /kroop/, a viral infection of the respiratory tract that occurs primarily in infants and young children. Croup occurs after another upper breathing tract infection. Symptoms include hoarseness, fever, a distinct "barking" cough, and breathing distress from bronchospasm and edema. Infection is carried by airborne particles or by contact with infected fluids. The acute stage starts rapidly, most often occurs at night and may be triggered by exposure to cold air.

crowing, high-pitched respiratory sound indicative of respiratory distress; a type of stridor. This sound usually presents in cases of partial upper-airway obstruction due to foreign bodies or epiglottitis. It is indicative of serious airflow obstruction and is easily audible without a stethoscope.

crown,   1. the upper part of an organ or structure, as the top of the head. **2.** the upper part of a human tooth that is covered by enamel.

crowning, the phase at the end of labor in which the baby's head is seen at the opening of the vagina. The labia are stretched around the head during crowning just before birth. *See also labor.*

cruciate ligament of the atlas /kroo´shē·āt/, a crosslike ligament that attaches the atlas to the base of the skull superiorly and connecting to the axis inferiorly.

cruise speed, the optimum speed at which an aircraft flies while in forward flight.

crush injury, trauma from exposure of tissue to a force of compression that interferes with the normal structure and function of the involved tissue.

crush syndrome, a life-threatening complication of prolonged compression or immobilization that causes alteration or destruction of muscle tissue. *See also rhabdomyolysis.*

crust, a solid, hard outer layer formed by the drying of body fluids; a scab. Crusts are common in skin conditions, such as eczema, impetigo, seborrhea, and during the healing of burns and sores.

Crutchfield tongs, a device put into the skull to hold the head and neck straight. The device is used in patients with cervical spine fractures.

cry,   1. a sudden, loud, willful, or automatic sound in response to pain, fear, or a startle reflex. **2.** weeping, because of pain or as a response to depression or grief.

cryocautery /-kô´tərē/, applying any substance, such as solid carbon dioxide, that destroys tissue by freezing. Also known as **cold cautery.**

cryogen /krī´əjən/, a chemical that causes freezing, such as carbon dioxide. It may be used to destroy diseased tissue without injury to nearby structures. **–cryogenic,** *adj.*

cryonics /krī·on´-/, the ways in which cold is applied for many treatments, as brief local anesthesia.

crypt, a blind pit or tube on a surface, as any of the small pits in the iris of the eye along its out-

side margin, known as **crypt of Fuchs.** *See also anal crypt.*

cryptitis /kriptī´-/, inflammation of a crypt, most often an anal crypt. Symptoms include pain, itching, and spasm of the sphincter.

cryptococcosis /krip´təkokō´-/, an infection caused by a fungus, *Cryptococcus neoformans.* It spreads through the lungs to the brain, skin, bones, and urinary tract. In North America it is most likely to affect middle-aged men in the southeastern states. Symptoms include respiratory difficulty, headache, blurred sight, and difficulty in speaking.

crystal, a solid substance with the atoms or molecules in a regular, repeating three-dimension pattern. The exact pattern marks the shape of the crystal. **–crystalline,** *adj.*

crystalline lens /kris´təlin, -līn/, a clear structure of the eye located between the iris and the vitreous humor. The lens is a biconvex structure with the back surface more convex than the front. It is attached to the ciliary body and retina by ligaments that adjust the shape of the lens. This allows the lens to keep an object focused on the retina. For distant sight the lens thins, and for near sight it thickens. *See also eye.*

crystalloid, a soluble substance, dissolved in a liquid, that can be diffused through a semipermeable membrane, such as lactated Ringer's solution.

CS gas, tear gas, consisting primarily of the compound orthochlorobenzilidine malanonitrile. This lacrimator is considerably more potent and causes more severe respiratory symptoms than CN (chloracetophenone) gas.

cuboid bone, the tarsal bone on the outside of the foot next to the calcaneus.

cul-de-sac,   1. a blind pouch. **2.** a dead-end street.

Culicidae, scientific classification for the mosquito family, of the order Diptera. This family includes the subfamilies Anophelinae and Culicinae.

Cullen's sign, ecchymosis around the umbilicus after trauma. This is an indication of intraabdominal or retroperitoneal hemorrhage that has usually occurred at least 12 hours previously.

culture-bound, referring to a health belief that is specific to a culture, as belief in certain kinds of prayer.

culture shock, the mental effect of a drastic culture change in the life of a person. There may be feelings of helplessness, discomfort, and confusion when trying to adapt to a different culture with unfamiliar practices, values, and beliefs.

cumulative, increasing by steps with an eventual total that may go past the expected result.

cumulative action, **1.** the increased action of a treatment or drug when given repeatedly, as the cumulative action of a regular exercise program. **2.** the increased effect of a drug when repeated doses build up in the body.

cumulative dose, the total dose that builds up from repeated exposure to radiation or a radioactive drug.

cuneiform /kyo͞one͞´əfôrm/, (of bone and cartilage) wedge-shaped.

CUPS system, a system of triage that assigns patients to one of the following four categories: **C**PR or **C**ritical, **U**nstable, **P**otentially Unstable, or **S**table.

cure, **1.** restoring the health of a patient with a disease or other disorder. **2.** the favorable result of treating a disease or other disorder. **3.** a course of treatment, a drug, or other method used to treat a medical problem.

curettage /kyo͞or´ətäzh´/, scraping material from the wall of a body cavity or other surface, done to remove abnormal tissue, or obtain tissue samples.

curie, the quantity of any radioactive nuclide such that 37 billion (3.7×10^{10}) disintegrations occur per second.

current, **1.** a mass of air or fluid moving in a certain direction. **2.** a flow of electrons along a conductor in a closed circuit; an electric current. Flow in one direction creates direct current, whereas flow in both directions in an alternating pattern creates alternating current.

current differential, difference in current flow within the same body of water, as where two currents flow near each other.

Cushing's disease (Harvey Cushing, American surgeon, 1869-1939), a disorder resulting from the excessive release of adrenocorticotropic hormone by the pituitary gland. The cause is often a tumor on the pituitary gland. Symptoms include fat pads on the chest, back, and face; high blood sugar; round "moon" face; muscle weak-

ness; purplish streaks on the skin; fragile bones; acne; and heavy growth of hair on the face. Also known as **hyperadrenalism.** Compare **Cushing's syndrome.**

Cushing's phenomenon, a compensatory rise in systemic blood pressure when intracranial pressure acutely increases, generally above 50% of the systolic pressure. Also known as **Cushing's effect, Cushing's response.**

Cushing's syndrome (Harvey Cushing, American surgeon, 1869-1939), a disorder resulting from excess adrenocorticotropic hormone made by the pituitary gland. It occurs when large doses of steroid drugs are given over a period of several weeks or longer. Symptoms include elevated blood sugar, overweight, a round "moon" face, muscle wasting, low potassium levels, and emotional change. The skin may be highly colored and fragile; minor infections may become severe and long-lasting. Children with the disorder may stop growing. Lowering or changing the drug may relieve the symptoms. Also known as **hyperadrenocorticism.** Compare **Cushing's disease.**

Cushing's triad, decreased pulse and respiratory rate, increased systolic blood pressure, and widened pulse pressure due to increased intracranial pressure.

cusp, **1.** a sharp or rounded projection that rises from the chewing surface of a tooth. **2.** any one of the small flaps on the valves of the heart.

custodial care, nonmedical care given on a long-term basis, most often for invalids and patients with long-term diseases.

cutaneous /kyo͞otā´nē·əs/, referring to the skin.

cutaneous horn, a hard, flesh-colored bulge of the skin, most often on the head or face. It may be a forerunner of cancer and is usually removed.

cutaneous papilloma. See **skin tag.**

cutdown, surgical access of a vein for purposes of intravenous cannulation. The skin is incised with a scalpel and the vein exposed and clamped. A catheter is inserted through the vein wall and sutured in place. Used in patients with small or constricted veins, as in hypovolemic shock, this technique allows placement of large-bore catheters for blood and/or fluid resuscitation. Also known as **venous cutdown.**

cuticle /kyo͞oˊtikəl/, **1.** skin. **2.** the sheath of a hair follicle. **3.** the thin edge of thick skin at the base of a nail.

cut sheet, the daily plan for a job foreman, which shows depth and grades for pipe to be laid at a building drainage site.

cutter. See **hydraulic-powered rescue tool.**

cutting sign, *(informal)* the act of animal or human tracking.

cutting torch, a gas (usually acetylene) cutting and welding tool, using an intense flame to perform the work required. It was a common rescue tool in the 1950s and 60s for removing victims from wreckage. The serious hazards that accompanied its use meant its fall into disfavor with the advent of hydraulic-powered rescue tools. Also known as **acetylene torch, welding torch.**

cyanide poisoning /sīˊənīd/, poisoning from swallowing or breathing in cyanide. It may be in substances such as bitter almond oil, wild cherry syrup, prussic acid, hydrocyanic acid, or potassium or sodium cyanide. Symptoms include tachycardia, seizures, and headache. Cyanide poisoning can result in death within 1 to 15 minutes.

cyanosis, a bluish-gray discoloration of the skin or mucous membranes due to deoxygenated hemoglobin.

cyclic, 1. occurring in cycles. **2.** a device that tilts the blades of the helicopter main rotor, causing backward, forward, and lateral movement of the aircraft. Usually located on the floor between the pilot's legs, it is one of three controls used to maintain the helicopter in flight. *See also collective.*

cyclone. See **tropical cyclone.**

cycloplegic /sīˊkləpleˊjik/, **1.** a drug or treatment that causes paralysis of the ciliary muscles. **2.** one of a group of drugs used to paralyze the ciliary muscles of the eye.

cyst, a closed sac in or under the skin lined with skin tissue and containing fluid or semisolid material, such as a **sebaceous cyst.**

cystic, pertaining to a cyst, the gallbladder, or the urinary bladder.

cystectomy /sistekˊtəmē/, surgical removal of all or a part of the bladder.

cysteine /sisˊtēn/, an amino acid found in many proteins in the body, including keratin. It is an important source of sulfur for the body.

cysticercosis /sisˊtisərkōˊ-/, an infection by the larval stage of the pork tapeworm (*Taenia solium*) or the beef tapeworm (*T. saginata*). See also *tapeworm infection.*

cystic fibroma, a fiberlike tumor in which cystic breakdown has occurred.

cystic fibrosis, an inherited disorder of the exocrine glands. It causes the glands to secrete very thick mucus. The glands most affected are those in the pancreas, lungs, and sweat glands. Cystic fibrosis is often diagnosed in infancy or early childhood. It occurs principally in whites. The earliest symptom is often a blockage of the small bowel. Other early signs are a long-term cough, and constant lung infections. There is no known cure.

cystine /sisˊtin/, an amino acid found in many proteins in the body, including keratin and insulin.

cystinosis /-ōˊsis/, a congenital disease with amino acid (cystine) deposits in the liver, spleen, bone marrow, and cornea. Symptoms include rickets and slowed growth. Also known as **cystine storage disease.**

cystinuria /-o͞orˊēˑə/, **1.** high amounts of the amino acid cystine in the urine. **2.** an inherited defect of the kidney filtering tubes, marked by excess urinary release of cystine and many other amino acids. In high amounts, cystine forms kidney or bladder stones.

cystitis /sistīˊ-/, an inflammation of the urinary bladder and ureters. Symptoms include bloody urine, pain, and the need to urinate often. It may be caused by a bacterial infection, stone, or tumor.

cystocele /sisˊtəsēl/, sagging of the urinary bladder through the wall of the vagina. A large cystocele may cause voiding difficulty or incontinence, urinary tract infection, and painful sexual union. Compare **rectocele.**

cystogram /-gramˊ/, x-ray films of the bladder and ureters.

cystoscopy /sistosˊkəpē/, the examination of the urinary tract with a cystoscope placed in the urethra. In addition, cystoscopy is used for obtaining samples of growths and for removing polyps.

cytochrome oxidase, an enzyme that transfers cytochrome electrons to oxygen, which allows oxygen to unite with hydrogen and form water.

cytocide /sī´təsīd/,   any substance that destroys cells. **–cytocidal,** *adj.*

cytoctony /sītok´tənē/,   destroying of cells, as in killing cells in culture by viruses.

cytogene /sī´təjēn/,   a particle in the cytoplasm of a cell that reproduces itself and can carry inherited data. **–cytogenic,** *adj.*

cytogenesis /sī´təjen´əsis/,   the beginning, growth, and division of cells. **–cytogenetic, cytogenic,** *adj.*

cytogenetics /-jənet´-/,   the branch of genetics that studies the cell parts that concern heredity, mainly the chromosomes.

cytogenic gland /-jen´ik/,   a gland that releases living cells, such as the testicles and ovaries.

cytology /sītol´-/,   the study of cells, their growth, structure, action, and diseases.

cytolysis /sītol´isis/,   the destruction of a living cell, primarily by breaking down the outer membrane.

cytomegalovirus /-meg´əlō-/,   a member of a group of large herpes-type viruses that can cause serious illness in newborns and in patients being treated with drugs that slow down the immune system, as after an organ transplant.

cytometry /sītom´ətrē/,   counting and measuring cells, such as blood cells. **–cytometric,** *adj.*

cytomorphosis /-môrfō´-/,   the many changes that occur in a cell during the course of its life cycle, from the first stage until death.

cyton /cī´tən/,   the cell body of a nerve, or the part of a nerve with the nucleus and its surrounding cytoplasm. Also known as **cytone** /sī´tōn/.

cytophoresis /-fôr´əsis/,   a process of removing red or white blood cells or platelets from patients with certain blood disorders.

cytoplasm.   See **cell.**

cytosine /si´təsin/,   a substance that is an important part of DNA and RNA. It occurs in small amounts in most cells.

cytotoxin,   a substance that has a harmful effect on some cells. Antibody may act as a cytotoxin. **–cytotoxic,** *adj.*

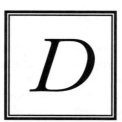

dacryocyst /dak´rē·əsist´/, a tear sac at the inner corner of the eye.

dacryocystitis /dak´rē·ōsistī´-/, an infection of the tear sac. It is caused by blockage of the duct that drains into the nose (nasolacrimal duct). Symptoms include tearing and discharge from the eye.

dactyl /dak´təl/, a digit (finger or toe).

Dalton's law (John Dalton, English scientist, 1766-1844), the total pressure exerted by a gas mixture is the sum of the individual pressures that create the given volume or gas mixture. Also known as **Dalton's law of partial pressures.**

damp, 1. moist. **2.** a noxious gas found in caves or underground mines. *See also afterdamp, black damp, cold damp, fire damp, stink damp, white damp.*

dander, dry scales shed from the skin or hair of animals or the feathers of birds. Dander may cause an allergic reaction in some persons.

dandruff, scaly material shed from the scalp. It is composed of dead skin. *See also seborrheic dermatitis.*

dark adaption, the process of vision adjustment that allows the eyes to develop dark, or night, vision. The modification of day into night vision requires approximately 30 minutes. In this time, the rods of the eye become 100,000 times more sensitive than they are in sunlight, while the cones develop 100 times increased sensitivity. Once adapted, the eyes must remain in low light conditions to retain their sensitivity. Ten seconds of other than dark or red light will negate night vision until adaption can again occur. *See also cone, rod.*

day blindness, an abnormal visual condition (hemeralopia) in which bright light causes blurring of vision. It may be a side effect of certain drugs used to prevent seizures.

DDT (dichlorodiphenyltrichloroethane), an effective insecticide that has fallen into disuse due to its environmental toxicity. Because of slow biological degradation, this chemical can build up to levels toxic to animals for which it was not intended. Now known as **chlorophenothane.**

deadman. See **snow anchor.**

dead reckoning, estimating position without astronomical sightings or other technological assistance. On land, this may depend on knowing the terrain or gathering clues as to location from the surrounding area. At sea, times and speed can give information about location or direction. *See also deduced reckoning.*

dead space, 1. that part of the airway from which no gas exchange with the body occurs. Included are all of the upper airway and all of the lower airway except the alveoli. **2.** area within maximum range of an observer or weapon, that cannot be covered by observation or fire due to intervening obstacles, terrain, or weapons limitations. **3.** area within range of a radio transmitter in which a signal is not reliably received. Also known as dead zone.

deaf-mute, a person who is unable to hear or speak.

deafness, a condition of partial or complete loss of hearing.

death, permanent cessation of all vital functions. *See also biological death, brain death, clinical death.*

death rate, the number of deaths per 1000 people in a given population over a particular time.

death rattle, *(informal)* the respiratory sounds heard in the later stages of pulmonary edema. The viscous, rattling sound is characteristic of air moving through fluid and is easily heard from the patient's mouth. Also known as **coarse, audible rhonchi.** *See also breath sounds.*

debility, feebleness, weakness, or loss of strength. *See also asthenia.*

debride /dibrēd´/, to remove dirt and damaged tissue from a wound or a burn. This prevents infection and aids healing. **—debridement,** *n.*

decalcification, loss of calcium salts from the teeth and bones, caused by malnutrition, malabsorption, or other factors. It may result, especially in older people, from a diet that lacks enough calcium.

decalescence, the decrease in temperature that marks a sudden increase in heat absorption by metals, when they are heated through critical temperatures.

decay, radioactive, the decrease in activity of any radioactive material with the passage of time as a result of the spontaneous disintegration of the material.

deceleration, to slow, or diminish, speed.

decerebrate, extension and rigidity of the arms and legs, with the palms of the hands rotated posteriorly. Unconscious patients who present with this posturing have a lesion below the upper brainstem and have a grave prognosis. Also known as **decerebrate posturing, decerebrating.** *See also decorticate.*

decibel, a unit of measure of the intensity of sound. A decibel is one tenth of a bel; an increase of 1 bel is approximately double the loudness of a sound. Also known as **db.**

Declaration of Geneva, an oath administered by some medical schools at graduation. This declaration is a statement of commitment to uphold certain standards in medicine. It was adopted in 1948 by the Second General Assembly of the World Medical Association. *See also Hippocratic Oath, Prayer of Maimonides.*

decoder, device that receives and recognizes unique codes or sounds transmitted electronically.

decompensation, the failure of a system, as cardiac decompensation in heart failure.

decomposition, the breakdown of a substance into simpler chemical forms.

decompression chamber, pressure container used to evaluate conditions of flight (and their effect on materials and test subjects) on exposure to pressures less than those experienced at sea level. *See also recompression chamber.*

decompression meter, a device carried or worn by a diver that electronically computes decompression status by integrating altitude, depth, temperature, and time with recognized decompression tables.

decompression sickness, syndrome occurring in the human body when nitrogen bubbles are formed in the bloodstream after rapid ascent from depth. Prolonged diving time at depths below 30 feet causes saturation of the blood with nitrogen. If appropriate periods of time are not spent at different levels of ascent, this nitrogen comes out of solution in the blood, forming bubbles, which cause blockage of various blood vessels. Symptoms include mild to severe joint pain (limb-bends), skin mottling and itching (cutaneous decompression sickness, or skin-bends), cyanosis, dyspnea, and substernal chest pain (pulmonary decompression sickness, or chokes). Nitrogen bubble formation in the spinal cord generally causes low back pain, followed by varying degrees of weakness and sensory and motor loss in the lower extremities (neurologic decompression sickness). Also known as **bends, caisson disease, compressed air illness, DCS, diver's paralysis.** *See also gas embolism.*

decongestant, a drug, substance, or procedure that reduces congestion or swelling, especially of the nasal passages.

decontamination, the process of making personnel, equipment, and supplies safe by the elimination of harmful substances.

decorticate, flexion of the arms and extension of the legs caused by a lesion at or above the upper brainstem. This type of posturing occurs in the unconscious patient as a result of head injury or tumor. Also known as **decorticate posturing, decorticating.** *See also decerebrate.*

decubitus, **1.** a patient's position in bed, as defined by a descriptor, such as left lateral decubitus. **2.** a bedsore. Also known as **pressure sore.** *See also ulcer.*

dedicated line, **1.** telephone circuit that is connected to specific points requiring frequent telephone communications. This line allows communication by simply lifting the handset from the receiver. **2.** a telephone with a specified purpose, such as at a paramedic base station or poison control. Also known as **direct line, hot line, straight line.**

deduced reckoning, estimating position without using electronic or manual direction-finding devices. On land, this may involve using a map, surrounding landforms, and/or time, to make a determination. At sea, aircraft or ship log information, estimated drift rate and time, and direction or position can be used. *See also dead reckoning.*

deep palmar arch, the end of the radial artery in the lower arm. It joins the end of the ulnar artery, which also travels down the lower arm, in the palm of the hand.

deep vein, one of the many veins that accompany the arteries. The vein and artery are usually wrapped together in a sheath. Compare **superficial vein.**

deep well system, pipe casings driven into the ground in areas of high groundwater content. Pumps are then used to continuously remove water from the area, so that a trench can be safely excavated. *See also dewatering.*

defecation, evacuation of feces from the bowel; a bowel movement.

defense mechanism, an unconscious reaction that offers protection from a stressful situation. Examples include conversion, denial, and dissociation. Also known as **ego defense mechanism.**

deferent duct /def´ərənt/. See **vas deferens.**

defibrillation, sudden electrical and/or pharmacological depolarization of fibrillating cardiac cells in cases of ventricular tachycardia without pulses or ventricular fibrillation. This uniform repolarization resets the cardiac electrical system, so that viable cardiac electrical activity is allowed to resume. Also known as **defib, unsynchronized cardioversion.** *See also cardioversion.*

deficiency disease, disease resulting from the lack of one or more essential nutrients in the diet. It can be caused by failure of the body to absorb the nutrients from food or digestive problems. Compare **malnutrition.**

deflagration, a thermal reaction that moves from burning gases to unburned material by conduction, convection, and radiation. The combustion rate is less than the speed of sound.

deformity, something distorted or flawed. A deformity may affect the body in general or just part of it. It may be the result of disease, injury, or birth defect.

degenerative disease /dijen´ərətiv/, any disease in which there is decay of structure or function of tissue. Some kinds of degenerative disease are **arteriosclerosis, osteoarthritis.**

degenerative joint disease. See **osteoarthritis.**

degeneration, the gradual decay of normal cells and body functions.

degloving, traumatic removal of extremity skin and muscle from bone, usually involving the hand or fingers.

degradation, physical destruction or deterioration of equipment or material due to ambient conditions, chemical exposure, or use.

degree of solubility, an indication of the solubility of the material—negligible, less than 0.1%; slight, 0.1% to 1%; moderate, 1% to 10%; appreciable, greater than 10%; complete, soluble at all proportions.

dehiscence /dihis´əns/, the separation of an incision or the opening of a closed wound.

dehydrated alcohol, a clear, colorless liquid containing at least 99.5% ethyl alcohol. Also known as **absolute alcohol.**

dehydration, **1.** the significant loss of water from the body tissues. Dehydration may occur after fever, diarrhea, vomiting, or any condition where there is rapid loss of body fluids. It is of particular concern in infants, young children, and the elderly. **2.** completely removing water from a substance.

déjà vu /dāzhävY´, -vē, -voo´/, the feeling that one has lived an event or been in a place before. It is normal in everyone, but occurs more often in some emotional and physical disorders. Déjà vu results from an unconscious connection with the present experience.

DeLee suction, neonatal and infant suction device, utilizing mouth suction or other external vacuum sources. This device allows manual regulation of suction to protect delicate oral and nasal tissue in newborns, though oral application of suction is not recommended by the Centers for Disease Control and Prevention. Also known as **DeLee trap suction.**

delegation of authority, the extension of authority for particular functions from the designated source to others. While authority may be delegated, responsibility for outcome usually remains with the original source, as with a physician for the paramedics who operate as his extension.

delirium tremens, a potentially life-threatening reaction to sudden withdrawal of alcohol in the alcoholic. The reaction may follow an alcoholic binge (during which no food was eaten). It can also be triggered by head injury, infection, or withdrawal of alcohol after extended drinking. Symptoms include tachycardia, excitement, confusion, hallucinations, tremors, fever, and chest pain. The episode may last from 3 to 6 days. Also known as **DT's.**

delivery, the birth of a child.

delivery room, a unit of a hospital for childbirth.

delta, land at the mouth of a river, usually composed of sand, silt, and pebbles.

delta cell, a structural component of the islets of Langerhans; delta cells secrete somatostatin.

delta wave, a slurred or widened upstroke at the beginning of the cardiac QRS complex, which causes prolongation of the complex. It indicates anomalous impulse conduction and is diagnostic of Wolff-Parkinson-White syndrome.

deltoid muscle, a large, thick muscle that covers the shoulder joint. It bends, extends, rotates, and moves the arm away from the body. The deltoid attaches to the clavicle, several points of the scapula, and the humerus.

delusion, a belief or perception held to be true even though it is illogical and wrong. Kinds of delusion include the **delusion of being controlled,** the false belief that one's feelings, thoughts, and acts are controlled by something else; the **delusion of grandeur,** a wild exaggeration of one's own importance, wealth, power, or talents; and the **delusion of persecution,** an extreme belief that one is being mistreated and harassed by unknown enemies. Delusions are seen in various forms of schizophrenia. Compare **illusion.**

demand valve, *(informal)* a manually controlled oxygen delivery device for use in patients with apnea, ineffective ventilations, or a need for high oxygen concentrations. A universal fitting (15/22 mm) allows use with a face mask, esophageal airways, or endotracheal tubes.

dementia, a deteriorated mental state that is incurable and, generally, terminal, such as alcoholic dementia, epileptic dementia, senile dementia, toxic dementia.

demineralization, a decrease in the amount of minerals or salts in tissues.

denatured alcohol, ethyl alcohol made unfit for drinking by adding poisonous chemicals.

dendrite /den´drīt/, a structure that extends from the neuron. It receives signals that are sent on to the cell body. Compare **axon.**

dengue fever /deng´gē, den´gā/, a viral infection transmitted to humans by mosquito. It occurs in tropical and subtropical regions. Symptoms include fever, a bright-red rash, and severe head, back, and muscle pain.

denial, **1.** refusal of something requested or needed. **2.** an unconscious defense mechanism in which thoughts and feelings that cause emotional conflict are avoided. It often involves failure to admit what is true or real.

dens, *pl.* **dentes** /den´tēz/, a tooth or toothlike structure. *See also dentition, tooth.*

density, the relative weight of a substance when compared with another substance of equal bulk. When the substance that is used for comparison is an equal volume of water, its density is known as **specific gravity.**

dental arch, the curve formed by the grouping of a normal set of teeth.

dentate fracture, any break that causes jagged bone ends that fit together like the teeth of gears.

dentin /den´tin/, the chief material of teeth. It surrounds the inner part of the tooth (pulp) and is covered by the enamel. It is harder and denser than bone.

dentistry, practice of preventing and treating diseases and disorders of the teeth and gums.

dentofacial anomaly /-fā´shəl/, a defect of the mouth structure in form, function, or position.

dentogingival junction /-jinjī´vəl/, the place of joining between the surface of the teeth and the gum.

denture /den´chər/, an artificial tooth or a set of teeth that are not permanently fastened in the mouth.

deoxyribonucleic acid, a large nucleic acid molecule, found mainly in the chromosomes of the nucleus of a cell. It is the carrier of genetic information. Also known as **desoxyribonucleic acid, DNA.** *See also nucleic acid, ribonucleic acid.*

dependence, the state of being addicted.

dependent, relying on someone or something for help, support, or other needs.

dependent lividity, the pooling of blood in areas of the body lower than the heart, commonly seen after a prolonged period of cardiac arrest. The skin develops darkened areas similar to ecchymosis. This is considered a sign of obvious death.

dependent personality, behavior in which there is an extreme need for attention, acceptance, and approval from other people.

depersonalization disorder, an emotional disorder in which there is a loss of the feeling of personal identity (depersonalization). Everything becomes dreamlike. The body may not feel like one's own, and important events may be watched with detachment. It is common in some forms of schizophrenia and in severe depression.

depot, **1.** any area of the body in which drugs or other substances, as fat, are stored as needed. **2.** a drug that is injected in the body and absorbed over a period of time into the blood. **3.** any storage area.

depressant, a drug that decreases the activity or function of a body or system.

depressed fracture, any fracture of the skull in which pieces of bone are below the surface of the skull.

depression, **1.** a depressed area or hollow; downward movement. **2.** a decrease of body activity. **3.** an emotional state in which there are extreme feelings of sadness, dejection, lack of growth, and emptiness. *See also bipolar disorder.* –**depressive,** *adj.*

depressor, any drug that reduces activity when applied to nerves and muscles. *See also depressant.*

depressor septi, one of the three muscles of the nose. It serves to narrow the nostril.

deprivation, the state of being denied economic, emotional, or nutritional support or the use of the senses.

depth hoar, snow that has been exposed to varying temperatures and pressures, causing a melting and reformation of snow crystals so that they become large, coarse, and well developed. These new crystals play a large part, due to limited cohesive properties, in avalanche formation. The temperature gradient necessary for crystal reformation is equal to or greater than 10° C per meter. Also known as **sugar snow.**

depth perception. See **perception.**

derivative, anything that is obtained from another substance, as penicillin is derived from a fungus.

dermatitis /dur´mətī´-/, an inflammation of the skin, marked by redness, pain, or itching. The condition may be chronic or sudden.

dermatofibroma /dur´mətō·fībrō´mə/, a papule on the skin. It is painless, round, firm, and gray or red. It is most commonly found on the arms and legs.

dermatology /dur´mətol´-/, the study of the skin. This includes the diagnosis and treatment of skin disorders by a **dermatologist,** a doctor specializing in the skin.

Dermatophagoides farinae /-fəgoi´dēz/, a common household dust mite. It causes allergic reactions in sensitive persons. The mites thrive on skin, hair, pet foods, carpets, and bedding, as well as house dust.

dermatophytid /-fī´tid, dur´mətof´itid/, an allergic skin reaction, marked by small blisters and linked to fungal infections.

dermatosis /dur´mətō´-/, any disorder of the skin that does not cause inflammation, as **dermatosis papulosa nigra,** a common skin condition with many noncancerous, dark papules on the cheeks. Compare **dermatitis.**

dermis, the layer of skin below the epidermis, comprised of dense, irregular, connective tissue; the layer of living skin tissue where blood vessels and nerves are found. Also known as **corium, true skin.** *See also epidermis.*

dermoid cyst, a tumor with a fiberlike wall. It is filled with fatty material and cartilage. More than 10% of all tumors on the ovary are dermoid cysts. They are most often noncancerous.

descend, moving downward.

desensitize, to decrease a person's reaction to any of the various antigens that might cause an allergy.

desiccant /des´ikənt/, any drug or treatment that causes a substance to dry up. Also known as **exsiccant.**

desmosis /dezmō´-/, any disease of the connective tissue.

desquamation /des´kwəmā´shən/, a process in which the top layer of skin flakes off in small pieces. Some conditions and medications speed up desquamation. Also known as **exfoliation.**

detached retina. See **retinal detachment.**

detection, phase of search and rescue using active procedures to seek out the lost persons or clues to their location. These procedures involve three types of actual search. The type I search involves trained searchers (aircraft, dogs, hasty teams) looking in areas of easy detection, such as drainage structures, ridges, roads, and trails, in a rapid, initial attempt to find a subject. Type II is a systematic procedure that searches areas using trained teams with wide spacing between them to follow up on clues or when a subject is still believed able to respond. Type III is a thorough, highly systematic search using trained and untrained personnel to closely examine a closed-grid search zone. Also known as **detection mode.** *See also attraction.*

detergent, a cleaning agent.

detonation, a vigorous exothermic chemical reaction that spreads faster than the speed of sound (release rate of less than 0.01 second) and produces an explosion. *See also deflagration.*

detoxification, removal of the poison from a substance or speeding up its removal from the body.

development, **1.** the gradual process of change from a simple to a more complex level. The ability of humans to adapt to surroundings and to function in society is gained through growth and learning. **2.** the series of events that occur in an organism from the time the egg is fertilized to the adult stage. **—developmental,** *adj.*

deviate /dē´vē·it/, a person or an event that varies from the normal standard.

dewatering, removing water from an area, particularly a trench or flooded compartment on a ship.

dew point, the temperature at which a vapor reaches saturation and starts to condense. In the atmosphere, fog will begin to form once this point is reached.

dexamethasone, an anti-inflammatory steroid used in the presence of allergy, head injury, and neurogenic shock. It decreases edema after histamine response and central nervous system injury. Although there are no side effects for field use, its onset of action is up to 2-6 hours. Also known as **Decadron.**

dextran, a plasma volume expander, containing large dextrose molecules, used in the presence of hypovolemic shock. Nausea and vomiting are the primary side effects. Contraindicated in patients taking anticoagulants, this agent also makes accurate blood typing difficult.

dextrose, a simple sugar that is highly soluble in water. Also known as **glucose.**

dextrose 50% in water, a carbohydrate solution used in patients with altered levels of consciousness and history of diabetes and/or low blood sugar. While there are no contraindications or side effects for field use, this solution can increase cerebral edema in patients with cerebrovascular accident (CVA). Also known as **D50, D50W, 50% dextrose.**

dextrose 5% in water, a carbohydrate solution used for dilution of intravenous drip drugs and as an intravenous lifeline for administration of drugs. There are no contraindications or side effects for field use.

dhobie itch /dō´bē/, a form of tinea cruris that occurs in tropical areas that is more intense than the form that occurs in temperate climates.

diabetes, multiple disorders of metabolism; most frequently used to refer to a disorder of carbohydrate metabolism that results from abnormal production or utilization of insulin. Types include diabetes mellitus, impaired glucose tolerance, and gestational diabetes. See Appendix 1-11.

diabetes insipidus, a disorder of metabolism caused by diminished production/secretion of antidiuretic hormone (vasopressin) or an inability of the kidneys to respond to it. This causes extreme thirst and urination.

diabetes mellitus, a disorder of metabolism that primarily results from absent or diminished insulin secretion by the pancreas or from defects of insulin receptors in the body. This causes an inability to utilize glucose properly.

diabetic /-bet´ik/, **1.** referring to diabetes. **2.** a person who has diabetes mellitus.

diabetic coma, altered level of consciousness due to an inability of the body to use glucose for metabolism, as a result of absent or decreased insulin production. Characterized by unconsciousness with dry, flushed skin and acetone breath odor, this condition generally requires 12-36 hours of decreased insulin levels before becoming obvious. Also known as **diabetic ketoacidosis, hyperglycemia.** *See also insulin shock.*

diabetic neuropathy, the nerve impairment that accompanies long-standing diabetes. Symptoms include loss of peripheral sensation, impaired motor function, and destructive changes to cerebral tissue. Although these changes may occur in any diabetic, those with brittle or unstable diabetes seem to be affected most frequently.

diabetic retinopathy, pathological changes in the retina accompanying diabetes.

diad, the combination of sarcoplasmic reticulum and T tubules.

diagnosis, the use of science and skill to establish the cause and nature of a patient's condition or disease. Done systematically, this evaluation assesses a patient's signs and symptoms, previous history, physical examination, and the tests necessary to reach a conclusion. This information provides a logical basis for patient treatment. *See also clinical diagnosis, diagnosis by exclusion, differential diagnosis, physical diagnosis.*

diagnosis by exclusion, reaching a diagnosis by eliminating other possibilities. *See also diagnosis.*

diagnostician /dī·əgnostish´ən/, a person skilled and trained in making diagnoses.

dialysate, **1.** *(informal)* dialyzing fluid used during renal dialysis, which, prior to use, contains small concentrations of calcium, potassium, sodium, and other essential electrolytes normally found in the blood. **2.** The dialyzing fluid after it has been in contact with the blood and contains waste products, such as creatinine and urea.

dialysis, the act of cleansing or purifying the blood, utilizing the principles of osmosis and diffusion across a semipermeable membrane. It is accomplished by the use of an artificial membrane, known as a dialyzer, and machine **(hemodialysis)** or the patient's own peritoneal membrane **(peritoneal dialysis).**

dialysis disequilibrium syndrome, a disorder caused by a rapid change in body fluid that sometimes occurs in dialysis. The condition may cause nervous system disorders, irregular heart rate, and pulmonary edema.

diapedesis /dī´əpədē´-/, the passage of red or white blood cells through the walls of blood vessels. This occurs without damage to the vessels.

diaper sling. See **seat harness.**

diaphoresis, increased skin moisture; sweating, usually excessively. Although strenuous exertion or warm weather are normal causes, epinephrine release can also provoke sweating. This can occur after myocardial infarction, trauma, infection, or any condition threatening the stability of the body's systems.

diaphragm /dī´əfram/, a dome-shaped muscle that separates the chest cavity from the abdominal cavity. The diaphragm aids breathing by moving up and down. When breathing in, it moves down and increases the space in the chest. When breathing out, it moves up, decreasing the volume.

diaphragm pump, a pump that uses a diaphragm instead of a piston, to create a positive displacement device that effectively moves water contaminated with particulate matter.

diaphragmatic breathing, breathing pattern identified by minimal abdominal movement without chest movement. This pattern of inadequate respirations is usually seen after injury to the cervical vertebrae between C3 and C7.

diaphragmatic hernia. See **hernia.**

diaphysis /dī·af´isis/, the shaft of a long bone.

diarrhea /dī´ərē´ə/, the frequent passage of loose, watery stools. It is usually the result of increased activity of the colon. The condition may be caused by stress and anxiety, diet, drugs, inflammation, irritation, faulty absorption of the bowel, the effects of poison, or radiation.

diastasis /dī·as´tə-/, the separation of two body parts that normally are joined together, as the separation of parts of a bone.

diastole, the period of relaxation during the cardiac cycle, when the cardiac muscle fibers lengthen, causing the heart to dilate and fill with blood. Coronary perfusion also occurs during this phase. *See also systole.*

diastolic blood pressure. See **blood pressure.**

diathesis /dī·ath´əsis, dī´athē´-/, *pl.* **diatheses,** a congenital condition in which the body is more susceptible to certain diseases or disorders than normal.

diazepam, a skeletal muscle relaxant used to terminate seizures and to decrease anxiety and awareness during cardioversion. Respiratory depression or arrest is a major side effect. There are no contraindications for field use. Also known as **Valium.**

dielectric, any material that is a nonconductor of electricity.

diencephalon, the portion of the brain that lies between the cerebral hemispheres and the mesencephalon. The structures included in this area are the epithalamus, hypothalamus, metathalamus, and thalamus.

diet, **1.** food and drink judged by nutritional value, composition, and effects on health. **2.** food and drink restricted in type and amount for treatment or other purposes. **3.** the usual amount of food and drink consumed. Compare **nutrition.** **–dietetic,** *adj.*

dietetics, the study of foods and their nutrients and how they relate to both health and disease.

Dietl's crisis /dē´təlz/, a sudden, severe pain in the kidney, caused by rapidly drinking very large amounts of liquid or by blockage in the ureter.

differential diagnosis, any condition having similar signs and symptoms that must be considered during patient evaluation.

differentiation, **1.** a process in development in which simple cells or tissues change to take on specific physical forms, functions, and chemical properties. **2.** taking on functions and forms different from those of the original. **3.** telling apart one thing or disease from another, as in differential diagnosis.

diffuse, widely spread, as through a fluid.

diffusion, the tendency of molecules of a substance to move from an area of high concentration to one of lower concentration. This process occurs with gaseous, liquid, or solid substances and results in an equalization of concentration.

digastricus /dīgas´trikəs/, one of the muscles of the mandible. It acts to open the jaw and to move the bone (hyoid) under the tongue.

digest, to convert food into a form that can be absorbed by the body. This is done by chewing food, adding water, and the action of stomach and intestinal fluids.

digestion, the changing of food into substances able to be absorbed by the body. This takes place in the stomach and intestines. **–digestive,** *adj.*

digestive gland, any of the many structures that releases substances that break down food so that it can be absorbed by the body. Some kinds of digestive glands are the salivary glands, gastric glands in the stomach, intestinal glands, liver, and pancreas.

digestive system, the organs, structures, and glands of the body through which food passes or is digested. The digestive system includes the mouth, throat, stomach, and small and large intestines. The digestive tube is a muscular tube, about 30 feet (9 meters) long, which extends from the mouth to the anus.

digital, **1.** referring to a finger or toe. **2.** an instrument that accepts data and/or produces output in the form of characters or digits. **3.** a signal formed as a series of electrical pulses that proceed in discrete jumps instead of gradual changes.

digital lock, an automotive security device that requires sequential input of a preset combination via a touchpad to unlock vehicle doors.

digitalis, a cardiac glycoside used to decrease the effect of congestive heart failure and rapid atrial dysrhythmias. It functions by increasing cardiac stroke volume and thereby cardiac output. Nausea and vomiting may be seen as side effects, particularly if the patient develops digitalis toxicity.

digitate /dij´itāt/, having fingers or fingerlike projections. *See also digital.*

diking, application of a barrier that prevents passage of a hazardous material to an area where it will produce more harm.

dilatation /dil´ətā´shən/, normal increase in the size of a body opening, blood vessel, or tube. An example is the widening of the pupil of the eye in dim light. Also known as dilation. **–dilatate, dilate** /dī´lāt/, *v.*

dilatation and curettage /dilətā´shən and kyurətäzh´/, artificially enlarging the cervical opening (or os) and scraping the endometrial lining of the uterus. This is usually done to diagnose disease of the uterus or to correct excessive or prolonged bleeding. Also known as **D&C.**

dilatator pupillae, a muscle that contracts the iris of the eye and widens the pupil.

dilutent, any substance that weakens a solution or mixture by diluting it.

dilution, making a less concentrated solution from a solution of greater concentration.

dioxin /dī´ok´sin/, a herbicidal ingredient used widely throughout the world to help control plant growth. Because of its high level of poison, it is no longer made in the United States. Dioxin was an ingredient of Agent Orange sprayed by the U.S. military aircraft over areas of Southeast Asia from 1965 to 1970 to kill concealing trees and shrubs. No safe exposure levels have been found. It has been strongly linked to many cancers and is very harmful to all living things.

diphenhydramine hydrochloride, an antihistamine used to counter allergic response and extrapyramidal reactions. This anticholinergic medication binds to histamine receptor sites to prevent further allergic reaction. Drowsiness and transient hypotension may be seen as side effects. There are no contraindications for field use. Also known as **Benadryl.**

diphtheria, an infectious bacterial disease that causes the formation of a false membrane on any mucous surface or the skin. Symptoms include low-grade temperature and sore throat with the presence of a yellow-white membrane adhering to the tonsils or other oral surfaces. Foul breath is common. With the development of antitoxin, this disease is rarely encountered in developed countries.

diplegia /dīple´jə/, paralysis affecting the same parts on both sides of the body.

diploë /dip´lō·ē/, the spongy tissue between the bones of the skull.

diplopia, double vision. Also known as **ambiopia.**

dip pipe, a pipe with a sunken outlet.

dipsomania /dip´sō-/, an uncontrollable craving for alcoholic beverages.

Diptera, the order of insects that are characterized by one pair of wings. Included are blackflies, deerflies, horseflies, mosquitos, and tsetse flies. These insects are the most significant carriers of human disease known.

direct contact, touching of two persons or organisms. Many communicable diseases may be spread by the direct contact between an infected and a healthy person.

direct current, electrical current of constant magnitude flowing in only a single direction. Also known as **DC.**

direct medical control, real-time communications between field personnel and a medical control physician. Many systems require this type of control in order to implement various advanced life support procedures. Also known as **on-line medical control.** *See also indirect medical control.*

direct pressure, generally used to describe the application of pressure by hand against a bleeding artery or vein, in order to control bleeding. It is the most reliable method of hemorrhage control with the least amount of damage to the area.

direttissima /dir´etis´imə/, a direct ascent of a mountain face.

disability, the loss or damage of physical or mental fitness. Compare **handicap.**

disaccharide /dīsak´ərid/, a sugar made up of two simple sugars, such as lactose and sucrose.

disaster, 1. a sudden, awful event. **2.** *(World Health Organization)* a sudden ecologic phenomenon of sufficient magnitude to require external assistance. **3.** any community emergency that seriously affects the lives and property of its citizens and that exceeds the capacity of the community to effectively respond to that emergency. *See also multiple casualty incident.*

disc. See **disk.**

discharge, 1. to release a substance or object. **2.** to release a burst of energy from or through a nerve. **3.** to release an electrical charge. **4.** a release of emotions. **5.** to release a patient from a hospital.

disease, 1. an unhealthy state of the body with signs and symptoms that distinguish one condition from another. **2.** a specific condition with a characteristic set of signs and symptoms. **Acute disease** has a rapid onset and a short course. **Chronic disease** persists for a prolonged period of time. **Functional disease** may be (1) a disorder that affects function or performance while not affecting tissue or (2) a condition with symptoms for which no physical cause can be found. An **intercurrent disease** develops while another disease is present and may alter the course of the first disease.

disengagement, 1. moving the part of the baby lowest in the pelvis in order to aid childbirth. **2.** the detachment of oneself from other persons or responsibilities.

disentanglement, the stage of extrication that frees a victim from wreckage, allowing further medical care and removal.

disequilibrium, unstable, off-balance.

disequilibrium syndrome, abnormal neurologic changes that can occur during or after hemodialysis. These symptoms include ataxia, confusion, and/or seizures, which are due to the rapid alteration in fluid and electrolyte levels in response to the dialysis treatment.

disinfectant, a chemical that can destroy bacteria.

disinfection, to remove infectious agents by chemical or physical means. Chemicals used include alcohols, ammonia, chlorine, iodides, and phenols. Washing is the most common physical method of disinfection.

disinfestation, the process of killing infesting insects and parasites, usually by chemical methods.

disk, 1. also spelled **disc.** A flat, round, platelike structure, such as a joint (articular) disk or an optic disc. **2.** the cartilage between the vertebrae. Also known as **discus.**

dislocation, the displacement of any part of the body from its normal position. This applies most often to a bone moved from its normal position with a joint. *See also subluxation.* **–dislocate,** *v.*

disorientation, a state of mental confusion as to place, time, or personal identity.

dispatch, the implementation of a decision to move a resource or resources from one place to another. Also known as **communications.**

dispatch center, a facility from which resources are directly assigned to an incident. Also known as the **communications center.**

displaced fracture, a bone break in which two ends of the bone are separated from each other.

displacement, 1. the state of being moved from the normal position. **2.** an unconscious defense mechanism to avoid emotional conflict. Emotions or ideas are transferred from one object or person to another that is less threatening.

disruptive functioning, an inability to adjust to a stressful situation.

dissecting aortic aneurysm, progressive dilatation of a portion of the aorta at a weak point between the middle (tunica media) and outer (tunica adventitia) layers of the vessel wall.

dissection, arterial wall separation.

disseminated intravascular coagulation, a disorder resulting in an increase of the body's clotting substance in response to disease or injury. This may be provoked by septicemia, hypotension, hypovolemia, childbirth, or injury. Also known as **DIC.**

dissemination, a phase of cancer in which cells spread (metastasize) to other parts of the body.

dissociation, 1. the act of separating into parts or sections. **2.** an unconscious defense mechanism by which an idea or emotion is separated from the consciousness. In this way it loses emotional significance.

dissociative disorder, a type of hysterical neurosis. Emotional conflicts are denied to the point that a split in the personality occurs. This causes a confusion in identity. Symptoms include amnesia, flight from reality, dream state, or multiple personality. The disorder is caused by failure to cope with severe stress or conflict. Compare **conversion disorder.**

distal /dis´təl/, away from or being the farthest from a point of origin, such a central point of the body, as the distal phalanx is the bone at the tip of the finger. Compare **proximal.**

distance regulation, behavior that is related to the control of personal space. Most humans need a certain space between themselves and others. This space offers security, but does not create a sense of isolation. The amount of social distance varies with different persons and in different cultures.

distend, to stretch or become inflated.

distribution, **1.** the dividing or spreading of any entity, as in oxygen to tissues. **2.** the presence of particular patterns, such as population density.

disturbed soil, soil that has been previously excavated.

diuresis, secretion of abnormally large amounts of urine. This may be due to diabetes, drug action, or ingestion of large quantities of fluids.

diuretic, a substance that stimulates the kidneys to excrete water.

diurnal /dī´ur´nəl/, occurring during the day. Compare **nocturnal.**

diurnal variation, the range of the release rate of a substance, such as urine, being collected for laboratory analysis over a 24-hour period.

diversion, **1.** controlled movement of a hazardous material to an area where it will produce less harm. **2.** a distraction.

diverticulitis /dī´vərtik´yəlī´tis/, inflammation of one or more diverticula in the wall of the colon. Inflammation and abcesses form in the tissues surrounding the colon. The opening of the colon narrows and may become blocked. The patient will experience pain, often in the lower abdomen, and fever. *See also colostomy.*

diverticulosis /-lō´sis/, a pouchlike bulging through the muscular layer of the colon without inflammation. This occurs most often in the sigmoid colon, primarily in people over age 50. Most patients with this condition have few symptoms except for occasional bleeding from the rectum, and vague abdominal distress.

diverticulum /dī´vərtik´yələm/, *pl.* **diverticula,** a pouchlike bulging through the muscular wall of a tubular organ. A diverticulum may occur in the stomach, in the small intestine, or, most commonly, in the colon.

division, **1.** the separation of something into two or more parts. A kind of division is **cell division. 2.** that organizational level having responsibility for operations within a defined geographic area or with functional responsibility. The division level is organizationally between the strike team and the branch. *See also group.*

dizygotic /dī´zīgot´ik/, referring to twins from two fertilized eggs. Compare **monozygotic.** *See also twin.*

dizziness. See **vertigo.**

dobutamine hydrochloride, a synthetic catecholamine used in the treatment of congestive heart failure. It improves cardiac output by increasing the force of systolic contraction. Side effects include palpitations and ventricular irritability. This agent should not be used in the presence of bradycardias.

Doctor of Medicine, Doctor of Osteopathy. See **physician.**

documentation, the recording of facts to supply information or evidence.

doll's eyes, the normal reflex where the eyes of an unconscious patient orient in one direction and attempt to maintain that direction even as the head is turned. An absence of this reflex is indicative of central nervous system impairment.

dominance, a basic genetic principle stating that not all genes operate with equal strength. If two genes produce a different trait, such as eye color, the gene that is expressed is dominant.

dominant gene. See **gene.**

donor, a human or other organism that gives living tissue to be used in another body, for example, blood for transfusion or a kidney for transplantation. *See also blood donor, transplant.*

Do not resuscitate, written physician order indicating that a patient is not to be resuscitated in cases of cardiac or respiratory arrest. Patients with terminal or end-stage disease may be placed in this status prior to an event that would normally require resuscitation. Also known as **DNR, no-code.**

dopamine hydrochloride, a natural catecholamine used in the presence of cardiogenic or low-resistance shock states. This sympathomimetic improves blood pressure by increasing the force of systolic contraction, while selectively dilating blood vessels in the brain, heart, kidney, and mesentery. Hypertension and ventricular irritability may be seen as side effects.

dope, *(slang)* morphine, heroin, marijuana, or another illegal substance.

doppler detector, a diagnostic device utilizing sound waves to locate gas bubbles within the bloodstream, as in arterial gas embolism or decompression sickness.

dorsal /dôr´səl/, referring to the back or posterior. Compare **ventral. –dorsum,** *n.*

dorsal digital vein, one of the veins along the sides of the fingers. The veins from both sides of the fingers unite to form three dorsal metacarpal veins, which end in a dorsal vein network on the back of the hand.

dorsal interventricular artery, the branch of the right coronary artery. It branches to supply both ventricles.

dorsalis pedis artery /dôrsā´lis pē´dis/, the continuation of the anterior tibial artery of the lower leg. It starts at the ankle joint, divides into five branches, and supplies various muscles of the foot and toes.

dorsal scapular nerve, one of a pair of nerve branches above the clavicle. It supplies the muscles of the shoulder blade (rhomboideus major and the rhomboideus minor) and continues to the levator muscle in the neck.

dorsiflexion, movement of a part so as to bend it toward the posterior aspect of the body, such as when the hand is bent backward.

dorsiflexor /-flek´sər/, a muscle causing backward flexion of a part of the body, such as the hand or foot.

dosage, the size, frequency, and number of doses of a drug to be given to a patient.

dose, 1. amount taken at one time, as with medication, radiation. **2.** *(slang)* venereal disease.

dose, radiation, an accumulated quantity of ionizing radiation. It is a measure of the energy absorbed per gram of absorbing material. The unit of absorbed dose is the rad. The term "dose" is often used in the sense of the exposure, expressed in "roentgens," which is a measure of the total amount of ionization that the quantity of radiation could produce in air. The absorbed dose in tissue is about 1 rad when the exposure in air is 1 roentgen.

dose equivalent, a quantity used in radiation protection. It expresses all radiation on a common scale for evaluating and comparing the effects of radiation in humans. It is defined as the product of the absorbed dose in rads and certain modifying factors. The unit of dose equivalent is the rem. For the most common forms of radiation (X, gamma, and beta), the dose equivalent in rems is numerically equal to the absorbed dose in rads.

dose threshold, the minimum amount of absorbed radiation that produces an effect.

dosimeter /dōsim´ətər/, an instrument to detect and measure total radiation exposure.

DOT hazard class, the designation for hazardous materials as found in the Department of Transportation regulations, CFR part 49.

double-blind study, an experiment made to test the effect of a treatment or drug. Groups of experimental and control subjects are used in which neither the subjects nor the investigators know the identity of the treatment being given to any group. In a double-blind test of a new drug, the drug may be identified to the investigators only by a code.

Down's syndrome, a disorder present at birth that causes mental retardation and physical defects. It is more frequent in infants born to women over 35 years of age. Infants with the disorder are small with weak muscles. They have a small head with a flat skull, depressed nose bridge, low-set ears, and a large, protruding tongue that is furrowed and lacks the central groove. Most significant is the mental retardation, which varies considerably, although the average IQ is in the range of 50 to 60. Also known as **mongolism.**

Downey cells, white blood cells (lymphocytes) identified in patients with infectious mononucleosis.

downstream, away from the oncoming flow; downriver.

downstream V, the clear passage in a rapids; a chute.

downwind, the direction in which the wind is blowing.

downwind leg, that part of an aircraft's traffic pattern in which it is traveling with the wind parallel to the runway.

D-post, the fourth roof support post from the front of a motor vehicle. It is normally present in the station wagon type of vehicle.

dracunculiasis /drakun´kyəlī´əsis/, a parasitic infection. It is caused by the worm (nematode) *Dracunculus medinensis.*

drainage, the free flow or withdrawal of fluids.

drainage tube, a heavy-gauge catheter used to remove air or a fluid from a cavity or wound in the body. The tube may be attached to a suction device or it may simply allow flow by gravity into a container.

dram, a unit of mass equivalent to an apothecaries' measure of 60 grains or 1/8 ounce and to 1/16 ounce or 27.34 grains avoirdupois.

drawing, *(informal)* a vague sensation of muscle tension.

dream, **1.** ideas, thoughts, emotions, or images that pass through the mind during the rapid eye movement stage of sleep. **2.** a creation of the imagination during wakefulness. **3.** the expression of thoughts, emotions, memories, or impulses repressed from the consciousness.

dream state, a condition of altered consciousness in which a person does not recognize the environment and reacts in a manner not like his or her usual behavior, as by flight or an act of violence. The state is seen in epilepsy and certain neuroses. *See also automatism, fugue.*

dressing, a covering for diseased or injured parts; a covering that is held in place by a bandage. Types of dressings include absorbent, dry, nonadherent, occlusive, pressure. *See also bandage.*

Dressler's syndrome, an inflammatory disorder that may occur several days after myocardial infarction. It results from the response of the body's immune system to a damaged heart. Symptoms include fever, pulmonary edema, joint pain, and inflammation of the pleura and pericardium.

drift, a change that occurs in a strain of virus so that variations appear periodically with alterations in the virus' qualities.

drift angle, the angle of the tire in relation to the road direction in a curve. When transiting a curve, a vehicle's tires must be turned to a greater angle than the curve, so that the necessary turning force is created. Also known as **slip angle.**

drip, **1.** *(informal)* an intravenous medication infusion. **2.** *(slang)* gonorrhea.

drip loop, a looped connection of electrical wire near the wire's entrance to a structure. The loop allows the wire to enter at an angle, which prevents rain or snow from entering the service conduit.

dromotropic, chemicals that affect the speed of conduction through the conducting tissue of the heart. Increased speed causes a positive effect. Slowing of conduction is referred to as a **negative dromotropic effect.** *See also chronotropic, inotropic.*

drop foot, a condition in which the foot is flexed downward and cannot voluntarily be flexed up; usually due to nerve damage.

droplet infection, an infection caused by inhaling germs that are in particles of liquid sneezed or coughed by an infected person or animal.

drowning, death by asphyxia after submersion. *See also near-drowning.*

drug, **1.** any substance taken by mouth, injected into a muscle, the skin, a blood vessel, or a cavity of the body, or applied to the skin to treat or prevent a disease. **2.** *(informal)* a narcotic substance.

drug abuse, the use of a drug for a nontherapeutic effect. Some of the most commonly abused drugs are alcohol, amphetamines, barbiturates, cocaine, methaqualone, and opium alkaloids. Drug abuse may lead to organ damage, addiction, and disturbed patterns of behavior. Some illegal drugs have no known therapeutic effect in humans. *See also drug addiction.*

drug action, the means by which a drug has a desired effect. Drugs are usually classified by their actions. For example, a vasodilator, which is prescribed to decrease the blood pressure, acts by dilating the blood vessels.

drug addiction, a condition marked by an overwhelming desire to continue taking a drug because it produces a desired effect, usually an altered mental activity, attitude, or outlook. *See also alcoholism, drug abuse.*

drug allergy, allergy to a drug shown by reactions ranging from a mild rash to anaphylaxis. The seriousness of the reaction depends on the person, the drug, and the dose.

drug dependence, a psychologic craving for or a physical dependence on a drug. It results from habituation, abuse, or addiction. *See also drug abuse, drug addiction.*

drug-drug interaction, a change of the effect of a drug when given with another drug. The effect may be an increase or a decrease in the action of either drug. The effect may also be a side effect that is not normally linked to either drug. *See also side effect.*

drug-protein complex, a complex molecular compound formed when a drug binds to a protein.

dry suit, a watertight diving suit that protects divers from the effects of very cold water and/or hazardous materials in the water. Air within the suit is warmed by the body and serves as insulation against the cold. Buoyancy can also be controlled by regulating the amount of air inside the suit. *See also wet suit.*

dry suit squeeze. See **squeeze.**

Duckworth's phenomenon, respiratory arrest prior to cardiac arrest as a result of intracranial disease.

duct, a narrow tubelike structure, especially one through which material is released.

duct carcinoma, a cancer developed from the lining of ducts, especially in the breast or pancreas.

ductless gland, a gland lacking a duct. Endocrine glands, which release hormones directly into blood or lymph, are ductless glands.

dumping syndrome, a disorder with profuse sweating, nausea, dizziness, and weakness, experienced by patients who have had a gastrectomy. Symptoms are felt soon after eating, when the contents of the stomach empty too rapidly into the duodenum. *See also gastrec-tomy.*

duodenal /dŌŌ´ədē´nəl/, the proximal portion of the small intestine (duodenum).

duodenal ulcer. See **peptic ulcer.**

duodenum /dŌŌ´ədē´nəm, dŌŌ·od´ənəm,/, *pl.* **duodena, duodenums,** the shortest, widest portion of the small intestine that joins the stomach at the pyloric valve. It is about 10 inches (25 cm) long. It is divided into superior, descending, horizontal, and ascending portions. Compare **jejunum, ileum.**

duplex, a communications system with the ability to transmit and receive traffic simultaneously. This capability is achieved by the use of two different frequencies within the same device, one for reception and the other for transmission.

dura mater /dŌŌr´ə mā´tər, dyŌŌ´rə/, the fiberlike, outermost of the three membranes surrounding the brain and spinal cord. The **dura mater encephali** covers the brain. The **dura mater spinalis** covers the cord. *See also meninges.*

duration of action, the time from onset of a drug's action until the end of its effect.

dust, any fine, particulate, dry matter. **Inorganic dust** refers to dry, finely powdered particles of an inorganic substance, especially dust. When inhaled, it can cause abnormal conditions of the lungs. **Organic dust** is dried bits of matter from plants, animals, fungi, or germs that are fine enough to be carried by the wind.

dust off, **1.** a medical evacuation mission performed by helicopter, particularly within the U.S. military. **2.** the helicopters that perform those missions.

duty to act, a legal relationship, between one or more individuals and an individual or private or public organization, that requires that the person or organization with the duty to act, possess, and bring to bear that degree of care, knowledge, and skill that is usually exercised by reasonable and prudent practitioners under similar circumstances, given prevailing knowledge and available resources.

dwarf, an abnormally short person, especially one whose bodily parts are not proportional.

dwarfism, the abnormal underdevelopment of the body with varying degrees of mental retardation. Dwarfism has numerous causes, including genetic defects, hormone lack involving either the pituitary or thyroid glands, chronic diseases (as rickets, kidney failure, and intestinal malabsorption defects).

dye, **1.** to apply coloring matter to a substance. **2.** a chemical compound that colors a substance to which it is applied. Various dyes are used to color drugs, to stain tissues, as therapeutic agents, and in tests.

dynamic pressure, the force that occurs in a medium in motion, such as the shock wave following a blast.

dysadrenia /dis´adrē´nē·ə/, abnormal adrenal gland function. It features decreased or increased production of gland hormones.

dysbarism /dis´bərizəm/, all pathologic changes that are caused by an environment of altered pressure. All disorders due to increased or decreased pressure extremes from that encountered at sea level are included, such as those of astronauts, aviators, and scuba divers. *See also specific entry.*

dyscholia /-kō´lyə/, any abnormal condition of the bile, either regarding the amount released or the condition of the contents.

dysconjugate gaze, failure of the eyes to track simultaneously in the same direction from their normal resting position. Brain stem dysfunction causes this abnormality.

dyscrasia /-krā´zhə/, an abnormal blood or bone marrow condition, such as leukemia, aplastic anemia, or Rh incompatibility.

dysentery /dis´inter´ē/, an inflammation of the intestine, especially of the colon. It may be caused by chemical irritants, bacteria, protozoa, or parasites. The symptoms are frequent and bloody stools, stomach pain, and straining. Dysentery is common when sanitary living conditions, clean food, and safe water are not available. **Amebic dysentery** is an inflammation of the intestine caused by *Entamoeba histolytica.*

dysfunctional, unable to function normally, as a body organ or system. **–dysfunction,** *n.*

dysfunctional uterine bleeding, a disorder of bleeding from the uterus caused by hormone imbalance rather than a disease.

dysgenesis /-jen´əsis/, **1.** defective formation of an organ or part, primarily during early fetal development. **2.** loss of the ability to reproduce.

dysgraphia, an inability to write correctly, usually due to a lesion in the brain.

dyshidrosis, **1.** disorder of the sweat glands. **2.** a skin disorder marked by recurrent eruption of vesicles on feet and hands. Also known as **pompholyx.**

dyskinesia /dis´kinē´zhə/, impaired ability to make voluntary movements. **–dyskinetic** /-et´ik/, *adj.*

dyslexia, disorders of learning, reading, or writing.

dysmaturity, **1.** the failure of an organism to develop or mature in structure or function. **2.** a fetus or newborn who is abnormally small or large for the length of pregnancy (age of gestation). *See also birth weight.*

dysmelia /-mē´lyə/, a birth defect marked by missing or shortened arms and legs. This is linked to abnormalities of the spine in some individuals. *See also phocomelia.*

dysmenorrhea /dis´menôrē´ə-/, pain linked to menstruation.

dysmorphophobia /dis´môrfō-/, **1.** a delusion of body image. **2.** the morbid fear of deformity or of becoming deformed.

dysostosis /dis´ostō´-/, an abnormal condition with defective bone formation (ossification), especially in fetal cartilages.

dyspareunia /dis´pərōō´nē·ə/, painful sexual intercourse. *See also vaginismus.*

dyspepsia /-pep´sē·ə/, a vague feeling of discomfort under the sternum after eating. There is an uncomfortable feeling of fullness, heartburn, bloating, and nausea. Dyspepsia is a symptom of an underlying disorder, such as peptic ulcer, gall-bladder disease, or appendicitis. **Cholelithic dyspepsia** refers to sudden indigestion linked to the dysfunction of the gallbladder. **Functional dyspepsia** results from a smooth muscle or nervous system dysfunction. Faulty digestion that is linked to a disease or a change in an organ other than an organ of digestion is termed **reflex dyspepsia.**

dysphagia /-fā´jə/, difficulty in swallowing, commonly linked to disorders of the esophagus.

dysphasia /-fā´zhə/, difficulty in speaking, usually resulting from an injury to the speech area of the brain. Symptoms include lack of coordination in speaking and getting words out of order. It may occur with other language disorders, such as inability to write (dysgraphia).

dyspnea, difficulty breathing.

dyspraxia /-prak´sē·ə/, a partial loss of the ability to perform skilled, coordinated movements. *See also apraxia.*

dysprosium, a rare earth metallic element. Radioactive isotopes of dysprosium are used in studies of the bones and joints.

dysproteinemia /-prō´tēnē´mē·ə/, an abnormality of the protein content of the blood.

dysreflexia /dis´riflek´sē·ə/, a nerve or muscle condition with abnormal reflexes.

dysrhythmia /-rith´mē·ə/, any abnormality in a normal rhythmic pattern. See Appendix 1-8. Compare **arrhythmia.**

dyssebacea /dis´ibā´shē·ə/, a skin condition marked by red, scaly patches on the nose, eyelids, scrotum, and lips. It results from a lack of vitamin B2 and is commonly seen in persons with alcoholism, liver disease, and protein malnutrition. Also known as **shark skin.**

dystocia, difficult labor.

dystonic reaction, an adverse effect seen in patients taking phenothiazine medications, which causes facial distortion, muscle spasm in the back, face, or neck, and speech alterations. Although not life-threatening, the condition can be very painful. Also known as **extrapyramidal reaction.** *See also extrapyramidal reaction.*

dystrophy /dis´trəfē/, any condition caused by defective nutrition. The term is often applied to a change in muscles that does not involve the nervous system, as in fatty breakdown linked to increased muscle size but decreased strength. *See also muscular dystrophy.*

dysuria /-yŏŏr´ē·ə/, painful urination, resulting from a bacterial infection of blockage in the urinary tract. Dysuria is a symptom of such conditions as cystitis, urethritis, prostatitis, tumors, and some gynecologic disorders. Compare **hematuria, pyuria.**

E

ear, the organ of hearing. The ear has three parts: the inner, middle, and outer ear. The outer ear is both the skin-covered cartilage **(auricle)** that protrudes from either side of the head, and the tube **(external auditory canal)** that extends from the outside of the head to the middle ear. The two parts of the outer ear focus sound waves on the eardrum, between the outer and middle ear. Also called the **tympanic membrane,** the eardrum carries sound vibrations to the inner ear by means of the bones of the middle ear. The **middle ear** is the space between the eardrum and the inner ear. It is filled with air carried from the back of the throat by the auditory (eustachian) tube. It holds three small bones called the hammer (malleus), anvil (incus), and the stirrup (stapes). These bones pick up the vibrations caused by sound waves hitting the eardrum. The bones pass the vibrations on to the inner ear. The **inner ear** (labyrinth) is filled with fluid, and holds two organs. One of the organs provides a sense of balance (vestibular apparatus), the other picks up the sound vibrations from the inner ear fluid and carries them to the nerve endings that sense sounds.

earthdam, dam constructed from compacted soil material.

earthquake, a pressure wave in the Earth's crust caused by movement of underlying rock strata (tectonic plates) along preexisting fault lines. These move against each other, creating cumulative strain, until the plate's slippage causes pressure waves.

ebb current, the horizontal motion of water away from land.

ebb tide, a falling or low tide; that which moves away from land.

eccentricity, behavior that is seen as odd or peculiar for a given culture or community, although not unusual enough to be considered dangerous.

ecchymosis, skin discoloration due to extravasation of blood into the tissues, which causes irregular shaped hemorrhagic areas. The color varies from blue-black to yellow, depending on the age of the discoloration.

eccrine /ek´rin/, fluid released through a duct to the surface of the skin. *See also exocrine.*

eccrine gland, one of two kinds of sweat glands in the skin. These glands are unbranched, coiled, and tubelike and are found throughout the skin. They cool the body by evaporation of the sweat they release, which is clear, has a faint odor, and contains water, sodium chloride, and traces of albumin, urea, and other compounds. Compare **apocrine gland.**

echelons of care, the distribution of military medical resources in various capabilities and locations. Most military medical care is provided in four echelons. The first level is essential emergency care provided by medics or corpsmen. The second level occurs at a clearing station or battalion aid station, where the patient is triaged and emergency care continued. A medical installation, equipped to provide initial wound surgery and resuscitation, provides the third level of care. The fourth level occurs in a general hospital that is staffed to provide definitive care.

echocardiography /ek´ōkär´dē·og´rəfē/, a method of diagnosis utilizing sound waves that studies the structure and motion of the heart. Sound waves (ultrasonic) directed through the heart are reflected backward when they pass from one type of tissue to another, such as from heart muscle to blood. Also known as **ultrasonic cardiography.**

echoencephalography /-ensef´əlog´rəfē/, the use of sound waves (ultrasonic) to study the brain.

echolalia /-lā´lyə/, the automatic and meaningless repeating of another's words or phrases, especially as seen in schizophrenia.

eclampsia, seizures due to toxemia of pregnancy, which may occur up to two weeks after delivery. *See also pre-eclampsia.*

ecthyma, a skin infection identified by shallow lesions with adherent crusts. This usually occurs in the presence of impetigo whose treatment has been neglected.

ectoparasite /-per´əsīt/, an organism that lives on the outside of the body of the host, such as a louse.

ectopic, **1.** in an abnormal position. **2.** a cardiac complex originating from somewhere other than the SA node. It may be early (premature) or late (escape) in nature. Also known as **ectopic beat, escape beat, extrasystole, premature beat.**

ectopic pregnancy. See **pregnancy.**

ectropion, eversion of an edge, such as an eyelid.

eczema /ek´simə/, inflammation of the outer layer of skin from an unknown cause. Eczema is not a distinct disease but a symptom. *See also dermatitis.*

eddy, a secondary current of water moving against the main current in a circular motion. A solid obstruction produces an eddy behind it when the water is forced around the obstruction. *See also eddy line.*

eddy line, demarcation between water flowing in an eddy and water flowing downstream.

edema, excessive fluid within the body's tissues. Also known as **anasarca, dropsy.**

edge roller, a device with multiple rollers, positioned over the edge of a cliff, over which rope is run. The primary purpose of this device is to prevent rope abrasion against edges, but it also facilitates upward rope movement when hauling is necessary.

edge tender, person(s) responsible for both rope care and situational observation at the edge of a precipice. Responsibilities include preventing rope abrasion and tangle, observing ascent and descent, and anticipating potential problems.

effacement, the shortening of the cervix and thinning of its walls as it is stretched and widened by the fetus during labor. *See also birth, labor.*

effective performance time, the amount of time an individual is able to perform useful duties in a flight environment of inadequate oxygen. Also known as **EPT.** *See also time of useful consciousness.*

efferent /ef´ərənt/, directed away from a center, such as certain arteries, veins, nerves, and lymph channels. Compare **afferent.**

efferent duct, any duct through which a gland releases its fluids.

efficacy /ef´əkəsē/, the greatest ability of a drug or treatment to produce a result, regardless of dosage.

effort syndrome, condition causing chest pain, dizziness, fatigue, and irregular tachycardia, often found in soldiers in combat. The symptoms of effort syndrome often mimic angina pectoris but are rarely anxiety states.

effusion, the escape of fluid into a cavity, such as a pericardial or pulmonary effusion.

ego /ē´gō, eg´ō/, **1.** the conscious sense of the self; those elements of a person, such as thinking and feeling, that mark the person as an individual. **2.** the part of the self that experiences and maintains conscious contact with reality and balances the drives and demands of the self with the social and physical needs of society.

ego boundary, a sense or awareness that there is a difference between the self and others. In some psychoses the person does not have an ego boundary and cannot tell the difference between his or her own personal feelings and other people's feelings.

egocentric, seeing the self as the center of all experience and having little regard for the needs, interests, ideas, and attitudes of others.

ego ideal, the image of the self that a person strives to be both consciously and unconsciously and against which he or she measures himself or herself. It is usually based on a positive identification with the important and influential figures of early childhood years. *See also identification.*

egomania, an extreme, long-term focus on the self and magnified sense of one's own importance.

ego strength, the ability to maintain the ego by a group of traits that together contribute to good mental health.

egotism /ēˊgətizm, egˊ-/, a magnifying of the importance of the self and the contempt of others. *See also egoism.*

egress /ēˊgres/, the act of moving forward or coming out of.

eight plate. See **figure eight descender.**

Einthoven's law /īntˊhoˊvənz/, on the electocardiogram, the potential in lead II is equal to the sum of potentials in leads I and III. Also known as **Einthoven's equation.** *See also Einthoven's triangle.*

Einthoven's triangle (Willem Einthoven, Dutch physiologist, 1860-1927), an electrical triangle formed by the patients' right arm, left arm, and left leg, used to position electrodes for EKG monitoring. This positioning is used to determine the direction of cardiac vectors to various leads.

ejaculation, the release of semen from the male urethra. –**ejaculatory** /ijakˊyələtôrˊē/, *adj.*

ejaculatory duct, the passage through which semen enters the urethra.

ejecta, material thrown by a natural force, such as matter thrown out of an erupting volcano.

ejection, **1.** forceful expulsion of blood from the cardiac ventricles. **2.** sudden propulsion of an unrestrained occupant from a vehicle, due to deceleration forces. This represents a major mechanism of injury during accidents. **3.** jettisoning a crew member from an aircraft via a rocket-propelled seat.

ejection fraction, the amount of blood that is released during each contraction of a ventricle compared with the total volume of blood released by both ventricles.

ejection seat, rocket-propelled seat that pushes an aircraft occupant away from a disabled aircraft at high speed. These devices present one of the major hazards during rescue from military aircraft.

elastic bandage, bandaging material that exerts continuous pressure on the applied area, due to its elasticity. Also known as **Ace, Ace wrap, Ace Bandage.**

elasticity, the physical property of returning to original size and shape after being stressed.

elastin /ilasˊtin/, a protein that forms the main part of yellow elastic tissue fibers.

elbow, the hinged joint of the arm. The humerus and the radius and ulna join at the elbow. The elbow allows the forearm to flex, extend, and rotate. The elbow is a common site of injury, especially from sports.

elder abuse, inflicting mental and/or physical pain or injury, unreasonable confinement, or willful deprivation of services necessary to maintain the mental and/or physical health of an elderly person.

elective, treatment that is done by choice but that is not required, as elective surgery.

electric burns, burn injuries sustained due to electric current passing through tissue. Severity is determined by the pathway taken by the current, the amount of current, and skin resistance. Burn injuries generally follow blood vessel, muscle, and nerve pathways, causing the majority of damage below the surface of the skin.

electric shock, the physical sensation sustained by the body with the passage of electrical current through it.

electrocardiograph, device used to record electrical variation within cardiac tissue. Also known as **ECG, EKG.**

electrocution, **1.** the delivery of electrical current into body tissue. **2.** the injury or death that may result from the passage of electricity through the body.

electrode /ilekˊtrōd/, **1.** a contact for inducing or recording electric activity. **2.** a substance that conducts an electric current from the body to measuring equipment.

electroencephalogram   /-ənsef´ələgram´/, a graph of electrical activity made by the brain cells, as is picked up by electrodes placed on the scalp. Changes in brain wave activity can show nervous system disorders and level of consciousness. Also known as **EEG.** *See also brain waves.*

electroencephalography /-ensef´əlog´rəfē/, the process of recording brain wave activity with an instrument called an **electroencephalograph.** Electrodes are attached to the patient's head and the patterns of electric activity received are then recorded on a chart. Used to aid in the diagnosis of seizures, brainstem disorders, tumors or clots, and impaired consciousness. *See also electroencephalogram.*

electrohemodynamics   /-hē´mōdīnam´-/, a method for measuring the efficiency of blood flow in the body. This measures blood pressure, the strength of nerve impulses, and the ability of the system to hold and direct flowing blood.

electrohydraulic heart /-hīdrôlik/, a type of artificial heart in which the ventricles are driven by the alternate pumping of a fluid rather than by compressed air. *See also artificial heart.*

electrolyte /ilek´trəlīt/, an element or compound that, when melted or dissolved in water or other solvent, dissociates into ions (atoms able to carry an electric charge). Electrolyte amounts vary in blood plasma, in tissues, and in cell fluid. The body must maintain electrolyte balance to use energy. Potassium (K^+) is needed to contract muscles and propagate nerve impulses. Sodium (Na^+) is needed to maintain fluid balance. Some diseases, defects, and drugs may lead to a lack of one or more electrolytes.

electromagnetic radiation, emitted energy in the form of a wave resulting from changing electric or magnetic fields. Familiar electromagnetic radiations range from x-rays (and gamma rays) at short wavelengths through the ultraviolet, visible, and infrared regions to radar and radio waves of relatively long wavelength.

electromechanical dissociation, phenomenon seen in a compromised heart where cardiac electrical activity does not produce cardiac mechanical activity (no blood flow). A rhythm is shown on EKG, but there is no corresponding pulse. This event is seen during cardiac arrest states and has many causes, including hypovolemia, trauma, and cardiac muscle hypoxia. Now known as **pulseless electrical activity.** Also known as **EMD.** *See also pulseless electrical activity.*

electromyogram /-mī´əgram/. See **electroneuromyography.**

electroneuromyography /-nyo͞or´ōmī·og´rəfē/, a method to test and record nerve and muscle function. The record created is known as an **electromyogram.**

electronic fetal monitor, a device that allows the fetal heartbeat and the contractions of the uterus to be observed.

electronic position indicator, device that measures distances ship-to-shore by measuring elapsed time for a radio echo. Also known as **EPI.**

electron microscopy, using an electron microscope, a beam of electrons is focused by a special lens onto very thin tissue or other sample. A second lens projects the image onto a screen. The image has a resolution 1000 times greater than with an optical microscope.

eleidin /elē´idin/, a clear protein substance that resembles keratin, found in the skin, mucous membrane, and other surface tissues.

element, one of 105 primary substances that cannot be broken down by chemical means.

elevation, **1.** lifting an extremity above the level of the heart as a method of controlling bleeding or swelling. **2.** height or altitude above a certain level, generally sea level.

elixir, a clear liquid made of water, alcohol, sweeteners, or flavors mainly in drugs that are taken by mouth.

elliptical, oval shaped.

El Niño /el nē´nyō/, warming of eastern Pacific surface water that affects agricultural and rainfall patterns worldwide. Shifts in ocean currents and wind can cause rainfall in normally arid locations and floods in areas used to moderate rain. Often beginning near Christmas, an occurrence can last months or years.

elongation, lengthening or stretching.

emaciation /imā´sē·ā´shən/, extreme leanness caused by disease or lack of nutrition.

emancipated, being set free. Children may assume adult lives and responsibilities earlier than the age of consent, if they meet the criteria for independence established by each state. These criteria include military service, marriage, or other living arrangements separate from the parents, with their consent.

embayment, a large bay formed by a river bend or depression in the shoreline.

embolectomy /em´bōlek´-/, an incision made in an artery to remove an embolus.

embolism, an obstruction of blood flow due to a mass of undissolved matter lodging in a blood or lymph vessel. The mass (embolus) may be clotted blood, pieces of tissue, fat globules, air or other gas, foreign bodies such as bullets, or sheared bits of intravenous catheter. An obstruction of blood flow that persists more than a few minutes usually leads to varying degrees of tissue compromise, including infarction. An **air embolism** may occur when air enters the circulation from a needle or puncture wound. **Cerebral embolism** obstructs blood flow to a portion of the brain, as sometimes occurs in cerebrovascular accident (CVA). **Fat embolism** may occur, as after a fracture forces fat globules into the circulation. Expanding gas may block multiple vessels in **gas embolism,** as occurs in arterial gas embolism in scuba divers after pneumothorax. **Pulmonary embolism** decreases or obstructs pulmonary artery blood flow.

embolotherapy /em´bəlō-/, a method of blocking a blood vessel with a catheter that balloons at one end. It is used to treat bleeding ulcers and blood vessel defects. During surgery it is used to stop blood flow to a tumor.

embolus /em´bələs/, *pl.* **emboli,** a foreign object such as a bubble of air or gas, a bit of tissue, or a blood clot that travels through the bloodstream until it becomes lodged in a vessel. *See also thrombus.*

embouchure /äm´boo͞oshoor´/, **1.** the point where a river valley opens out onto a plain. **2.** the mouth of a river.

embryo /em´brē·ō/, in humans, the stage of growth between the time the fertilized egg is implanted in the uterus, which occurs about 2 weeks after conception, until the end of the seventh or eighth week of pregnancy. The period involves early growth of the major organ systems, and of the main external features. Compare **fetus.**

embryologic development, the stages in the growth and development of the embryo from the time of fertilization of the egg until about the eighth week of pregnancy. The stages are divided into two periods. The first is the formation of the embryo **(embryogenesis).** It occurs during the 10 days to 2 weeks after fertilization until the embryo is implanted in the wall of the uterus. The second period **(organogensis)** involves the growth of organs and organ systems during life in the womb. This stage occurs from about the end of the second week to the eighth week of pregnancy.

embryology /em´brē·ol´-/, the study of the origin, growth, and function of an organism from the time it is fertilized to birth.

embryonic layer /em´brē·on´ik/, one of the three layers of cells in the embryo: the endoderm, the mesoderm, and the ectoderm. From these layers, all of the structures and organs of the body grow.

emergency, an unexpected situation that arises suddenly and threatens the life or welfare of one or more persons (Latin, *emergere,* to raise up). *See also true emergency.*

emergency childbirth, childbirth that occurs unexpectedly and under less than optimum conditions. Maternal hypovolemia and infant hypothermia are major considerations. Risk of infection is also increased.

emergency department, section of a hospital that cares for medical and trauma emergencies. Staffed by physicians, nurses, and other technical staff, this department accepts both ambulance and walk-in patients. Whereas the department's primary focus is emergency care, it also serves as a referral area for primary physicians, an entrance for admission to the hospital, and occasionally a follow-up care center. It often has laboratory, surgical, and x-ray capabilities within the department. Also known as **ED, emergency room, ER.** *See also emergency room.*

emergency locator transmitter, an aircraft electronic device that, when activated, transmits a signal on emergency frequencies 121.50 and 243.0 megahertz. This signal alerts other aircraft and air traffic control towers to the presence of an aircraft emergency and general location of the aircraft in distress. Transmitter activation is manual or automatic (after an impact exceeding 4 g of force). Also known as **ELT.**

emergency medicine, medical specialty encompassing diagnosis and treatment of medical and trauma emergencies.

Emergency Medical Services, 1. concept of providing medical care during an emergency. This concept encompasses not only on-scene and transport medical care, but also includes 911/call screening, call dispatch, public education, vehicle maintenance, and hospital facilities. **2.** (informal) the systems organized to provide care during a medical or trauma emergency. Also known as **EMS.**

Emergency Medical Services System, the network of systems organized to provide all the services required for handling of out-of-hospital medical and trauma emergencies. These systems are organized at the local, regional, state, or national level. Important system components are communications, primary response (first response, basic, and advanced life support), transport, available hospital facilities, and public education. Also known as **EMSS.**

Emergency Medical Technician, 1. medical provider who generally performs prehospital medical care. The provider's level of medical capability is generally delineated by a qualifier added to the title, such as Emergency Medical Technician—Basic (National Registry). The Basic level of care is generally noninvasive and includes such skills as airway management, hemorrhage control, splinting, and patient packaging. The Intermediate-level caregiver provides all Basic skills plus intravenous infusion, noncardiac medications, and advanced airway skills. The Paramedic provider has additional capabilities, including cardiac rhythm interpretation, advanced pharmacology, and advanced-level assessment skills. Also known as **EMT.** See also paramedic. **2.** (informal) any provider of prehospital medical care.

emergency room, area of a hospital that cares for emergencies. This term is still in common usage, but it is usually inaccurate. Predating emergency departments, this location was not usually staffed full-time, those working there had no emergency medical education, and it was often no more than a holding area for admission to the hospital. Also known as **ER.** See also emergency department.

emergency telephone number. See 911, page 235.

emergent, 1. acute, sudden, unexpected. **2.** growing from a cavity, orifice, or other location.

emesis, 1. vomiting. See also emesis gravidarum, irritation emesis, nervous emesis, reflex emesis. **2.** the substance vomited.

emesis gravidarum /em´əsis grävidär´o͞om/, vomiting due to and/or during pregnancy.

emetic /imet´ik/, a substance that causes vomiting.

emissary veins /em´əser´ē/, the small vessels that connect the spaces in the dura with the veins on the outside of the skull.

emmetropia /em´ətrō´pē·ə/, the state of normal (20/20) vision. Compare **amblyopia, hyperopia, myopia. —emmetropic,** adj.

emotion, the feeling part of awareness as compared with thinking. Physical changes, such as illness, can come with changes in emotion, whether the feelings are conscious or not.

emotional abuse, harassment, humiliation, intimidation, and verbal assault.

emotional need, a psychologic need centered on such basic feelings as love, fear, anger, sorrow, anxiety, frustration, and depression. Such needs occur in everyone and become greater during times of stress and physical and mental illness, and at various stages of life, such as infancy, early childhood, and old age.

emotional response, a response to a certain feeling. It occurs with physical changes that may not be obvious. An example is crying as a response to death of a loved one.

emotional support, the sensitive, understanding approach that helps patients accept and deal with their illnesses. See also stages of dying.

empathy /em´pəthē/, the ability to know and, to some extent, share the emotions of another and to understand the meaning of that person's behavior. **–empathize,** v.

empennage /äm´pənäzh´, em´pənäzh´/, tail assembly of an aircraft, which includes elevators, rudders, and stabilizer.

emphysema, pulmonary overinflation and alveolar destruction, which causes loss of lung elasticity and poor exchange of gases. This condition is one of several chronic obstructive lung diseases. *See also asthma, asbestosis, black lung, bronchitis, chronic obstructive lung disease.*

emprosthotonos /em´prosthot´ənəs/, a position of the body in which it is stiffly bent forward at the waist. It is the result of long-term muscle spasm, most often seen with tetanus infection or strychnine poisoning.

empyema /em´pī·ē´mə/, purulent material in a body cavity, especially in the pleural space. It is caused by an infection, such as pleurisy or tuberculosis.

emulsify, to mix a liquid into another liquid, making a suspension that has globules of fat. Bile is an emulsifier in the digestive tract. An **emulsion** is a mix of two liquids, made so that small droplets are formed, as oil and water.

enamel, a hard white substance that covers a tooth.

enanthema /en´anthē´mə/, a sore on the surface of a mucous membrane.

encapsulated, referring to arteries, muscles, nerves, organs, and other body parts that are enclosed in fiber or membrane sheaths.

encapsulated source, radioactive material sealed in a container (needle, tube) that has sufficient strength to prevent breakage or leakage under the conditions of use for which it was designed. Also known as **sealed source.**

encephalitis /ensef´əlī´-/, *pl.* **encephalitides** /-tidēz/, an inflammation of the brain, primarily from infection that results from the bite of an infected mosquito. It may also be caused by lead or other poisoning, or bleeding.

encephalomyocarditis /-mī´əkärdī´-/, an infection of the brain, spinal cord, and cardiac tissue caused by a group of viruses. Rodents are a major source of the infection. Symptoms are generally similar to those of poliomyelitis.

encephalopathy /ensef´əlop´əthē/, any defect of the structure or function of brain tissues. It often refers to chronic defects in which there is a breakdown or death of tissue. **Acute necrotizing hemorrhagic encephalopathy** is a disorder that leads to brain tissue death. Typical signs are severe headache, fever, and vomiting. Seizures may occur.

encoder, a device that generates unique or unusual electrical signals, so as to be recognized by other receivers, as a means of activating or alerting particular devices or personnel.

encopresis /en´kōprē´-/, inability to control bowel movements. **–encopretic,** *adj.*

encyst /ensist´/, to form a cyst or capsule. *See also cyst.* **–encysted,** *adj.*

endarterectomy /en´därtərek´-/, a surgical procedure to remove the tunica intima of an artery that has become thickened by artherosclerosis.

endarteritis /en´därtərī´-/, a disease in which the inner layer of one or more arteries becomes inflamed. The arteries may be partially or completely blocked.

endemic /endem´ik/, a disease or infection common to a geographic area or population. *See also epidemic, pandemic.*

endocardial fibroelastosis /fī´brōē´lastō´-/, a defect in which the wall of the left ventricle becomes thick and fibrous. This often makes the capacity of the ventricle larger, but it may also make it smaller.

endocarditis /-kärdī´-/, a defect in which the endocardium and the heart valves become inflamed. **Bacterial endocarditis** is caused by various types of *Streptococcus* or *Staphylococcus*. This disease affects equal numbers of men and women of all ages. It causes heart murmurs in about 30% of the cases, and tends to affect the valves on the left side of the heart.

endocardium /-kär´dē·əm/, *pl.* **endocardia,** the lining of the atria and ventricles of the heart. It contains small blood vessels and smooth muscle. Compare **epicardium, myocardium.**

endocervix /-sur´viks/, the membrane lining the canal of the uterine cervix.

endocrine, **1.** an internal secretion. **2.** referring to a ductless gland that secretes directly into the bloodstream.

endocrine system, the network of ductless glands and other structures that secrete hormones into the bloodstream. Glands of the endocrine system include the thyroid and the parathyroid, the pituitary, the pancreas, the adrenal glands, and the gonads. The pineal gland is also thought of as an endocrine gland because it lacks ducts, although its precise function is not known. The thymus gland, once thought of as an endocrine gland, is now classed with the lymph system. Secretions from the endocrine glands affect a number of functions in the body, as in metabolism and growth, and secretions of other organs.

endocrinology /-krinol´-/, the study of the form and function of the endocrine system and the treatment of its problems.

endogenous /endoj´ənəs/, coming from inside the body, as a disease that is caused by failure of an organ. Compare **exogenous. —endogenic,** *adj.*

endolymph /en´dəlimf/, the fluid in the ducts of the inner ear. The endolymph carries sound waves to the ear drum and helps maintain balance.

endometrial /-mē´trē·əl/, referring to the cavity or lining of the uterus.

endometriosis /-mē´trē·ō´-/, a growth of endometrial tissue outside the uterus. The most typical symptom of endometriosis is pain, especially severe menstrual cramp and with bowel movements.

endometritis /-mitrī´-/, an inflammation of the endometrium often caused by infection. Symptoms include fever and abdominal pain. It occurs most often after childbirth or abortion and in women using an intrauterine contraceptive device. Endometritis may cause sterility because scars block the fallopian tubes. *See also pelvic inflammatory disease.*

endometrium /-mē´trē·əm/, the mucous membrane lining of the uterus, consisting of three layers. The endometrium changes thickness during the menstrual cycle. Two of the layers are shed with each menstrual flow. The third layer provides the surface for the placenta to attach to during pregnancy.

endomorph /en´dəmôrf/. See **somatotype.**

endophthalmitis /endof´thalmī´-/, inflammation of the inner eye. The eye becomes red, swollen, and painful. The vision is often blurred. There may be vomiting, fever, and headache. The cause may be bacterial or fungal, injury, allergy, or vascular disease.

endoplasmic reticulum, the circulatory system of the cell, consisting of canals throughout a cell's cytoplasm. Also known as **ER.**

endorphin /endôr´fin/, a substance of the nervous system. Endorphins are composed of amino acids. They are made by the pituitary gland and act on the nervous system to reduce pain. They produce effects like that of morphine. Compare **enkephalin.**

endoscopy /endos´kəpē/, examination of the inside of organs and cavities of the body with a special lighted device (endoscope).

endothelium /-thē´lē·əm/, the layer of cells that lines the heart, blood and lymph vessels, and fluid-filled cavities of the body. It is well supplied with blood and heals rapidly.

endothermic, 1. absorption of heat. **2.** storing up potential energy or heat.

endotracheal /-trā´kē·əl/, within or through the trachea.

endotracheal intubation, advanced airway management technique utilizing an endotracheal tube inserted through the mouth or nose into the trachea. This technique provides a patent airway, to allow the free flow of gases from outside the body into the lungs. It also permits medication administration, positive pressure ventilation, and suctioning, while preventing aspiration of blood or stomach contents. Types include digital (tactile), fiberoptic, oral, nasotracheal, retrograde, and transilluminated tracheal intubation. Also known as **ET intubation, intubation.**

endotracheal tube, plastic tube used to secure a patient's airway. Placed through the mouth or nose, this device may be used in conjunction with a laryngoscope and/or Magill forceps. A balloon located at the distal end of the tube is inflated to provide a seal between the lungs and outside environment. Also known as **ET tube.** *See also endotracheal intubation.*

endotracheal suctioning, removal of debris and foreign bodies from the bronchi though the use of suction via an endotracheal tube.

end tidal CO$_2$ detector, sensor device attached to an endotracheal tube, which detects the presence of carbon dioxide in expired air and records its presence. Adequacy of ventilation and proper placement of the endotracheal tube can generally be determined by this measurement, although it should not be the sole determinant of proper placement.

energy, the capacity to do work or to perform activity. **—energetic,** *adj.*

enervation, **1.** lack of energy; weakness. **2.** removal of a complete nerve or of a section of nerve.

engine, a firefighting vehicle designed to pump water at a fire scene. Although it may carry some water onboard, this apparatus receives most of its water from other sources, such as hydrants, lakes, pools, and tankers. *See also truck.*

engine company, a fire department unit consisting of an engine and at least two personnel.

engorgement, swelling or congestion of body tissues.

engulfment, the spread of a hazardous material after its release.

enhanced automaticity, accelerated cardiac depolarization, usually due to abnormal leakage of sodium ions into cardiac cells. Rapid rate dysrhythmias usually result.

enhanced 911, emergency telephone communications system utilizing a three-digit number that, when answered, provides an immediate computer listing of the address to which the number is listed.

enkephalin, a peptide in the central nervous system that acts as an analgesic.

enophthalmos /en´ofthal´məs/, a receding of the eye into the orbit. It is caused by an injury or birth defect.

enriched material, material in which the relative amount of one or more isotopes (naturally occurring) has been increased.

enteric coating /enter´ik/, a coating added to drugs taken by mouth that need to reach the intestine. The coating resists the effects of gastric acid, which can destroy certain drugs.

enteric infection, a disease of the intestine caused by any infection. Symptoms include diarrhea, stomach pain, nausea and vomiting, and loss of appetite. There may be a great loss of fluid from vomiting and diarrhea.

entericoid fever, a typhoidlike disease that causes fever and inflammation in the stomach and intestine. *See also typhoid fever.*

enteritis /en´tərī´-/, inflammation of the intestinal lining. Causes include bacteria, viruses, and some functional disorders. Compare **enterocolitis, gastroenteritis.**

Enterobacteriaceae /en´tərōbaktir´ē·ā´si·ē/, a family of bacteria that includes Salmonella.

enterocolitis /-kōlī-/, an inflammation of both the large and small intestines. *See also necrotizing enterocolitis.*

enterokinase /-kī´nās/, a substance in the intestine that helps the body absorb protein.

enterolithiasis /-lithī´əsis/, the presence of stones (enteroliths) in the intestine.

enterostomy, a surgically created permanent opening into the intestine through the abdominal wall.

enterovirus, a virus that lives primarily in the intestinal tract. Kinds of enteroviruses are **coxsackievirus, echovirus, poliovirus.**

entrapment, the state of being caught or trapped. Also known as **pinned.**

entropion /entrō´pē·on/, a turning inward of the edge of the eyelid toward the eye.

enucleation /ēnōō´klē·ā´shən/, **1.** removal of an organ or tumor in one piece. **2.** removal of the eye.

enuresis /en´yōōrē´-/, inability to control the need to urinate, especially in bed at night.

envenomation, poisoning caused by an animal bite, typically a snake or jellyfish.

environmental hazard, condition capable of posing an unreasonable risk to air, plant, soil, water, and/or wildlife quality.

environmental health, all of the aspects in and around a community that affect the health of the population.

environmental information, the label of a hazardous material may provide information on both the storage and disposal of the product and the environmental or wildlife hazards that could occur. This information can be most useful when planning cleanup and disposal after a fire or spill.

enzyme, a protein produced in the cells that causes chemical reactions in organic matter.

enzyme poisons, those substances that inhibit cellular reactions by competing with or altering the enzymes necessary to catalyze those reactions.

eosinophil /ē´əsin´əfil/, a two-lobed white blood cell (leukocyte). Eosinophils make up 1% to 3% of the white blood cells of the body. They increase in number with allergy and some infections. Compare **basophil, neutrophil.**

eosinophilia /-fil´yə/, an increase in the number of eosinophils in the blood. This occurs in allergies and many conditions with inflammation.

eosinophilic leukemia, a cancer of white blood cells, mainly eosinophils. It resembles chronic myelocytic leukemia but is more acute. *See also leukemia.*

EPA establishment number, the location where a hazardous material product was manufactured.

EPA registration number, required for all pesticide products marketed in the United States. It is one of three ways to positively identify a pesticide. The others are by the product name or chemical ingredient statement. The registration number will appear as a two- or three-section number. A U.S. Department of Agriculture number may appear on products registered before 1970.

ephapse /ef´aps/, a point of side-to-side contact between nerve fibers. Nerve signals may be passed through the walls of the nerves rather than the synapse between the ends of two nerves. This may be a factor in epileptic seizures. Compare **synapse.**

epicanthus /ep´ikan´thəs/, a vertical fold of skin over the inner corner of the eye. It may be slight or marked. Also known as **epicanthal fold.**

epicardium /-kär´dē·əm/, the outer layer of tissue that forms the wall of the heart. *See also myocardium.*

epicondyle /-kon´dəl/, a projection at the end of a bone.

epicranium /-krā´nē·əm/, the complete scalp, including the skin, muscles, and tendon sheets.

epicranius /-krā´nē·əs/, the muscle and tendon layer covering the superior and lateral skull from the posterior head to the eyebrows. It consists of broad, thin muscles connected by an extensive tendon sheet. Branches of the facial nerves can draw back the scalp, raise the eyebrows, and move the ears.

epidemic, a disease that occurs clearly in excess of the normal incidence of the disease, as at a military base or in a town. Compare **endemic, pandemic.**

epidemiologist /-dem´ē·ol´-/, a physician or scientist who studies the frequency and distribution, prevention, and control of disease in a community or a group of persons.

epidermis /-dur´mis/, the outer layers of the skin. It is made up of an outer, dead portion and a deeper, living portion. Epidermal cells gradually move outward to the skin surface, changing as they go. Also known as **cuticle. –epidermal, epidermoid,** *adj.*

epididymis /-did´imis/, *pl.* **epididymides,** one of a pair of long, tightly coiled tubes that carry sperm from the testicles to the tip of the penis. An **appendix epididymidis** is a cyst sometimes found on the epididymis.

epididymitis /-did´imī´-/, inflammation of the tubes (epididymides) that carry sperm from the testicles to the penis. It may result from venereal disease, urinary tract infection, or removal of the prostate.

epididymoorchitis /-did´imō·ôrkī´-/, inflammation of the testicles and the tubes (epididymides) that carry sperm from the testicles to the penis.

epidural /-door´əl/, outside the dura mater.

epigastric node /-gas´trik/, a lymph node in one of the groups that serve the stomach, intestine, and pelvis. *See also lymphatic system, lymph node.*

epiglottis, leaf-shaped structure located posterior to the base of the tongue. It covers the tracheal entrance as swallowing occurs but generally remains open to allow free passage of air into the lungs.

epiglottitis /-glotī´-/, inflammation of the epiglottis. **Acute epiglottitis** affects mostly children, usually between 2 and 7 years of age. Symptoms include fever, sore throat, croupy cough, an inability to swallow, drooling, and shortness of breath.

epilepsy. See **seizure disorders.**

epinephrine, a natural catecholamine used in the presence of allergic reaction and anaphylaxis, asthma, and such cardiac dysrhythmias as asystole, bradycardias, and ventricular fibrillation. This agent causes bronchodilation, increased AV conduction, contractility, heart rate, and vasoconstriction. Side effects include supraventricular tachycardia and ventricular irritability.

epiphyseal fracture /-fiz´ē·əl/, a fracture at the end of a long bone where bone growth occurs. This results in separation of the head of the bone.

epiphyseal line, the junction of epiphysis and bone. *See also epiphyseal plate.*

epiphyseal plate, the location of bone growth between the head and shaft of a bone. Once the bone stops growing, the plate is obliterated.

epiphysis /ipif´isis/, *pl.* **epiphyses,** the rounded head of a long bone, as in the arm or leg. During childhood it is separated from the shaft of the bone by the growth plate where bone growth occurs. When the bone stops growing, the growth plate becomes solid. Compare **diaphysis. –epiphyseal,** *adj.*

episcleritis /-sklerī´-/, inflammation of the outer layers of the sclera.

episiotomy /epē´zē·ot´əmē/, an incision performed to enlarge the opening of the vagina. This is done during childbirth to aid in delivery and prevent stretching of the mother's muscles and connective tissues. Such stretching is thought to cause the bladder and uterus to relax and so decrease their ability to function. The incision is closed after the baby is delivered.

episode, an incident that stands out from everyday life, as an episode of illness.

episodic care, a type of medical service in which care is given to a person for a certain problem. The patient does not remain for continued care. Emergency departments provide episodic care.

epistaxis, nosebleed.

epithalamus /-thal´əməs/, a part of the brain that transmits nerve signals for the senses and movement.

epithelium, the layer of cells that covers external and internal body surfaces, such as epidermis, mucous membrane. This layer protects surfaces and allows absorption and secretion of necessary substances.

epizootic /ep´izō·ot´ik/, an animal living as a parasite on the surface of another animal.

Epstein-Barr virus, the herpes virus that causes mononucleosis ("kissing disease"). Also known as **EBV.**

equilibrium, **1.** a state of balance caused by the equal action of opposing forces, such as calcium and phosphorus in the body. **2.** a state of mental or emotional balance. **3.** the ability to maintain the sense of balance.

Erb's palsy, a kind of paralysis caused by injury to the nerves of the brachial plexus. It occurs most often in infants during delivery. Symptoms include numbness in the arm and paralysis and wasting of the muscles.

erectile /irek´til/, capable of being raised to an erect position.

ergonomics, the science of designing job tasks and equipment so as to enhance human efficiency and health. Traits of human anatomy, physiology, and psychology are factored into design considerations.

ergot alkaloid, one of a large group of alkaloids found in the common fungus *Claviceps purpurea.* This fungus grows on rye and other grains.

erosion, the wearing away or slow destruction of a tissue. Erosion may be caused by infection, injury, or other disease. It usually occurs with an ulcer. Also known as **sloughing.** *See also necrosis.*

eructation, the act of bringing up air from the stomach with a typical sound. Also known as **belching.**

eruption, the rapid growth of a skin rash, especially one caused by a virus or by a drug reaction.

erysipelas /er´isip´ələs/, a skin infection (cellulitis) with redness, swelling, blisters, fever, pain, and swollen lymph nodes. It is caused by streptococci.

erysipeloid /-loid/, an infection of the hands marked by red and blue-red patches. It is caused by handling meat or fish infected with *Erysipelothrix rhusiopathiae.* Also known as **fish-handler's disease.**

erythema /er´ithē´mə/, reddening of the skin or mucous membranes. It is the result of dilation of capillaries near the skin surface. Examples of erythema are nervous blushes and mild sunburn.

erythema infectiosum, an acute infection, primarily of children. Symptoms include fever and a rash beginning on the cheeks and appearing later on the arms, thighs, buttocks, and trunk. As the rash spreads, previous areas fade. Sunlight worsens the rash. It usually lasts about 10 days. Also known as **fifth disease.**

erythema multiforme, an allergic condition with a rash on the skin and mucous membranes. A variety of sizes and shapes appear on the patient (multiforme) and include nodules, blisters, and bull's-eye-shaped areas.

erythema nodosum, an allergy causing vascular inflammation. It causes reddened, tender nodes on both legs, mild fever and pains in muscles and joints. This condition occurs with streptococcal infections, tuberculosis, sarcoidosis, drug allergy, ulcerative colitis, and pregnancy.

erythrasma /er´ithraz´mə/, a bacterial skin infection of the axilla or groin regions. There are irregular, reddish-brown raised patches. It is more common in diabetics.

erythroblastosis fetalis /irith´rəblastō´sis fētā´lis/, a type of anemia that occurs in newborns who have Rh positive blood, but whose mothers are Rh negative. *See also Rh factor.*

erythrocyte /irith´rəsīt´/, a red blood cell. It is a concave disk, microscopic in size, and contains hemoglobin. As the main component of the circulating blood, its main function is to transport oxygen, which is carried by the hemoglobin. Kinds of erythrocytes include **burr cell, discocyte, macrocyte, meniscocyte, spherocyte.** Also known as **red blood cell, red cell, red corpuscle.**

erythrocytosis /-ō´sis/, an abnormal rise in the number of circulating red cells. *See also polycythemia.*

erythroleukemia /-lo͞okē´mē·ə/, a malignant blood disorder marked by an excess production of red blood cells in bone marrow. Also known as **diGuglielmo's disease.**

erythropoiesis /-pō·ē´sis/, the process of red blood cell (erythrocyte) production. The bone marrow produces cells with nuclei. These cells mature into erythrocytes without nuclei that contain hemoglobin. *See also erythrocyte, hemoglobin.*

erythropoietin /erith´rōpō·ē´tin/, a hormone produced in the kidneys. It is released into the bloodstream in response to low oxygen levels. The hormone controls the production of red blood cells (erythrocytes) and is thus able to raise the oxygen-carrying capacity of the blood. *See also erythropoiesis.*

escape beat, an automatic electrical discharge from a natural pacemaker site when the dominant cardiac rhythm pauses for a period of time longer than the inherent rate of slower cardiac pacemaker cells. The EKG will show a QRS complex occurring after the time the normal cardiac complex should have occurred.

escape rhythms, cardiac electrical rhythms that result when a higher (faster) cardiac pacemaker site fails to discharge regularly. Junctional and ventricular rhythms may be seen when sinus and atrial pacemakers are affected. *See also escape beat.*

eschar /es´kär/, a scab or dry crust resulting from a burn, infection, or skin disease.

Escherichia coli /esh´irī´kē·ə kō´lī/, a species of bacteria of the family Enterobacteriaceae. *E. coli* normally lives in the intestines and is common in water, milk, and soil. It causes urinary tract and wound infection.

eskimo roll, a self-rescue technique practiced by kayakers to allow righting of a capsized boat.

esophageal gastric tube airway, an airway device that occludes the esophagus and allows airflow into the trachea. Air is prevented from entering the stomach, and gastric contents are prevented from entering the lungs. A nasogastric tube may be inserted through the device to decompress the stomach of air and fluids. Also known as an **E.G.T.A.**

esophageal obturator airway, an airway device that occludes the esophagus and allows airflow into the trachea. Air is prevented from entering the stomach, and gastric contents are prevented from entering the lungs. Also known as an **EOA.**

esophageal varices, a network of twisted veins at the lower end of the esophagus. It is enlarged and swollen as the result of high pressure within the portal vein in the abdomen. These vessels often form open sores and bleed. This is often a complication of cirrhosis of the liver.

esophagectomy /ēsof´əjek´-/, an operation in which all or part of the esophagus is removed. This may be required to treat severe, recurrent, bleeding esophageal varices.

esophagitis /-jī´tis/, inflammation of the lining of the esophagus. Causes include gastric reflux, infection, and irritation. *See also reflux.*

esophagoscopy /-gos´kəpē/, examination of the esophagus with an endoscope.

esophagus /ēsof´əgəs/, the muscular canal, 9½ inches long (about 24 cm), extending from below the tongue to the stomach. The esophagus is fibrous and muscular and is lined with mucous membrane. **–esophageal,** *adj.*

esophoria /es′əfôr′ē·ə/, deviation of one eye toward the other eye when the eyes are not focused on an object. Compare **strabismus.**

ester /es′tər/, a class of chemical compounds formed by an alcohol bonding to one or more organic acids. Fats are esters, formed by the bonding of fatty acids with the alcohol glycerol.

estrogen /es′trojən/, one of a group of hormonal steroid compounds that aid in the development of female secondary sex traits (such as breast development). Human estrogen is produced in the ovaries, adrenal glands, testicles, and both the fetus and placenta. Estrogen prepares the wall of the uterus for fertilization, implantation, and nutrition of the embryo after each menstrual period. **–estrogenic,** *adj.*

ethanol, ethyl alcohol, a colorless, flammable liquid that is a product of grain fermentation and distillation. Also known as **ETOH.**

ethmoid bone /eth′moid/, the spongy bone at the base of the skull that forms the walls of the superior portion of the nasal cavity.

ethyl alcohol. See **alcohol.**

ethyl oxide, a colorless liquid solvent similar to diethyl ether, widely used in pharmaceutical production.

etiology /ē′tē·ol′-/, the study of all factors that may be involved in the development of a disease. This includes the condition of the patient, the cause, and the way in which the patient's body is affected.

eukaryocyte /yoōker′ē·əsīt′/, a cell with a true nucleus. These cells are formed in all higher organisms and in some microorganisms.

eukaryon /yoōker′ē·on/, **1.** a nucleus in a cell that is very complex, organized, and surrounded by a nuclear membrane. Eukaryons usually occur only in higher organisms. **2.** an organism containing a very complex, organized nucleus surrounded by a nuclear membrane. This is typical of all organisms except bacteria, viruses, and blue-green algae.

euphoretic /yoō′fəret′ik/, **1.** a substance or event tending to produce a condition of euphoria, such as LSD, mescaline, and marijuana.

euphoria /yoōfôr′ē·ə/, **1.** a feeling of well-being or elation. **2.** a greater than normal sense of physical and emotional well-being. It is not based on reality, is out of proportion to its cause, and is inappropriate to the situation. This is commonly seen in some forms of mental disorders, poisoning, and in drug-induced states.

euploid /yoō′ploid/, **1.** referring to a person, organism, or cell with a chromosome number that is an exact multiple of the normal (haploid) number of the species. Diploid refers to two sets of chromosomes, triploid to having three, tetraloid to four, and polyploid to over two sets.

eupnea, normal respiration.

eustachian tube /yoōstā′shən, -stā′kē·ən/, a tube lined with mucous membrane that joins the nasopharynx and the inner ear. This tube allows air pressure in the inner ear to be equalized with the outside air pressure. Also known as **auditory tube.**

euthanasia /yoō′thənā′zhə/, deliberately bringing about the death of a person who is suffering from an incurable disease. Euthanasia can be performed actively, such as by giving a lethal drug, or by allowing the person to die by not giving treatment. Also known as **mercy killing.**

evacuate, **1.** to empty. **2.** to move patients or victims to a place of safety.

evaporation, the change of a substance from a solid or liquid state to a gas. *See also boiling point.* **–evaporate,** *v.*

eversion, turning outward.

Eve's method (F. C. Eve, British physician, 1871–1952), *(historical)* now obsolete method of manual artificial respiration. The victim was laid facedown with wrists and ankles tied to the stretcher, arms above the head. The stretcher was suspended approximately 34 inches (77 cm) above the ground so that the head and feet could be alternately lowered to a 45° angle at a rate of twelve cycles per minute. *See also artificial respiration.*

evisceration /ivis′ərā′shən/, **1.** the removal of the viscera from the abdominal cavity; disembowelment. **2.** the removal of the contents from an organ or an organ from its cavity. **3.** bulging of an internal organ through a wound or incision, especially in the abdominal wall. **–eviscerate,** *v.*

evocator, a specific chemical or hormone that is produced by embryonic tissue. The substance stimulates the embryo to grow and change.

evolution, 1. cycle; job; mission; procedure; step. **2.** an orderly, continual process involving gradual change or development from a simple to a complex state.

exacerbation /igzas´ərbā´shən/, an increase in the seriousness of a disease or disorder. It is marked by greater intensity in the symptoms.

exanthema /ig´zanthē´mə/, a rash that often has the specific features of an infectious disease. Chickenpox, measles, roseola infantum, or rubella usually have particular types of exanthema.

excavation, 1. a depression or hollow. **2.** the formation of a cavity. **3.** an opening in the ground that results from digging.

excise /iksīz´/, to remove completely, as surgically removing the tonsils.

excitability, the property of a cell that allows it to react to irritation or stimulation.

excoriation /ekskôr´ē·ā´shən/, an injury to the surface of the skin or other part of the body caused by scratching or scraping. **–excoriate,** v.

excreta /ekskrē´tə/, any waste matter discharged from the body; feces or urine.

excrete /ekskrēt´/, to remove a waste substance from the body, often through normal secretion, such as a drug excreted in urine. **–excretion,** n.

excretion, 1. elimination of waste products from the body. **2.** the waste products eliminated from the body.

excretory /eks´kretôr´ē/, relating to the process of excretion.

excretory duct, a duct that conducts waste substances.

exercise, any action or skill that exerts the muscles and is performed repeatedly in order to condition the body, improve health, or maintain fitness. *See also aerobic exercise, anaerobic exercise.*

exfoliation, peeling and flaking of tissue cells. This is a normal process of the skin that occurs constantly. Exfoliation may be often seen in certain skin diseases or after a severe sunburn. *See also desquamation.*

exfoliative dermatitis, any skin inflammation in which there is too much peeling or shedding of skin. Causes include drug reactions, scarlet fever, leukemia, and lymphoma.

exhale, to breathe out. **–exhalation,** n.

exhibitionism, the flaunting of oneself or one's abilities in order to attract attention.

exocrine /ek´səkrin/, referring to the process of releasing outwardly through a duct to the surface of an organ or tissue or into a vessel. Compare **endocrine system.** *See also eccrine.*

exocrine gland, any of a group of glands that open on the surface of the skin, organ, or into a vessel through ducts. These glands secrete specialized substances. Examples are the sweat and sebaceous glands of the skin, and the salivary glands in the mouth. Exocrine glands are also found in the kidney, digestive tract, and mammary glands. *See also apocrine gland.*

exogenous /igzoj´ənəs/, beginning outside the body or an organ of the body or produced from external causes. For example, a disease caused by bacteria or a virus is exogenous. Compare **endogenous. –exogenic,** adj.

exophoria /ek´səfôr´ē·ə/, deviation of one eye to the side. This occurs when the eyes are at rest. When focusing on an object, the deviation disappears. *See also strabismus.* **–exophoric,** adj.

exophthalmia /ek´softhal´mē·ə/, bulging of the eyes (exopthalmos). Causes include a tumor pushing outward, bleeding or edema of the brain or eye, paralysis or injury to the eye muscles, an overactive thyroid gland, and varicose veins in the orbit.

exophytic /-fit´ik/, the tendency to grow outward, as an exophytic tumor grows on the surface of an organ or structure.

exothermic, a chemical reaction that produces heat.

exotropia /-trō´pē·ə/. See **strabismus.**

expected date of confinement, the predicted date of a pregnant woman's delivery. Also known as **due date, EDC.**

expectorant, referring to a substance that aids in coughing up mucus or other fluids from the lungs. Also known as **mucolytic. –expectorate,** v.

expectoration, removing mucus, sputum or fluids from the throat and lungs by coughing or spitting.

expiration, **1.** breathing out. Compare **inspiration.** **2.** termination or death. –**expire,** *v.*

expiratory reserve volume /ekspī´rətôr´ē/, the largest amount of air that can be forced out of the lungs after a normal breath. Also known as **ERV.**

explosion, any sudden, violent release of chemical, mechanical, thermal, or nuclear energy.

explosive limit, the point above or below which a vapor will not explode. Above the upper explosive limit, the mixture is too rich to burn or explode. Below the lower explosive limit, its concentration is too lean. Also known as **explosive range, flammable limit, flammable range.**

exposure, **1.** illness due to prolonged contact, without adequate protection, with environments that are too cold or hot for normal human activity. **2.** in the vicinity of disease or other hazards without having necessarily been in contact with the organism or substance. **3.** the structures that face, but are not necessarily involved in, a fire. **4.** the face of a cliff or mountain from which a climb or rescue must take place.

exposure hazard, hazard existing from the inhalation, ingestion, or absorption of the material involved.

expressed consent, informed consent. *See also consent.*

expression, **1.** the indication of a physical or emotional state through facial appearance or tone of voice. **2.** the act of pressing or squeezing in order to expel something.

exsanguination, **1.** deprivation of blood. **2.** death from hemorrhage.

extended care facility, an institution devoted to providing medical, nursing, or custodial care over a long period of time. Also known as **convalescent home, nursing home.**

extended family, a family group consisting of the parents, their children, the grandparents, and other family members. The extended family is the basic family group in many societies.

extension, an increase in the angle between two adjoining bones, as extending the leg increases the angle between the thigh and the calf. Compare **flexion.**

extensor, one of the muscles of the forearm or of the calf of the leg.

external, **1.** being on the outside of the body or an organ. **2.** acting from the outside. **3.** referring to the outward or visible appearance. Compare **internal.**

external cardiac massage, technique of artificial circulation, in which blood flow is produced in limited amounts by compression of the anterior chest wall. Done manually or mechanically, the increase in intrathoracic pressure can move up to 33% of the body's normal blood flow. When combined with artificial respiration, these techniques constitute cardiopulmonary resuscitation. Also known as **ECM.** *See also cardiac massage, cardiopulmonary resuscitation.*

external exposure, exposure of a person by radiation originating from a radiation source outside the body.

external jugular vein, one of a pair of large blood vessels in the neck that drain most of the blood from the surface of the skull and deep tissues of the face. Also used as an intravenous insertion site when more peripheral veins are inaccessible. Also known as **EJ, XJ.**

external pacing, the use of an artificial pacemaker to provide electrical cardiac stimulation via electrodes placed on the chest and back. This technique may be used in cases of asystole, symptomatic bradycardia or heart block, and pacemaker failure. Also known as **transcutaneous pacing.**

exteroceptive /eks´tərōsep´tiv/, stimulation that comes from outside the body. The term also refers to the nerves that are stimulated by outside events. Compare **interoception, proprioception.**

extracellular /-sel´yələr/, outside a cell in spaces between cell layers. *See also cell, interstitial.*

extracellular fluid, the part of the body fluid outside the tissue cells. This includes interstitial fluid and blood plasma. The adult body contains nearly 3 gallons (11.2 liters) of interstitial fluid. This accounts for about 16% of body weight. In addition, there are about 3 quarts (2.8 liters) of plasma, which is about 4% of body weight.

Plasma and interstitial fluid are very similar chemically and help control the movement of water and electrolytes throughout the body.

extracorporeal /-kôrpôr´ē·əl/, outside the body, as extracorporeal circulation in which venous blood is routed outside the body to a heart-lung machine and returned to the body through an artery.

extract, 1. to pull or remove forcibly. 2. a preparation made by removing the soluble part of a compound, by using alcohol or water, and then evaporating the solution. 3. the active portion of a drug that was obtained by chemical process or distillation; can be a powder or liquid.

extraction, the process of leaving, removing, or withdrawing. *See also insertion 2.*

extradural /-do͞or´əl/, outside the dura mater.

extraocular /-ok´yələr/, outside the eye.

extraocular muscle palsy, paralysis of the eye muscles. This may affect the following muscles: the superior, inferior, medial, and lateral rectus muscles, and the superior and the inferior oblique muscles. *See also strabismus.*

extraperitoneal /-per´itōnē´əl/, occurring or located outside the peritoneal cavity. The peritoneal cavity is formed by a membrane (peritoneum) lining the abdominal and pelvic walls and covering the organs.

extrapyramidal disease, any of a large group of conditions with uncontrolled movement and changes in muscle tone and abdominal posture. Disorders such as tardive dyskinesia, chorea, athetosis, and Parkinson's disease are extrapyramidal diseases.

extrapyramidal reaction, sudden impairment of muscle tone due to an adverse reaction to neuroleptic medications. Primary symptoms involve rigidity or distortion of head, face, and/or neck musculature. Although painful, the impairment is not life-threatening, but it can be mistaken by the inexperienced for psychotic behavior. The medications that are usually responsible include the phenothiazines (chlorpromazine, promethazine, thioridazine) and butyrophenones (haloperidol). Also known as **acute dystonia, acute dystonic reaction, phenothiazine reaction.**

extrapyramidal system, the part of the nervous system that controls movement. These nerves include the basal ganglia, substantia nigra, subthalamic nucleus, part of the midbrain, and the motor neurons of the spine.

extrapyramidal tracts, the tracts of nerves from the brain to the spinal cord that coordinate and control movement. Within the brain, the extrapyramidal tracts are nerve relays between the many motor areas of the brain. The extrapyramidal tracts are functional rather than anatomic units. They control and coordinate posture, position, support, and locomotor mechanisms. The tracts cause contractions of muscle groups in sequence or at the same time. Compare **pyramidal tract.**

extrasystole, a premature cardiac complex originating somewhere in the heart other than in the SA node. Also known as an **ectopic,** a **PAC, PJC, premature atrial contraction, premature junctional contraction, premature ventricular contraction, PVC.** *See also ectopic, premature atrial contraction, premature junctional contraction, premature ventricular contraction.*

extrauterine /-yo͞o´tərin/, occurring or located outside the uterus, as is an ectopic pregnancy.

extravasation, the escape of fluid into surrounding tissue.

extremity, 1. the terminal portion of anything. 2. an arm or leg.

extrication, 1. accessing and removing, through use of force, a patient who is actively restrained by an object, such as fallen material or the structural components of machinery or vehicles. 2. to free from confinement or danger. *See also rescue.*

extrication collar, a semirigid immobilization device, made of stiffened plastic and foam, that encircles the neck and serves to provide head support and to restrain neck movement when spinal injury is suspected. One part of a complete immobilization system, this device is inadequate for total spinal immobilization. *See also immobilization.*

extrication officer, the person in the incident command system responsible for supervising the removal of entrapped victims.

extrication sector, the section within the incident command system responsible for removal of trapped victims.

extroversion /-vurˊzhən/, **1.** the tendency to direct one's interests and energies toward things outside the self. A person who is outgoing is known as an **extrovert. 2.** the state of being primarily concerned with what is outside the self. Compare **introversion.**

extubation, removal of a tube from the orifice it occupies.

exudate /eksˊyədāt/, fluid, cells, or other substances that have been slowly discharged though small pores or breaks in cell membranes. Perspiration, purulent drainage, and serum are sometimes called exudates.

exudative /igzo͞oˊdətiv/, relating to the oozing of fluid and other materials from cells and tissues, usually as a result of inflammation or injury.

eye, one of a pair of organs of sight, located in bony hollows at the front of the skull. The eyes are embedded in fat and supplied by one pair of optic nerves from the forebrain. Structures associated with the eye are the muscles, fascia, eyebrow, eyelids, conjunctiva, and the lacrimal gland. The eye has three layers that enclose two spaces separated by the lens. The smaller space in front of the lens is divided by the iris into two chambers, both filled with aqueous humor. The posterior chamber is larger than the anterior chamber and contains the jelly-like vitreous body. The outside layer of the eye consists of the transparent cornea in the front, which makes up one fifth of the layer. The lens, which is just behind the cornea, and the cornea focus images onto the retina. The sclera makes up the other five sixths of the outer layer. The middle layer is supplied with blood and consists of the choroid under the sclera, the ciliary body which focuses the lens, and the iris which controls the amount of light entering the eye. The inner layer of nervous tissue is the retina. Light waves passing thorough the lens strike a layer of rods and cones in the retina, creating impulses that are carried by the optic nerve to the brain.

eyebrow, **1.** the arch of bone over the eye that separates the eye socket from the forehead. **2.** the arch of hairs growing along the ridge of the bony arch.

eyeground, the posterior (fundus) of the eye. *See also funduscopy.*

eyelid, a moveable fold of skin over the eye.

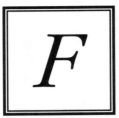

Fab fragment, portion of an immunoglobulin molecule that binds a specific antigen. Several specific antidotes for drug toxicity are being developed from this material. Also known as **Fab piece.**

face, **1.** anterior portion of the head from forehead to chin and laterally to the ears. **2.** to turn toward a specific direction. **3.** the exposed portion of a mountain, usually sheer in nature and composed of rock. **4.** the smooth, upright surface of a dam.

face presentation, presentation of a fetus's forehead as the first part of the body to enter the birth canal, during delivery.

facial artery, one of a pair of arteries that arise from the external carotid arteries. They divide into four neck and five facial branches, and supply the tissues in the head.

facial muscle, the five groups of facial muscles which include the muscles of the scalp, ear, nose, eyelid, and mouth. Also known as **muscle of expression.**

facial nerve, either of a pair of sensory and motor nerves that arise from the brainstem. Also known as **seventh cranial nerve.**

facial vein, one of a pair of veins that drain blood from the facial surface.

facies /fā´shi·ēz/, *pl.* **facies,** **1.** the face. **2.** the surface of any body structure, part, or organ. **3.** the face's expression or appearance.

facilitated diffusion, biochemical process that selectively moves substances across semipermeable membranes from a higher to a lower concentration via catalyst proteins.

factor of safety, the ratio between the breaking stress of a material and the greatest stress to which it will be subjected.

factor I. See **fibrinogen.**

factor II. See **prothrombin.**

factor III. See **thromboplastin.**

factor IV, a term for calcium as an element in the process of blood clotting.

factor V, a blood clotting factor that occurs in normal plasma but is lacking in patients with parahemophilia. It is needed to change prothrombin to thrombin. Also known as **proaccelerin.**

factor VII, a clotting factor in the blood plasma and broken down in the liver when vitamin K is present. Also known as **proconvertin.**

factor VIII, a clotting factor in normal plasma but lacking in patients with hemophilia A. It is composed of two separate substances. The lack of one substance results in hemophilia A, and the lack of the other results in Von Willebrand's disease. Also known as **antihemophilic globulin.** *See also antihemophilic factor.*

factor IX, a blood clotting factor in normal plasma but lacking in patients with hemophilia B. Also known as **Christmas factor.**

factor X, a clotting factor that occurs in normal plasma. Factor X is made in the liver when vitamin K is present. Also known as **Stuart-Power factor.**

factor XI, a blood clotting factor in normal plasma. A lack of it results in a blood clotting disease (hemophilia C). Also known as **plasma thromboplastin antecedent.**

factor XII, a blood clotting factor in normal plasma. Also known as **activation factor.**

factor XIII, a blood clotting factor in normal plasma. It acts with calcium to make protein (fibrin) clot. Also known as **fibrinase, fibrin stabilizing factor.**

faculty, any normal function or ability of a living organism, as being able to sense and recognize sense stimulations.

Fahrenheit (Gabriel D. Fahrenheit, German-Dutch physicist, 1686-1736), scale for measuring temperature, in the English system of weights and measures, in which the boiling point of water is 212° and the freezing point is 32° at sea level (1 atmosphere of pressure). Also known as **F.** Compare **Celsius.**

failure to thrive, inadequate growth of an infant (or elderly person). Causes include birth defects, major organ system defects, sudden illness, malnutrition and psychologic or social factors, as maternal deprivation syndrome.

faint, *(informal)* to lose consciousness, as in fainting (psychogenic shock). *See also syncope.*

fallopian tube /fəlō´pē·ən/, one of a pair of tubes opening at one end into the uterus and at the other end into the cavity over the ovary. Each tube is the passage through which an egg (ovum) is carried to the uterus and through which sperm travel toward the ovary. Also known as **oviduct, uterine tube.**

fallout, the spread of radioactive waste after the release of radioisotopes.

false imprisonment, confining someone without their consent or following proper legal procedure.

false labor, irregular tightening of the pregnant uterus that begins during the first three months of pregnancy. The contractions increase in time, length, and strength as pregnancy continues. Near the end of pregnancy, strong false labor may be confused with the contractions of true labor. Also known as **Braxton Hicks contraction.**

false negative, an incorrect result of a medical test or procedure that fails to indicate the presence of the condition or disease being tested for.

false positive, a test result that incorrectly shows the presence of a disease or other condition.

familial, referring to the prevalence of a disease in some families and not in others, usually but not always hereditary. Compare **acquired, congenital, hereditary.**

family, 1. a group of people related by heredity, as parents, children, and brothers and sisters. The term sometimes includes persons living in the same household or those related by marriage. 2. a category of animals or plants. Humans are members of the genus *Homo,* which is a part of the hominid family which, in turn, is a part of the primate order of mammals. *See also genetics, heredity.*

family history, the health of the members of the patient's family, used to determine diseases for which the patient may be at high risk.

family medicine, the branch of medicine that is concerned with the diagnosis and treatment of health problems in people of either sex and any age. Physicians who practice family medicine are often called family practice physicians, family physicians, or, formerly, general practitioners.

Fanconi's syndrome, a group of disorders including kidney disease, marked by weakened bones, excess acid in the urine, and low blood potassium. One form, idiopathic Fanconi's syndrome, is inherited and usually appears in early middle age. Another is acquired and is usually the result of poisoning from many sources, including the use of outdated tetracycline.

fantasy, 1. the completely free play of the imagination; fancy. 2. the mental process of changing undesirable experiences into imagined events to fulfill a wish, need, or desire, or to express unconscious conflicts, as a daydream.

farmer's lung, a pulmonary disorder caused by breathing dusts from moldy hay. It is a form of pneumonitis affecting individuals who have developed an allergy to mold spores. Symptoms include coughing, nausea, chills and fever.

farsightedness, an eyesight disorder caused by an error of refraction in which vision of distant objects is sharper, more focused than that of near objects. Also known as **hyperopia.**

fascia /fash´ē·ə/, *pl.* **fasciae,** fiberlike connective tissue of the body that may be separated from other structures, as the tendons and the ligaments. It varies in thickness and weight and in the amounts of fat, fiber, and tissue fluid it contains. **–fascial,** *adj.*

fascia bulbi, a thin membrane that surrounds the eye from the optic nerve to the pupil and allows the eye to move freely.

fascial compartment, a part of the body that is walled off by fiberlike (fascial) membranes. It usually contains a muscle or group of muscles or an organ, as the heart is contained in the mediastinum.

fasciculation, uncontrollable muscle tremor, classically seen in snake envenomations. Less commonly, these tremors may be noted in cold injuries, seizures, and toxic drug ingestion.

fasciculus /fəsik´yələs/, *pl.* **fasciculi,** a small bundle of muscle, tendon, or nerve fibers. The shape of fasciculi in a muscle is related to the power of the muscle and its range of motion. **–fascicular,** *adj.*

fascioliasis /fas´ē·əli´əsis/, an infection with a liver fluke *(Fasciola hepatica).* Symptoms include abdominal pain, fever, jaundice, and diarrhea. One becomes infected by swallowing forms of the fluke found on water plants, as raw watercress. The disease is common in many parts of the world, including southern and western United States.

fat, **1.** a substance made up of lipids or fatty acids and occurring in many forms ranging from oil to tallow. **2.** a type of body tissue made up of cells containing stored fat (depot fat). Stored fat is usually called white fat, which is found in large cells, or brown fat, which consists of lipid droplets. Stored fat contains more than twice as many calories per gram as sugars and is a source of energy. *See also fatty acid, lipid.*

fatal funnel, a narrow entrance, such as a hallway, that provides violent persons with an absolute focus for their field of vision, while restricting the visual capability and safe exit for those who are entering.

fatigue, **1.** a state of exhaustion or a loss of strength or endurance, as may follow extreme physical activity. **2.** an inability of tissues to respond to stimulations that normally cause muscles to contract or other activity. Muscle cells generally need a recovery period after activity. During this time cells restore their energy supplies and release waste products. **3.** a sense of weariness or tiredness. **4.** an emotional state linked to extreme or extended exposure to psychic pressure, as in battle or combat fatigue.

fat metabolism, the process by which fats are broken down and used by the cells of the body. Before use can occur, fats must be changed into fatty acids and glycerol. The body builds only saturated fatty acids. Certain hormones, as insulin and the glucocorticoids, control fat metabolism.

fatty acid, any of several acids found in fats. An **essential fatty acid** is one that cannot be produced by the body but is needed for its proper growth and functioning. It must therefore be included in the diet. Sources include natural vegetable oils, wheat germ, seeds (pumpkin, sesame, and sunflower), poultry fat and fish oils. **Saturated** and unsaturated fatty acids differ mainly in how viscous they are. The more saturated a fatty acid the more solid it is. **Polyunsaturated fatty acids** are rich in liquid vegetable oils. An unsaturated fatty acid is one that is generally found in vegetables. Saturated fatty acids are found mainly in meat. A diet high in saturated fatty acids may lead to a high level of cholesterol in the blood, and in some patients is linked to heart disease.

fatty liver, a buildup of fats in the liver. Causes include alcoholic cirrhosis, intravenous drug use, and exposure to poisonous substances, as carbon tetrachloride and yellow phosphorus. Fatty liver is also seen in kwashiorkor and is a rare problem of late pregnancy. Symptoms include loss of appetite, enlarged liver, and abdominal distress. *See also cirrhosis.*

fauces /fô´sēz/, the opening of the mouth into the throat.

fax, **1.** electronic transmission of an image over telephone lines. **2.** the bit-mapped rendition of a document. Also known as **facsimile.**

fax modem, computer device capable of transmitting a fax. *See also fax.*

fear, a feeling of dread that may result from anticipation of/or actual pain or other negative phenomena.

febrile /fē´bril, feb´ril/, referring to high body temperature, as a feverish reaction to an infection.

feces /fē´sēz/, mostly solid waste from the digestive tract. It is formed in the intestine and released through the rectum. Feces consists of water, food remains, bacteria, and fluids of the intestines and liver. Also known as **stool**. *See also defecation.* **–fecal,** *adj.*

fecundity /fəkun´ditē/, the ability to produce offspring, especially in large numbers and rapidly; fertility. **–fecund,** *adj.*

feeding, the act or process of taking or giving food. **Forced feeding** is the giving of food by force, as nasal feeding, to persons who cannot or will not eat.

feet dry, *(aviation, special operations)* radio code meaning over land or on land.

feet wet, *(aviation, special operations)* phrase meaning over water or on water.

felon, **1.** a purulent or open sore near the nail or distal finger or toe. **2.** *(law enforcement)* a person who has been convicted of a felony.

Felty's syndrome, a spleen disorder occurring with adult rheumatoid arthritis. *See also hypersplenism.*

female, referring to the sex that bears children; feminine.

feminization, **1.** the normal growth or beginning of female sex characteristics. **2.** the beginning of female sex characteristics in a male. Causes include tumors, advanced alcoholism, or the use of estrogen therapy for cancer.

femoral /fem´ərəl/, referring to the femur.

femoral artery, the major artery of the leg that begins in the groin and ends posterior to the knee, where it becomes the popliteal artery. This artery is important as a pressure point for bleeding control and as an alternative site for checking pulses and obtaining blood gases.

femoral nerve, the main nerve of the thigh.

femoral vein, a large blood vessel in the upper leg that originates at the end of the popliteal artery and terminates at the external iliac vein. This vein empties the leg and is located near the femoral artery.

femur /fē´mər/, the thigh bone.

fenestra /fənes´trə/, *pl.* **fenestrae,** an opening in a bandage or cast that is created to reduce pressure or to provide skin care.

fenestration, a surgical opening made to gain access to the space within an organ or a bone. Also known as **window. –fenestrate,** *v.*

ferritin /fer´itin/, an iron compound found in the intestine, spleen, and liver. It contains over 20% iron and is essential for red blood cells.

fertile, **1.** able to reproduce or bear offspring. **2.** able to be fertilized. **3.** fruitful; not sterile.

fertilization, the union of male and female gametes to form a zygote from which the embryo develops. The process takes place in the fallopian tube of the female when a sperm unites with the egg (ovum).

fetal age /fe´təl/, the age of the embryo from the time since fertilization. Also known as **fertilization age.** Compare **gestational age.**

fetal circulation, the pathway of blood flow in the fetus. Oxygenated blood from the placenta travels through the umbilical cord to the liver. The blood then flows to the heart. It goes through a hole between the right and left atria of the heart. Oxygenated blood is available for circulation through the left ventricle to the head and upper body area. The blood returning from the head and arms enters the right ventricle and is pumped through the pulmonary artery and into the aorta for circulation to the lower parts of the body. The blood is returned to the placenta through the umbilical cord arteries.

fetal distress, hypoxia of a fetus as noted by persistent fetal tachycardia in the early stages (greater than 20 to 30 beats above that fetus's normal rate or fetal heart rate above 160) and by fetal bradycardia (less than 100) as hypoxia becomes severe. Causes of distress include carbon dioxide retention, hypoxia, and metabolic acidosis.

fetal position, the relationship of the body of the fetus to the mother's pelvis, as the head directed to the back of the mother's right side, results in a fetal position called **right occiput posterior.**

fetal presentation, the body part of the fetus that first appears in the pelvis at birth.

fetal souffle /fe´təl soo͞´fəl/, whistling sound, heard when auscultating the fetal heartbeat, due to the movement of blood through the umbilical vessels. It is synchronous with the heartbeat. Also known as **funic souffle.** *See also uterine souffle.*

fetish, any object or idea given unreasonable attention or worth.

fetoscope /fē´təskōp´/, a stethoscope for auscultating the fetal heart beat through the mother's abdomen. A fetoscope may also be an instrument with a light on one end and is used to observe the fetus through an incision in the abdomen.

fetotoxic /fē´tōtok´sik/, referring to anything that is poisonous to the fetus.

fetus, an unborn baby, from the ninth week of conception to birth.

fever, an elevated temperature above 98.6° F (37° C). Infection, nerve disease, and many drugs may cause fever. Fever speeds up metabolism 7% per °C. Seizures may occur in children whose fevers tend to rise quickly. Delirium is seen with high fevers. *See also seizures.*

fiberoptic, a flexible material that allows light to be transmitted along its length by reflecting the light along the wall of the fiber. The glass or plastic material thereby allows the transmission of light (visual images) around corners.

fibril /fī´bril/, a small threadlike structure that often is part of a cell.

fibrillation, spontaneous contraction of individual muscle fibers. *See also atrial fibrillation, ventricular fibrillation.*

fibrin /fī´brin/, strands of protein that give structural strength to blood clots. Compare **fibrinogen.** *See also blood clotting.*

fibrinogen /fībrin´əjən/, a protein in the blood clotting process that is converted into protein (fibrin) by thrombin when calcium is present. Also known as **factor I.** Compare **fibrin.** *See also blood clotting.*

fibrinolysin /fī´brinol´isin/, an enzyme that dissolves protein (fibrin). Also known as **plasmin.**

fibrocartilage /-kär´tilij/. See **cartilage.**

fibroma /fībrō´mə/, a tumor largely made up of fiberlike or fully developed connective tissue.

fibromyositis /-mī´əsī´-/ stiffness and joint or muscle pain, with inflammation of the muscle tissues and the fiberlike connective tissues. The condition may develop after infection or injury. Kinds of fibromyositis include **lumbago, torticollis.** *See also rheumatism.*

fibrosing alveolitis, a lung disorder (alveolitis) with breathlessness and air hunger, occurring in rheumatoid arthritis and other diseases. *See also alveolitis.*

fibrosis /-sī´tis/, **1.** a fiberlike connective tissue that occurs normally in the growth of scar tissue. It replaces normal tissue lost through injury or infection. **2.** the spread of fiberlike connective tissue over normal smooth muscle or other normal organ tissue. *See also cystic fibrosis.*

fibrositis /-sī´tis/, an inflammation of fiberlike connective tissue. Symptoms include pain and stiffness. Compare **fibromyositis, myositis.**

fibrous capsule /fī´brəs/, **1.** the layer of tissue surrounding the joint between two bones. **2.** the tough envelope of membrane surrounding some organs, as the liver.

fibula /fib´yələ/, a bone of the lower leg, posterior to and smaller than the tibia. In relation to its length, it is the narrowest of the long bones.

Fick principle, the oxygen concentration difference between arterial and mixed venous blood is equal to (1) the amount of oxygen uptake per unit of blood as it passes through the lungs, (2) the percentage dissolved in the circulation, and (3) the percentage off-loaded to the tissues. Cardiac output can be calculated from this information when heart rate and respiratory rate are included.

fight or flight reaction, the theory that, in situations of danger, an organism has a mechanism that readies it to meet emergencies with maximum energy. Also known as **emergency theory.**

figure eight descender, rope descent and/or rescue device. Composed of cast metal, the device consists of two rings, joined to resemble the number eight **(simple or recreational eight).** The **rescue eight** has an additional two tines (ears) that radiate from the top of the device, preventing rope jam or tangle in a critical situation. Also known as **eight plate, figure eight plate.**

filament /fil´əmənt/, a fine threadlike fiber. Filaments are found in most tissues and cells of the body.

filariasis /fil´ərī´əsis/, a disease caused by the presence of *Filaria* worms in the tissues of the body. After many years, the last stage occurs (**elephantiasis**), in which an arm or leg may become greatly swollen and the skin coarse and tough.

film badge, a pack of photographic film used for approximate measurement of radiation exposure for personnel-monitoring purposes. The badge may contain two or three films of differing sensitivity, and it may contain filters that shield parts of the film from certain types of radiation for determining the types and energies of the radiation.

fimbria, 1. any structure that resembles a fringe. 2. the fringelike structures located at either end of the fallopian tubes.

fin, 1. swimming device worn on the feet to increase the surface area of the foot, thereby making underwater propulsion faster and more efficient. 2. a fixed or adjustable aircraft surface that provides directional stability, such as a tail fin, vertical stabilizer.

final approach, that portion of an aircraft's landing pattern in which it is lined up with the runway and heading straight in to land. *See also base leg.*

finance section, the division of the incident command system that is responsible for all costs and financial considerations of an incident. The section may be composed of a compensation and claims unit, cost unit, procurement unit, and time unit. *See also incident command system.*

financial abuse, misuse or theft of funds and/or property of the elderly or impaired.

finger, any of the digits of the hand. The fingers are composed of the metacarpal bone and three phalanges. Some count the thumb as a finger, although it has one less bone. The digits of the hand are numbered 1 to 5, starting with the thumb.

finger sweep, technique for clearing the oropharynx of emesis or foreign objects, sweeping from one side to the other, utilizing one or two fingers. A **blind finger sweep** is one that is utilized without visualizing the oropharynx or seeing any debris in the mouth.

fire blanket, fire-resistant material that is used to protect a victim from fire hazard, as during vehicle rescue, or stored in high-risk fire locations (skyscrapers), ready to be applied over a victim whose clothes are burning, in an effort to suffocate the flames.

fire damp, 1. combustible gas consisting primarily of methane formed by the decomposition of coal in mines. 2. the explosive mixture formed by coal gases and air. *See also damp.*

fire entry suits, suits that offer protection for short duration entry into a flame environment. Designed to withstand exposures to radiant heat levels as high as 2000° F (1093° C), entry suits consist of a coat, pants, and separate hood assembly. They are constructed of several layers of flame-retardant materials, with the outer layer often aluminized. Also known as **crash-rescue suit, flame suit.**

FIRESCOPE, *(historical)* a committee, Firefighters of Southern California Organized for Potential Emergencies, that met during the early 1970s to standardize the management of wildland firefighting. One of this group's accomplishments was the creation of the incident command system, used by EMS, fire, and police departments across the United States as the command structure for smooth scene organization.

fire shelter, a sheet of aluminized material, carried by wildland firefighters, in which they can wrap themselves as last-resort protection when trapped by rapidly moving wildland fire.

firewall, 1. the partition separating a vehicle's engine compartment from the passenger compartment. 2. a bulkhead that separates two compartments of an aircraft.

firmware, computer memory chips that hold their data without electrical power, as do those utilized with read-only memory (ROM).

firn, an intermediate level in ground ice formation, in which high pressures compress degenerating snow crystals (grains) and seal off airspaces between grains of snow. The next level sees the creation of glacier or water ice. Also known as **névé.**

first aid, initial emergency assistance, usually by nonmedical personnel, administered to individuals who have become ill or injured, prior to the arrival of a first responder, EMT, or paramedic unit. Provision of warmth and direct pressure on bleeding vessels are examples of this type of care.

first-degree AV block, prolonged conduction of atrial impulses through the atrioventricular (AV) node, which causes consistent EKG prolongation of the PR interval without dropped beats. Although this dysrhythmia is not life-threatening itself, it may be a sign of an impending higher level of heart block. Also known as **first-degree block, first-degree heart block.** *See also second-degree AV block, Stokes-Adams attack, third-degree AV block.*

first responder, 1. the initial unit or person at a scene who is trained in emergency care. Such a responder is part of an organized system of emergency medical care for the locality. 2. a category of emergency medical training established by the U.S. Department of Transportation (DOT). This training consists of approximately 40 hours of basic emergency care procedures, such as airway management, hemorrhage control, and CPR.

first stage of labor, the stage of the birthing that begins with the onset of regular contractions and ends with complete dilation of the cervix.

fishnet suit. See **soft transport vehicle.**

fissile radioactive material, material that has the capability of undergoing fission and thus requires controls to assure nuclear criticality safety during transport. Fissile materials include plutonium-238, plutonium-239, plutonium-241, uranium-233, and uranium-235.

fission /fish´ən/, the act of splitting into parts.

fission, nuclear, the splitting of a nucleus into at least two nuclei, which releases a relatively large amount of energy.

fission products, a general term for the complex mixture of substances produced as a result of nuclear fission.

fissure, 1. a natural groove on the surface of an organ, occasionally marking anatomical divisions of the organ, as with the lobes of the lung. 2. a separation or tear in the skin or a membrane. 3. a narrow opening in the ground.

fist pacing, *(historical)* precordial thumping technique used in cases of brady-asystolic arrest, (asystole, prolonged sinus arrest, or sinus bradycardia with a very slow rate) prior to the development of portable transcutaneous pacemakers. A sharp blow to the lower half of the sternum was performed in a rhythmic fashion at a rate of 1 per second. Occasionally successful, this procedure was thought to generate electrical impulses in the cardiac tissue, stimulating the ventricles to contract. If there was no success after 30 seconds, external cardiac compressions would be initiated.

fistula /fis´chələ/, an abnormal passage from an internal organ to the body surface or between two internal organs.

Fitz-Hugh and Curtis Syndrome (T. Fitz-Hugh Jr., American M.D., 1894-1963; A. H. Curtis, American M.D., 1881-1955), pelvic peritonitis due to discharge of purulent drainage from the fallopian tubes. This complication of pelvic inflammatory disease causes acute, sharp, right-upper quadrant abdominal pain and rebound tenderness, days or weeks following initial pelvic inflammatory disease. Also known as **gonococcal perihepatitis.**

fixation, stopping at a certain stage of psychologic growth, as oral fixation.

fixative, any substance used to bind, glue, or keep rigid.

fixed line flyaway. See **long-line haul, short haul.**

fjord /fē·ōrd´/, a deep, narrow inlet of the sea between high, steep cliffs.

flaccid /flak´sid/, weak, lacking muscle tone.

flagellate /flaj´əlāt/, a microorganism that moves by waving whiplike, thready fibers (filaments), as *Trypanosoma, Leishmania, Trichomonas,* and *Giardia. See also protozoa.*

flagellation /flaj´əlā´shən/, the act of whipping, beating, or flogging.

flail chest, a defect in the chest wall caused by trauma, which fractures two or more adjacent ribs in two or more places. The segment created by this injury moves opposite the rise and fall of the chest, creating a paradoxical chest motion. Flail segments can cause significant hypoventilation and hypoxia and may be accompanied by significant pulmonary contusion.

flammable, easily ignited and capable of burning with great rapidity.

flammable range. See **explosive limit.**

flare, 1. enlarge. 2. a sudden emission of bright flame. 3. an area of flush or redness that surrounds a line drawn across the skin by a pointed instrument, due to dilation of arterioles. 4. to suddenly become angry. 5. a sudden worsening of illness or disease. 6. an illumination device, used to bring attention to road or rail hazards or to illuminate or target a position. Also known as **parachute flare, pop-up flare, railroad flare, road flare.**

flare path, a brightly illuminated area, usually a landing strip, that is used to guide aircraft.

flaring, widening of the nostrils while breathing, as a sign of air hunger or dyspnea.

flash burn, burns caused by momentary exposure to a source of intense heat, as in an explosion.

flash flood, sudden, violent flood of water after a dam break, downpour, tidal wave, or wind-driven wave surge. Damage, injury, or death is due to fast-moving water that carries debris, such as mud, rocks, trees. Flash floods account for the majority of flood fatalities in the United States. *See also flood.*

flashover, the simultaneous ignition of highly heated combustibles.

flash point, the minimum temperature at which a liquid gives off enough vapors to ignite and flashover, but not continue burning without additional heat; the point of spontaneous combustion.

flatulence /flach´ələns/, an excess amount of air or gas in the stomach and intestine. It may cause mild to moderate pain.

flexion /flek´shən/, a movement allowed by certain joints of the skeleton. It decreases the angle between two connecting bones, as bending the elbow. Compare **extension.**

flexor carpi radialis, a muscle of the forearm that flexes the hand.

flexor carpi ulnaris, a muscle of the forearm. It flexes the hand.

flexor digitorum superficialis, a large muscle of the forearm.

flight following, the procedure followed by aviation communications specialists that allows continuous tracking of an aircraft's position via radioed position reports at regular intervals. Electronic tracking devices may also be incorporated as part of the process.

flight of ideas, a stream of talk in which the patient switches quickly from one topic to another, each subject unrelated to the one before it. The condition is often a symptom of sudden manic states and schizophrenia.

floater, a spot that drifts in front of the eye. It is made by a shadow cast on the retina from material within the eyeball. Most floaters are leftovers of blood vessels that were in the eye

before birth. The cause may be injury, diabetes mellitus, high blood pressure, cancer, detachment of the retina or other eye diseases.

floating kidney, a kidney that is not securely fixed in position because of a birth defect or injury. Compare **ptotic kidney.**

floating rib. See **rib.**

flood, the covering of dry land by a large quantity of water; the most common natural disaster. It affects more people and causes more fatalities than any other natural disaster. Seventy percent of all flood deaths occur in the Bangladesh-India region. *See also flash flood.*

flooding, **1.** anxiety reduction from phobias, by exposing the patient to that phobia until it can be resisted. **2.** profuse uterine bleeding. **3.** covering or immersing with water.

flood tide, a tide at its highest point; incoming or rising tide. *See also ebb tide.*

floppy disk, a round disk made of flexible material and contained in a square, rigid cartridge, this device is used to store computer data. Removable from the computer floppy drive, it is made to be reused multiple times. Also known as **diskette.** Compare with **hard disk.**

floppy infant syndrome, a general term for some childhood muscle diseases (juvenile spinal muscular atrophies).

flotation, **1.** buoyant support. **2.** distribution of weight over a larger area than normal.

flowmeter, device for measuring flow, such as an oxygen flowmeter (measured in liters per minute).

flu, *(informal)* **1.** influenza. **2.** any viral infection of the respiratory or intestinal system. See **influenza.**

fluid, a liquid or gas that flows and adjusts to the shape of its container.

fluke, a parasitic flatworm of the class Trematoda, some of which can live in humans, infecting the liver, the lungs, and intestine, as the organism that causes **schistosomiasis.** Also known as **trematode.**

fluoride, the chemically combined form of the element fluorine (F) added to toothpaste and the water supply of many areas to harden tooth enamel and decrease cavities.

fluoroscope, a device consisting of a radiation source and a viewing screen that is used for examining internal structures. Although the picture obtained is similar to an x-ray, movement is also visualized, allowing procedures to be done during visualization.

fluorosis /flo͞oro͞-/,   excess fluorine in the body.

flush,   1. sudden redness of skin. **2.** irrigation of a body part or cavity with copious amounts of water. **3.** a type of blood pressure, taken in infants and young children, where capillary refill of the distal portion of an extremity is used, in conjunction with a blood pressure cuff, to obtain a systolic reading.

flutter waves,   P waves, seen in atrial flutter, that occur so rapidly that they create a sawtooth pattern between the QRS complexes. These waves, occurring at between 250 and 350 times per minute, represent abnormal atrial depolarization followed by repolarization. The patient will usually be symptomatic. Also known as **F waves.** *See also atrial flutter.*

foaming agents,   firefighting liquids that consist of a mixture of finely divided gas bubbles interspersed in a liquid. These agents are used to provide an oxygen-excluding blanket over flammable material to prevent an ignition source from starting a fire.

focal infection,   a persistent infection of an organ or region of the body.

focus,   a specific location, as the site of an infection or the point at which rays of light converge.

folic acid /fo͞-lik, fol´ik/,   a vitamin of the B complex group needed for cell growth and reproduction. It functions with vitamin B_{12} and C in the breakdown of proteins and in the production of hemoglobin. It also increases the appetite and stimulates production of hydrochloric acid in the stomach. Rich sources include spinach and other green leafy vegetables, liver, kidneys, and whole-grain cereals.

folie /fole´/,   a mental disorder. **Folie du doute** /dYdo͞ot´/is one of doubting, repeating a certain act or behavior, and not being able to make a decision.

folinic acid /folin´ik/,   an active form of folic acid used to treat some anemias (megaloblastic). Also known as **leucovorin.**

follicle /fol´ikəl/,   a pouchlike recessed spot, as the hair follicles within the skin. **–follicular,** *adj.*

follicle stimulating hormone,   pituitary gland hormone that stimulates the growth and aging of follicles (graafian) that contain the ovum in the ovary. It also stimulates the production of sperm in the male. Also known as **menotropins.**

folliculitis /folik´yəli͞-/,   inflammation of hair follicles.

following distance,   the distance between a vehicle and one in front of it. Safe following distance requires adequate reaction and stopping time, which varies with road surface, speed, and driver capability. *See also braking distance, three-second rule.*

fomentation,   a treatment for pain or inflammation with a warm, moist application to the skin.

fomites,   substances capable of harboring and transmitting pathogenic organisms.

fontanel/fon´tənel´/,   a space between the bones on an infant's skull covered by tough membranes. The front fontanel, roughly diamond-shaped, remains soft until about 2 years of age. The back fontanel, triangular in shape, closes about 2 months after birth. Increased pressure may cause a fontanel to become tense or bulge. A fontanel may be soft and sunken if the infant is dehydrated.

food,   1. any substance, usually of plant or animal origin, made up of carbohydrates, proteins, fats, and minerals and vitamins. It is used by the body to provide energy, growth, repair, and good health. **2.** nourishment in solid form.

Food and Drug Administration,   a federal agency responsible for enforcing laws covering food, drugs, and cosmetics, as protection against the sale of unsafe or dangerous substances.

food poisoning,   a condition resulting from eating food contaminated by toxins. **Bacterial food poisoning** results from eating food contaminated by bacteria. Symptoms of illness include fever, chills, nausea, vomiting, diarrhea, and general discomfort beginning 8 to 48 hours after the contaminated food is eaten and continuing for several days.

foot,   the distal portion of the leg.

foot-candle,   brightness, or luminous intensity, equal to 1 lumen per square foot; replaced in the SI system by the candela.

foramen /fôrā´mən/, *pl.* **foramina,**   an opening (aperture) in a membrane or bone, the **foramen magnum** is a passage in the occipital skull through which the spinal cord enters the spinal column, the **foramen ovale** is an opening in the wall between the atria in the fetal heart.

force, energy applied so that it begins motion, changes the speed or direction of motion, or changes the size or shape of an object.

forced expiratory volume, the volume of air that can be forced out in 1 second after taking a deep breath. Also known as **fev.** Compare **vital capacity.**

forceps, any surgical instrument which has two sides. Forceps are used to grasp, handle, press, pull, or join tissue, equipment, or supplies.

forcible entry, forceful building or vehicle entry by use of tools or techniques that break, chop, cut, hammer, pry, or spread.

ford, a shallow portion of a river or stream that is suitable for crossing.

foreign body, any object or substance found in a cavity, organ, or tissue in which it does not belong.

foreign body obstruction, complete or partial blockage of the airway due to a foreign object, such as food. Partial obstruction is characterized by respiratory difficulty and, when severe, cyanosis and wheezing. Complete obstruction rapidly leads to loss of consciousness and cyanosis due to absence of air exchange. *See also airway.*

forensic medicine /fôren´-/, a branch of medicine that deals with criminal investigation and analysis.

foreskin, a loose fold of skin that covers the end of the penis or clitoris. Also known as **prepuce.**

forest penetrator. See **jungle penetrator, rigid transport vehicle.**

formaldehyde /fərmal´dəhīd/, a poisonous, colorless, noxious gas that is used as a preservative.

formula, a simple statement, generally using numbers and symbols, showing the contents of a chemical compound, or a method for preparing a substance.

formulary /fôr´myələr´ē/, a list of drugs. Hospitals keep formularies that list all drugs commonly stocked in the hospital pharmacy.

fornication /fôr´nəkā´shən/, sexual intercourse.

foul, to become immovable, jammed, or twisted.

Fowler's position (George R. Fowler, American surgeon, 1848-1906), position assumed by the patient when the head of the gurney or bed is

elevated. **High Fowler's** position places the patient in a sitting position with the head elevated to approximately 90°. Semi-sitting positioning with the head at approximately a 45° angle is referred to as **semi-Fowler's position.**

fracture, 1. a broken bone. Divided into simple (closed) and compound (open) injuries, they may also be classed by the type of break that the bone sustains: **comminuted, greenstick, impacted, linear, oblique, spiral, transverse. 2.** breaking of bone.

fracture-dislocation, a broken bone involving the bony structures of any joint, with dislocation of the same joint.

fragmentation, blowing or breaking into fragments.

frazil, crystals of ice that have formed on the surface of a fast-flowing river. The speed of the water movement prevents the ice from forming into a sheet.

freckle, a brown or tan spot on the skin usually caused by exposure to sunlight.

freeboard, the portion of a boat's sides that are above the waterline.

freestanding time, the period of time during which trench walls remain standing unsupported after excavation.

fremitus, tremors of vibration, particularly those felt through the chest wall by palpation. Types include bronchial, friction, pericardial, pleural, tactile (vocal).

French scale, a measurement system used to size tubular instruments and catheters, based on a scale of ⅓ millimeter equaling 1 French (or 1 millimeter equaling 3 French). Grading is done with a metal plate with sized holes. Also known as **Charrière scale, Fr.**

frenotomy /frenot´əmē/, surgically repairing a defective band of tissue.

Frenzel maneuver, a swallowing movement against a closed glottis with lips closed and nostrils pinched. The technique is used to prevent ear squeeze (barotitis) and rupture of the eardrum while descending to depth; it is an attempt to equalize the pressure between the middle ear and external environment. *See also Valsalva's maneuver.*

frequency, 1. the number of repetitions of a phenomenon that occurs in a certain period of time. **2.** the number of cycles per second, especially electrical or radio waves. **3.** a condition characterized by urination in short, recurrent intervals.

frequency modulation, a radio wave that varies (modulates) its frequency while maintaining a constant amplitude. Also known as **FM.** *See also amplitude modulation.*

Freudian /froi´dē·ən/, referring to Sigmund Freud (1856-1939), his psychology, ideas, and rules. These ideas stress the early years of childhood as the basis for later neurotic disorders.

friction, the act of rubbing one object against another. *See also attrition.*

friction burn, tissue injury caused by rubbing the skin. *See also abrasion.*

friction coefficient, 1. the amount of force needed to move an object, divided by the weight of the object. **2.** the maximum traction created by a tire, on a particular road surface, divided by the weight on the tire. Variables of this traction include present weather conditions, tire characteristics, type of road surface, and speed of vehicle.

friction rub, a dry, grating sound heard with a stethoscope. It is normal when heard over the liver and spleen. When auscultated over the heart, this suggests inflammation of the sac that surrounds the heart; a pleural friction rub may also be present in the lungs during conditions which would cause inflammation.

frôlement /frôlmäN´/, the rustling type of sound auscultated in the chest in diseases of the pericardium.

frontal lobe. See **brain.**

frontal lobe syndrome, behavior and personality changes seen following cancer or injury of the frontal lobe of the brain. The patient may show off, then burst into a rage or become irritable. In other cases the person may become depressed and not care about personal appearance.

frontal plane, an imaginary anatomical plane through the middle of the body that divides the body into front and back, or anterior and posterior. Also known as **coronal plane.**

frost line, the depth of frost penetration of the soil in a given area.

frostbite, localized tissue damage due to exposure to freezing or near-freezing temperatures.

The extremities are the most frequently involved tissues. Injury has traditionally been categorized into four degrees of damage, although recent studies favor division of injury into mild (no tissue loss) and severe (tissue loss). The four degrees of injury are first (numbness, erythema), second (superficial blisters surrounded by numbness and erythema), third (deep blisters with dark, bloody fluid), and fourth (full-thickness dermal freezing). *See also chilblain, cold urticaria, frostnip, immersion foot.*

frostnip, a mild form of cold injury that occurs without loss of tissue.

fructose /fruk´tōs, fro͞ok´-/, a form of sugar that is sweeter than sucrose. It is found in honey, in fruits, and combined in many carbohydrates. Also known as **fruit sugar, levulose.**

fuel tender, any vehicle capable of supplying fuel to ground or airborne equipment.

fugue /fyo͞og/, a mental condition with amnesia and physical flight from an undesired situation. The person appears normal and acts as though aware of activities and behavior. Later, the person cannot remember the actions or behavior.

fulcrum, the point on which a lever is supported or turns.

fulminating /ful´minā´ting/, rapid, sudden, severe, as an infection or edema.

fumarole, a hole in an active volcanic area from which gas and vapor are ejected.

fumes, fine dust or vapor dispersed in air.

fumigation, the use of poisonous fumes or gases to destroy living organisms, particularly those that harbor germs dangerous to humans.

function, an act, process, or series of processes that serve a purpose.

functional residual capacity, the amount of air still in the lungs at the end of a normal exhalation.

fundus /fun´dəs/, the base or most interior part of an organ; the part farthest from the mouth of an organ, as the fundus of the uterus or the fundus of an eye.

funduscopy /fundus´kəpē/, the examination of the fundus of the eye by means of an ophthalmoscope.

fungemia /funjē´mē·ə/, the presence of fungi in the blood.

fungicide /fun´jisīd/, a drug that kills fungi.

fungus /fung´gəs/, *pl.* **fungi** /fun´jī/, a simple parasitic plant that lacks chlorophyll. A simple fungus reproduces by budding; many-celled fungi reproduce by making spores. Of the 100,000 known species of fungi, about 10 cause diseases in humans. *See also fungal infection.*

funicular, referring to cable or rope or the tension applied to it.

funiculitis /fənik´yəlī´-/, any inflammation of a cordlike structure of the body, as the spinal cord or spermatic cord.

funiculus /fənik´yələs/, a division of the white matter of the spinal cord.

funnel, **1.** a cone-shaped device, ending as a tube at its base, used to pour liquid or powder into a small opening. **2.** a lighting or ventilating shaft. **3.** the smokestack of a ship or steam engine.

furosemide, a diuretic agent used in the presence of congestive heart failure with pulmonary edema. Sodium chloride is prevented from reabsorbing in the kidneys, allowing increased excretion of potassium, sodium chloride, and water. This agent also produces vasodilation of blood vessels. Side effects include transient hypotension. Contraindications for field use are hypotension, pregnancy, and renal dialysis patients. Also known as **Lasix.**

fuselage, main body of an aircraft to which engines, rotors, wings, and/or tail are attached.

fusible, **1.** having a low melting point. **2.** able to be fused.

fusion, process of uniting or joining together.

fusion beat, an EKG complex that occurs as a result of two ventricular impulses occurring simultaneously. The resulting waveform is usually smaller than either impulse alone would have generated, because the depolarization energy that occurs from two different directions cancels out much of the normal electrical signature seen on EKG.

fusion point, melting point.

F waves. See **flutter waves.**

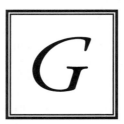

gag reflex, a response to stimulation of the upper palate or posterior oropharynx, causing gagging and/or vomiting in many people. Although occasionally used as a determinate of level of consciousness, it can be absent in the otherwise normal patient.

gait, the manner or style of walking, including rhythm and speed.

galactokinase deficiency /gəlak´təkī´nas/, an inherited disorder of carbohydrate metabolism.

galactose /gəlak´tōs/, a sugar found in lactose, nerve cells, sugar beets, and seaweed.

Galen's bandage /gā´lənz/, a bandage for the head, composed of a strip of cloth with each end divided into three pieces.

gall /gôl/. See **bile.**

gallbladder, a pear-shaped sac, near the right lobe of the liver, which holds bile. During digestion of fats, it contracts, secreting bile into the duodenum. Obstruction of the system may lead to jaundice and pain. It is a common condition in overweight, middle-aged women.

gallop, three heart sounds, instead of the usual two. When auscultated, the combination resembles the sound made by a running horse and is indicative of serious cardiac disease. Also known as **gallop rhythm.** *See also heart sounds.*

gallstone, a mineral deposit (calculus) formed in the biliary tract, consisting of bile pigments and calcium salts. Gallstones may cause flank pain and inflammation of the gallbladder. Increased amounts of cholesterol in the blood (as occurs in obesity), diabetes, underactive thyroid gland, biliary stasis, and inflammation of the biliary system promote the formulation of gallstones.

gamete /gam´ēt/, **1.** a mature male or female germ cell that is able to function in fertilization and that contains the haploid number of chromosomes. **2.** the egg (ovum) or sperm (spermatozoon). *See also haploid.*

gamma-aminobutyric acid, an amino acid that carries nerve impulses. It is found in the brain, heart, lungs, kidneys.

gamma-efferent fiber, any of the motor nerve fibers that carry impulses from the central nervous system to the fibers of the muscles. The gamma efferent fibers are responsible for deep tendon reflexes, spasms, and stiffness.

gamma globulin. See **immune gamma globulin.**

gamma radiation, electromagnetic radiation of high energy originating in atomic nuclei and accompanying nuclear reactions such as fission, radioactive decay, and neutron capture. Physically, gamma rays are identical with x-rays of high energy, the only essential difference being that the x-rays are produced in other ways, e.g., by slowing down electrons of high energy. These constitute the most penetrating type of radiation and are a major external hazard. Symbol: γ.

Gamow bag, a lightweight, portable hyperbaric chamber used for on-site treatment of high-altitude cerebral and pulmonary edema. The device can generate a pressure of 2 pounds per square inch (103 torr) above ambient pressure, so as to simulate a descent. Victims affected have recovered, in some cases, enough to walk unassisted back to lower altitudes.

ganglion /gang´glē·on/, *pl.* **ganglia,** **1.** a knot, or knotlike mass. **2.** one of the nerve cells collected in groups outside the central nervous system. The two types of ganglia are sensory and autonomic.

gangrene /gang´grēn/, necrosis or death of tissue, usually the result of loss of blood supply or bacterial invasion. The arms and legs are most often affected, but gangrene can occur in the intestine, gallbladder, or other organs. Gangrene may spread rapidly and result in death in a few days. Types include: **dry, moist, and gas.**

gap junction, small channel between cells that allows passage of ions and small molecules.

Gardner-Diamond syndrome, a disorder with large areas of ecchymosis that appear without apparent cause but often occur with emotional upsets or abnormal processing of protein.

gas, state of matter distinguished by an ability to diffuse rapidly, a tendency to distribute evenly in its container, and a very low density—with its volume determined by pressure and temperature. *See also liquid, solid.*

gas main, a large-diameter underground pipeline that carries natural gas.

gas service line, a small-diameter pipe underground that connects a gas main to the user.

gastrectomy /gastrek´-/, surgical removal of part or all of the stomach. It may be done to remove a peptic ulcer, to stop bleeding of an ulcer, or to remove cancer.

gastric /gas´trik/, referring to the stomach.

gastric distention, swelling of the abdomen due to an influx of air or fluid. Mouth-to-mouth and other basic life support ventilation techniques may cause this as a common side effect, increasing the chance of vomiting and subsequent aspiration. Decreased ability of the diaphragm to move downward may also hamper ventilatory efforts.

gastric fistula, an abnormal passage into the stomach, usually opening on the outer surface of the abdomen. A gastric fistula may be created

surgically to provide tube feeding for patients with severe disease of the esophagus.

gastric intubation. See **nasogastric intubation.**

gastric juice, digestive fluids of the stomach, including hydrochloric acid. Excess release may lead to irritation of the stomach lining and peptic ulcer.

gastric lavage. See **lavage.**

gastric motility, the movements of the stomach that aid in digestion, moving food through the stomach and into the duodenum.

gastric node, any of the lymph glands associated with an organ in the abdomen or pelvis.

gastrin /gas´trin/, a hormone, released by the opening to the stomach (pylorus). It causes the flow of gastric juice and causes bile and pancreatic enzyme release.

gastritis /gastrī´-/, an inflammation of the lining of the stomach. The symptoms—loss of appetite, nausea, vomiting, and discomfort after eating—usually subside after the cause has been removed. Types include: **acute, chronic, atrophic, hemorrhagic, and hypertrophic.**

gastrocnemius /gas´trok·nē´mē·əs/, a muscle in the posterior lower leg.

gastrocolic reflex, a wavelike movement of the colon that often occurs when food enters the stomach.

gastroenteritis /-en´tərī´-/, inflammation of the stomach and intestine. Symptoms include loss of appetite, nausea, vomiting, abdominal pain, and diarrhea. The disorder could be caused by bacterial or viral infections, chemical irritants, or other conditions, such as lactose intolerance.

gastroenterostomy /-en´təros´təmē/, an operation to form an artificial opening between the stomach and the small intestine, usually at the jejunum. Compare **gastrectomy.**

gastroesophageal /-ēsof´əjē´əl/, the stomach and the esophagus.

gastrointestinal /-intes´tinəl/, referring to the organs of the gastrointestinal tract, from mouth to anus.

gastrointestinal bleeding, any bleeding from the stomach or intestine. Vomiting of blood, called **hematemesis** indicates rapid bleeding of the upper digestive tract. It is often linked to esophagal varices or peptic ulcer. Coffee-ground-colored emesis also indicates bleeding from the esophagus, stomach, or duodenum. The passage of red blood through the rectum, called **hematochezia,** is usually from bleeding in the colon or rectum, but it can result from the loss of blood higher in the digestive tract. Blood passed from the stomach or small intestine generally loses its red color because of contact with enzymes. Cancer, colitis, and ulcers are among causes of hematochezia. Abnormal, black, tarry stools containing digested blood are called **melena.** This usually results from bleeding in the upper bowel or stomach and is often a sign of peptic ulcer. Also known as **GI bleed.** *See also coffee ground emesis.*

gastrointestinal obstruction, any blocking of the movement of intestinal contents. Symptoms include vomiting and abdominal pain. Bowel sounds are softer than normal or absent.

gastroscopy /gastros´kəpē/, visualization of the inside of the stomach by means of a device inserted through the esophagus. *See also endoscopy.*

gastrostomy /gastros´-/, an operation which creates an opening into the stomach through the abdominal wall. This may be done to feed a patient with cancer of the esophagus or one who is expected to be unconscious for a prolonged period of time. *See also colostomy, ostomy.*

gauge pressure, the amount of pressure greater than atmospheric pressure. When a pressure gauge is calibrated to read zero at sea level, it will always be 1 atmosphere less than absolute pressure. *See also absolute pressure.*

gauze, a thin fabric of open-weave cotton or linen, used for wound cleaning, dressing, and bandaging.

gavage /gäväzh´/, the process of feeding through a tube. *See also nasogastric feeding.*

gay, referring to homosexuality.

Geiger counter (Hans Geiger, German physicist, 1882-1945), device for measuring intensity of radiation, consisting of a detection tube (Geiger-Müller tube) attached or enclosed in a case with electronic recording equipment. When high-energy, ionizing radiation passes through the tube, gas contained inside the tube is ionized, allowing a pulse of current to be conducted.

gel, a colloidal substance that is firm, though containing a large amount of liquid.

gene /jēn/, the unit that carries physical characteristics from parent to child. The gene is a nucleic acid within a DNA molecule that structures and regulates the way body cells and tissues develop.

general adaptation syndrome, the defense response of the body or mind to injury or prolonged stress. It begins with a stage of shock or alarm, followed by resistance or adaptation, and ends in a state of adjustment and healing or of exhaustion and disintegration. Also known as **adaptation syndrome.** *See also stress reaction.*

general anesthesia, the total lack of sensation and consciousness brought on by anesthetic agents.

general gas law, gas flows from an area of greater concentration or pressure to an area of lower concentration or pressure. Also known as **Boyle's law.** *See also Boyle's law.*

general paresis. See **paresis.**

general practitioner, *(historical)* a family practice physician. *See also family medicine.*

general staff, the group of incident management personnel comprised of: incident commander, operation chief, planning chief, logistics chief, and finance chief.

generation, 1. the act or process of producing young; procreation. **2.** the period of time between the birth of one individual or organism and the birth of its offspring.

generic, nonspecific name pertaining to a class or group, as in the noncommercial name for a pharmaceutical agent.

generic equivalent, a drug sold under its generic name, identical in chemical composition to a drug sold under a trademark.

generic name, the official name assigned to a drug. A drug is licensed under its generic name, and all manufacturers of the drug list it by its generic name. However, a drug is usually marketed under a trademark chosen by the manufacturer. *See also trade name.*

genesis /jen´əsis/, **1.** the origin, generation, or developmental evolution of anything. **2.** the act of producing or procreating. **–genetic,** *adj.*

gene splicing, the process by which a piece of DNA is attached to or inserted in a strand of

DNA from another source. *See also genetic engineering.*

genetic code /jənet´ik/, information carried by DNA molecules that decides the physical traits of offspring, such as eye color or hair color. The code fixes the pattern of amino acids that build body tissue proteins in a cell. An error in the code can result in a wrong arrangement of the amino acids in the protein, causing a birth defect.

genetic engineering, the process of manipulating DNA molecules. Enzymes are used to break the DNA molecule into pieces so that genes from another organism can be put into the chromosomes of another species. Through genetic engineering, such human proteins as the growth hormone, insulin, and interferon have been produced in bacteria.

genetics, 1. the science that studies the principles and mechanics of heredity, or the means by which traits are passed from parents to offspring. **2.** the total genetic makeup of a particular individual, family, group, or condition.

Geneva convention, *(historical)* an agreement among the major nations of 1864 and 1906 that lead to the establishment of the Red Cross Society. Among the convention's many topics of agreement were those related to the safety of combat wounded and those who care for them.

geniculate neuralgia /jənik´yəlāt/, a severe inflammation of the facial nerve. Symptoms include pain, loss of the sense of taste, paralysis of the face, and a decrease in saliva and tears. It sometimes follows herpes zoster infection.

geniohyoideus /jē´nē·ōhī·oi´dē·əs/, one of the muscles rising from the lower jaw. It acts to pull the hyoid bone in the neck and the tongue forward.

genitals, the reproductive organs.

genitourinary /jen´itōyo͞or´iner´ē/, referring to the sexual and urinary systems of the body, either the organs, their function or both. Also known as **GU, urogenital.**

genome /jē´nōm/, the complete set of genes in the chromosomes of each cell of a particular individual.

genotype /jē´nōtīp´/, the complete set of genes of an organism or group, as determined by the combination and location of the genes on the chromosomes. Compare **phenotype. –genotypic,** *adj.*

genus /jē´nəs/, *pl.* **genera** /jen´ərə/, a subdivision of a family of animals or plants. A genus usually is made up of several closely related species. The genus *Homo* has only one species, humans *(Homo sapiens).*

geographic tongue, small white-to-yellow plaques that develop on the tongue. They gradually leave red patches surrounded by thickened white borders. The patches grow together, forming figures with curved outlines. The condition may persist for months or years.

geotrichosis /jē´ōtrikō´-/, a condition, linked with the fungus *Geotrichum candidum,* which may cause diseases of the mouth, throat, and intestine. Pulmonary infections may produce a cough with thick, bloody sputum. Geotrichosis most often occurs in people with poor disease resistance and in diabetics.

geriatrics /jer´ē·at´-/, the branch of medicine dealing with aging and the diagnosis and treatment of diseases affecting the aged.

germ, 1. any microorganism, especially one that causes disease. **2.** a unit of living matter able to develop into a self-sufficient organism, as a seed, spore, or egg. **3.** a sexual reproductive cell as a sperm or egg.

German measles. See **rubella.**

germ cell, 1. a sexual reproductive cell in any stage of development. **2.** an egg or sperm or any of their preceding forms.

germicide, a drug that kills disease causing microorganisms.

germinal stage, the space of time in which the egg becomes fertilized, undergoes cell division several times, travels to the womb, and, as in a blastocyst, begins to implant itself in the lining of the womb (endometrium). The germinal stage is over at about 10 days of gestation.

germination, the first growth and development of an organism from the time of fertilization to the forming of the embryo. **–germinate,** *v.*

germ layer. See **embryonic layer.**

germ plasm, the material of the germ cells that holds the basic reproductive and hereditary codes; the sum total of the DNA in a particular cell or organism.

gerontology /jer´ontol´-/, the study of aging, including medical, mental, social, and other aspects as they effect both the individual and society.

gestate /jes´tāt/, **1.** to carry a growing fetus in the womb. **2.** to grow and develop slowly toward maturity, as a fetus in the womb.

gestation, the period of time from the fertilization of the egg until birth. Gestation varies with the species; in humans the average length is 266 days or approximately 280 days from the beginning of the last menstrual period. *See also pregnancy.*

gestational age, the age of a fetus or a newborn, usually stated in weeks dating from the first day of the mother's last menstrual period.

g-force, that force produced by acceleration or gravity. One g is the equivalent of the pull of gravity at sea level of the earth's surface at latitude 45° North (32.1725 ft/sec^2; 980.621 cm/sec^2).

Gibbs ascender, an aluminum alloy mechanical device, designed as a type of rope clamp to be used to move up a rope. The design of this type allows it to work well on dirty or wet rope. *See also hard ascender.*

gibbus /gib´əs, jib´əs/, **1.** a swelling on a body surface, usually on just one side. **2.** an abnormal curving of the spine.

gigantism /jīgan´-/, an abnormal condition marked by excess height and weight. Causes include excess release of growth hormone and some genetic disorders. *See also acromegaly.*

Gilbert's syndrome, an inherited condition with excessive bile color in the blood and liver disease.

Gilles de la Tourette syndrome /zhēl´dəlä-tŌŌret´/, a condition marked by twitches, tics, and uncontrolled arm and shoulder motion. Obscene speech often develops. Also known as **Tourettes, Tourettes syndrome.**

gingiva /jinjī´və/, *pl.* **gingivae,** the gum of the mouth, a mucous membrane and its supporting fiberlike tissue that surrounds the teeth.

gingivostomatitis /-stō´mətī´-/, painful ulcers on the gums and mucous membranes of the mouth. It is the result of a herpesvirus infection. *See also herpes simplex.*

glabella /gləbəl´ə/, the flat triangular area of bone of the forehead.

gland, specialized cells that release substances for use in the body.

glans /glanz/, *pl.* **glandes** /glan´dēz/, **1.** a general term for a small, round mass or body. **2.** tissue that can swell and harden.

Glasgow coma scale, system for assessing the degree of conscious impairment in seriously ill or injured victims and for predicting duration and outcome of coma in the unconscious.

glass, a brittle, but solid transparent material composed of silica and other materials. Types include polarized (exiting light waves vibrate in only one direction), safety (laminated, so that it breaks without shattering), tempered (treated with heat to make it more resistant to breakage).

glaucoma /glôkō´mə, gloukō´mə/, elevated pressure within an eye. It is caused by blockage of the normal flow of the fluid in the space between the cornea and lens of the eye (aqueous humor). Types include: **acute (angle-closure, closed-angle,** or **narrow-angle)** and **chronic (open-angle** or **wide-angle).**

glaze, 1. becoming glassy or uncomprehending. **2.** ice that is formed by rain falling on objects that are cooled below freezing. **3.** an area of icy ground.

gliding, a smooth, continuous movement, the simplest allowed by various joints of the skeleton. It is common to all moveable joints and allows one surface to move smoothly over the next surface, no matter what shape. Compare **angular movement, circumduction and rotation.**

gliding joint, a joint in which facing bones allow only gliding movements, as in the wrist and the ankle. The ligaments or other tissues around each gliding joint limit motion.

glioma /glī·ō´mə/, any of the largest group of cancers of the brain, composed of certain nerve cells (glial cells). Types of gliomas are **astrocytoma, ependymona, medulloblastoma** and **oligodendroglioma.** Also known as **gliosarcoma.**

glissade /glisäd´/, a controlled slide down a steep slope, usually related to movement over ice or snow.

globule /glob´yōol/, a small round mass.

globulin, simple proteins that are insoluble in pure water, but soluble in neutral solutions of strong acid salts. Types include fibrinogen, lactoglobulin, and serum globulin.

globus hystericus, a feeling of a lump in the throat that cannot be swallowed or coughed up. It often accompanies emotional conflict or acute anxiety.

glomangioma /glōman´jē·ō´mə/, a tumor that develops from a group of blood cells in the skin. Also known as **angioneuroma.**

glomerular disease /glōmer´yələr/, any of a group of diseases that affect the glomerulus of the kidney.

glomerular filtration rate, amount of plasma filtered through Bowman's capsules in the nephron of a kidney per minute.

glomerulonephritis /glōmer´yəlōnəfrī´-/, an inflammation of the glomerulus of the kidney. Symptoms include blood in the urine and edema.

glomerulus, mass of capillary loops at the beginning of each nephron in the kidney.

glossitis /glosī´-/, inflammation of the tongue.

glossodynia /glos´ədin´ē·ə/, pain in the tongue, caused by inflammation, infection, or an open sore.

glossophytia /-fit´ē·ə/, a condition in which a black patch develops on the tongue. The usually painless condition may be caused by heavy smoking or the use of antibiotics.

glossopyrosis /-pīrō´-/, a burning sense in the tongue caused by inflammation or by exposure to extremely hot or spicy food.

glottis, **1.** a slitlike opening between the vocal cords (plica vocalis). **2.** the voice apparatus made up of the true vocal cords and the opening between them (rima glottidis). –**glottal, glottic,** *adj.*

glucagon, **1.** a hormone produced in the islets of Langerhans that stimulates the conversion of glycogen to glucose in the liver. Secretion is induced by low blood sugar and by growth hormone. **2.** a polypeptide used with known or suspected hypoglycemic diabetics, in whom an intravenous line cannot be started. This agent increases blood glucose by inducing the liver to convert stored glycogen into glucose. Side ef-

fects include nausea and vomiting. It can be given via only the intramuscular route.

glucocorticoid /glōō´kōkôr´tikoid/, a hormone that aids carbohydrate processing, acts to lessen inflammation and affects many body functions. Glucocorticoids aid the release of amino acids from muscle, take fatty acids from fat stores, and increase the ability of muscles to tighten and avoid fatigue. The most important of these is cortisol.

glucose /glōō´kōs/, a sugar found in foods, especially fruits, and a major source of energy in body fluids. Glucose, when eaten or produced by the digestion of carbohydrates, is taken into the blood from the intestine. Excess glucose in circulation is stored in the liver and muscles as glycogen and converted to glucose and released as needed. *See also dextrose, glycogen.*

glucosuria /-sōor´ē·ə/, abnormal levels of glucose in the urine from the eating of large amounts of carbohydrate or from a kidney disease, as nephrosis, or a processing disease, as diabetes mellitus. –**glucosuric,** *adj.*

glue sniffing, the act of breathing the vapors of a compound (toluene) used as a solvent in certain glues. Intoxication and dizziness result. Long-term exposure may damage a number of organ systems.

glutamate /glōō´təmāt/, a salt of glutamic acid.

glutamic acid /glōōtam´ik/, an amino acid occurring widely in a number of proteins.

glutamine, an amino acid found in many proteins in the body. It helps remove ammonia from the body.

gluteal tuberosity, a ridge on the surface of the femur to which is attached the gluteus maximus muscle.

glycerol /glis´ərôl/, an alcohol contained in fats.

glycine /glī´sin/, an amino acid found in many animal and plant proteins.

glycogen /glī´kəjən/, the major carbohydrate stored in animal cells. It is made from glucose and stored primarily in the liver and, to some extent, in muscles. Glycogen is changed to glucose and released into circulation as needed by the body for energy. *See also glucose.*

glycolic acid, a substance in bile that aids in digestion and absorption of fats.

glycolysis, glucose converted to pyruvic acid anaerobically.

glycoside /-sīd/, any of several carbohydrates that yield a sugar and a nonsugar when broken down. The plant *Digitalis purpurea* yields the glycoside digitalis.

glycosuria /-sŏŏr´ē·ə/, abnormal presence of a sugar, especially glucose, in the urine. It is usually linked with diabetes mellitus. **–glycosuric,** *adj.*

glycosuric acid, a compound that is made by the body as it processes tyrosine. It is found in the urine of people who have alkaptonuria.

goblet cell, one of the many special cells that release mucus and form glands of the lining of the stomach, the intestine, and parts of the respiratory tract.

goiter, an enlarged thyroid gland, usually seen as a swelling in the neck. The enlargement may be linked to disordered thyroid function. *See also Graves' disease.* **–goitrous,** *adj.*

gold, a yellowish, soft metallic element.

golden hour, the critical period of time after trauma during which surgical intervention provides the highest survival rates and lowest complications achieveable.

Golgi apparatus /gôl´jē/ (Camillo Golgi, Italian histologist, 1843-1926), one of many small structures found in the cytoplasm of most cells. It is linked to the forming of carbohydrate units of various substances. Also known as **Golgi body.**

Golgi-Mazzoni corpuscles, a number of thin capsules that circle the nerve endings in the tissue under the skin of the fingers. They are special sensory end organs.

gonad /gō´nad/, a gland that releases gametes, as an ovary or a testis. **–gonadal,** *adj.*

gonadotropin /gon´ədōtrop´in/, a hormone that causes the testes and the ovaries to function.

gonococcus /gon´əkok´əs/, *pl.* **gonococci** /-kok´sī/, a bacterium of the species *Neisseria gonorrhoeae,* the cause of gonorrhea.

gonorrhea /gon´ərē·ə/, a common sexually carried disease. It most often affects the sex organs, bladder, and kidneys, and sometimes the throat, eye, or rectum. It is transmitted by contact with the infected person or by contact with body fluids containing *Neisseria gonorrhoeae.* Symptoms include difficult urinating, greenish-yellow drainage from the urethra or vagina, and itching, burning, or pain around the vagina or urethra.

good samaritan laws, legal protection for anyone who aids another voluntarily and without compensation in an emergency. As long as the rescuer acts in good faith and performs as a reasonable person would in similar circumstances, he or she is held immune from prosecution by the victim or the victim's family.

Goodpasture's syndrome, a chronic disorder usually linked to an inflammation of the kidneys. Symptoms include coughing of blood, breathing difficulty, anemia, and kidney failure.

Gordon's reflex (Alfred Gordon, American physician, 1874-1953), extension of the great toe when sudden pressure is applied to the deep flexor muscles of the lower leg. The reflex is present in pyramidal tract disease. *See also Babinski's reflex.*

gout, a disease of uric acid processing. Excess uric acid is converted to sodium urate crystals that settle into joints and other tissues. Men are more often affected than women. The condition can result in painful swelling of a joint.

graafian follicle /graf´ē·ən/, a baglike structure in the ovary that ruptures during ovulation to release an egg. Under the influence of the follicle-triggering hormone, one ovarian follicle matures into a graafian follicle during each menstrual cycle. The cells that form the graafian follicle are arranged in a layer 3 to 4 cells thick around a fluid. Within the follicle the egg triples in size and, when the follicle ruptures, is swept into the opening of a fallopian tube. The hollow of the follicle collapses when the egg is released, and the cells enlarge to become the corpus luteum.

grade, degree of descent or rise on a surface.

grade crossing, a highway-level railroad crossing.

grade pole, a fiberglass or wood pole, cut or marked to a particular length and used by workers setting pipes on a grade.

graft. See **transplant.**

grain, the smallest unit of mass of the avoirdupois, apothecary, and troy weight scales, with a mass of 4.79891 milligrams in all three scales. The avoirdupois ounce contains 437.5 grains, and the apothecary and troy ounce contains 480 grains. Also known as **gr.**

grain itch, skin sores due to a mite that lives in grain or straw.

gram, a unit of mass in the metric system equal to 1/1000 of a kilogram, 15.432 grains, and 0.0353 ounce avoirdupois. Also known as **g, gm.**

gram-molecular weight, the weight of a substance expressed in grams, 6.023×10^{23} molecules.

grand mal seizure /gräNmäl´/. See **seizure.**

grand multipara, a female with seven or more deliveries.

granular /gran´yələr/, **1.** looking or feeling like sand. **2.** appearing under the microscope to have particles within or on the surface. **–granularity,** *n.*

granulation tissue, projections of tissue formed on the surface of an open wound that has not properly closed. This tissue later becomes fibrous scar tissue.

granulocyte /gran´yələsīt´/, a white blood cell (leukocyte) containing granule in the cytoplasm. Kinds of granulocytes are **basophil, eosinophil, neutrophil.**

granulocytosis /-sītō´-/, an increase in the number of granulocytes in the blood.

granuloma /gran´yəlō´mə/, a tumor of the granulation tissue that forms during wound healing. It may result from inflammation, injury, or infection.

grapnel, a multipronged hook, usually used as a throwing attachment from which rope is hung or as a grasping device for underwater objects (dragging).

grasp reflex, a reflex stimulated by stroking the palm or sole causing the fingers or toes to flex in a grasping motion. The reflex occurs in diseases of brain tissue. In young infants the tonic grasp reflex is normal: When one strokes the infant's palms, the stroking fingers are grasped so firmly that the child can be lifted into the air.

gravel bars, gravel accumulation due to a slowing of current in a portion of river.

Graves' disease, a disorder of excess thyroid hormone production. It is usually linked to an enlarged thyroid gland and bulging eyes (exophthalmia). Graves' disease, which is more common in women than in men, occurs most often between the ages of 20 and 40 and often follows an infection or physical or emotional stress. Symptoms include nervousness, weight loss, fatigue, palpitations, heat intolerance and stomach pain. There may be an enlarged thymus, overgrowth of the lymph nodes, and heart and bone disorders. If poorly controlled, infection or stress may cause a life-threatening thyroid storm. Also known as **toxic goiter.** *See also goiter.*

gravid, pregnant; carrying fertilized eggs or a fetus.

gravity, the heaviness or weight of an object caused by the universal effect of attraction between objects. The force of the gravity depends on the masses of the objects and on the distance between them.

gray (Louis H. Gray, British physician, 1905-1965), a measurement (in the International System of Units) of the intensity of ionizing radiation equivalent to 100 rads (radiation absorbed dose) or 1 joule per kilogram of tissue. The gray is replacing the rad as a unit of scientific measurement. *See also sievert.*

gray matter, the gray tissue that makes up the core of the spinal cord. It is arranged in two large side-by-side masses linked by a band of fibers. Each portion of the gray matter spreads, forming the horns of the spinal cord. The horns consist mostly of cell bodies of neurons. The quantity of gray matter varies greatly at different cord levels. Nuclei in the gray matter of the spinal cord function as centers for all spinal reflexes. *See also spinal cord.*

great auricular nerve, one of the nerves branching from a network of nerves in the neck. One branch spreads to the skin of the face over the parotid gland. The other branch supplies the skin of the mastoid process and the posterior ear.

greater trochanter, the large bulge of the femur to which are attached various muscles of the thigh.

great saphenous vein, one of the longest veins in the body. It contains 10 to 20 valves along its course through the leg and the thigh before joining the femoral vein.

great vessels, the aorta, pulmonary arteries and veins, and superior and inferior venae cavae.

Greene splint, *(historical)* a split frame scoop-type stretcher that could be divided into halves, slid under the patient and reconnected. Utilizing rigid wire struts instead of flat metal plates, it was an early forerunner of the scoop stretcher. Also known as **Greene stretcher, Robinson, Sarole.** *See also scoop stretcher.*

Grey-Turner's sign, ecchymosis of the flanks associated with retroperitoneal hemorrhage. This sign occurs 12 to 24 hours after initial injury. *See also Cullen's sign.*

grid, an outline of numbered or lettered squares, superimposed on a map, to be used as a reference.

grid team, a group of trained search and rescue personnel who are assigned a search area within a particular map grid. This technique can be used to intensively cover small areas of ground, generally in search of small clues or pieces of evidence (close-grid search) or wide areas in search of lost or missing victims. Also known as **grid searchers.**

grief, a pattern of physical and emotional responses to separation or loss. The effects are similar to those of fear, hunger, rage, and pain. The emotions proceed in stages from alarm to disbelief and denial, to anger and guilt, to finding a source of comfort, and, finally, to adjusting to the loss. The way in which a grieving person acts is greatly affected by the culture in which the person has been raised.

gripes /grīps/, intermittent, severe pain in the large and small intestine. Also known as **colic.**

grippe, *(historical)* influenza. Also known as **grip.**

grivation, the difference between grid north and magnetic north on a map. Also known as **grid magnetic angle, grid variation.**

groin, each of two areas where the abdomen joins the thighs.

groove, a shallow furrow in various structures of the body. For example, grooves along the bones form channels for nerves.

Groshong catheter, a thin, silicone catheter with an injection port on the external end, a blind (closed) internal end, and a pressure-sensitive two-way valve in the catheter wall. As a central venous catheter that is placed into a jugular or subclavian vein, it is used in patients who require venous feeding, medication, or blood withdrawal for prolonged periods of time. Saline solution is flushed into the catheter weekly to keep it patent. In some emergency medical systems, it is used as a reliable venous route for medication, in the critical patient for whom no other intravenous access is possible. *See also Hickman catheter.*

gross, **1.** referring to the study of tissue without magnification (macroscopic). **2.** large or obese. Compare **microscopic.**

ground, the background of a visual field that can affect the ability of a patient to focus on an object.

ground control approach, an aircraft landing technique, used when the ground is totally obscured, in which the controlling ground facility, using radar, guides the aircraft to the runway. Also known as **GCA, IFR approach, IFR landing.** *See also instrument flight rules, instrument landing system.*

ground cover, a tarpaulin placed on the ground to provide a location for laying out equipment.

ground effect, the supporting cushion of air under a helicopter (or hovercraft), created by the main rotor wash, when hovering close to the ground. The height of this air cushion is influenced by air temperature, altitude, atmospheric pressure, and aircraft type and weight. When the ground effect supports a helicopter, it is referred to as **hovering in ground effect (HIGE).** When it does not, it is said to be **hovering out of ground effect (HOGE).** Much more aircraft power is required to hover out of ground effect.

ground itch, skin inflammation due to hookworm (Ancylostoma or Necator) larvae.

ground pads, full sheets of plywood placed near the edge of a trench to evenly distribute weight over the surface and minimize the possibility of cave-in.

ground swell, wide, slow waves in a heavy sea, due to a distant earthquake, explosion, or storm.

ground wave, radio waves transmitted along the earth's surface.

ground wire, a wire connecting to the ground.

ground zero, the surface point on ground or water, above, at, or below which a nuclear weapon is exploded.

group, an incident command system's organizational level that is responsible for a specific function at an incident, such as air support, extrication, salvage, triage.

growing pains, 1. pains that occur in the muscles and joints of children or teenagers, often due to different rate of growth where bones elongate. They may result from fatigue, posture problems, and other causes that are not linked to growth. **2.** emotional problems felt during adolescence.

growth, 1. the normal development of body, organs, and mental powers from infancy to adulthood. In childhood, growth is measured according to age at which physical changes usually appear and at which mental tasks are achieved. Such stages include the prenatal period, infancy, early childhood, middle childhood and adolescence. **2.** an increase in the size of an organism or any of its parts.

growth hormone, a hormone released by the pituitary gland, which promotes protein building in all cells, increases use of fatty acids for energy and reduces use of carbohydrate. Growth effects depend on the presence of thyroid hormone, insulin, and carbohydrates. More than half the total daily amount is released during early sleep. A lack causes dwarfism; an excess results in gigantism or acromegaly. *See also acromegaly, dwarfism, gigantism.*

grunting, expiratory sound made in patients with significant respiratory distress, particularly newborns. The grunting pushes air into small (terminal) airways and helps to keep them inflated.

guaiac test /gwī´ak/, a test using a special solution (guaiac) on feces and urine (or emesis) to detect blood in the intestinal and urinary tracts.

guanine /gwan´ēn/, a basic component of DNA and RNA. It occurs in trace amounts in most cells.

guarding, voluntary or involuntary abdominal muscle contraction in the presence of severe abdominal pain.

Guérin's fracture /gāraNs´/, a fracture of the maxilla. Also known as **LeFort I fracture.**

Guillain-Barré syndrome /gēyaN´bärā´/ (G. Guillian, French physician, 1876-1961; J. Barré, French physician, 1880-1979), peripherial nerve disease involving two or more nerves. Also known as **infectious neuronitis, Landry-Guillain-Barré syndrome, polyneuronitis.**

gulf, a section of sea surrounded in part by land and larger in area than a bay, but with a relatively smaller opening.

gum. See **gingiva.**

gunwales, the upper edge of a boat's side. Also known as **gunnel.**

gurney (Sir Goldsworthy Gurney, British physician, 1793-1875), any stretcher with wheels; originally, one with a fixed height.

gut, 1. intestine. **2.** *informal.* stomach and bowel. **3.** surgical thread made from the intestines of sheep.

gynandrous /gīnan´drəs/, describing a man or a woman who has some of the physical characteristics usually found in the other sex, as a female pseudohermaphrodite. Compare **androgynous.**

gynecology /gī´nəkol´-, jī´-, jin´-/, a branch of medicine that deals with the health care of women. It is usually practiced along with obstetrics.

gynecomastia /gī´nəkōmas´tē·ə/, a swelling of one or both breasts in men. It may be due to hormonal imbalance, tumor of the testis or pituitary, drugs containing estrogen or steroids, or failure of the liver to dissolve estrogen in the bloodstream,

gynephobia /gī´nə-/, a deathly fear of women or an intense dislike of the company of women. It occurs almost exclusively in men.

gyrus /jī´rəs/, *pl.* **gyri** /jī´rī/, one of the spiral twists of the surface of the brain caused by the folding in of the outer layer.

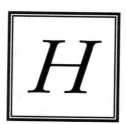

habit, **1.** a usual way of behaving. **2.** an unwilled pattern of behavior or thought. **3.** the habitual use of drugs or narcotics.

habituation, dependence on a drug, tobacco, or alcohol caused by repeated use, but without the addictive, physiologic need to increase the dose. Compare **addiction.**

habitus /hab´itəs/, a person's looks or physique, such as an athletic habitus. *See also somatotype.*

hail, ice formed by prolonged contact with clouds at low temperature and reaching the earth's surface as particles or pieces.

hair, a threadlike protein formed in the skin.

hairy tongue, a dark, colored coating of the tongue that is a harmless and frequent side effect of some antibiotics. The condition improves without treatment. *See also glossitis.*

Haldane, John S. (British biologist, 1892-1964), *(historical)* scientist who published, in 1908, the first set of decompression tables for diving.

half-life, **1.** the time necessary for one-half of an initial quantity of a substance to disintegrate or disappear by means of a chemical or nuclear reaction. **2.** the time required for one-half of a substance to be eliminated or metabolized from an organism.

half-thickness, the amount of absorbing material necessary to reduce the radiation energy that passes through it by one-half.

halitosis /hal´itō´-/, bad breath caused by poor oral hygiene, certain foods, such as garlic or alcohol, and some diseases, such as the odor of acetone in diabetes and ammonia in liver disease.

Halley, Sir Edmund (British astronomer, 1656-1742), *(historical)* scientist who devised a method of providing diving bells with surface air to a depth of 60 feet.

hallucination, something sensed that is not caused by an outside event. It can occur in any of the senses and is named accordingly: auditory (hearing), gustatory (taste), olfactory (smell), tactile (feeling), or visual hallucination. **–hallucinate,** *v.*

hallucinogen /həlōō´sənəjən´, hal´əsin´əjən/, a substance that excites the brain, causing hallucination.

hallucinosis /-ō´sis/, a mental state in which one is primarily aware of hallucinations. **Alcoholic hallucinosis** is a disorder caused by serious alcoholism after stopping or reducing alcohol intake.

hallux /hal´əks/, *pl.* **halluces** /hal´yesēg/, the great toe.

hallux rigidus, a painful deformity of the great toe that limits motion at the joint where the toe joins the foot.

hallux valgus, a deformity in which the great toe is bent to the outside toward the other toes; in some cases the great toe rides over or under the other toes.

halo, cerebrospinal fluid (lighter serous color) that may be found around a blood stain on light-colored material when the hemorrhage is due to skull fracture. Also known as **target.**

Halon, halogenated hydrocarbon used as a fire-extinguishing agent for the protection of aircraft engines and computer or electrical equipment. It is nonconducting of electricity, leaves little residue, is rapidly vaporized in fire, and is heavier than air. It is toxic if inhaled.

hamate bone /ham´āt/, a bone in the wrist, superior to the fourth and fifth fingers.

Hamman's sign (John Hamman, American surgeon, 1877-1954), systolic crunching sound that may be auscultated over the heart in the presence of air in the mediastinal space. This phenomenon may be seen during esophageal and/or tracheal perforation, left-sided pneumothorax, or any other condition that causes pneumomediastinum. Also known as **Hamman's crunch.**

hammertoe, a toe permanently bent at the middle joint, causing a clawlike appearance. It may be present in more than one toe but is most common in the second.

hamstring muscle, any one of three muscles at the back of the thigh.

hamstring tendon, one of three tendons that originate from the hamstring muscles in the posterior thigh and connect those muscles to the knee.

hand, the part of the upper limb distal to the forearm. It is the most flexible part of the skeleton and has a total of 27 bones.

hand crew, predetermined individuals who are supervised, organized, and trained principally for clearing brush as a fire suppression measure.

handedness, willed or unwilled preference for use of either the left or right hand. The preference is related to which side of the brain is dominant, with left-handedness occurring when the right side of the brain is dominant and vice versa. Also known as **chirality, laterality.**

handicap, referring to a congenital or acquired mental/physical defect that interferes with normal function of the body or the ability to be self-sufficient. Compare **disability.**

hand winch, a chain or steel cable pulling tool, used during vehicular and structural extrication and lifting operations. Two lengths of chain or cable are pulled together by a hand-operated winch, creating the lifting or pulling action. For rescue, one-and-a-half tons is the minimum tool capacity that should be used. Also known as a **come-along.**

hangman's fracture, an unstable fracture of the bony protuberances of C2, often accompanied by dislocation of C2 or 3 and disruption of the spinal cord. This fracture is found in victims of hanging and is generally not compatible with life.

hangnail, a piece of partially torn skin of the cuticle or nail fold.

Hansen's disease. See **leprosy.**

haploid /hap´loid/, having a single set of chromosomes, as in sex cells. Also known as **monoploid.** *See also euploid.* –**haploidy,** *n.*

haptoglobin /hap´təglō´bin/, a blood protein. The amount of haptoglobin is increased in some disorders with inflammation, and is decreased or absent in some kinds of anemia.

hard ascender, any mechanical device designed as a rope clamp and used to move up rope, or as a safety device on raising and lowering systems. Types include Clog, CMI, Hiebeler, Jumar. *See also ascender, Gibbs ascender.*

hard disk, a metallic disk, usually incorporated into the central processing unit of a computer, on which large amounts of information are stored and retrieved for data processing. The disk is covered with magnetic recording material and can store 1000 or more megabytes of data. The unit that houses the hard disk is known as a **hard drive.** Also known as **fixed disk, hard drive.** Compare with **floppy disk.**

hardening of the arteries. See **arteriosclerosis.**

hard palate, the bony part of the roof of the mouth, behind the soft palate and bounded in front and on the sides by the gums and teeth. Compare **soft palate.**

hard pulse, pulse that forcibly strikes against the finger when palpated and is compressed with difficulty. It is suggestive of hypertension. Also known as **pulsus duras.**

hard-slab avalanche, an avalanche composed of hard, dense snow (>24 hours old) that begins its slide as a cohesive mass. This type of avalanche develops in the presence of a strong wind that blows snow into a dense, hard pack, which later breaks loose from its base. *See also avalanche.*

harness-cutting knife,   V-blade knife used for cutting seat belts, webbing, parachute straps, and clothes. Its curved, blunted end allows it to be safely inserted and used without danger of cutting the victim.

Hartmann's Solution (Alexis F. Hartmann, American physician, 1898-1964), *(historical)* Ringer's solution. Also known as **lactated Ringers, Ringer's lactate.**

Harvey, William (British physician, 1578-1657), *(historical)* scientist who first described the circulation of blood, in 1628.

hasty pit,   a trench dug in a snowpack for the purpose of examining the layers of snow to determine cohesiveness and danger of avalanche in the area of that snowpack. The pit should be deep enough to reach at least to the permanent snowpack, if not the ground.

hasty search,   a type I search (rapid search of small, high-probability areas) by hasty teams for information or location of lost and/or missing persons. *See also hasty team.*

hasty team,   a rapidly assembled group of experienced searchers, who attempt to locate, treat, and extricate lost or trapped victim(s). Because many of these circumstances are time dependent, such teams utilize a minimum number of rescuers required (usually three per team), travel lightly (enough equipment for 24 hours), and move rapidly.

hauling line,   a length of rope used for raising or lowering. These ropes should be at least 9 millimeter or ½ inch, depending on load.

haversian canal (Clopton Havers, British physician, 1650-1702), small bone perforation through which blood vessels, connective tissue, and nerves pass into bone.

haversian system,   circular section of bone tissue around a central (haversian) canal, interconnected with other canals, which forms part of the structure of bone. *See also haversian canal.*

hawser,   a cable, usually of steel, that is used for hauling or mooring a ship.

hay fever,   *(informal)* an acute seasonal allergic irritation of the nose and sinuses caused by tree, grass, or weed pollens. Also known as **pollinosis.** *See also allergy, rhinitis.*

hazard,   1. danger, risk, peril. The dangers may be sight hazards (those that are obvious) or intelligence hazards (those that may not be obvious or that only potentially exist). **2.** to expose to danger, risk, or chance. **3.** to attempt.

hazard analysis,   any examination of risks present during a response.

hazard area,   a geographically identifiable area in which a specific hazard presents a potential threat to life and property.

hazardous atmosphere,   any gaseous environment that can harm unprotected personnel.

hazardous material,   any substance that causes or may cause adverse effects on the health or safety of employees, the public, or the environment.

hazardous materials incident,   the release, or potential release, of a hazardous material from its container into the environment.

hazardous materials response team,   specially trained persons responsible for directly managing hazardous materials incidents. They may include personnel from emergency services, private industry, governmental agencies, or any combination of these. They generally perform more complex and technical functions than the initial responding units.

hazardous materials specialists,   specially trained and equipped members of the hazardous materials response community who possess both the technical and manipulative skills to function as the hazard sector officer or incident safety officer. In addition these specialists perform advanced hazard and risk assessment and implement advanced control procedures.

hazardous materials technicians,   specially trained members of the response community who are responsible for identification, basic hazard and risk assessment, implementation of basic control procedures, and use of specialized equipment (including personal protective equipment and basic decontamination procedures).

hazardous waste,   any waste or combination of wastes that poses a substantial present or potential hazard to human health or living organisms, because such wastes are nondegradable or persistent in nature, because they can biologically magnify, or because they may otherwise cause or tend to cause detrimental cumulative effects.

haze, a cloudy or misty appearance in the atmosphere, in a liquid, or on a solid surface. Atmospheric haze is usually due to suspended dust or vapor particles or to intense heat that causes irregular densities between layers.

headache, a pain in the head from any cause. *See also migraine.*

headbed, *(informal)* lateral cervical immobilizer. *See also cervical immobilization device.*

header, **1.** a large-diameter pipe with suction hose inlets. These are used in water removal operations prior to subsurface/trench construction and operations. **2.** a column or plume of smoke seen in the distance as an indication of fire. **3.** *(informal)* a headfirst fall or dive; to land on one's head.

heading, **1.** direction of travel. **2.** a large horizontal cut into a body of rock for purposes of extracting ore or enlarging an underground mining area; a passageway between two tunnels.

head tilt, hand pressure on the forehead of a supine patient, utilized when manually opening an airway. Use of the chin as a lift point is often combined with the head tilt to create maximum hyperextension of the head. The procedure is then known as **head-tilt chin lift.**

head-to-toe survey. See **secondary survey.**

healing, the act or process in which the normal, healthy structures and functions are restored to parts of the body that were diseased, damaged, or not functioning.

health, a state of physical, mental, and social well-being and the absence of disease or other disorder. It involves constant change and adaptation to stress.

health maintenance organization, a group or entity that provides for the delivery of necessary health care to a group of pre-enrolled individuals within a particular area or region. The cost of providing that care is paid via predetermined periodic payments by the participants. Also known as **HMO.**

health physics, the study of the effects of radiation on the body and the methods for protecting people from those effects. Also known as **medical physics.**

health risk, a factor that increases one's chances for illness or death. These factors may include social or income levels, certain individual behaviors, family and individual histories, and certain physical changes.

hearing, the sense or perception of sound. *See also deafness.*

hearing aid, an electronic device that increases the volume of sound for persons with damaged hearing. The device consists of a microphone, a battery power supply, an amplifier, and a receiver.

heart, the hollow muscular organ that provides the pumping capability necessary to circulate blood throughout the body. At an average rate of 72 times per minute, the heart beats 104,000 times per day. The heart is divided into four chambers (right and left atria, right and left ventricles) that involve two distinct pumps (the right, or pulmonary, side and the left, or systemic, side). The atria are the receiving chambers, for blood returning to the heart, and the ventricles are pumping chambers, for sending blood into the systems. The cardiac tissue is composed of three layers: epicardium (outer), myocardium (middle), and endocardium (inner). The organ is entirely enclosed in a sac called the **pericardium.** Self-generated nerve impulses are conducted through the cardiac conduction system, causing an overall contraction of the muscle which results in blood flow.

heart block. See **bundle branch block, third-degree heart block.**

heartburn, *(informal)* a burning sensation in the chest or epigastric area due to hyperacidity, indigestion, reflux (stomach contents flowing back into the esophagus), or ulcer. Also known as **pyrosis.** *See also hernia, reflux, ulcer.*

heart failure, failure of the heart to pump enough blood to meet the needs of body tissue. Common causes include arteriosclerosis, congenital defects, electrolyte imbalance, hypertension, myocardial infarction, pulmonary disease, and valvular disease. **Left-sided failure** causes dyspnea and pulmonary edema. **Right-sided failure** causes fatigue and pedal edema. Most heart failure consists of varying combinations of right- and left-side failure. **Congestive heart failure** is the acute form of this condition with life-threatening hypoxia due to decreased cardiac output and pulmonary edema. Also known as **congestive heart failure.**

heart murmur, sustained cardiac sounds that are heard during contraction, relaxation, or both. These diastolic and/or systolic sounds may be produced by restricted blood flow, high rates of flow, or vibration of loose structures.

heart sounds, characteristic cardiac noises caused by cardiac movement, blood flow, or disease processes. The first heart sound (S1) occurs at the beginning of ventricular contraction when ventricular blood volume is greatest. These sounds are caused by the closure of the mitral and tricuspic valves. The second heart sound (S2) occurs at the end of ventricular contraction and is due to the closure of the aortic and pulmonic valves. Other sounds that may be heard include S3, S4, murmurs, and rubs.

heart valve, one of the four structures in the heart that control the flow of blood by opening and closing with each heart beat. The valves permit the flow of blood in only one direction. The **aortic valve** is between the left ventricle and the aorta. It has three cusps that close when the heart beats to prevent blood from flowing back into the heart from the aorta. The **mitral valve,** also called **bicuspid valve,** is between the left atrium and left ventricle. It is the only valve with two small cusps. The mitral valve allows blood to flow from the left atrium into the left ventricle. Narrowing of the ventricle forces the blood up against the valve. This closes the two cusps so the flow of blood is directed from the ventricle into the aorta. The **pulmonary valve** is composed of three cusps that grow from the lining of the pulmonary artery. The cusps close during each beat to keep blood from flowing back into the right ventricle. The **tricuspid valve** is between the right atrium and the right ventricle. The tricuspid valve has three cusps. As the right and the left ventricles relax during diastole the tricuspid valve opens, allowing blood to flow into the ventricle. In systole both ventricles contract, pumping out their contents, while the tricuspid and mitral valves close to prevent any backflow. Also known as **cardiac valve.**

heat cramp, any cramp in the arm, leg or stomach due to decreased water and salt in the body. It usually occurs after vigorous physical exertion in very hot weather or under other conditions that cause heavy sweating and loss of body fluids and salts.

heat edema, swelling of feet and ankles in individuals not acclimated to tropical or subtropical climates. There is usually some correlation to prolonged periods of sitting or standing. This is a benign condition that is not related to cardiac dysfunction or thrombophlebitis.

heat exhaustion, a heat-related illness characterized by weakness, thirst, nausea and/or vomiting, and muscle cramps. Moderate elevation of core temperature (<104° F [40° C]) occurs. There are two types of heat exhaustion: that occurring from salt depletion and that occurring from water depletion. Most cases of the illness are combinations of both. Compare **heat stroke.** *See also heat cramps, heat edema, heat syncope.*

heat lightning, sheet lightning without thunder, seen near the horizon at dusk or nighttime, believed to be distant lightning reflected from high clouds.

heat rash, papules caused by blockage of sweat ducts during periods of heat and high humidity. Tingling and prickling sensations are common. Also known as **miliaria, prickly heat.**

heat stroke, the life-threatening failure of the body's temperature-regulating mechanisms after exposure to high or prolonged heat stress. Signs include altered levels of consciousness and/or bizarre behavior, body temperature above 105° F (40.5° C), tachycardia, and seizures with a history of having been exposed to heat stress. **Classic (or epidemic) heat stroke** occurs during high outdoor humidity and temperature, usually involving the aged and poor. Contributing factors include decreased access to water, lack of air-conditioning, poor living-space ventilation, and medications that decrease ability to withstand heat. Sweating was absent in most victims of this condition. **Exertional heat stroke** occurs after temperature regulation fails due to heat production within the body, as may occur with athletes and soldiers. Hypoglycemia and acute renal failure may be seen in these patients, but sweating is usually present in approximately half of them. Also known as **heat hyperpyrexia, sunstroke.** Compare **heat exhaustion.**

heat syncope, /sin´kəpē´/, fainting due to increased or extreme environmental temperatures combined with venous pooling and volume loss. Initial symptoms include diaphoresis, dizziness, nausea, tunnel vision, and weakness. Compare **heat exhaustion, heat stroke.**

heaves, (informal) vomiting and retching.

heavy metal, a metallic element with a specific gravity five or more times that of water. The heavy metals are antimony, arsenic, bismuth, cadmium, cerium, chromium, cobalt, copper, gallium, gold, iron, lead, manganese, mercury, nickel, platinum, silver, tellurium, thallium, tin, uranium, vanadium, and zinc. Small amounts of many of these elements are common and necessary in the diet. Large amounts of any of them may cause poisoning.

Heberden's node /hē´bərdənz/, an enlargement of bone or cartilage in a joint of a finger. This most often occurs in wasting diseases of the joints.

heel, the posterior portion of the foot, formed by the largest tarsal bone, the calcaneus.

Hegg sled, commercially produced litter, used to remove victims from broken rock (scree) in ice and snow environments. This metal litter is usually carried via mounted shoulder handles or pulled by skiers, over snow.

Heimlich maneuver (Henry Heimlich, American physician, 1920), technique for removing an airway obstruction caused by a foreign object. Using the hands to create pressure over the epigastrium, the obstruction can often be forced out of the trachea by the back pressure created. This obstruction, in adults, is usually food that completely blocks the passage of air from the mouth to lungs. This procedure requires no equipment and can effectively be taught to a nonmedical population. *See also airway obstruction.*

helibase, a location within the general incident area for parking, fueling, maintenance, and loading of helicopters.

helibase crew, a crew of three or more individuals who may be assigned to support helicopter operations.

helicopter rappelling, descending from a hovering helicopter by static rope. This technique is used whenever a landing site or helicopter hoist is not available and/or speed is essential.

helicopter tender, a ground service vehicle capable of supplying fuel and support equipment to helicopters.

helipad, a designated helicopter landing area of permanent construction. Fueling and hanger facilities may be available. Also known as **heliport.**

heliport, a designated helicopter landing area that is accessible by road. Also known as **helipad.**

helispot, a designated helicopter landing area that does not have road access.

helitack, the initial attack phase of fire suppression using helicopters and trained airborne teams to achieve immediate control of wildfires.

helitanker, a helicopter equipped with a fixed tank or a suspended bucket-type container that is used for aerial delivery of water or fire retardants.

helix /hē´liks/, a coiled, spiral-like formation typical of many organic molecules, as deoxyribonucleic acid (DNA).

helminthiasis, a class of disease caused by worms (helminths) that may penetrate the skin, muscles, or intestines. These include flukes, tapeworms, and roundworms. Ascariasis, bilharziasis, filariasis, hookworm, and trichinosis are common types of this disease.

hemagglutination /hem´əglo͞otinā´shən, hē´mə-/, a clumping together of red blood cells. This is a reaction of the body's defenses and may be caused by antibodies (as **hemagglutinin**), viruses, and other substances.

hemangioma /hēman´jē-ō´mə/, a benign tumor composed of a mass of blood vessels.

hematemesis /hem´ətem´əsis/, vomiting blood or bloody material. *See also gastrointestinal bleeding.*

hematocrit /hēmat´əkrit/. See **blood count.**

hematogenous /hem´ətōj´ənəs/, coming from or carried in the blood.

hematology /hem´ətol´-, hē´mə-/, the study of blood and blood-forming tissues. A physician who specializes in the study of blood and its diseases is called a **hematologist.**

hematoma /hem´ətō´mə/, a collection of blood in a localized area within an organ, space, or tissue. A degree of edema is usually present. This mass forms in an area that has been traumatized and will resolve in 1 to 3 weeks.

hematomyelia /hem´ətōmē´lyə/, the appearance of blood in the fluid of the spinal cord.

hematopoiesis /-pō·ē´sis/, the normal formation and development of blood cells in the bone marrow. In severe anemia and other blood disorders, cells may be produced in organs outside the marrow (extramedullary hematopoiesis).

hematuria /hem´ətoŏr´ē·ə/, presence of blood in the urine. Hematuria can be caused by many kidney diseases and disorders of the genital and urinary systems.

heme /hēm/, the colored, nonprotein part of the hemoglobin molecule in the blood that contains iron. Heme carries oxygen in the red blood cells, releasing it to tissues that give off excess amounts of carbon dioxide. *See also hemoglobin.*

hemeralopia /hem´ərəlō´pə·ə/. See **day blindness.**

hemianesthesia /hem´i-/, a loss of sensation on one side of the body.

hemianopia /-anō´pē·ə/, defective vision or blindness in one half of the visual field. **Homonymous hemianopia** is blindness or defective vision in the right or left halves of the visual fields of both eyes.

hemicrania /-krā´nē·ə/, **1.** a headache, usually migraine, that affects only one side of the head. **2.** a birth defect in which one half of the skull in the fetus is missing.

hemiectromelia /-ek´trəmē´lyə/, a birth defect in which the limbs on one side of the body are not fully formed.

hemihyperplasia /-hī´pərplā´zhə/, excessive growth of one half of a specific organ or body part, or of all the organs and parts on one side of the body.

hemihypoplasia /-hī´pōplā´zhə/, partial or incomplete development of one half of a specific organ or body part, or of all the organs and parts on one side of the body.

hemikaryon /-ker´ē·on/, a cell nucleus that contains the halved (haploid) number of chromosomes, or one half of the diploid number, such as that of the sex cells.

hemiparesis /-pərē´-/, muscular weakness of one half of the body.

hemiplegia /-plē´jə/, paralysis of one side of the body. Also known as **unilateral paralysis.** –**hemiplegic,** *adj.*

Hemiptera, an order of insects characterized by a beaklike mouth used for sucking. This large group of insects includes assassin bugs, bedbugs, and water scorpions.

hemisphere, **1.** one half of a sphere or globe. **2.** the lateral half of the brain. –**hemispheric, hemispherical,** *adj.*

hemochromatosis /hē´məkrō´mətō´-/, a rare disease in which iron deposits build up throughout the body. Hepatomegaly, skin discoloration, diabetes mellitus, and heart failure may occur. The disease most often develops in men over 40 years of age and as a result of some anemias requiring multiple blood transfusions.

hemoconcentration, an increase in the number of red blood cells resulting either from a decrease in the liquid content of blood or from increased production of red cells.

hemodialysis /-dī·al´isis/. See **dialysis.**

hemodynamics /-dīnam´-/, the study of factors affecting the force and flow of circulating blood.

hemoglobin /-glō´bin/, a complex protein-iron compound in the blood that carries oxygen to the cells from the lungs and carbon dioxide away from the cells to the lungs. Each red blood cell contains 200 to 300 molecules of hemoglobin. Each molecule of hemoglobin contains several molecules of heme, each of which can carry one molecule of oxygen. **Hemoglobin A,** also called adult hemoglobin, is a normal hemoglobin. **Hemoglobin F** is the normal hemoglobin of the fetus, (most of which is broken down in the first days after birth and replaced by hemoglobin A). It can carry more oxygen and is present in increased amounts in some diseases, including sickle cell anemia, aplastic anemia, and leukemia. Small amounts are produced throughout life.

hemoglobinopathy /-glō´binop´əthē/, any of a group of inherited disorders known by changes in the structure of the hemoglobin molecule. Kinds of hemoglobinopathies include **hemoglobin C disease** and **sickle cell anemia.** Compare **thalassemia.**

hemoglobinuria /-oŏr´e·ə/, the presence in the urine of hemoglobin that is unattached to red blood cells. Hemoglobinuria can result from various diseases of the body's defense system or certain blood disorders. **March hemoglobinuria** occurs after excess physical exercise or prolonged exercise, as marching or long-distance running.

hemolysin /hēmel´isin/, any of the many substances that dissolve red blood cells. Hemolysins are produced by many kinds of bacteria, including some of the staph and strep germs. They are also found in venoms and in some vegetables. Hemolysins appear to aid bacteria in invading blood cells.

hemolysis /hēmol´isis/, the breakdown of red blood cells and the release of hemoglobin. It occurs normally at the end of the life span of a red cell. However, it may occur under other circumstances, as when fighting off disease or as a side effect of hemodialysis. Circulatory volume overload can also precipitate hemolysis. *See also dialysis.* –**hemolytic,** *adj.*

hemopericardium /-per´ikär´dē·əm/, blood within the sac surrounding the heart.

hemoperitoneum, blood in the peritoneal space.

hemophilia /-fil´yə/, a group of hereditary bleeding disorders in which there is a lack of one of the factors needed to clot blood. **Hemophilia A** is the classic type of hemophilia. **Hemophilia B,** also known as **Christmas disease,** is similar to but less severe than hemophilia A. **Hemophilia C,** also called **Rosenthal's syndrome,** is also similar to but less severe than hemophilia A.

hemoptysis /hēmop´tisis/, coughing up of blood from the respiratory tract.

hemorrhage /hem´ôrij/, a loss of blood internally or externally. Hemorrhage may be from arteries, veins, or capillaries. –**hemorrhagic,** *adj.*

hemorrhoid, an enlarged varicose vein in the lower rectum or anus.

hemosiderosis /hē´mōsid´ərō´-/, an increased deposit of iron in a variety of tissues, usually without tissue damage. It is often linked to diseases involving extensive destruction of red blood cells, such as thalassemia.

hemostasis /hēmos´təsis, hē´mōstā´sis/, the control of hemorrhage by mechanical or chemical means or by the clotting process of the body. *See also blood clotting.*

hemostatic, having to do with a procedure, device, or substance that stops the flow of blood. Direct pressure, tourniquets, and hemostats are mechanical hemostatic measures.

hemothorax /-thôr´aks/, blood and fluid in the chest cavity, usually due to injury. It may also be caused by blood vessels that rupture as a result of inflammation from pneumonia, tuberculosis, or tumors.

Henry's Law, *(regarding the solution of gases in liquids)* at a given temperature, the mass of gas dissolved in a given volume of solvent is proportional to the pressure of the gas with which it is in equilibrium.

hepatic /həpat´ik/, having to do with the liver.

hepatic coma, altered level of consciousness, caused by acute or chronic liver failure. This failure prevents the liver from removing toxic waste products from the blood. Symptoms include weakness, memory loss, jaundice, unconsciousness, seizures, and hypotension.

hepatic fistula, an abnormal passage from the liver to another organ or body structure.

hepatic node, a lymph gland found in the lower trunk and the pelvic organs supplied by branches of the celiac artery.

hepatitis, inflammation of the liver, commonly due to alcohol, bacterial or viral infection, drugs, parasites, and poisons. Signs include clay-colored stool, dark urine, enlarged liver, and jaundice. **Cholestatic hepatitis** is due to infection that disrupts the flow of bile from the bile ducts. **Viral hepatitis** results from infection with hepatitis virus A, B, C, D, or E. Symptoms include right-upper quadrant abdominal pain, diarrhea, fever, nausea, and vomiting. Hepatitis A is a slow-onset virus spread by direct contact or through fecal-infected food or water. Hepatitis B (serum) is a rapid-onset type of viral infection caused by contaminated blood or unsterile needles or instruments. Hepatitis C is a post-transfusion type of hepatitis that is frequently seen in renal dialysis patients. The form of viral hepatitis known as D may be either acute or chronic. It is caused by a defective RNA virus that requires hepatitis B virus to reproduce. The chronic type may be the most severe of the viral forms. Hepatitis E is a waterborne, epidemic type that principally occurs in Africa and Asia. This variation appears to be intestinally transmitted.

hepatization, the changing of lung tissue into a solid mass. In early pneumonia the gathering of red blood cells in the alveoli produce **red hepatization.** In later stages of pneumonia, when white blood cells fill alveoli the process becomes **gray hepatization,** or **yellow hepatization** when fat deposits are added.

hepatocyte /hep´ətōsīt´/, the most basic liver cell that performs all the functions of the liver.

hepatoduodenal ligament /hep´ətōdo͞o·ədē´nəl, -do͞o·od´ənəl/, part of the membrane that lines the abdomen between the liver and the small intestine. A fiber-like capsule between the two layers of the ligament contains the hepatic artery, the common bile duct, the portal vein, lymphatics, and a network of nerves.

hepatojugular reflux /-jug´ələr/, a distention of the jugular vein when pressure is applied for 30 to 60 seconds over the stomach, suggestive of right-sided heart failure.

hepatoma /hep´ətō´mə/, a cancer of the liver. Symptoms include pain, hypotension, anorexia, and ascites.

hepatomegaly /-meg´əlē/, enlargement of the liver. It is often found by palpation when the liver can easily be palpated below the ribs and is tender to the touch. Hepatomegaly may be caused by hepatitis, alcoholism, obstruction of bile ducts, or cancer.

hepatotoxic /-tok´sik/, destroying liver cells.

hepatotoxicity /-toksis´itē/, the tendency of a substance to have a harmful effect on the liver.

hereditary, having to do with a feature, condition, or disease passed down from parent to offspring; inborn; inherited. Compare **acquired, congenital, familial.**

heredity, **1.** the process by which particular traits or conditions are passed along from parents to offspring, causing resemblance of individuals related by blood. It involves the division and rejoining of genes during cell division and fertilization. **2.** the total genetic makeup of an individual; the sum of the features inherited from ancestors and the possibilities of passing on these qualities to offspring.

Hering-Breuer reflex (Carl E. K. Hering, German physiologist, 1834-1918; Josef Breuer, German physician, 1842-1925), inhibition of respiratory inspiration due to a reflex triggered by inflation of the lungs. Pressure receptors in the lungs prevent an overfill of alveoli and stimulate expiration.

hermaphroditism /hərmaf´rəditizm/, a rare condition in which both male and female sex organs exist in the same person. The condition results from a chromosomal abnormality. Also known as **hermaphrodism.** Compare **pseudohermaphroditism.**

hernia, the protrusion of an organ through a weakness in the muscle wall that surrounds it. A hernia may be present at birth or may be acquired later in life because of overweight, muscular weakness, surgery, or illness. An **abdominal hernia** is a loop of bowel that pushes through the muscles of the abdomen. A protrusion of the stomach through an opening in the diaphragm is a **diaphragmatic hernia.** This occurs most often at the point where the esophagus passes through the diaphragm. A kind of diaphragmatic hernia is **hiatal hernia,** a protrusion of a portion of the stomach upward through the diaphragm. Symptoms usually include heartburn after meals, when lying down, and on exertion. There may be vomiting and a dull pain below the sternum that radiates to the shoulder. A **femoral hernia** is one in which a loop of intestine pushes into the groin. With an **inguinal hernia,** a loop of intestine pushes into the inguinal canal, sometimes filling, in a male, the entire scrotal sac. Of all hernias, 75% to 80% are inguinal hernias. An **umbilical hernia** is a bulging of intestine through a weakness in the abdominal wall around the umbilicus.

herniated disk, rupture of the pad between vertebrae, usually between the lumbar vertebrae. Also known as **herniated nucleus pulposus, ruptured disk, slipped disk.**

herniation, the protruding of a body organ or part of an organ through a tear in a membrane, muscle, or other tissue. *See also hernia.*

herniation syndrome, pressure on the brainstem (medulla) and obstruction of cerebrospinal fluid flow after increased intracranial pressure forces the brain downward into the foramen magnum. Altered levels of consciousness, decorticate and/or decerebrate posturing, and respiratory arrest will follow if the pressure is not relieved. It can be caused by any condition causing increased intracranial pressure, but typically occurs following acute subdural hemorrhage.

herniorrhaphy /hur´nē·or´əfē/, the surgical repair of a hernia.

heroin, an opiate derivative with no currently acceptable medical use in the United States. Heroin is controlled by law in the Comprehensive Drug Abuse Prevention and Control Act of 1970. It may not be prescribed to patients but only used for research and teaching or for chemical analysis.

herpes genitalis /hur´pēz/, an infection caused by Type 2 herpes simplex virus, usually transmitted by sexual contact, that causes painful blebs on the skin and moist lining of the sex organs of males and females.

herpes simplex, an infection caused by a herpes simplex virus, which attacks the skin and nervous system and usually produces small, short-lasting, irritating, and sometimes painful fluid-filled blebs on the skin and mucous membranes. Oral herpes (herpes labialis) infections tend to occur in the facial area, particularly around the mouth and nose; herpes genitalis infections are usually limited to the genital area.

herpesvirus, any of five related viruses including herpes simplex viruses 1 and 2, varicella-zoster virus, Epstein-Barr virus, and cytomegalovirus.

herpes zoster, infection caused by the varicella-zoster virus, affecting mainly adults. It causes painful skin blebs that follow the route of nerves infected by the virus. The pain and blebs usually occur on only one side of the body, and any sensory nerve may be affected. Early symptoms may include digestive system disturbances, vague discomfort, fever, and headache.

herpetiform /hərpet´ifôrm/, having clusters of blebs, resembling the skin sores of some herpesvirus infections.

hertz (Heinrich R. Hertz, German physicist, 1857-1894), a unit of frequency equal to 1 cycle per second.

hesitation marks, *(informal)* scratches or minor lacerations, usually seen on the wrists or arms, after an attempt at suicide.

hetastarch, a colloid (carbohydrate starch derivative) that acts as a volume expander, increasing circulating blood volume by pulling fluid from the cells. Anaphylaxis is an occasional side effect of this drug. Also known as **Hespan.**

heterogamy /het´ərog´əmē/, sexual reproduction in which there is joining of dissimilar sex cells, usually differing in size and structure. The word primarily refers to the reproductive processes of humans and mammals as opposed to certain lower plants and animals.

heterogeneous /het´ərōjē´nē·əs/, **1.** consisting of unlike elements or parts. **2.** not having a uniform quality throughout. Compare **homogeneous. –heterogeneity,** *adj.*

heterogenous /het´əroj´ənəs/, derived or developed from another source or from two different sources.

heteroploid /-ploid´/, **1.** an individual, organism, strain, or cell that has fewer or more whole chromosomes in its body cells than is normal for its species. **2.** such an individual, organism, strain, or cell. *See also euploid.*

heterosexual, **1.** a person whose sexual preference is for people of the opposite sex. **2.** sexual preference for people of the opposite sex. **–heterosexuality,** *n.*

hiatal hernia. See **hernia.**

hiatus /hī·ā´təs/, a usually normal opening in a membrane or other body tissue. **–hiatal,** *adj.*

hiccup, a sound that is produced by contraction or spasm of the diaphragm, followed by reflex closure of the vocal cords. Hiccups have a variety of causes, including indigestion, rapid eating, surgery, and displaced pacemaker. Most episodes do not last longer than a few minutes, but long-lasting or repeat attacks sometimes occur. The condition is most often seen in men. Also known as **hiccough.**

Hickman catheter, an in-dwelling central venous catheter used for blood withdrawal, intravenous therapy, and medication administration. This soft, double-lumen catheter is left in place for prolonged periods of time for patients who are receiving large amounts of intravenous medications. Forcing fluid through the catheter is contraindicated because of the danger of catheter rupture. *See also Groshong catheter.*

hidrosis /hidrō´-/, sweating. **Anhidrosis** is an abnormal lack of sweating. **Dyshidrosis** is a condition in which abnormal sweating occurs. **Hyperhidrosis** is a state of increased sweating. It may be caused by heat, overactive thyroid, menopause, or infection.

high-altitude cerebral edema, neurological impairment that develops during ascent to altitudes greater than 5000 ft (about 1500 m) in otherwise healthy but unacclimatized individuals. Symptoms involve a rapid onset with altered levels of consciousness, apathy, and difficulty with motor movements. Also known as **HACE.** *See also acute mountain sickness.*

high-altitude pulmonary edema, respiratory difficulty that develops during ascent to altitudes above 5000 ft (about 1500 m) in otherwise healthy but unacclimatized subjects. Symptoms occur after several hours or days at altitude and vary from a dry cough to the crackles and rhonchi of pulmonary edema. Also known as **HAPE.** See Appendix 1-16.

high blood pressure. See **hypertension.**

highest intercostal vein, one of a pair of veins that drain the blood from the superior chest.

high-pressure nervous syndrome, involuntary tremors and seizures during mixed-gas diving at depths greater than 600 ft (about 200 m). It is believed to be due to a combination of inert gas tissue saturation and cell compression due to the pressures at great depth. Also known as **HPNS.**

high-risk infant, any newborn, regardless of birth weight, size or length of time in the womb, who has a greater than average chance of sickness or death, especially within the first 28 days of life.

high velocity, weapons that fire ammunition at speeds of 2000 feet per second or faster. *See also low velocity.*

hinge joint, a fluid-filled joint in which bone surfaces are closely molded together in a way that permits extensive motion in one plane. The joints of the fingers are hinge joints. Compare **gliding joint, pivot joint.**

hipbone. See **innominate bone.**

hip joint, the ball-and-socket joint of the hip. It consists of the head of the femur in the acetab-

ulum. These are attached by seven ligaments which permit very extensive movement. Also known as **coxal articulation.**

hippocampus, structure in the lower brain that integrates mood, emotions, and concentration.

Hippocrates (Hippocrates of Cos, Greek physician, 460-360 B.C.), *(historical)* known as the father of medicine, he first introduced the scientific approach to healing.

Hippocratic oath, a vow taken by Hippocrates' students as they became physicians. It is given today at some medical schools on graduation and is a standard by which physicians can judge their ethics.

hippus, rapid contraction and dilatation of the pupils, even in the presence of a light source. **Respiratory hippus** is pupillary contraction during expiration and dilatation while inspiring. Also known as **iridodonesis.**

hirsutism /hur´sōōtizm/, excessive body hair as a result of heredity, hormonal imbalance, or medication.

His-Purkinje system (Wilhelm His, Jr., German physician, 1863-1934; Johannes E. von Purkinje, Bohemian physiologist, 1787-1869), two components of the cardiac electrical conduction system, which transmits impulses from the AV node into the ventricles. The bundle of His conducts impulses from the AV node to the bundle branches. The Purkinje system transmits impulses from the bundle branches to the myocardial cells of the ventricles.

histamine /his´təmin, -mēn/, a compound, found in all cells, produced by the breakdown of histidine. It is released in allergic reactions and causes vasodilatation.

histidine /his´tidin/, a basic amino acid found in many proteins and the substance from which histamine is produced. It is an essential amino acid in infants.

histology /histol´-/, **1.** the science dealing with the microscopic identification of cells and tissue. **2.** the structure of organ tissues, including the makeup of cells and their organization into various body tissues.

histone /his´tōn/, any of a group of proteins, found in the cell nucleus, especially of glandular tissue. They help regulate gene activity but interfere with clotting of the blood.

histoplasmosis /-plazmō´-/, an infection caused by breathing in spores of the fungus *Histoplasma capsulatum*. It is common in the Mississippi and Ohio valleys. The fungus, spread by airborne spores from soil infected with the droppings of infected birds, acts as a parasite on the cells of the body's defense system.

histotoxin /-tok´sin/, any substance that is poisonous to the body tissues. It is usually produced within the body. **–histotoxic,** *adj.*

histrionic personality disorder /his´trē·on´ik/, a disorder having intensely exaggerated behavior, which is typically self-centered and results in severe disturbance in the patient's relationships with others. This can lead to psychosomatic disorders, depression, alcoholism, and drug dependency. Symptoms include emotional excitability, such as irrational angry outbursts or tantrums; abnormal craving for activity and excitement; overreaction to minor events; inconsistency; and continuous demand for reassurance because of feelings of helplessness and dependency. *See also narcissistic personality disorder.*

hives. See **urticaria.**

Hodgkin's disease /hoj´kinz/, a malignant disorder with painless, steady enlargement of lymph glands and spleen. Symptoms include anorexia, low-grade fever, and night sweats. Clusters of cases have been reported, but there is no definite evidence of an infectious agent.

hole. See **hydraulic.**

Holger-Nielsen method. See **back-pressure arm-lift method.**

holistic health care, a system of total patient care that considers the physical, emotional, social, economic, and spiritual needs of the patient. It also considers the patient's response to the illness and the impact of the illness on the patient's ability to meet self-care needs.

hologynic /-jin´ik/, **1.** designating genes located on attached X chromosomes. **2.** of or pertaining to traits or conditions passed on only from the mother (the maternal line).

Homan's sign, pain in the calf that occurs with bending the foot back, indicating thrombophlebitis.

home care, a health service provided in the patient's home for the purpose of promoting, maintaining, or restoring health or reducing the effects of illness and disability. Service may include medical, dental, or nursing care, speech or physical therapy, the homemaking services of a home health aide, or transportation service.

homeodynamics /hō´mē·ōdīnam´-/, the process of constantly changing body functions while keeping an overall balance of systems and health.

homeopathy /hō´mē·op´əthē/, a system of healing based on the theory that "like cures like." The theory was advanced in the late eighteenth century by Dr. Samuel Hahnemann, who believed that a large amount of a particular drug may cause symptoms of a disease and a mild dose may reduce those symptoms; thus, some disease symptoms could be treated by very small doses of medicine. In practice, homeopathists (physicians who practice homeopathy) dilute drugs to achieve the smallest dose of a drug that seems necessary to control the symptoms in a patient. They also prescribe only one medication at a time. Compare **allopathy. –homeopathic,** *adj.*

homeostasis /-stā´-/, a relatively constant state within the body, naturally maintained. Various sensing, feedback, and control systems bring about this steady state, especially the reticular formation in the brainstem and the hormone-producing glands. Some of the functions controlled by homeostatic mechanisms are heart rate, blood pressure, body temperature, respirations, and glandular secretion. **–homeostatic,** *adj.*

homicide, the death of one human being caused by another human. Homicide is usually intentional and often violent.

homiothermic /hō´mē·ōthur´-/, referring to the ability of warm-blooded animals to keep a relatively stable body temperature regardless of the temperature of the environment. This ability is not fully developed in newborn humans.

homogeneous /-jē´nē·əs/, **1.** consisting of similar elements or parts. **2.** having a uniform quality throughout. Compare **heterogeneous. –homogeneity,** *adj.*

homogenesis /-jen´əsis/, reproduction by the same process in succeeding generations so that offspring are similar to the parents. Compare **heterogenesis.**

homogenous /hōmoj´ənəs/, having a likeness in form or structure because of a common ancestral origin. Compare **heterogenous.**

homolateral /-lat´ərəl/, pertaining to the same side of the body.

homolog /hom´əlog/, any organ corresponding in function, origin, and structure to another organ, as the flippers of a seal corresponds to human hands.

homologous chromosomes /hōmol´əgəs/, any two chromosomes in the doubled set of the body cell that are identical in size, shape, and gene placement. In humans there are 22 pairs of homologous chromosomes and one pair of sex chromosomes, with one member of each pair coming from the mother and the other from the father. Any difference in the size, number, or genetic makeup of the chromosomes leads to defects or disorders from mild to severe in the affected individual.

homoplasty /hō´məplas´tē/, likeness in form or structure because of similar environmental conditions or parallel evolution rather than because of common ancestral origin.

homosexual, **1.** pertaining to, or denoting the same sex. **2.** a person, generally male, who is sexually attracted to members of the same sex. Compare **heterosexual.** *See also lesbian.*

homunculus /hōmung´kyələs/, *pl.* **homunculi,** **1.** a dwarf in whom all the body parts are in proportion and in whom there is no deformity or abnormality. **2.** *(in psychiatry)* a little man created by the imagination who possesses magical powers.

hood, a cloth device made of fire-resistant material that covers the head, neck, and ears for protection during extrication and firefighting operations.

hookah. See **surface supplied diving equipment.**

hookworm infection, a condition resulting from a spread of hookworms of the genera *Ancylostoma, Necator,* or *Uncinaria* in the small intestine. Infection may be prevented by keeping soil free of fecal matter and by wearing shoes.

hopelessness, a psychologic condition in which one believes that all efforts to change one's life situation will be fruitless.

hordeolum /hôrdē´ələm/. See **sty.**

hormone, a chemical substance produced in one part or organ of the body that starts or runs the activity of an organ or a group of cells in another part of the body. Hormones from the endocrine glands are carried through the bloodstream to the target organ. Release of these hormones is regulated by other hormones, by the nervous system, and by a signal from the target organ indicating a decreased need for the stimulating hormone.

Horner's syndrome, a condition with narrowed pupils, drooping eyelids, and unusual facial dryness resulting from an injury to the cervical spinal cord.

horse collar, a padded horseshoe-shaped rescue device that is attached to a hoist and used for lifting conscious victims vertically into a helicopter. This device requires victim training for safe use and cannot be used to lift those with upper-body trauma or altered levels of consciousness.

horsepower, a unit of power equal to 550 footpounds per second, or 745.7 watts.

horse serum, any vaccine prepared from the blood of a horse, especially tetanus antitoxin. Because many people are allergic to horse serum, human tetanus serum is preferred.

horseshoe fistula, an abnormal, semicircular passage in the area around the anus with both openings on the surface of the skin.

hospice /hos´pis/, a system of home-centered care designed to assist the patient with a long-term illness to be comfortable and to maintain a satisfactory lifestyle through the last phases of dying. Hospice care includes home visits, professional medical care, teaching and emotional support of the family, and physical care of the patient. Some hospice programs provide care in a center, as well as in the home. *See also stages of dying.*

host, **1.** an organism that is a victim of parasitic invasion. A **primary** or **definitive host** is one in which the adult parasite lives and reproduces. Humans are definitive hosts for pinworms and tapeworms. A **secondary** or **intermediate host** is one in which the parasite exists in its nonsexual, larval stage. Humans are intermediate hosts for malaria parasites. A **reservoir host** is a primary animal host for organisms that are sometimes parasitic in humans and from which humans may become infected. A **dead-end host** is any animal from which a parasite cannot escape to continue its life cycle. **2.** the recipient of a transplanted organ or tissue. Compare **donor.**

hostility, the tendency of an organism to threaten harm to another or to itself. The hostility may be expressed passively and actively.

hot, 1. elevated temperature. **2.** any location that has dangerous levels of contamination. **3.** *(aviation)* any operation performed with engines running and/or loaded weapons. **4.** any location with active weapons fire or explosives. **5.** actively conducting electrical current.

hot flash, a short-term feeling of warmth. Hot flashes result from blood flow disturbances caused by hormone changes. The exact cause is not known. Also known as **hot flush.**

hot line, a means of contacting a trained counselor or specific agency for help with a particular problem, as a rape hot line or a battered-child hot line. Such services are usually staffed by volunteers who answer phones 24 hours a day, 7 days a week.

hot stick. See **clampstick.**

hot zone, an area in which contamination or other danger exists or may occur. Also known as **inner perimeter.** *See also inner perimeter.*

hourglass uterus, a womb with a segment of circular muscle fibers that contract during labor, causing lack of progress in the birth despite adequate labor contractions. The baby is pushed in rather than out during contractions.

hovercraft, a vehicle designed to transit bodies of water on a cushion of air. Many hovercraft do not actually touch the water while in operation and can be used for short distances on land. Also known as **ACV, air cushion vehicle, GEM, ground effect machine, skim.** *See also air cushion vehicle.*

hover jumping, stepping from the skid of a hovering helicopter when landing is not possible or timely. The technique requires that the helicopter hover near the ground. Also known as **hover stepping.**

huddle, water survival technique that conserves body heat by gathering a group of people into a tight circle, facing each other.

huffing, *(informal)* the intentional breathing in of noxious or toxic substances to obtain a feel-

ing of euphoria. Most commonly seen with glue or paint sniffing from a paper or plastic bag.

human chorionic somatomammotropin, a hormone produced during pregnancy that regulates carbohydrate and protein processing in the mother to ensure that the fetus receives glucose for energy and protein for growth.

human immunodeficiency virus, a virus (retrovirus) that infects and kills body cells, particularly those of the human immune system, which may then lead to acquired immune-deficiency syndrome (AIDS), AIDS-related complex (ARC), or other fatal diseases that capitalize on the body's inability to fight disease. It is easily killed by heat and common disinfectants, such as 1:10 household bleach solution, hydrogen peroxide, Lysol, and 35% isopropyl alcohol. Although found in many body fluids, it has only been proven to be transmitted via blood and/or blood products, semen, the uterus (into the placenta), and vaginal secretions. Also known as **HIV.**

humerus /hyōō´mərəs/, *pl.* **humeri,** the largest bone of the upper arm. The lower end has several grooves that connect with the radius and ulna. –**humeral,** *adj.*

humidifier lung, a fungal pulmonary condition common among workers involved with refrigeration and air conditioning equipment. Symptoms include chills, cough, fever, nausea, and vomiting. Also known as **air conditioner lung.** *See also pneumonitis.*

hurricane. See **tropical cyclone.**

Hurst tool. See **hydraulic-powered rescue tool.**

hyaline membrane disease /hī´əlin/. See **respiratory distress syndrome of the newborn.**

hybrid /hī´brid/, **1.** an offspring produced from mating plants or animals from different species, varieties, or genotypes. **2.** pertaining to such a plant or animal.

hydatid /hī´dətid/, a cyst or cystlike structure that, usually, is filled with fluid.

hydatid cyst, a cyst in the liver that contains larvae of the tapeworm *Echinococcus granulosus,* whose eggs are carried from the intestinal tract to the liver via the blood. Patients generally lack symptoms, except for an enlarged liver and a dull ache over the right upper quarter of the abdomen. Anaphylaxis may occur if the cyst ruptures.

hydatid mole. See **molar pregnancy.**

hydatidosis /-ō´sis/, infection with the tapeworm *Echinococcus granulosus. See also hydatid cyst.*

hydradenitis /hī´dradənī´-/, an infection or inflammation of the sweat glands.

hydramnios /hīdram´nē·əs/, an abnormal condition of pregnancy with an excess of fluid surrounding the fetus. It is linked to maternal disorders, including toxemia of pregnancy and diabetes mellitus. Some fetal disorders may interfere with normal exchange of amniotic fluid, resulting in hydramnios. The chances of premature labor and stillbirth are increased.

hydraulic, disruption of water flow when water curls upward and back on itself after flowing over an object beneath the surface. This water hazard develops into a circular motion that can trap a victim under water. Also known as **hole, reversal.** *See also keeper hydraulic.*

hydraulic jack tool, hand-operated jacks that use a pump to create pressure on a plunger via fluid (usually oil). Plunger movement causes the pushing or spreading that makes the jack useful during vehicular and structural extrication. Jack capacities range from 2 to 500 tons. Also known as **Porto-power, railroad jack.** Compare **hydraulic-powered rescue tool.**

hydraulic-powered rescue tool, engine- or electrically operated system that uses hydraulic fluid under pressure to operate various types of hydraulic rescue tools. Primary components of this system are the power plant, power spreader, power cutter, and power ram. Although these tools have many applications, they are primarily used during vehicular and structural extrication. Also known as **jaws, Hurst tool.** Compare **hydraulic jack tool.**

hydraulic shoring, jacks or shoring, powered by the action of hydraulic fluid, used to stabilize an unstable or unsecured wall. Also known as **speed shores.**

hydroa /hīdrō´ə/, a skin condition of childhood that occurs each summer after exposure to sunlight, sometimes accompanied by itching and thickening of the skin. Hydroa usually disappears soon after puberty.

hydrocarbon, any of a group of chemical compounds (organic) that contain hydrogen and carbon. They are found in living matter, and many are derived from petroleum.

hydrocele /hī´drəsēl/, a buildup of fluid in any saclike cavity or duct, specifically in the membrane surrounding the testicles or along the spermatic cord.

hydrocephalus /hī´drōsef´ələs/, a disorder in which an abnormal amount of spinal fluid causes widening of the cerebral ventricles. The condition may be congenital with rapid onset of symptoms, or it may progress slowly so that neurologic signs do not come until late childhood or even early adulthood. In infants, the head grows at an abnormal rate.

hydrochloric acid, a compound of hydrogen and chlorine, which forms a strong acid that is the primary component of gastric juice.

hydrogen, a gaseous element that is normally colorless, odorless, and highly inflammable.

hydronephrosis /-nefrō´-/, distention of the kidney caused by urine that cannot flow past an obstructed ureter. The cause may be a tumor, a stone lodged in the ureter, inflammation of the prostate gland, or a urinary tract infection. The patient may have pain in the flank.

hydropenia /-pe´nē·ə/, lack of water in the body tissues.

hydrophobia, 1. rabies. 2. a morbid, extreme fear of water.

hydroplane, loss of tire contact with the road as water trapped beneath the tire forms a wedge of water onto which the tire begins to ride.

hydrops /hī´drops/, an abnormal amount of clear, watery fluid in a body tissue or cavity, such as a joint, fallopian tube, middle ear, or gallbladder. Hydrops in the entire body may occur in infants born with thalassemia or severe Rh sensitization. **Hydrops fetalis** is a massive fluid buildup in the fetus or newborn.

hydrosalpinx /-sal´pingks/, an infection of a fallopian tube that is enlarged and filled with clear fluid. It results from infection that has caused a blockage of the tube.

hydrostatic pressure, the pressure exerted by a liquid at rest.

hydrostatic test, a periodic test of compressed gas cylinders to determine whether they can safely contain compressed gases. Testing is generally required every five years.

hydrothorax /-thôr´aks/, fluid in the chest cavity without inflammation.

Hydrozoa, an order of invertebrate marine organisms that possess venomous stinging cells called *nematocysts*. This group of coelenterates includes the Portuguese man-of-war, Pacific bluebottle, and fire coral. *See also nematocysts.*

hymen /hī´mən/, a fold of tissue at the vaginal entrance.

Hymenoptera, the order of venomous insects that includes ants, bees, and wasps.

hyperacidity /hī´pərasid´itē/, excess acidity, as in the stomach.

hyperactivity, abnormally increased activity.

hyperalimentation /-al´imentā´shən/, feeding of a large amount of nutrients.

hyperammonemia /-am´ōnē´mē·ə/, increased ammonia in the blood. Ammonia is produced in the intestine and absorbed into the blood, and its poisonous effect is detoxified in the liver. If there is overproduction or a decreased ability to detoxify it, levels in the blood may increase.

hyperbaric chamber. See **decompression chamber.**

hyperbaric oxygenation /-ber´ik/, giving oxygen at high atmospheric pressure. It is done in pressure chambers that permit the delivery of pure oxygen and air at pressures up to five times normal. Hyperbaric oxygenation is used to treat carbon monoxide poisoning, air embolism, smoke inhalation, cyanide poisoning, decompression sickness, and wounds.

hyperbilirubinemia /-bil´iro͞o´binē´mē·ə/, excess bilirubin in the blood. Symptoms include jaundice, lack of appetite, and fatigue. The disorder is most often linked to liver disease or blockage of bile.

hypercalcemia /-kalsē´mē·ə/, increased calcium in the blood. It most often results from bone loss and release of calcium, as occurs in bone tumors and osteoporosis. Patients with hypercalcemia are confused and have abdominal and muscle pains and weakness.

hypercalciuria /-kal´sēyo͞or´ē·ə/, increased calcium in the urine, resulting from conditions such as certain types of arthritis, marked by large amounts of bone loss. Concentrated amounts of calcium in the urinary tract may form kidney stones.

hypercapnia /-kap´nē·ə/, increased carbon dioxide in the blood. Also known as **hypercarbia.**

hyperchloremia /-klôrē´mē·ə/, increased chloride in the blood.

hyperchlorhydria /-klôrhid´rē·ə/, increased release of hydrochloric acid by cells lining the stomach.

hypercholesterolemia /-kōles´tərōle´mē·ə/, increased cholesterol in the blood. High levels of cholesterol and other lipids may lead to arteriosclerosis.

hyperdynamic syndrome, a cluster of symptoms that signal the onset of septic shock. It often includes a rapid rise in temperature, flushing of the skin, tachycardia, and alternating rise and fall of blood pressure. *See also shock.*

hyperemesis gravidarum /-em´əsis/, an abnormal condition of pregnancy marked by long-term vomiting, weight loss, and fluid and electrolyte imbalance. If the condition is severe, liver and kidney failure may result.

hyperemia /-ē´mē·ə/, increased blood flow to an area of the body, as in the inflammatory response, local relaxation of small blood vessels, or blockage of the outflow of blood from an area. Skin in the area usually becomes reddened and warm. **–hyperemic,** *adj.*

hyperextension, a position of maximum extension.

hyperflexia, the forcible overbending of a limb.

hyperfunction, increased function of any organ or system.

hypergenesis /-jen´əsis/, excess growth; overdevelopment. The condition may involve parts of the body or the entire body. It may even result in the formation of extra parts, as the development of additional fingers or toes. **–hypergenetic,** *adj.*

hyperglycemia /-glīsē´mē·ə/, increased glucose in the blood, most often linked to diabetes mellitus. Diabetic ketoacidosis may result. Compare **hypoglycemia.**

hypergolic materials, any substances that ignite spontaneously on contact with one another without requiring a source of ignition.

hyperimmune, having an unusual abundance of antibodies, producing a greater than normal immunity.

hyperkalemia /-kəlē´mē·ə/, increased potassium in the blood. This condition often occurs in kidney failure. Symptoms include nausea, muscle weakness, and cardiac dysrhythmias.

hyperkeratosis /-ker′ətō′-/,   formation of skin overgrowth, as a callus.

hyperlipidemia /lip′idē′mē·ə/,   an excess of fats (lipids) in the blood.

hyperlipoproteinemia /-lip′ōprō′tēnē′mē·ə/, any of a group of disorders that cause an increase of certain protein-bound fats lipids and other fatty substances in the blood. *See also lipoprotein.*

hypermagnesemia /-mag′nēsē′mē·ə/,   increased magnesium in the blood. Symptoms include fatigue, weakness and cardiac conduction anomalies.

hypermetria /-mē′trē·ə/,   decreased ability to control the range of muscular action, causing movements that overreach the intended goal of the affected person. Compare **hypometria.**

hypermorph /hī′pərmôrf/,   **1.** a person whose arms and legs are too long in relation to the trunk. **2.** *(in genetics)* a mutant gene that shows increased activity in the expression of a trait.

hypernatremia /-natrē′mē·ə/,   increased sodium in the blood, usually caused by an excess loss of water and electrolytes resulting from diarrhea, excessive sweating, or too little water intake. Patients may develop altered levels of consciousness and seizures. *See also diabetes insipidus.*

hyperopia /-ō′pē·ə/.   See **farsightedness.**

hyperosmia /-oz′mē·ə/,   increased sensitivity to odors. Compare **anosmia.**

hyperparathyroidism /-per′əthī′roidizm/,   overactivity of one or more of the four parathyroid glands. Too much parathyroid hormone (PTH) is made. Calcium is drawn from the bones, and much of it is then absorbed by the kidneys, stomach, and intestines. Kidney failure, peptic ulcers, bone fractures, and weak muscles may develop. Other symptoms may include nausea, anorexia, and altered levels of consciousness.

hyperphenylalaninemia /fen′ilal′əninē′mē·ə/,   an abnormally high amount of the amino acid, phenylalanine, in the blood. This may result from one of several defects in the process of breaking down phenylalanine. *See also phenylketonuria.*

hyperphoria /-fôr′ē·ə/,   the tendency of an eye to deviate upward.

hyperpigmentation /-pig′məntā′shən/,   unusual darkening of the skin. Causes include heredity,

drugs, and exposure to the sun. Compare **hypopigmentation.**

hyperplasia /-plā′zhə/,   an increase in the number of cells of a body part. Compare **hypertrophy.**

hyperploidy /-ploi′dē/,   any increase in chromosome number that involves individual chromosomes rather than entire sets, resulting in more than the normal number characteristic of the species, as in Down's syndrome. Compare **hypoploidy.** *See also euploid.*

hyperpnea /-pnē′ə/,   increased respiratory rate.

hyperprolactinemia /-prōlak′tinē′mē·ə/,   too much of the hormone prolactin in the blood.

hyperpyrexia /pīrek′sē·ə/,   an extremely high temperature sometimes occurring in serious infectious diseases, especially in young children. Marked by a rapid rise in temperature, tachycardia, tachypnea, diaphoresis, and cyanosis. *See also fever.*

hyperreflexia /-riflek′sē·ə/,   markedly increased reflex reactions.

hypersensitivity,   an increased tendency to overreaction to a particular stimulus. *See also allergy.* **–hypersensitive,** *adj.*

hypersensitivity pneumonitis,   lung inflammation caused by exposure to a foreign substance (allergen). The allergen may be from a fungus, bird droppings, animal fur or as a result of a drug. Symptoms include fever, difficulty in breathing, fatigue, and pulmonary edema. The symptoms usually develop 4 to 6 hours after exposure.

hypersensitivity reaction,   the excessive response of the immune system to a sensitizing antigen. The antigenic stimulant is an allergen and the response may be immediate or delayed. Several factors determine the strength of an allergic response: responsiveness of the host to the allergen, amount of allergen, kind of allergen, the timing of the exposures, and the site of the allergen-immune mediator reaction.

hypersomnia /-som′nē·ə/,   **1.** very deep or long sleep, usually caused by mental rather than physical factors. **2.** great drowsiness.

hypertelorism /-tel′ərizm/,   a developmental defect marked by an abnormally wide space between two organs or parts. Compare **hypotelorism.**

hypertension, marked high blood pressure persistently exceeding 140/90. **Essential hypertension,** also called **primary hypertension** (the most frequent), has no one known cause, but its risk is increased by overweight, high sodium, high cholesterol, and a family history of high blood pressure. **Secondary hypertension** is linked to diseases of the kidneys, lungs, glands, and vessels, such as **pulmonary hypertension. Systolic hypertension** shows only an elevation of systolic pressure. Hypertension is more common in men than in women and is twice as common in blacks as in whites. Persons with mild or moderate hypertension may have no symptoms or may experience headaches and tinnitus. High blood pressure is often accompanied by rapid or irregular heart rates, diophoresis, nausea, and pulmonary edema. **Malignant hypertension** (most life-threatening form) is very high blood pressure (a diastolic pressure higher than 120) that may damage the tissues of small vessels, the brain, eyes, heart, and kidneys. Symptoms include severe headaches, blurred vision, and altered levels of consciousness. *See also blood pressure.*

hypertensive emergencies, a clinical situation in which a patient has severe elevation of blood pressure (diastolic pressure greater than 115 mmHg) with neurologic symptoms or other progressive organ involvement. Signs include altered levels of consciousness, pulmonary edema, and/or seizures. Previously known as **hypertensive crisis.**

hypertensive encephalopathy, neurologic dysfunction, including headache, altered levels of consciousness, and seizures, associated with hypertensive emergencies.

hyperthermia /-thur´mē·ə/, a much higher than normal body temperature. **Habitual hyperthermia** is a condition of unknown cause that occurs in young females, in which body temperatures of 99° to 100.5° F occur off and on for years. Fatigue, vague aches and pains, loss of sleep, and headaches also occur. **Malignant hyperthermia** is an inherited disorder that features an often fatal high body temperature.

hyperthyroidism /-thī´roidizm/, a disorder with increased activity of the thyroid gland. The gland is usually swollen, releasing greater than normal amounts of thyroid hormones, which speeds up the body processes. Symptoms include nervousness, tremor, constant hunger, weight loss, fatigue, heat intolerance, and irregular heart beat. Antithyroid drugs are usually given. *See also Graves disease.*

hypertonic, **1.** higher solute concentration on one side of a semipermeable membrane than on the other. **2.** greater than normal solute concentration, with normal usually being compared to that of the human body. **3.** increased muscle tone or tension. Compare **hypotonic.**

hypertrophic catarrh /-trof´ik/, a chronic condition marked by inflammation and discharge from a mucous membrane, with thickening of the mucous and submucous tissue.

hypertrophy /hīpur´trəfē/, an increase in the size of an organ or other part of the body, due to an increase in the size of the cells rather than the number of cells. Compare **atrophy.** –**hypertrophic,** *adj.*

hyperventilation, **1.** rapid respirations. **2.** rapid ventilation (>30/min) with a positive pressure ventilation device, such as bag-valve mask, demand valve. This technique is used when high levels of oxygenation or low levels of carbon dioxide are necessary, as in head injury or ingestion of tricyclic antidepressants. **3.** *(informal)* a syndrome consisting of rapid respirations brought on by stress, which causes numbness and tingling in the face and extremities, a sense of shortness of breath, and carpopedal spasms. Although stressful for the victim, the condition is generally benign.

hypervolemia /-vōlē´mē·ə/, an increase in the amount of fluid outside the cells, particularly in the volume of circulating blood.

hypesthesia /hī´pesthē´zhə/, decreased level of sensation in response to stimulation of the sensory nerves. Touch, pain, heat, and cold are poorly perceived.

hyphema /hīfē´mə/, bleeding into the anterior chamber of the eye, usually caused by trauma.

hypnagogue /hip´nəgog/, an agent or substance that tends to induce sleep. *See also hypnotics.* –**hypnagogic,** *adj.*

hypnosis, a passive, trancelike state that resembles normal sleep during which perception and memory are changed, resulting in increased responsiveness to suggestion. The condition is usually caused by the monotonous repetition of words and gestures while the subject is completely relaxed. Hypnosis is used in some forms of psychotherapy and psychoanalysis or in medicine to reduce pain and aid relaxation.

hypnotic, a drug used as an aid in sleep.

hypnotism, the study or practice of producing hypnosis. One who practices hypnotism is a **hypnotist.**

hypoacidity /hī´pō·asid´itē/, a lack of acid.

hypoactivity, diminished activity of the body or its organs, such as lowered cardiac output, thyroid gland activity, or intestinal activity.

hypoalimentation, inadequate nourishment.

hypocalcemia /-kalsē´mē·ə/, decreased calcium in the blood. Severe hypocalcemia causes irregular cardiac rate, muscle spasms, and burning or prickling feelings of the hands, feet, lips, and tongue. Causes include hypoparathyroidism, kidney failure, severe inflammation of the pancreas, or decreased magnesium and protein in the blood. *See also tetany.*

hypocapnea, decreased carbon dioxide in the blood.

hypochlorhydria /-klôrhid´rē·ə/, decreased hydrochloric acid in the stomach.

hypochondria /-kon´drē·ə/, a condition with extreme anxiety, depression, and the belief that certain real or imagined physical symptoms are signs of a serious illness or disease despite medical evidence to the contrary. The cause may be an unresolved mental problem and may involve a specific organ, such as the heart, lungs, or eyes or several body systems at various times or at the same time.

hypodermic needle /dur´mik/, a hollow needle that attaches to a syringe for injecting medication into the body or for withdrawing fluid, such as blood, for examination.

hypodermoclysis /-dərmok´lisis/, the injection of a solution beneath the skin to supply fluid, nutrients, and other substances.

hypofibrinogenemia /-fī´brōjənē´mē·ə/, decreased fibrinogen, a blood clotting factor, in the blood. The condition may occur as a side effect of early detachment of the placenta in pregnancy.

hypoglossal nerve /-glos´əl/, either of a pair of nerves needed for swallowing and for moving the tongue.

hypoglycemia /-glīsē´mē·ə/, decreased glucose in the blood, usually caused by excessive insulin or low food intake. Symptoms include weakness, headache, hunger, and altered levels of consciousness. *See also diabetes, insulin, insulin shock.*

hypoglycemic agent, any of a large group of drugs, including insulin, prescribed to decrease the amount of sugar in the blood.

hypokalemia, low potassium levels in the blood, which causes weakness and cardiac dysrhythmias.

hypomagnesemia /-mag´nēsē´mē·ə/, decreased magnesium in the blood. Symptoms include nausea, vomiting, muscle weakness, tremors, and muscle spasms.

hypomania, a mentally unhealthy state of optimism, excitability, a marked hyperactivity and talkativeness, heightened sexual interest, quick anger and irritability, and a decreased need for sleep.

hypometria /-mē´trē·ə/, an inability to control muscular action, resulting in movements that fall short of the intended goals of the affected person. Compare **hypermetria.**

hypomorph /hī´pōmôrf/, a person whose legs are too short in relation to the trunk and whose sitting height is too great a fraction of standing height.

hyponatremia /-natrē´mē·ə/, decreased circulating sodium caused by diminished excretion or increased retention of water in the bloodstream. Symptoms include muscle spasms, altered consciousness, and seizures.

hypoparathyroidism /per´əthī´roidism/, lowered parathyroid function, which can be caused by the gland itself or by raised blood calcium levels.

hypoperfusion, decreased or inadequate perfusion, as due to hypovolemia.

hypoplasia /-plā´zhə/, incomplete or underdeveloped organ or tissue, usually the result of a decrease in the number of cells.

hypoploidy /-ploi´dē/, any decrease in chromosome number that involves individual chromosomes rather than entire sets, resulting in fewer than the normal number characteristic of the species, such as in Turner's syndrome. The unbalanced sets of chromosomes are referred to as hypodiploid, hypotriploid, hypotetraploid, and so on, depending on the number of multiples of the basic number of chromosomes they contain. Compare **hyperploidy.** *See also euploid.*

hypopnea, decrease in depth of respirations.

hypoproteinemia /-prō´tēnē´mē·ə/, a disorder with a decrease in the amount of protein in the blood. Symptoms include edema, nausea, vomiting, diarrhea, and abdominal pain. It may be caused by too little protein in the diet, intestinal diseases, or kidney failure.

hypoprothrombinemia /-prōthrom´binē´mē·ə/, an abnormal reduction in the amount of prothrombin (factor II) in the blood. There is poor clot formation, increased bleeding time, or uncontrolled bleeding. The condition is usually the result of severe liver disease or anticoagulant therapy with dicumarol. *See also blood clotting.*

hypoptyalism /hī´pōtī´əlizm/, a decrease in the amount of saliva released by the salivary glands.

hypopyon /hīpō´pē·on/, purulent material in the front chamber of the eye, appearing as a gray fluid between the cornea and the iris. It may occur as a side effect of conjunctivitis, herpetic keratitis, or corneal ulcer.

hyposensitive, reduced ability to respond to stimuli.

hypospadias /-spā´dē·as/, an inherited defect in which the urinary opening is on the underside of the penis. Compare **epispadias.**

hypotelorism /-tel´ərizm/, a condition with an abnormally decreased distance between two organs or parts.

hypotension, **1.** lowered systolic and diastolic blood pressure. **2.** decreased muscle tone.

hypothalamus /-thal´əməs/, a portion of the brain that controls and integrates part of the nervous system, the endocrine processes, and many bodily functions, as temperature, sleep, and appetite. **–hypothalamic,** *adj.*

hypothermia, lowered body core temperature. It is considered both a symptom and a syndrome. Most hypothermia is divided into primary (due to environment) and secondary (due to specific diseases) classifications. **Accidental hypothermia** is an unintentional drop in the

normal body core temperature (99.6 to 100° F or 37.6 to 38° C) of approximately 3.5° F (about 2° C) that is not due to central nervous system disease. See Appendix 1-17.

hypothyroidism /-thī´roidism/, decreased thyroid gland activity. Removal or atrophy of the thyroid gland may be responsible. Weight gain, arthritis, and slowed body metabolism may occur.

hypotonic, **1.** lower solute concentration on one side of a semipermeable membrane than on the other. **2.** less than normal solute concentration, with normal usually being compared to that of the human body. **3.** decreased muscle tone or tension. Compare **hypertonic.**

hypoventilation, decreased rate or depth of breathing.

hypovolemia /-vōlē´mē·ə/, low circulating blood volume due to hemorrhage. See Appendix 1-12.

hypovolemic shock. See **shock.**

hypoxemia /hī´poksē´mē·ə/, decreased circulating oxygen in the blood. Symptoms include cyanosis, tachycardia, and altered levels of consciousness.

hypoxia /hīpok´sē·ə/, decreased oxygen in the cells. Symptoms include cyanosis, tachycardia, and altered levels of consciousness. The tissues most sensitive to hypoxia are the brain, heart, and liver. Compare **hypoxemia.** *See also anoxia.*

hysterectomy /-ek´-/, surgical removal of the uterus. Types include **total,** in which the uterus and cervix are removed, and **radical,** in which ovaries, fallopian tubes, and lymph glands are removed with the uterus and cervix. Menstruation ceases after either type is performed. In an **abdominal hysterectomy,** the uterus is removed through the abdomen. **Colpohysterectomy** refers to removal of the uterus vaginally. A **panhysterectomy** is the removal of the uterus and cervix.

hysteria, a state of tension or excitement in a person or group, marked by unmanageable fear and short-term loss of control over the emotions.

hysteric neurosis, an emotional disorder in which extreme excitability and anxiety caused by conflict are changed into physical symptoms having no organic basis or into states of changed consciousness or identity. Kinds include **conversion disorder** and **dissociative disorder.**

I

iatrogenic /ī´atrōjen´ik, yat´-/, caused by treatment or diagnostic procedures. An iatrogenic disorder is a condition caused by medical personnel or procedures or through exposure to the environment of a health care facility.

ice ax, mountaineering pickax used for cutting footholds in ice or snow. Also known as **ice axe.**

iceboat, a boat used for traveling on ice, designed with runners to allow smooth movement over the surface.

icebreaker, a ship designed to create a passage through ice by using its strong bow and powerful engines to ride up onto the ice and break it.

icecap, a permanent ice cover over an area of land, such as a glacier.

icefall, an unstable collection of ice blocks and deep crevasses, formed by glacier movement around or over an obstruction. *See also bergschrund.*

ice field, a continuous sheet of floating ice. Also known as an **icecap.**

ice floe, a large mass of floating ice, though smaller than an ice field.

ice foot, the belt of ice that edges a frozen or polar coast between the high- and low-water mark.

ice needle, a thin ice crystal found floating in the air during clear, cold weather.

ice out, the thawing process of the surface of a body of water.

ice pack, 1. ice in a bag or towel that is used to decrease temperature or swelling of a body part.

2. a large area of pack ice, though more stable than an ice floe.

ice piton /pē´ton, pētōN´/, metal spike with threads that is used as an anchor point in ice and hard snow. It is generally driven in and unscrewed out of ice.

ice point, the temperature at which air-saturated water and ice are in equilibrium, generally at 32° F (0° C) at standard atmospheric pressure.

ice screw, metal spike with threads that is used as an anchor in ice and hard snow. It is generally driven in until the threads catch and then screwed into and out of the ice.

ice-up, the process of freezing.

ichthyosis /ik´thē·ō´-/, any of several congenital skin conditions in which the skin is dry and cracked. It usually appears at or shortly after birth and may be part of several rare disorders. Also known as **fish skin disease, xeroderma.**

ictal, referring to a sudden, sharp onset, as a seizure.

icteric, relating to or marked by jaundice.

id, *(in psychoanalysis)* the part of the psyche working in the unconscious that is the source of instinctive energy and has strong tendencies to self-preservation.

ID number, the four-digit identification number assigned to a hazardous material by the Department of Transportation: may include the prefix UN (United Nations) or NA (North American).

idea, thought, concept, intention, or impression that is in the mind as a result of awareness or understanding. A returning, irrational thought that persists in the mind is called a **compulsive idea.** It often results in a compelling need to do some improper act. A **fixed idea** is a continuous, single-minded thought or one that controls mental activity and continues despite evidence or logical proof that it is false. An **idea of influence** is an obsessive delusion, often seen in paranoid disorders, that external forces or persons are controlling one's thoughts, actions, and feelings. An **idea of persecution,** seen often in paranoid disorders, is a belief that one is threatened, discriminated against, or mistreated by others or by outside forces. An **idea of reference** is an obsessive delusion that the statements or actions of others refer to oneself, usually viewed as negative.

identification, an unconscious defense mechanism by which a person patterns his or her personality on that of another person, assuming the person's nature and actions. The process is a normal function of personality growth and learning. It adds to the gaining of interests and ideals. **Competitive identification** is done in order to outdo the other person. **Positive identification** is a patterning of one's personality on that of another for whom one has much respect.

identity crisis, a time of being confused about one's sense of self and role in society, occurring most often in the change from one stage of life to the next.

ideophobia /ī´dē·ō-/, an anxiety disorder marked by the irrational fear or distrust of ideas or reason. *See also phobia.*

idiopathic disease /id´ē·ōpath´ik/, a disease that develops without an apparent or known cause although it may have a recognizable pattern of signs and symptoms and may be curable.

idiopathy /id´ē·op´əthē/, any primary disease with no apparent cause. **–idiopathic,** *adj.*

idiosyncrasy, 1. physical or behavioral characteristics that are unique to an individual or group. **2.** an idea, action, or substance that makes one react differently than others. *See also allergy.*

idiot savant /ēdē·ō´säväN´, savant´/, a person with severe retardation who is able to perform unusual mental feats, primarily those involving music, puzzle-solving, or the use of numbers.

idioventricular rhythm, a ventricular escape rhythm, characterized by an absent P wave, a QRS complex of greater than 0.12 second, and a rate of 40 or less.

id reaction, an allergy caused by a fungal infection.

igloo space, storage area designed for ammunition and explosives, in an earth-covered concrete/steel bunker.

ignition point. See **ignition temperature.**

ignition temperature, minimum temperature to which a substance must be heated in order to initiate or cause self-sustained combustion, independent of the heat source. Also known as **auto ignition temperature, ignition point.**

ileitis /il´ē·ī´-/, inflammation of the distal portion of the small intestine. *See also Crohn's disease.*

ileocecal valve /il´ē·ōsē´kəl/, the valve between the inferior small intestine and the superior large intestine. The valve has two flaps that project into the large intestine, allowing the contents of the intestine to pass only in a forward direction.

ileostomy /il´ē·os´-/, surgical procedure which forms an opening of the ileum onto the surface of the abdomen, through which fecal matter is emptied. *See also colostomy, enterostomy, ostomy.*

ileum /il´ē·əm/, *pl.* **ilea,** the distal portion of the small intestine that opens into the large intestine. **–ileac, ileal,** *adj.*

ileus, 1. intestinal obstruction. Symptoms include abdominal distention, abdominal pain (initially spasmodic, then continuous), fecal vomiting. **2.** *(historical)* the colic and pain from intestinal obstruction.

iliac crest, the superior margin of the ilium.

ilium, superior and widest of the three bones of the pelvis.

illness, 1. a state of abnormal emotional, mental, physical, or social function, a state altered and diminished from the one that existed previously or from the norm. **2.** ailment, disease.

illusion, a false understanding of an external sensory stimulus, usually visual or auditory, as a mirage in the desert or voices on the wind. Compare **delusion, hallucination.**

image,   **1.** a person or thing that looks like another. **2.** a mental picture, idea, or concept of an objective reality. **3.** *(in psychology)* a mental representation of something seen before and later changed by other events. *See also body image, tactile image.*

imagery /im´ijrē´/,   *(in psychiatry)* the forming of mental concepts, figures, ideas; any product of the imagination.

imbricate /im´brikāt/,   to build a surface with overlapping layers of material.

immature baby,   a term sometimes used for an infant weighing less than 1134 g (2.5 lb) and underdeveloped at birth.

immediately dangerous to life and health,   any atmosphere that poses an immediate hazard to life or produces immediate, irreversible, debilitating effects on health. These concentrations represent concentrations at which respiratory protection is required and are expressed in parts per million or milligrams per cubic meter. Also known as **IDLH.**

immersion,   the placing of a body or an object into water or other liquid so that it is completely covered by the liquid. –**immerse,** *v.*

immersion foot,   neurovascular damage to the feet without actual freezing of tissue. This condition generally develops over a period of hours or days by exposing wet feet to temperatures between 32 and 50° F (0 and about 10° C). Symptoms include paresthesia, leg cramps, edema, and mottling. Gangrene can result. Also known as **trench foot.** *See also frostbite.*

immersion hypothermia,   decreased body temperature brought on by submersion in cold water. Seriousness of the condition is determined by water temperature, length of exposure, and physical condition of the patient.

immiscible /imis´ibəl/,   not able to be mixed, as oil and water.

immobilization,   procedure that involves placing the body in an immobile supine position to protect the spinal cord when injury is suspected. When the victim is found in a sitting position, initial efforts are directed to maintain the cervical spine in a position of neutrality until such time as the patient can be removed. Completion of the procedure requires that an extrication collar, spineboard or scoop stretcher (or equivalent), lateral immobilization device, straps, and tape be applied.

immune response,   the defensive response by the body to an antigen. *See also immunity.*

immune system,   a related group of responses of various organs that protects the body from disease organisms and other foreign bodies. The main organs of the immune system are the bone marrow, thymus, lymphoid tissues, spleen, and the lymphatic vessels. The system includes the humoral immune response and the cell-mediated response.

immunity,   the quality of being unaffected by a certain disease or condition. **Natural immunity** is a congenital and permanent form of immunity to a specific disease. **Acquired immunity** is any form that is obtained after birth. It may be natural or not. With **naturally acquired immunity** the body is able to fight off infections successfully after having the disease. Immunity is inherited from the mother during pregnancy. **Artificially acquired immunity** is obtained by vaccination. **Active immunity** is a form of long-term, gained immunity. It protects the body from new infection. **Passive immunity** is not permanent and does not last as long as active immunity. It results from antibodies that are carried through the placenta to a fetus or through colostrum from a mother to an infant. Passive immunity is also caused by injecting antiserum for treatment or prevention. **Autoimmunity** is an abnormal condition in which the body reacts against its own tissues. Autoimmunity may result in allergy and autoimmune disease. **Cellular immunity** refers to the growth of special white blood cells (T lymphocytes) after exposure to an antigen. Cellular immunity helps the body to resist infection caused by viruses and some bacteria and also plays a role in delayed allergic responses. **Humoral immunity** results from the development and the continuing presence of circulating antibodies which are produced by the body's defense system.

immunization,   a process by which resistance to an infectious disease is caused or increased.

immunodeficient,   decreased immunity and resistance to infection.

immunogen /imyōō´nəjən/, any agent or substance able to provoke an immune response or cause immunity.

immunoglobulin /im´yōōnōglob´yəlin/, any of five distinct antibodies in the serum and external secretions of the body. In response to certain antigens, immunoglobulins are formed in the bone marrow, spleen, and all lymphoid tissue of the body except the thymus. **Immunoglobulin A** (IgA) is the most common. It protects body tissues by seeking out foreign microorganisms and starting an antigen-antibody reaction. **Immunoglobulin D** (IgD) is a specialized protein found in small amounts in serum tissue. The precise function is not known, but it increases in quantity during allergic reactions to milk, insulin, penicillin, and various toxins. **Immunoglobulin E** (IgE) provides the main defense against antigens from the environment and is believed to be stimulated by immunoglobulin A. **Immunoglobulin G** (IgG) is a specialized protein produced by the body in response to invasions by bacteria, fungi, and viruses. **Immunoglobulin M** (IgM) is the largest in structure. It is the first immunoglobulin the body produces when challenged by antigens and triggers increased production of immunoglobulin G and antibody response.

immunology /-ol´-/, the study of the reaction of tissues of the immune system of the body to stimulation by antigens. A specialist in immunology is known as an **immunologist.**

immunomodulator /-mod´yəlā´tər/, a substance that acts to alter the body's immune response by increasing or decreasing the ability of the immune system to produce modified blood antibodies or cells that recognize and react with the antigen that caused their production. **–immunomodulation,** *n.*

immunosuppression, 1. the administration of agents that reduce the ability of the immune system to respond to stimulation by antigens. Immunosuppression may be deliberate, as when preparing for bone marrow or other transplants to prevent rejection of the donor tissue, or an accidental byproduct, as often results from chemotherapy for the treatment of cancer. **2.** a markedly lowered ability to respond to stimulation by antigens.

immunosuppressive, pertaining to a substance or procedure that lessens or prevents an immune response.

impacted, tightly or firmly wedged.

impacted fracture, a fracture in which the adjacent ends of the bone are wedged together.

impact force, the energy that results from forceful contact or collision. This forceful energy exchange results in trauma.

impact wrench, extrication tool that utilizes compressed air to turn a socket. The socket is used to unscrew bolted parts during an extrication.

impairment, any disorder in structure or function resulting from abnormalities that interfere with normal activities.

impaled object, an object forcefully thrust into a victim without subsequent removal prior to medical care. The foreign body is usually left in place until it can be safely removed. Projectiles, such as bullets and small pieces of shrapnel, are not usually considered impaled objects.

impedance, opposition to the flow of current in an electrical circuit or component. This includes all the effects of capacitance, inductance, and resistance.

imperforate /impur´fərit/, lacking a normal opening in a body organ or passageway.

impermeable, preventing passage of a substance or object; impenetrable.

impetigo, bacterial skin disease characterized by isolated pustules around mouth and nose. The pustules rupture and drain, causing crusted lesions. *See also ecthyma.*

implant, material inserted or grafted into an organ or structure of the body. The implant may be natural, as in a blood vessel graft, or artificial, as a pacemaker.

implantable cardioverter defibrillator, a self-contained electrical device, implanted under the skin, that is capable of sensing cardiac rhythm disturbances and delivering electrical shock, when appropriate. This device is desirable in patients with a risk or previous history of lethal rhythm disturbance.

implied consent, presumed consent. *See also consent.*

implosion, forcefully collapsing inward; the reverse of an explosion. Seen with object under an external pressure greater than its internal pressure.

impotence, **1.** weakness. **2.** inability of the adult male to achieve erection or, less commonly, to ejaculate having achieved an erection. Also **impotency. –impotent,** *adj.*

impregnate, **1.** to make pregnant; to fertilize. **2.** to saturate or mix with another substance. **–impregnable,** *adj.,* **impregnation,** *n.*

impression, **1.** an examiner's diagnosis or assessment of a problem, disease, or condition. **2.** a strong sensation or effect on the mind.

impulse, **1.** moving forward with sudden force. **2.** a sudden or unpremeditated act. **3.** a force transmitted through tissue that results in activity or inhibition, such as an ectopic or nervous impulse. **4.** the output of an artificial pacemaker.

inanition /in'ənish'ən/, **1.** an exhausted condition from lack of food and water or a defect in digestion; starvation. **2.** a slow-moving state from a loss of vitality or vigor.

inborn, acquired or occurring during life in the uterus; innate. *See also congenital, hereditary.*

inborn error of metabolism, one of many conditions caused by an inherited defect of an enzyme or other protein. Kinds of inborn errors of metabolism include **phenylketonuria, Tay-Sachs disease, galactosemia.**

incarcerate /inkär'sərāt/, to trap, imprison, or confine. *See also hernia.*

incest, sexual intercourse between close relatives, as members of the same family. Intercourse is incest only when those participating could not legally marry. **–incestuous,** *adj.*

incidence, **1.** the number of times an event occurs. **2.** *(in epidemiology)* the number of new cases in a particular period of time.

incident, an occurrence or event that requires action to prevent or minimize loss of life or damage to property and/or natural resources.

incident action plan, plan reflecting overall incident strategy and specific action plans for the next operational period.

incident base, that location at which the primary logistics functions are coordinated and administered. (Incident name or other designator will be added to the term "base.") The incident command post may be colocated with the base. There is only one base per incident.

incident commander, the individual responsible for overall management of all operations at an incident in which the incident command system has been implemented. Also known as **IC.**

incident command post, that location at which the primary command functions are executed and usually colocated with the incident base. Also known as **ICP.**

incident command system, the combination of facilities, equipment, personnel, procedures, and communications operating within a common organizational structure to effectively accomplish stated objectives pertaining to an incident. Also known as **ICS.**

incident management system. See **incident command system.**

incipient, beginning; the earliest stage.

incision, a surgical opening into an organ or space in the body.

incoherent, **1.** disordered; without logical connection. **2.** unable to express one's ideas in an orderly way.

incompatible, unable to coexist.

incompetence, lack of ability.

incontinence, the inability to control urination or defecation, common in the aged. **–incontinent,** *adj.*

increment, an increase or gain **–incremental,** *adj.*

incubation period, the time between exposure to a disease-causing organism and the onset of symptoms of a disease.

incus /ing'kəs/, *pl.* **incudes** /ing-kōō'dēz/, one of the three small bones in the middle ear. *See also ear.*

indentation, a notch or depression in the surface of an object. **–indent,** *v.*

indication, a reason to prescribe a medication or perform a treatment. **–indicate,** *v.*

indigenous /indij'ənəs/, native to or found naturally in a specified area or environment, as certain species of bacteria in the human digestive tract.

indigestion. See **dyspepsia.**

indirect medical control, utilization of standing orders and written protocols that do not require physician or base hospital contact in order to provide out-of-hospital advanced life support. Also known as **off-line medical control,**

standing orders. Compare **direct medical control.**

induce, to cause or stimulate the start of an activity –**inducer, induction,** *n.*

induction system, mixing system by which air and gasoline are supplied in appropriate proportions to an engine.

induration, hardening of a tissue, particularly the skin, because of excess fluid retention, inflammation, or growth of a tumor. –**indurated,** *adj.*

inert /inurt´/, **1.** not moving or functioning. **2.** (of a medical ingredient) not medically active; serving only a non-medical use in a drug. **3.** (of a chemical substance) not taking part in a chemical reaction or acting as a catalyst, as an inert gas.

inertia /inur´shə/, **1.** the tendency of a body at rest or in motion to remain at rest or in motion unless acted on by an outside force. **2.** a state of general inactivity in an organ or body.

in extremis, in a dire situation; close to death.

infant, a child who is in the earliest stage of life outside the womb. Infancy covers the time extending from birth to about 12 months of age, when the baby is able to assume an erect posture.

infant death, the death of a live-born infant before 1 year of age.

infanticide /infan´tisīd/, the killing of an infant or young child.

infantile, **1.** relating to or typical of infants or infancy. **2.** lacking maturity, or reasonableness. **3.** being in a very early stage of development.

infantile paralysis. See **poliomyelitis.**

infantilism /in´fantəlizm, infant´-/, **1.** a condition in which various body and mental traits of childhood persist in the adult. **2.** a condition, usually of psychologic rather than organic origin, with speech and voice patterns in an older child or adult that are typical of very young children.

infant mortality, the statistical rate of infant death during the first year after live birth. It is expressed as the number of such births per 1000 live births in a given geographic area in a given period of time. Neonatal mortality accounts for 70% of infant mortality.

infarct /infärkt´/, an area of decay in a tissue, vessel, organ, or part resulting from an interrup-

tion in the blood supply to the area, or, less often, by the blockage of a vein that carries blood away from the area. –**infarcted,** *adj.*

infarct extension, a decay in tissue that has spread beyond the original area, usually as a result of the death of neighboring cells.

infarction /infärk´shən/, the development and formation of an infarct. *See also myocardial infarction.*

infect, to transmit a germ that may cause an infectious disease in another person.

infection, **1.** the invasion of the body by germs that reproduce and multiply, causing disease by local cell injury, release of poisons, or germ-antibody reaction in the cells. **Endogenous infection** is caused by an organism that has remained in the body from a previous illness. After a time of being dormant, it has become active again, as tuberculosis, which often occurs again. **Mixed infection** is caused by several different microorganisms, as in pneumonia and wounds. Many combinations of bacteria, viruses, and fungi may be involved. **Retrograde infection** spreads along a tube or duct against the flow of fluids or wastes, as in the urinary and lymph systems. **Secondary infection** is caused by a microorganism that develops after an initial infection. **2.** a disease caused by the invasion of the body by germs. Compare **infestation.**

infectious, **1.** capable of causing an infection. **2.** caused by an infection.

infectious mononucleosis, an acute herpesvirus infection caused by the Epstein-Barr virus. Symptoms include fever, sore throat, and enlarged lymph glands. The disease is usually transmitted by droplet infection.

inferior, **1.** (*anatomical*) below (or toward the feet of) a given point of reference, as the feet are inferior to the legs. **2.** of poorer quality or value. Compare **superior.**

inferiority complex, a feeling of fear and resentment resulting from a sense of being inadequate.

inferior mesenteric vein, the vein in the lower body that returns the blood from the rectum and the colon. Compare **superior mesenteric vein.**

inferior phrenic artery, a small branch of the abdominal aorta, arising from the aorta itself, the renal artery, or the main abdominal artery. It supplies the diaphragm with blood.

inferior radioulnar joint, the pivot joint connecting the ulna and radius at the wrist. The joint allows the wrist to rotate the lower arm.

inferior sagittal sinus, a venous pathway that drains blood from the brain into the internal jugular vein.

interior thyroid vein, vein that drains blood from the veins of the thyroid gland.

inferior ulnar collateral artery, one of a number of branches of the deep brachial arteries in the arm, arising near the elbow and carrying blood to the muscles of the forearm.

infertile /infur´təl/, not being able to produce offspring. Compare **sterile. –infertility,** *n.*

infest, to attack, invade, and live on the skin or in the organs of a body. Compare **infect.**

infestation, the presence of animal parasites in the environment, on the skin, or in the hair.

infiltration, the process whereby a fluid passes into the tissues, as when an intravenous fluid catheter comes out of the vein.

inflammation, the response of the tissues of the body to irritation or injury. Inflammation may be acute or chronic. Signs are erythema, edema, and pain, accompanied by loss of function. The severity of any inflammation depends on the cause, the area affected, and the condition of the person.

influenza, a contagious infection caused by a virus and transmitted by airborne particles. Symptoms include sore throat, cough, chills, fever, muscular pain, and weakness. The incubation period is from 1 to 3 days and the onset is usually sudden. Also known as **grippe,** *(informal)* **flu.**

information officer, the command staff officer in the incident command system responsible for interface with the media and other agencies that require information direct from the incident scene.

informed consent, expressed consent. *See also consent.*

infrared, invisible light, generated from heated objects, that has a wavelength longer than (beyond) the red end of the spectrum, but shorter than microwaves. Useful in the detection, observation, and/or rescue of humans or animals and in many medical procedures, such as pulse oximetry.

infrared groundlink, a capability through the use of a special mobile ground station to receive air to ground infrared imagery for interpretation.

infundibulum, any funnel-shaped body part, such as that connecting the brain and pituitary gland.

infusion, **1.** the introduction of a substance, as a fluid, nutrient, or drug, into a vein. **2.** the substance introduced into the body by infusion. **–infuse,** *v.*

infusion pump, a device that delivers measured amounts of a drug through injection over a period of time. Some types of infusion pumps may be implanted surgically.

ingestion, the introduction of a substance into the body through the mouth.

ingredient statement, pesticide labels that list chemical ingredients by their relative percentages or as pounds per gallon of concentrate. "Active" ingredients are the active chemicals within the mixture. They must be listed by chemical name, and their common name may also be shown. "Inert" ingredients have no pesticide activity and are usually not broken into specific components, only total percentage.

inguinal /ing´gwinəl/, pertaining to the groin.

inguinal canal, the tubular passage through the abdominal wall. It is a common site for hernias. **Inguinal ring** refers to either of the two openings of the inguinal canal.

inguinal falx, a tendon that helps to strengthen the anterior wall of the groin. Also known as **conjoined tendon.**

inguinal hernia. See **hernia.**

inguinal node, a lymph node in the groin.

inhalation, the introduction of substances into the body by way of the respiratory system.

inhalation injuries, damage sustained from the breathing in of noxious gases or heat. The trachea and lungs are most frequently affected.

inhale, to breathe in. **–inhalation,** *n.*

inherent, inborn, innate; natural to an environment.

inherent rate, rate of impulse formation in the cardiac conduction system, as with 60-100 per minute in the sinoatrial node, 40-60 per minute in the atrioventricular node, 20-40 per minute in the ventricle.

inheritance, the acquiring by an offspring of genetic material from its parents; the total genetic makeup of the fertilized ovum. Traits or conditions are transmitted in this way from one generation to the next.

inherited disorder, any disease or condition that is genetically determined. Also known as **genetic disorder, hereditary disorder.**

inhibition, **1.** the act or state of inhibiting or of being inhibited, restrained, prevented, or held back. **2.** *(in psychology)* the unconscious restraint of a certain behavior, usually resulting from the social or cultural forces; the condition causing this restraint. **3.** *(in physiology)* restraining, checking, or arresting the action of an organ or cell. **4.** *(in chemistry)* the stopping or slowing down of the rate of a chemical reaction.

inhibitory, tending to stop or slow a process. Compare **induce.**

inion /in′ē·on/, the most prominent point of the occipital bone.

initial attack, resources initially committed to an incident.

injection, **1.** the act of forcing a liquid into the body with a syringe. Injections are named according to where they are given. **2.** the substance injected. **3.** erythema and swelling observed in the physical examination of a part of the body, caused by enlargement of the blood vessels from inflammation or infection. **–inject,** *v.*

Injury Severity Score, one of three components of a retrospective scoring system, used to determine the seriousness of injuries sustained from blunt or penetrating trauma. The system is more sensitive for use with blunt trauma. The scale runs from 1 (minor) to 75 (nonsurviveable). Generally, any patient with a score higher than 15 is considered to be major trauma. Also known as **ISS.** *See also Abbreviated Injury Scale, TRISS methodology.*

inlet, a passage leading into a cavity, as the pelvic inlet that marks the brim of the pelvic cavity.

in loco parentis /in lō′kō pəren′tis/, Latin meaning "in the place of the parent": the taking on by a person or institution of the parental obligations of caring for a child without adoption.

innate, **1.** existing in or belonging to a person from birth; inborn; hereditary; congenital. **2.** referring to a natural and essential trait of something or someone. **3.** originating in or produced by the mind.

inner cell mass, a cluster of cells around a central part of a fertilized ovum. The embryo develops from it. *See also trophoblast.*

inner perimeter, the restricted area of a tactical operation within which the objective must be secured. Only those personnel absolutely essential for securing the objective operate in this area. For law enforcement or military special operations, this will include any area that is subject to live weapons fire. Within the inner perimeter can be found hostile forces, hostages or prisoners, weapons or explosives, or stolen property. Also known as **hot zone, kill zone, restricted perimeter.** Compare **outer perimeter.**

innervation, the distribution or supply or nerve fibers or nerve impulses to a part of the body.

innocent, **1.** benign, healthy; not malignant. **2.** not guilty.

innominate artery /inom′ināt/, one of the three arteries that branch from the arch of the aorta. It divides into the right common carotid and the right subclavian arteries.

innominate bone, the hipbone. It consists of the ilium, ischium, and pubis. It joins with the sacrum and coccyx to form the pelvis.

innominate vein, a large vein on the lateral neck. It is formed by the union of the internal jugular and subclavian veins and drains blood from the head and neck.

inoculate /inok′yəlāt/, to introduce a substance into the body to cause or increase immunity to a disease or condition. It is introduced by making multiple scratches in the skin after placing a drop of the substance on the skin, by puncture of the skin with an implement bearing multiple short tines, or by injection.

inoculum /inok′yələm/, *pl.* **inocula,** a substance introduced into the body to cause or increase immunity to a given disease or condition. Also known as **inoculant.** *See also immunity.*

inotropic, a substance that improves the contractility of muscle, particularly the heart.

inpatient, a patient who has been admitted to a hospital or other health care facility for at least an overnight stay. It also refers to the treatment or care of such a patient.

in personam rights,   a demand that one person can make upon another; legal rights. *See also in rem rights.*

in rem rights,   a claim against the state for recognition and enforcement of a legal right. *See also in personam rights.*

insect bite,   the bite of any arthropod, such as a louse, flea, mite, tick, or spider. Many arthropods inject venom that produces poisoning or severe local reaction. Others inject saliva that may contain viruses, or substances that produce mild irritation. The degree of irritation of an insect's bite is affected by the shape of its mouth parts.

insertion,   1. the point of attachment (by a tendon) of a muscle to the bone it moves. Compare **origin. 2.** *(special operations)* placing personnel and equipment into a specific (often hostile) area, as required to complete a tactical operation or rescue. Compare **extraction.**

insidious /insid´ē·əs/,   describing a change that is gradual, subtle, or not noticed. Certain chronic diseases, such as glaucoma, are insidious. Their symptoms are not detected by the patient until the disorder is established. Compare **acute.**

insight,   1. the capacity of grasping the true nature of a situation or a deep truth. **2.** an instance of penetrating or comprehending a deep truth, primarily through intuitive understanding. **3.** *(psychology)* a type of self-understanding. Along with integration, it leads to change in faulty behavior. *See also integration.*

in situ /in sī´tōō, sit´ōō/,   **1.** in the natural or usual place. **2.** describing a cancer that has not spread or invaded neighboring tissues, as carcinoma in situ.

insomnia,   chronic inability to sleep or to remain asleep through the night. The condition is caused by a variety of physical and psychologic factors including emotional stress, physical pain and discomfort, disorders in brain function, drug abuse, and drug dependence.

inspection,   visually examining a patient. Compare **auscultation, palpation, percussion.**

inspiration,   the act of drawing air into the lungs; breathing in. The major muscle of inspiration is the diaphragm, the contraction of which creates a negative pressure in the chest,

causing the lungs to expand and air to flow inward. Since expiration is usually a passive process, the muscles of inspiration alone perform normal respiration. Compare **expiration.**

inspiratory capacity,   the maximum volume of air that can be inhaled into the lungs from the normal resting position after exhaling. It is measured with a device called a spirometer.

inspiratory reserve volume,   the maximum volume of air that can be further inspired from the normal resting position after inhaling.

instillation,   a technique in which a fluid is slowly placed into a cavity of the body and allowed to remain for a specific length of time before being withdrawn. It is done to expose the tissues of the area to the solution, to warmth or cold, or to a drug or substance in the solution. Compare **infusion, injection, insufflate. –instill,** *v.*

instrument flight rules,   those requirements that govern air travel when visual flight is not possible, usually due to overcast or other poor flying weather. The total navigation of an aircraft is accomplished by the information provided by its instruments and radios. Also known as **IFR.** *See also ground approach control, visual flight rules.*

instrument landing system,   an airport landing system that can guide an aircraft, flying under instrument flight rules, to safety through the use of directional radio beacons. *See also instrument flight rules.*

insufficiency,   inability of an organ or other body part to perform a necessary function adequately. A type of insufficiency is **vascular insufficiency.**

insufflate /insuf´lāt/,   to blow a gas or powder into a tube, cavity, or organ. It is done to allow visual examination, to remove an obstruction, or to apply medication. **–insufflation,** *n.*

insulin /in´soolin, in´syəlin/,   **1.** a naturally occurring hormone released by the pancreas in response to increased levels of sugar in the blood. The hormone acts to regulate the body's use of sugar and some of the processes involved with fats, carbohydrates, and proteins. Insulin lowers blood sugar levels and promotes transport and entry of sugar into the muscle cells and other tissues. **2.** a preparation of the hormone given in treating diabetes mellitus. **Human insulin** is made from bacteria found naturally in the human digestive tract. Human insulin does not cause the allergic reactions that animal insulins do, especially in patients who only require insulin on a short-term basis.

insulin kinase, an enzyme, assumed to be present in the liver, that activates insulin.

insulinoma /-ō´mə/, a benign tumor of the insulin-secreting cells of the pancreas.

insulin pump, mechanical device that delivers insulin into the bloodstream at a metered rate in diabetics who cannot produce adequate amounts of the hormone.

insulin reaction, the ill effects caused by high levels of circulating insulin.

insulin shock, altered level of consciousness and metabolism, resulting from an excess of insulin. This excess may be due to high insulin intake, increased metabolism, or inadequate carbohydrate intake, and it results in hypoglycemia. Signs include altered levels of consciousness; pale, wet skin; and rapid onset of symptoms. Compare **diabetic coma.** *See also diabetes, hyperglycemia, hypoglycemia.*

Integrated Emergency Management, a (U.S.) federal management system that encourages government and private resources to plan together for coordinated disaster response. Also known as **IEM.**

integration, **1.** the act or process of unifying or bringing together. **2.** *(in psychology)* the organization of all elements of the personality into a functional whole. *See also insight.* –**integrate,** *v.*

integument /integ´yəmənt/, a covering or skin. –**integumentary,** *adj.*

integumentary system, the skin and its extensions: hair, nails, and sweat and sebaceous glands.

intellect, **1.** the power and ability of the mind to know and understand. Intellect is contrasted with feeling. **2.** a person having a great capacity for thought and knowledge. –**intellectual,** *adj., n.*

intellectualization, *(in psychiatry)* a defense mechanism in which reasoning is used to block an unconscious conflict and the emotional stress linked to it.

intelligence, the ability to acquire, retain, and apply experience, understanding, knowledge, reasoning, and judgment in coping with new experiences.

intensive care, health care given for various acute life-threatening conditions. Also known as **critical care.**

intensive care unit, a hospital unit for patients needing close monitoring and intensive care. A **neonatal intensive care unit** is a hospital unit with special equipment for the care of premature and seriously ill newborn infants. *See also coronary care unit.*

intention, a healing process. Healing by **first intention** is the union of the edges of a wound to complete healing without scar formation or granulation. Healing by **second intention** is wound closure in which the edges are separated, granulation develops to fill the gap, and, finally, tissue quickly grows in over the granulations, producing a thin scar. Healing by **third intention** is wound closure in which granulation fills the gap with tissue growing over the granulation at a slower rate and producing a larger scar.

intercellular /-sel´yələr/, between or among cells.

intercostal /-kos´təl/, pertaining to the space between ribs.

intercostal node, a lymph node in one of three groups in the posterior intercostal spaces. Such nodes are associated with lymphatic vessels that drain the lateral sides of the chest. *See also lymph node.*

intercourse, *(informal)* sexual intercourse. See **coitus.**

interior mesenteric artery /mes´enter´ik/, a branch of the abdominal aorta. It arises just above the division into the common iliacs and supplies much of the colon and rectum.

interlobular duct /-lob´yələr/, any duct connecting or draining the small lobes of a gland.

intermediate care facility, a health facility that provides intermediate care, a level of medical care for certain chronically ill or disabled individuals. Medical-related services are offered to persons with a variety of conditions requiring institutional facilities. The degree of care is less than what is necessary in a hospital or skilled nursing facility.

intermediate cuneiform bone, the smallest of the three cuneiform bones of the foot.

intermenstrual, pertaining to the time between menstrual periods.

intermittent, alternating between periods of activity and inactivity, as rheumatoid arthritis, which is marked by periods of symptoms and periods of remission.

intermittent mandatory ventilation, ventilator setting that allows the patient to breathe spontaneously between ventilator breaths, while delivering a predetermined number of ventilations per minute. This occurs regardless of the number of patient inspiratory efforts. Also known as **IMV.**

intermittent positive pressure breathing, ventilation, under positive pressure, of a spontaneously breathing patient, who requires aerosol medication or increased pulmonary pressure to force fluid back into the circulation. Also known as **IPPB.**

intern, **1.** a physician in the first postgraduate year. **2.** a student enrolled in a training program that requires out-of-classroom training time, such as a paramedic intern.

internal, within or inside. **–internally,** *adv.*

internal ear. See **ear.**

internal exposure, exposure to hazardous materials that have entered the body.

internal fixation, any method of holding together fractured bone without external appliances. Various devices, as smooth or threaded pins, wires, screws, or plates, may be used to stabilize the fragments. Compare **external pin fixation.**

internalization, the process of adopting, either unconsciously or consciously, the attitudes, beliefs, values, and standards of someone else or, more generally, of the society or group to which one belongs.

internal jugular vein, one of a pair of neck veins that collects blood from the brain, face, and neck. Compare **external jugular vein.**

internal medicine, the branch of medicine concerned with study of the physiology and pathology of internal organs and with medical diagnosis and treatment of disorders of organs.

International Red Cross Society, an international charity organization, based in Geneva, Switzerland. It provides humane treatment to victims of war and disaster. It assures neutral hospitals and medical personnel during war. *See also American Red Cross.*

International River Scale, a measurement of the difficulty required to traverse a river. More uniformly adapted to the east coast of the United States, the scale runs from easy (class 1) to most difficult (class 6).

International System of Units, the standardization of measurement of substances, including some antibiotics, vitamins, enzymes, and hormones. An **International Unit** of substance is the amount that produces a specific biologic result and has the same strength and action as another unit of the same substance. *See also centimeter-gram-second system, SI units.*

internist, a physician specializing in internal medicine.

interoceptor /in´tərōsep´tər/, any sensory nerve ending in cells in the internal organs that responds to stimuli from within the body regarding their function, such as digestion, excretion, and blood pressure.

interphase, the stage in the cell cycle when the cell is not dividing.

interpolated, the firing of an ectopic beat between two normal beats without interruption of the underlying rhythm's regularity.

intersexuality, the state in which a person has male and female body features to varying degrees or in which the appearance of the external genitals is unclear or differs from the gonadal or genetic sex.

interstitial /-stish´əl/, referring to the space between cells.

intertrigo /-trī´gō/, an irritation of opposing skin surfaces caused by friction. Common sites are the axilla, breasts, and inner thighs. Infection may occur if the area is also warm and moist.

intervention, any act to prevent harm to a patient or to improve the mental, emotional, or physical function of a patient.

intervertebral /-vur´təbrəl/, of the space between any two vertebrae, such as the disks.

intervertebral disk, one of the fibrous disks located between spinal vertebrae. The disks vary in size, shape, thickness, and number depending on the vertebrae they separate.

intestinal fistula, an abnormal passage from the intestine to an outside abdominal opening. It may also refer to one created surgically after removal of a malignant or severely ulcerated segment of the bowel. *See also colostomy.*

intestinal flu, *(informal)* gastroenteritis. Symptoms include cramps, diarrhea, nausea, and vomiting. *See also gastroenteritis.*

intestinal obstruction, any blockage of the intestinal contents. Common causes include adhesions, impacted feces, tumor of the bowel, hernia, and bowel disease. *See also hernia, intussusception, volvulus.*

intestinal strangulation, diminished blood flow to the bowel, causing cyanosis and gangrene of the affected loop of bowel. This state is often caused by a hernia, intussusception, or volvulus. Early signs of intestinal strangulation are like those of intestinal obstruction, but peritonitis, shock, and the presence of a tender mass in the abdomen are important in making a correct diagnosis. Also known as **intestinal infarction.**

intestine, the canal from the stomach to the anus. The **large intestine** is the portion of the digestive tract made up of the cecum; the appendix; the ascending, transverse, and descending colons; and the rectum. The ileocecal valve separates the cecum from the ileum, preventing a reverse flow into the small intestine. The **small intestine** is the longest part of the digestive tract, extending for about 7 m (23 feet) from the opening of the stomach to the cecum. It is divided into the duodenum, jejunum, and ileum. Decreasing in width from beginning to end, it is surrounded by large intestine. **–intestinal,** *adj.*

intima, the innermost layer of a structure, such as a tunica intima.

intolerance, a state marked by an inability to absorb or make use of a nutrient or medicine. Exposure to the substance may cause an adverse reaction, as in lactose intolerance. Compare **allergy.**

intoxication, **1.** the state of being poisoned by a drug or other substance. **2.** the state of being drunk because of drinking too much alcohol. **3.** *(informal)* a state of high mental or emotional excitement, usually happiness.

intraaortic balloon pump /in´trə·ā-ôr´-/, a device that assists in the management of cardiogenic shock. The balloon is attached to a catheter inserted in the aorta and is automatically inflated and deflated to aid in pumping blood. Also known as **IABP.**

intraarticular /-ärtik´yələr/, in a joint.

intraatrial /-ā´trē·əl/, in an atrium in the heart.

intracardiac injection, injection of medication into the cardiac ventricles via needle and syringe directly through the chest wall.

intracellular fluid /-sel´yələr/, fluid in cell membranes of most tissues, with dissolved substances essential to healthy functioning of the body.

intracerebral /-ser´əbrəl/, in the brain tissue, inside the bony skull.

intracranial pressure, the force within the skull exerted by blood and cerebrospinal fluid. Generally used when referring to the pressure on the brain tissue.

intractable, having no relief, as a symptom or disease that is not helped by treatment.

intracutaneous /-kō͞otā´nē·əs/, in the layers of the skin.

intraocular /-ok´yələr/, in the eye.

intraocular pressure, the internal pressure of the eye, regulated via the trabecular meshwork. In older persons, the meshwork may block, causing higher intraocular pressure. *See also glaucoma.*

intraosseous, within the substance of the bone.

intraosseous infusion, technique of fluid and medication administration via a needle placed into the cavity within the proximal tibia or distal femur. This route can be used with patients through six years of age with any fluid and/or medication suitable for intravenous infusion.

intrapartal care, care of a pregnant woman from the start of labor to the end of the third stage of labor with the release of the placenta.

intrathecal /-thē´kəl/, referring to a structure, process, or substance in a sheath, as the spinal fluid in the theca of the spinal canal.

intrauterine device, a birth control device consisting of a bent strip of plastic or other material that is put in the uterus to prevent pregnancy. Also known as **intrauterine contraceptive device, IUD,** *(informal)* **coil, loop.**

intrauterine fracture, a fracture during fetal life.

intravenous (IV) /-vē´nəs/,   into or inside a vein.

intravenous controller,   any device that automatically delivers IV fluid at selectable flow rates.

intravenous feeding,   the giving of nutrients through a vein.

intravenous infusion,   1. a solution administered into a vein. **2.** the process of administration of intravenous fluids or medications.

intravenous peristaltic pump,   any of several devices for administering IV fluids by pressure on the tubing rather than on the fluid itself.

intravenous piggyback.   See **piggyback.**

intravenous piston pump,   any of several devices that control the infusion of IV fluids by piston action. Compare **intravenous controller, intravenous syringe pump.**

intravenous push,   the technique of intravenous drug administration via syringe into an intravenous line. It places drugs into the circulation faster than intravenous infusion. Also known as **IVP, IV push. Direct intravenous push** is medication administration via syringe directly into the venous system without benefit of an intravenous line. Also known as **direct IVP, direct IV push.**

intravenous syringe pump,   any of several devices that automatically compress a syringe plunger at a certain rate. Such devices are used with syringes that can deliver blood, medications, or nutrients by IV, arterial, or subcutaneous routes.

intravenous therapy,   the administration of fluids or drugs in the venous circulation through an intravenous catheter. Also known as **intravenous infusion.**

intraventricular /-ventrik´yələr/,   referring to the space in a ventricle.

intrinsic,   1. natural or inherent. **2.** originating from within an organ or tissue.

intrinsic factor,   a substance released by the gastric mucosa that is needed for the absorption of vitamin B_{12} and the normal growth of red blood cells. *See also nutritional anemia.*

introspection,   1. the act of examining one's own thoughts and emotions by focusing on the inner self. **2.** a tendency to look inward at the inner self. **–introspective,** *adj.*

introversion,   the tendency to direct one's interests, thoughts, and energies inward or to things concerned only with the self. Compare **extroversion.**

introvert,   a person whose interests are directed inward and who is shy, withdrawn, emotionally reserved, and self-absorbed. Compare **extrovert.**

intubation /in´tyōōbā´shən/,   passing a tube into a body aperture. Kinds of intubation are **endotracheal intubation** and **nasogastric intubation.**

intussusception /in´təsəsep´shən/,   the entering of one portion of intestine into another portion, causing intestinal obstruction. Symptoms include abdominal pain and vomiting. Also known as **invagination.**

inunction /inungk´shən/,   **1.** the rubbing of a drug mixed with oil or fat into the skin, with absorption of the active agent. **2.** any compound so applied.

invagination /invaj´inā´shən/,   **1.** a state in which one part of a structure telescopes into another, as the intestine during peristalsis. If the invagination is extensive or involves a tumor or polyps, it may cause blockage. **2.** surgery to repair a hernia by replacing the contents of the hernial sac in the abdominal cavity. *See also hernia, intestinal obstruction, peristalsis.* **–invaginate,** *v.*

invasion,   the process by which cancer cells move into deeper tissue and into blood vessels and lymph channels.

invasive,   1. a tendency to spread. **2.** procedures or treatments that penetrate the body.

inverse square law,   the relationship that the radiation intensity is inversely proportional to the square of the distance from the source.

inversion,   1. an abnormal state in which an organ is turned inside out, as a uterine inversion. **2.** a chromosomal defect in which two or more parts of a chromosome break off and separate. They rejoin the chromosome in the wrong order.

invert,   to turn something upside down or inside out.

investigational new drug,   a drug not yet approved by the Food and Drug Administration; only for use in experiments to evaluate its safety and effectiveness.

in vitro /in vē´trō/,   *(of a biologic reaction)* occurring in laboratory apparatus.

in vivo /in vē´vō/, *(of a biologic reaction)* occurring in a living organism.

involuntary, without conscious control or direction.

involution, a normal process marked by decreasing size of an organ, as involution of the uterus after birth.

iodine, an essential trace element. Almost 80% of the iodine present in the body is in the thyroid gland. A lack of iodine can result in goiter or cretinism. Iodine is found in seafoods, iodized salt, and some dairy products.

iodism /ī´ōdizm/, a state caused by too much iodine. Symptoms include increased saliva, rhinitis, weakness, and skin eruption.

iodize /ī´ōdīz/, to treat or saturate with iodine.

iododerma /ī´ōdōdur´mə/, a skin rash caused by an allergy to iodides in the diet.

ion /ī´on, ī´ən/, an atom or group of atoms with an electric charge.

ionization /ī´ōnīzā´shən/, the process in which a neutral atom or molecule gains or loses electrons. Ionization can cause cell death or change.

ionization chamber, a device that consists of two oppositely charged electrodes and is used to measure radioactivity.

ionizing radiation, electromagnetic radiation (x-ray and gamma ray photons) or particulate radiation (alpha particles, beta particles, electrons, positrons, protons, neutrons, and heavy particles) capable of producing ions by direct or secondary processes.

ionosphere, the region of the earth's atmosphere that lies between approximately 30 and 250 miles above the surface. This area contains gases ionized by the sun. The ionization allows radio waves to be refracted back to earth, allowing worldwide radio transmission.

ipecac, an emetic used in selected cases of drug ingestion in conscious patients where vomiting is desirable. It irritates the lining of the stomach and stimulates the vomiting center in the medulla. Contraindications usually include altered levels of consciousness and the ingestion of acids, alkalis, chlorinated hydrocarbons (Kwell), drugs that cause rapid onset of seizures (as tricyclic antidepressants, camphor, theophylline), and petroleum distillates. Also known as **syrup of ipecac.**

iridectomy /i´ridek´-/, surgical removal of a portion of the iris of the eye, often to restore drainage of the fluid to treat glaucoma or to remove a foreign body or tumor.

iridotomy /i´ridot´-/, an incision in the iris of the eye.

iris /ī´ris/, a circular, contracting disc suspended between the cornea and the crystalline lens of the eye. Dark pigment cells under the clear tissue of the iris produce different colored irises. In blue eyes the pigment cells are only on the posterior surface of the iris, but in gray, brown, and black eyes the pigment cells appear in the anterior layer.

iritis /īrī´-/, an inflammatory condition of the iris of the eye. Symptoms include pain, tearing, sensitivity to light, and, if severe, lessened visual sharpness. On examination the eye looks cloudy, the iris bulges, and the pupil is contracted.

iron, a common metallic element needed to make hemoglobin. **Total iron** refers to the total iron concentration in the blood.

iron deficiency anemia. See **nutritional anemia.**

iron metabolism, processes involved in the entry of iron into the body through its absorption, transport, and storage; formation of hemoglobin; and eventual excretion.

iron poisoning, poisoning caused by overdose of ferric or ferrous salts, marked by vomiting, hematochezia, cyanosis, and abdominal pain.

irradiation, exposure to radiant energy, such as heat, light, or x-ray. –**irradiate,** *v.*

irreducible, unable to be returned to the normal position or state, as an irreducible hernia. *See also incarcerate.*

irreversible shock, the point during inadequate cell perfusion when the cells become injured beyond the point of repair, even if adequate glucose and oxygen flow are restored. Death is the result.

irrigation, the process of washing out a body cavity or wounded area with a stream of water or other fluid. *See also lavage.* –**irrigate,** *v.*

irrigator, an apparatus with a flexible tube for flushing or washing out

irritable bowel syndrome, abnormally increased movement of the small and large intestine, often found with emotional stress. Young adults are often affected. Symptoms include diarrhea and pain in the lower abdomen. Also known as **mucous colitis, spastic colon.**

irritating material, any liquid or solid substance that upon contact with air or fire gives off dangerous or intensely irritating fumes, generally not including class A poisonous materials.

irritation emesis, vomiting due to brain tumors, medications, nephritis, or uremia.

ischemia /iskē´mē·ə/, poor blood supply to an organ or part, often marked by pain, as in ischemic heart disease. Some causes of ischemia are atherosclerosis and thrombus. **Ischemic pain** refers to the painful feeling associated with ischemia.

ischium /is´kē·əm/, most inferior of the three bones that make up the pelvis.

islet cell tumor, any tumor of the islets of Langerhans.

islets of Langerhans, cell clusters within the pancreas. Of the three types of cells (alpha, beta, delta) that exist, the greatest number are beta cells, which produce insulin. Disease or other impaired function of the islets can result in diabetes or hypoglycemia. Also known as **islands of Langerhans.**

isobar, **1.** a line on a meteorological map that connects the areas having the same barometric pressure at a particular time. **2.** an isotope. See **isotope.**

isoimmunization /īsō-/, the development of antibodies in a species with antigens from the same species, such as the development of anti-Rh antibodies in an Rh-negative person.

isogenesis /-jen´əsis/, development from a common origin and according to similar processes.

isolation, the separation of a patient from others to stop the spread of infection or protect the patient.

isoleucine (Ile) /-loo¯´sēn/, an amino acid in most dietary proteins. It is essential for proper growth in infants and nitrogen balance in adults. *See also amino acid.*

isopropyl alcohol /-prō´pil/, a clear, colorless, bitter aromatic liquid that can be mixed with water, ether, chloroform, and ethyl alcohol. A solution of 70% isopropyl alcohol in water is used as a rubbing compound. *See also alcohol.*

isoproterenol hydrochloride, a pure beta catecholamine that is used in cases of heart blocks with a palpable pulse, symptomatic bradycardias refractory to atropine, and torsades de pointes when a transcutaneous (external) pacemaker is not available. It increases heart rate and electrical conduction, bronchodilates and vasodilates, but increases myocardial oxygen consumption. Side effects include ventricular dysrhythmias, hypotension, and vomiting. Also known as **Isuprel.**

isoseismal, **1.** a line on a map that connects earthquake shock points of equal intensity. **2.** experiencing or indicating equal magnitudes of earthquake shock.

isotherm, a line, joining places on a map, of equal temperature or of equal mean temperature.

isotonic, **1.** having an equal amount of solute dissolved in a concentration; equal osmotic pressure. The concentration of substances in blood serum is usually used for comparison. **2.** equal tone or tension.

isotope, one of two or more forms of an element with different atomic weights, but the same atomic number. This difference is due to one or more extra neutrons in the nucleus. The changes in weight (mass) from the original element are specified by including the difference as part of the name, as in *carbon 14*. Also known as **isobar.**

isotopic tracer /-top´ik/, an isotope of an element put into a sample to permit observation of the course of the element through a chemical, physical, or biologic process.

isthmus /is´mus/, a narrow strip of land bordered by water that connects two larger bodies of land.

itch mite, any of the parasitic mites that burrow into the skin, such as the one that causes scabies (*Sarcoptes scabiei*).

Ixodes /iksō´dēz/, parasitic hard-shelled ticks that carry infections, as Rocky Mountain spotted fever.

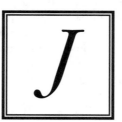

jack, a lifting and/or stabilizing device that is mechanical, pneumatic, or hydraulic in operation. Generally used in structural extrication and trench rescue, jacks also have limited application in vehicle extrication. Hydraulic jack tools, pneumatic shoring jacks, and mechanical jacks are examples of these devices.

Jackson's rule, after a seizure, simple and automatic functions are less affected and recover more quickly than complex ones.

jacksonian progression (John Hughlings Jackson, British physician, 1835-1911), seizure activity that begins in a localized muscle mass and moves or enlarges to include additional muscles without involving the whole body. *See also seizure.*

jacksonian seizure. See **jacksonian progression, seizure, Todd's paralysis.**

Jake's litter, rigid aluminum/plastic transport device, similar in design to a Stokes's litter (without a leg divider), that can be broken down into three pieces for ease of storage or transport to a victim. Positively buoyant for use in water rescue situations, its design also allows it to slide over ice, rock, or snow. A canvas cover with a clear plastic strip is available that can be stretched over the top for use in inclement weather or external helicopter transport situations. *See also rigid transport vehicle.*

jamais vu /zhämävY´, -vē´, -vo͞o´/, the feeling of being a stranger when with a person one knows or when in a familiar place. It occurs sometimes in normal people but more often in people who have epilepsy (temporal lobe). The phrase means "never seen." Compare **déjà vu.**

Janeway lesion (Edward G. Janeway, American physician, 1841-1911), a small, reddish blemish found on the palms or soles. It is a sign of subacute bacterial endocarditis.

Jarisch-Herxheimer reaction, a sudden fever and worsening of skin lesions seen a few hours after the giving of penicillin or other antibiotics to treat spirosis, or relapsing fever. It lasts less than 24 hours and requires no treatment.

jaundice, a yellow discoloration of the skin, mucous membranes, and eyes, caused by increased bilirubin in the blood. Persons with jaundice may also have nausea, vomiting, and abdominal pain. Jaundice is a symptom of many disorders, including liver diseases, biliary obstruction, and some anemias. *See also hepatitis.*

jaw, *(informal)* the mandible.

jaw reflex, an abnormal reflex elicited by tapping the chin while the mouth is open and the jaw relaxed. Rapid closure of the jaw implies damage to the cerebral cortex.

jaws. See **hydraulic-powered rescue tool.**

jaw thrust, displacing the lower jaw forward by pushing anteriorly on the angles of the jaw. This airway maneuver is used when head-tilt chin-lift is inadequate or spinal injury is suspected. Originally described (1858) and then modified by J. F. Esmarch, it was previously known as the **triple jaw thrust** (when part of the maneuver included tilting the head back). Also known as **modified jaw thrust, triple jaw thrust.**

Jefferson fracture,   a fracture marked by bursting of the atlas ring of the spine.

jejunum /jəjoo´nəm/,   one of the three portions of the small intestine, connecting the duodenum and the ileum. The jejunum has a slightly larger diameter and a thicker wall than the ileum. Compare **ileum. –jejunal,** *adj.*

jellyfish sting,   a wound caused by skin contact with a jellyfish, a sea animal with a bell-shaped body and long tentacles with stingers.

jet insufflation,   positive pressure ventilation technique, utilizing high-pressure oxygen delivered at high ventilation rates, generally through a catheter placed through the cricothyroid membrane or trachea. Although first developed in 1954, the technique is not widely popular due to the increased availability of endotracheal intubation. Also known as **percutaneous transtracheal ventilation, transtracheal jet ventilation.**

jet lag,   a condition marked by fatigue, sleeplessness, and decreased body functions caused by disruption of the normal biological clock (circadian rhythm) because of air travel across several time zones.

jogger's heel,   foot pain common among joggers and distance runners. Symptoms include bruising and bursitis caused by repetitive and forceful strikes of the heel on the ground.

johnboat,   a small rectangular boat with a flat bottom. Usually found on smaller bodies of inland water and used for fishing, it is occasionally used as a rescue device to retrieve victims who have fallen through ice. Also known as a **Jonboat.**

joint,   any of the connections between bones. Each is classified according to structure and ability as in fibrous, cartilaginous, or synovial. A cartilaginous joint is one that can move slightly. In it, the cartilage joins the bone. Typical slightly moveable joints connect the vertebrae and the pubic bones. A fibrous joint is an immoveable joint, as those of the skull segments, in which a fiberlike tissue may connect the bones. A synovial joint is a freely moveable joint in which touching bony surfaces are covered by cartilage and connected by ligaments lined with synovial membrane. Kinds of synovial joints are ball and socket, condyloid, gliding, hinge, pivot, saddle, and uniaxial. Most of the joints in the body are freely moveable. Also known as **articulation.**

joint capsule.   See **capsule.**

joint chondroma,   a mass of cartilage that develops in the synovial membrane of a joint.

joule (James P. Joule, British physicist, 1818-1889),   amount of work done in 1 second by a current of 1 ampere against 1 ohm of resistance. Used to describe current flow during defibrillation and cardioversion, 1 joule is equal to 1 watt-second.

Joule's law,   **1.** *(gas physics)* at a constant temperature the internal energy of a gas does not vary with its volume. Also known as **ideal gas law. 2.** *(electrical physics)* the higher the resistance of a tissue to a flow of current, the greater the potential to transform electrical energy to thermal energy (square of the current's strength times tissue resistance times current flow duration).

J point.   See **J wave.**

judgment,   *(in psychiatry)* seeing the relation of ideas and experience and forming the correct conclusions from them.

jugular notch,   superior margin of the manubrium. Also known as **suprasternal notch.**

Jumar ascender.   See **hard ascender.**

junctional rhythm,   EKG rhythm originating from the area of the atrioventricular (AV) node (junction); with an inverted, absent, or retrograde P wave; a shortened P-R interval (less than 0.12 second), and a rate of 40 to 60 per minute. The QRS complex is 0.12 second or less and the R-R interval is constant. Although this may be seen as a normal variation, it can also be symptomatic of low cardiac output due to the slow rate. Also known as **AV rhythm, junctional escape rhythm, nodal rhythm.**

junctional tachycardia,   EKG rhythm with an inverted, absent, or retrograde P wave; a shortened P-R interval (less than 0.12 second); and a rate of greater than 100. The QRS is 0.12 second or less and the R-R interval is constant. This rhythm disturbance is due to an irritable atrioventricular (AV) node (junction) overriding the normal cardiac pacemaker, as during digitalis toxicity, myocardial infarction, or myocarditis. The patient may be symptomatic due to the rapid rate causing a decrease in cardiac output (and therefore in blood flow). Also known as **junctional tach.**

jungle penetrator, an encapsulated helicopter hoist device used to retrieve victims located under a canopy of trees. Approximately three ft (about 1 meter) long, it is lowered to the ground at the end of a hoist cable, the seats are extended, and a safety belt is placed around each person being hoisted. Originally developed for combat search-and-rescue missions over thick jungle terrain, it is equally effective over less-dense forest. This device has a capacity for three persons but is difficult to use with injured victims. Also known as **forest penetrator.** *See also rigid transport vehicle.*

jurisdiction, an area of responsibility covering a specific geographic area.

jurisdictional agency, the agency having jurisdiction and responsibility for a specific geographical area.

juvenile, 1. a young person; child. **2.** referring to or suitable for a young person; youthful. **3.** physiologically immature.

juvenile delinquency, antisocial or illegal acts by children or adolescents. Such behavior is marked by aggression, destruction, hostility, and cruelty. It occurs more often in boys than girls. **Juvenile delinquent** refers to a person who acts illegally and who is not old enough to be treated as an adult under the laws of the community.

J wave, a deflection at the junction of the QRS complex and ST segments of the EKG. Although the etiology is unknown, this phenomenon may be seen in hypothermia, local cardiac ischemia, sepsis, and in pediatric patients. It is classically seen in hypothermia below 86° F (30° C) and is most common in leads II and V6. Size of the wave increases as body temperature becomes more depressed. Also known as **hypothermic hump, J point, Osborn wave.**

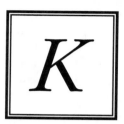

kalemia, potassium in the blood.

kaliuresis, excretion of potassium in the urine.

Kallmann's syndrome, a condition with the absence of the sense of smell and poorly developed reproductive glands.

Kaposi's sarcoma /kap´əsēz/, a cancer that begins as soft, brownish or purple papules on the feet and slowly spreads through the skin to the lymph nodes and abdominal organs. It occurs most often in men and is frequently associated with acquired immune deficiency syndrome, diabetes, and lymph cancer.

karst, geographic terrain characterized by sink holes, underground streams, and multiple layers of limestone. This terrain produces solution caves, the most common on earth.

karyon /ker´ē·on/, the nucleus of a cell.

karyosome /ker´ē·əsōm´/, a dense, irregular mass of genetic material in the cell nucleus that may be confused with the nucleolus.

karyotype /-tīp´/, **1.** the total portrait of the chromosomes in a body cell of an individual or species, as photographed through a microscope lens. It shows the number, form, size, and arrangement of chromosomes within the nucleus. **2.** a diagram of the chromosomes in a body cell of an individual or species, arranged in pairs in descending order of size. *See also chromosome.*

keeper hydraulic, water that recirculates uniformly backward, after flowing over an object below the surface, such that it is capable of trapping even buoyant objects. Also known as a **hydraulic.**

Kehr's sign, referred pain to the left side of the neck and/or shoulder due to irritation of the diaphragm. Generally a late finding, this irritation is commonly caused by injury to the spleen and may be increased when placing the patient in Trendelenburg position.

keloid /kē´loid/, overgrowth of scar tissue at the site of a wound of the skin. The new tissue is elevated, rounded, and firm, with irregular, claw-like margins. Young women and blacks are most likely to develop keloids. **Keloidosis** is a condition of habitual or multiple formation of keloids.

kelvin (William Thomson, First Baron Kelvin of Largs, British physicist, 1824-1907), unit of measurement for temperature where zero is −273.15° Celsius. Each kelvin is the same as a Celsius degree. Also known as **Celsius absolute.**

keratectomy /ker´ətek´-/, surgical removal of a portion of the cornea of the eye.

keratin /ker´ətin/, a fibrous, sulfur-containing protein found in human skin, hair, nails, and tooth enamel. It is often used as a coating for pills that must pass through the stomach unchanged to be dissolved in the intestine.

keratinization, a process by which skin cells exposed to the environment lose their moisture and are replaced by horny tissue.

keratinocyte /ker´ətinōsīt´/, a cell of the epidermis that produces keratin and other proteins.

keratitis /ker´ətī´-/, any inflammation of the cornea of the eye.

keratoconjunctivitis /-konjungk´tivi´-/, inflammation of the cornea and conjunctiva.

keratoconjunctivitis sicca, dryness of the cornea because of a lack of tear secretions. The eye feels gritty and irritated.

keratoconus /-kō´nəs/, a conelike bulge on the cornea of the eye. It may result in severe astigmatism.

keratolysis /ker´ətol´isis/, an abnormal loosening and shedding of the epidermis, which usually involves the palms of the hands or soles of the feet.

keratopathy /ker´ətop´əthē/, any disease of the cornea without inflammation. Compare **keratitis.**

keratosis /ker´ətō´-/, any skin condition in which there is overgrowth and thickening of the outer skin layers.

kernicterus /kernik´tərəs/, a buildup in central nervous system tissues of bilirubin.

kernmantle, a type of rope construction that consists of a braided outer sheath (mantle) and an inner core (kern, providing 85-90% of rope strength). Nylon fibers laid alongside one another allow only an approximately 5% stretch under load and constitute the bulk of **static kernmantle.** This design has minimal stretch with routine weight loading and is commonly used for rescue, rappelling, caving, and hauling. **Dynamic kernmantle** uses woven nylon fibers that allow rope stretch of up to 15% when under a load.

ketoacidosis /kē´tō·as´idō´-/, an excessive level of acid in the blood, accompanied by an increase of ketones in blood. Ketones are substances normally processed by the liver from fats. The condition may occur as a complication of diabetes mellitus. Symptoms are a fruity odor of the breath, altered levels of consciousness, nausea, vomiting, and dehydration. **Alcoholic ketoacidosis** refers to the condition in alcoholics.

ketoaciduria /-as´idoor´ē·ə/, presence in the urine of excessive amounts of ketones. It results from uncontrolled diabetes mellitus, starvation, or any other condition in which fats are consumed as body fuel instead of carbohydrates. Also known as **ketonuria.** *See also ketosis.*

ketone bodies /kē´ton/, a group name for ketones, substances produced in the body through a normal change fats undergo in the liver. Also known as **acetone bodies.**

ketosis /kētō´-/, an abnormal buildup of ketones in body tissues and fluid.

kidney, one of a pair of urinary filtration organs posterior to the abdomen and lateral to the spine. The kidneys are on a level with the border of the lowest ribs. Each kidney is about 11 cm long, 6 cm wide, and 2.5 cm thick. Each kidney weighs from 115 to 170 g. The kidneys produce and eliminate urine through a complex system with more than 2 million tiny filters (nephrons). The nephrons filter blood under high pressure, removing urea, salts, and other soluble wastes, forming urine. Collecting tubules take urine to the renal pelvis, which is at the center of the kidney. All of the blood in the body passes through the kidneys about 20 times every hour but only about one fifth is filtered by the nephrons during that period. Hormones control the function of the kidneys in regulating the water content of the body. The pituitary gland produces the most important, the antidiuretic hormone, which stimulates the reabsorption of water into the blood.

kidney dialysis. See **hemodialysis.**

kidney disease, any of a large group of conditions including infectious, inflammatory, obstructive, circulatory, and cancerous disorders of the kidney. Signs and symptoms of kidney disease include hematuria, edema, dysuria, and back pain. Specific symptoms vary with the type of disorder.

kidney failure, the inability of the kidneys to function. The condition may be acute or chronic.

kidney stone, a mineral buildup (stone) in the kidney. If the stone is large enough to block the ureter and stop the flow of urine from the kidney, it must be removed. Also known as **renal calculus.**

kill zone, *(special operations)* a designated area where live weapons fire is permitted, in order to secure a tactical objective.

kilogram (kg) /kil´əgram/, a unit for the measurement of mass in the metric system. One kilogram is equal to 1000 grams or to 2.2046 pounds avoirdupois.

Kimmelstiel-Wilson syndrome, degeneration of the glomerulus of the kidney, seen in diabetics.

kinematics /kin´əmat´-, kī´nə-/, the study of the motion of the body without regard to the forces acting to produce the motion. Kinematics considers the motions of all body parts relative to the part involved in the motion. Knowledge of these motions help to determine where a patient may have injuries after trauma. Compare **kinetics.**

kinesics /kinē´siks/, the study of body position and movement in communication between people.

kinesiology /kinē´sē·ol´-/, the scientific study of muscular activity and of the anatomy, physiology, and mechanics of body movement.

kinetics /kinet´-/, the study of forces that produce or modify motion. Compare **kinematics.**

KKK specifications, federal (U.S.) Department of Transportation criteria for acceptable ambulance design. Having ambulances that meet these design specifications is often a minimum requirement for approval of bids, grants, and loans related to emergency medical services operations and research.

Klebsiella /kleb´zē·el´ə/, a kind of bacteria that causes several respiratory diseases.

Kleine-Levin syndrome /klīn´-/, a disorder often associated with psychotic conditions, with symptoms of drowsiness, hunger, and excessive activity. Compare **narcolepsy.**

kleptolagnia /klep´təlag´nē·ə/, sexual excitement or satisfaction produced by stealing.

kleptomania /klep´tə-/, a neurosis with an uncontrollable urge to steal. Objects are not taken for their monetary value, immediate need, or use but for their symbolic meaning, which may be associated with an emotional conflict. **–kleptomaniac,** *n.*

knee, a joint that connects the femur with the tibia and fibula. It consists of three condyloid joints, 12 bands of ligaments, 13 bursae, and the patella. The largest bursa is the prepatellar bursa between the patellar ligament and the skin.

kneecap, (*informal*) a flat, triangle-shaped bone at the front of the knee joint. Also known as **patella.**

knee-hip flexion, body movement that allows the passage of body weight over the supporting leg while walking.

knife, a sharp-bladed instrument used for cutting or stabbing. Single-edged knives have some use in rescue applications, and single- and double-edged weapons are used during tactical operations.

knot, a distortion of rope or line, created by passing the free end through a loop and drawing it tight.

koilonychia /koi´lōnik´ē·ə/, spoon nails; a condition in which fingernails are thin and curved inwardly from side to side. Usually inherited, it may also occur with iron deficiency anemia and Raynaud's phenomenon.

Koplik's spots (Henry Koplik, American physician, 1858-1927), small red spots with bluish-white centers found on the inside of the mouth of persons with measles. The rash of measles usually erupts 1 or 2 days after the appearance of Koplik's spots.

Korotkoff sounds (Nikolai S. Korotkoff, Russian physician, 1874-1920), sounds of blood flow heard while auscultating blood pressure. The beginning and ending (change) of these sounds provide the parameters for blood pressure determination. *See also blood pressure, diastole, sphygmomanometer, systole.*

Korsakoff's psychosis /kôr´səkôfs/ (Sergei Korsakoff, Russian physician, 1853-1900), a form of memory loss seen in chronic alcoholics. The patient is disoriented due to decreased levels of thiamine. *See also Wernicke's encephalopathy.*

Krause's corpuscles, nerve endings sensitive to temperature.

Krebs' citric acid cycle /krebz/, a series of enzyme reactions in which the body uses carbohydrates, protein, and fats to yield carbon dioxide, water, and energy.

Kupffer's cells /koop´fərz/, liver cells that filter bacteria and other foreign proteins out of the blood.

Kussmaul breathing /koos´moul/, deep, rapid respirations with sighing. It occurs in diabetic ketoacidosis.

Kussmaul's pulse (Adolph Kussmaul, German physician, 1822-1902), a reduction or disappearance of the pulse during inspiration.

Kussmaul's sign, **1.** a pulse that rises in rate when exhaling and falls when inhaling. **2.** seizures and unconsciousness associated with toxin ingestion.

L

label, a substance, usually radioactive, with a special attraction for a specific organ, tissue, or cell, in which it may become deposited. The radioactivity can be followed through various body processes, making it useful in diagnosis.

labia /lā´bē·ə/, *sing.* **labium,** the liplike edges of an organ or tissue, such as the folds of skin at the opening of the vagina.

labia majora /majôr´ə/, *sing.* **labium majus,** two folds of skin, one on each side of the vaginal opening, that form the border of the vulva.

labia minora /minôr´ə/, *sing.* **labium minus,** two folds of skin between the labia majora, extending from the clitoris backward on both sides of the vaginal opening.

labile /lā´bil/, **1.** unstable; having a tendency to change or to be easily altered. **2.** describing a personality with rapidly shifting or changing emotions.

labile pulse, a pulse with frequent large changes in rate.

labor, the time and processes that occur during childbirth from the beginning of cervical dilatation to the delivery of the placenta. In the early stage of childbirth, called the **latent phase** or **prodromal labor,** there are irregular, few, and mild contractions of the uterus. Little or no dilation of the cervix or descent of the fetus occurs. During the **active phase** of labor, the cervix widens from about 5 cm to 10 cm (2 to 4 inches). The **acceleration phase** is the first part of active labor. The cervix opens more quickly during this time.

Known as **transition,** the last phase of the first stage of labor is sometimes shown by the cervix dilating 8 to 10 cm. When the cervix is fully widened, the contractions occur every 1 ½ to 3 minutes and last from 40 to 90 seconds. **Engagement** refers to the point in childbirth when the part of the fetus descending first comes down into the mother's pelvis. This occurs roughly halfway through labor. The **expulsive stage of labor** is the second stage, during which contractions of the uterus are accompanied by an urge to bear down. It begins after the cervix is completely widened. This stage ends with the complete delivery of the infant. **Premature labor** refers to labor that occurs earlier in pregnancy than normal, either before the fetus has reached a weight of 2000 to 2500 grams (5 to 5.5 pounds) or before the thirty-seventh week of pregnancy. **Cardinal movements of labor** refers to the sequence of movements by the infant as it comes down through the pelvis during labor and birth. **Dry labor** is labor in which the water (amniotic fluid) has already escaped. *See also birth.*

labored breathing, increased effort in breathing, including use of accessory muscles, grunting, or flaring of the nostrils.

labyrinth. See **ear.**

labyrinthitis /lab´ərinthī´-/, inflammation of the fluid-filled canals of the inner ear, resulting in dizziness.

laceration /las´ərā´shən/, a torn, jagged wound. **–lacerate,** *v.,* **lacerated,** *adj.*

lacrimal /lak´riməl/, pertaining to tear ducts.

lacrimal bone, one of the smallest bones of the face, located anterior of the inner wall of the eye socket.

lacrimal duct, one of two channels through which tears pass from the inner corner of the eye to the lacrimal sac. *See also lacrimal sac.*

lacrimal fistula, an abnormal channel from a tear duct to the surface of the eye or eyelid.

lacrimal gland, one of a pair of oval-shaped glands situated above the eye. The watery secretion from the gland consists of the tears that moisten the eye. The **lacrimal papilla** is the small elevation on the margin of each eyelid, through which tears emerge from the lacrimal gland.

lacrimal sac, one of two sacs lodged in a groove formed between the inner corners of the eyes and the nose. Tears from the eyes fill the sacs and drain down into the cavity of the nose.

lacrimation /lak´rima´shən/, **1.** the normal continuous secretion of tears by the lacrimal glands above the eyes. **2.** an excessive amount of tear production, as in crying or weeping.

lacrimators, chemical agents that cause intense tearing and blurred vision. These agents are used to distract or disperse groups of people and are hand-delivered, thrown, or fired from a weapon.

lactalbumin /lak´talbyo͞o´min/, a highly nutritious protein found in milk. It is similar to serum albumin. *See also serum albumin.*

lactase /lak´tās/, an enzyme that increases the rate of metabolism of lactose to glucose and galactose, carbohydrates needed by the body for energy. Lactase is concentrated in the kidney, liver, and intestinal lining.

lactated Ringer's. See **Ringer's lactate.**

lactation, the process of production and release of milk from the breasts for the feeding of an infant. *See also breast feeding.*

lacteal /lak´tē·əl/, pertaining to milk.

lacteal gland, one of the many lymph capillaries in the villi of the small intestine wall. The capillary is filled with a fluid (chyle) that turns milky white during the absorption of fat.

lactic, referring to milk and milk products.

lactic acid, an organic acid normally present in tissue. One form of lactic acid in muscle and

blood is a product of the change of the carbohydrates glucose and glycogen to energy during physical exercise.

Lactobacillus, any of a group of rod-shaped bacteria that produce lactic acid from carbohydrates.

lactogen /lak´təjən/, a drug or other agent that stimulates the production and release of milk. **–lactogenic,** *adj.*

lactose /lak´tōs/, a sugar found in the milk of all mammals. Also known as **milk sugar.**

lactose intolerance, a disorder resulting in the inability to digest lactose because of lactase deficiency. Symptoms include nausea, diarrhea, and cramps. *See also lactase deficiency.*

lactosuria /-o͞or´ē·ə/, the presence of lactose in the urine. This may occur in late pregnancy or during breast milk production (lactation).

ladder company, fire department unit consisting of three to four firefighters assigned to a vehicle whose primary purpose is to provide ventilation, lighting, rescue, and other services at the scene of a fire. The primary equipment of the vehicle to which they are assigned is generally one large mounted ladder or articulating arm, along with an assortment of other ladders and rescue equipment. Also known as **truck company.**

ladder splint, splinting device that consists of a wire mesh that can be bent to accommodate angulations and distortions but retain the rigidity necessary to support a fracture. The device originally resembled a small ladder. Also known as **wire ladder splint.** *See also SAM splint.*

lagophthalmos /lag´ofthal´məs/, a condition in which an eye cannot be fully closed because of a nervous system or muscle disorder. Also known as **hare's eye.**

lahar /lä´här/, volcanic debris flow or mudflow that forms when ash and ash fragments combine with water on downhill slopes. The often destructive flow can inundate towns and rivers. A **primary lahar** is due to volcanic activity, as in water formed by the heating of snow. **Secondary lahars** occur after saturation of debris by rainfall.

laked blood /lākt/, blood in which hemolysis of red blood cells has occurred, as may happen in poisoning or burns.

lallation /lalā´shən/, **1.** babbling, repetitive, unintelligible speech, like that of an infant. **2.** a speech disorder with a defective pronunciation of words containing the sound /l/ or the use of the sound /l/ in place of the sound /r/.

Lamaze method /ləmäz´/, a system of preparation for childbirth developed in the 1950s by a French obstetrician, Fernand Lamaze. The Lamaze method has become the most often used means of teaching natural childbirth, without the use of drugs. *See also natural childbirth.*

lamella /ləmel´ə/, *pl.* **lamellae**, **1.** a thin leaf or plate, as of bone. **2.** a medicated disk.

lamina /lam´inə/, *pl.* **laminae**, a thin, flat plate or layer, such as the lamina of the thyroid cartilage that overlays the structure on each side.

laminectomy /lam´inek´-/, the surgical removal of the thin bony arches (laminae) of one or more vertebrae, done to relieve compression of the spinal cord.

lancet, a short, pointed blade used to obtain a drop of blood for a sample.

lancinating, pertaining to a sensation that is sharply piercing or tearing, as a pain may be.

Landau reflex /lan´dou/, a normal response of infants when lying on the back to maintain an arc with the head raised and the legs slightly flexed. The reflex is poor in those with floppy infant syndrome and exaggerated in other disorders.

landing gear, the weight-bearing understructure that supports and cushions an aircraft, allowing it to take off and land. These structures are generally supported by wheels or skids.

landslide, masses of material that have broken away from and slide down an elevated geographical feature, such as a hill or mountain. Although the movement of the material can be slow or fast, there is always a danger to people and inhabited areas until the movement ceases. The most common landslides involve mud, snow, ice, dirt, and mixed debris.

lanugo /lanoo´gō, lanyoo´gō/, **1.** the soft hair covering a normal fetus, beginning with the fifth month of life in the uterus and almost entirely shed by the ninth month. **2.** the fine, soft hair covering all parts of the body except palms, soles, and areas where other types of hair are normally found. Also known as **vellus hair.**

laparoscopy /lap´əros´kəpē/, the examination of the abdominal cavity. An instrument consisting of a lighted tube with magnifying lenses (laparoscope) is inserted through a small incision in the abdominal wall. Also known as **abdominoscopy.**

laparotomy /-ot´-/, a surgical incision into the abdomen. Some types of laparotomy are **appendectomy, cholecystectomy, colostomy.**

large intestine. See **intestine.**

laryngectomy /ler´injek´-/, surgical removal of the larynx.

laryngismus /-jiz´məs/, uncontrolled spasm of the larynx. A crowing sound is made when breathing. The skin may become cyanotic. The larynx of the infant and child is particularly affected by infection or irritation and may become obstructed.

laryngitis /-jī´-/, inflammation of the mucous membrane lining the larynx, accompanied by swelling of the vocal cords with hoarseness or loss of voice.

laryngopharyngitis /lering´gōfer´injī´-/, inflammation of the larynx and pharynx. *See also laryngitis, pharyngitis.*

laryngoscope, instrument consisting of a handle and blade that is used for examining the larynx and assisting in the completion of procedures related to airway and pulmonary maintenance, as foreign body removal and endotracheal intubation. *See also endotracheal intubation, Magill forceps.*

laryngospasm /-spazm/, a sudden, temporary closure of the larynx. *See also laryngismus.*

laryngotracheobronchitis /-trā´kē·ōbrongkī´-/, an inflammation of the throat, larynx, and bronchi. Symptoms are hoarseness, a dry cough, and shortness of breath. *See also croup.*

larynx /ler´ingks/, the portion of the airway connecting the throat with the trachea. It produces the protrusion on the neck called the Adam's apple. The larynx, lined with mucous membrane, forms the inferior portion of the front wall of the throat. It is composed of rings of cartilages, connected together by ligaments and moved by muscles. **–laryngeal,** *adj.*

laser, acronym for *light amplification by stimulated emission of radiation,* a source of intense radiation of the visible, ultraviolet, or infrared portions of the light spectrum.

latent, pertaining to a condition that is inactive or existing as a potential problem, as tuberculosis may be latent for a long period of time and then become active under certain conditions.

latent period, an interval between the time of exposure to an injurious dose of radiation and the response of the body tissues to the radiation.

lateral, **1.** on the side. **2.** away from the midline of the body or body part.

lateral collision, an impact into the side of a vehicle. Also known as **T-bone accident.**

lateral pelvic displacement, one of the major leg muscle actions produced by the horizontal shift of the pelvis. It helps to synchronize the movements of walking.

lateral recumbent, position with the patient lying on his or her side, with the knees and thighs drawn up.

latissimus dorsi, one of a pair of large triangular muscles of the back. The base of the triangle is at the level of the lower four ribs. The latissimus dorsi moves the arm, draws the shoulder back and down, and helps draw the body up when climbing.

lava cave, tube formed underneath volcanic material, when the liquid magma cools on the surface, but continues to flow underneath. These caves are generally shallow and subject to erosion, making them unstable.

lavage /ləväzh´/, the process of washing out an organ for treatment, as when a poison has been swallowed. **Gastric lavage** is the washing out of the stomach with sterile water or saline. This is done to remove irritants and swallowed poisons. *See also dialysis, irrigation.*

Lawrence, Thomas Edward (British scholar/soldier, 1888-1935), *(historical)* early inventor of air and sea rescue equipment and techniques, especially the rescue speedboat. Also known as **Lawrence of Arabia, T. E. Lawrence.**

laxative, a substance that causes evacuation of the bowel. Compare **cathartic.**

lead, **1.** an electrical connection attached to the body for the purpose of monitoring physiological electrical activity. These are generally used to record cerebral or cardiac electrical activity. In prehospital, emergency department, and critical care areas, cardiac electrical activity is usually observed and recorded in lead II, although leads I, III, and MCL1 are also used. **2.** a poisonous metallic element with a specific gravity of 11.35.

leading edge, the forward or front part of an aerodynamic surface.

lead poisoning /led/, a condition caused by swallowing or breathing substances containing lead. Many children have developed the condition as a result of eating flakes of lead paint peeling from walls or furniture. Poisoning also occurs from drinking water carried in lead pipes, lead salts in some foods and wines, the use of pewter or earthenware dishes covered with lead glaze, and the use of leaded gasoline. Breathing of lead fumes is common in industry. Symptoms of chronic lead poisoning are extreme irritability, loss of appetite, and anemia. Symptoms of the acute form of lead poisoning are a burning sensation in the mouth and esophagus, constipation or diarrhea, mental disturbances, and paralysis of the arms and legs.

leather bottle stomach, a thickening of the wall of the stomach, resulting in a rigid, shrunken organ. Causes include cancer, syphilis, and Crohn's disease involving the stomach.

lecithin /les´ithin/, any of a group of phosphorus-rich fats common in plants and animals. Lecithins are found in the liver, nerve tissue, bile, and blood. They are essential for transforming fats in the body.

Le Fort fracture (Léon Le Fort, French surgeon, 1829-1893), facial fractures classified into three types: Le Fort I (Guerin's fracture) is a fracture involving the maxilla. Le Fort II (pyramidal fracture) involves the maxilla, nasal bones, and medial eye orbits. Le Fort III (craniofacial dysjunction) encompasses fractures of the maxilla, nasal bones, ethmoids, zygoma, vomer, and all the smaller bones of the base of the cranium.

left ventricular assist device, a mechanical pump that is used to aid the natural pumping action of the left ventricle of the heart. Also known as **LVAD.**

Legionnaires' disease, an acute pneumonia caused by infection with a germ (*Legionella pneumophilia*). There is an influenza-like illness followed by pleurisy. Symptoms include fever, chills, muscle aches, headache, dry cough, and diarrhea. Usually the disease is self-limited, but the death rate has been 15% to 20% in a few localized epidemics. Contaminated air conditioning cooling towers and moist soil may be a source of organisms. Person-to-person transmission has not occurred.

leishmaniasis /lēsh´mənī´əsis/, infection with a protozoan parasite of the *Leishmania* group that is transmitted to humans by sand flies. The diseases caused by these microorganisms may involve the skin or abdominal organs, causing ulcers or a skin disorder that resembles leprosy.

Lenegre's disease, chronic degenerative changes in the cardiac conduction system of the elderly, which leads to third-degree atrioventricular (AV) block. These changes are not normally associated with increased parasympathetic tone. Also known as **Lev's disease.**

lentigo /lentī´gō/, *pl.* **lentignes** /lentij´ənēz/, a tan or brown spot on the skin brought on by sun exposure, usually in a middle-aged or older person. Another variety, called **juvenile lentigo** and unrelated to sunlight, appears in children 2 to 5 years of age. Compare **freckle.**

Lepidoptera, an order of insects made up of the butterflies and moths, which begin their lives as caterpillars. Some of these caterpillars are venomous in nature, but most of the injuries inflicted are minor.

leprosy /lep´rəsē/, a chronic disease, caused by *Mycobacterium leprae*, that may take either of two forms. **Tuberculoid leprosy** appears as a thickening of nerves of the skin with saucer-shaped skin lesions. **Lepromatous leprosy** involves many systems of the body, with widespread skin lesions, eye inflammation, destruction of nose cartilage and bone, and atrophy of the testicles. Blindness may result. The disease occurs mostly in undeveloped tropical and subtropical countries. Also known as **Hansen's disease.**

leptocytosis /lep´tōsītō´-/, a condition in which abnormal red blood cells are present in the blood. Thalassemia, some kinds of liver disease, and absence of the spleen are linked with leptocytosis.

leptospirosis /-spīrō´-/, an acute infectious disease caused by a microorganism, *Leptospira interrogans,* transmitted through infected animals, especially rodents or dogs. Human infections come from direct contact with the urine or tissues of the infected animal or indirectly from contact with contaminated water or soil. Symptoms include jaundice, bleeding into the skin, fever, chills, and muscular pain. The most serious form is known as **Weil's disease.**

Leriche's syndrome /lərēshs´/, gradual obstruction of the abdominal aorta. Symptoms include pain in buttocks, thighs, or calves and absence of pulses in the legs.

lesbian, **1.** a female homosexual. **2.** referring to the sexual preference or desire of one woman for another. –**lesbianism,** *n.*

Lesch-Nyhan syndrome /lesh´-nī´han/, a hereditary disorder affecting males, in which there is an excess production of uric acid, normally present in blood and urine. Symptoms include mental retardation, self-mutilation of the fingers and lips by biting, impaired kidney function, and abnormal physical development.

lesion, **1.** a wound, injury, or other damage in body tissue. See Appendix 1-1.

lesser occipital nerve, one of a pair of nerves that runs along the side of the head behind the ear.

lethal /lē´thəl/, capable of causing death.

lethal concentrations-50%, the concentration of a substance that results in the death of 50% of the test populations; expressed in parts per million (ppm), milligrams per liter, or milligrams per cubic meter. (The lower the value, the more toxic the substance.) Also known as **LC-50.**

lethal dose-50%, the concentration of an ingested or infected substance that results in the death of 50% of the test populations; an oral or dermal exposure expressed in milligrams per kilogram. (The lower the dose, the more toxic the substance.) Also known as **LD-50.**

lethargy /leth´ərjē/, the state or quality of being indifferent or sluggish, as in **lucid lethargy,** a state in which there is a loss of will and an inability to act, even though the patient is conscious.

Letterman, Jonathan, *(historical)* Union major during the American Civil War who developed one of the first systems of triage and perfected the concept of issuing similar medical equipment items to all military units. This **Letterman exchange system** simplified the restocking of medical equipment and is the same concept used today in military and civilian medical systems.

leucine /loo´sin/, an amino acid essential for growth in infants and nitrogen balance in adults. It cannot be synthesized by the body and is obtained by the conversion of protein during digestion. A congenital inability of the body to use leucine properly is called **maple syrup urine disease.** *See also amino acid.*

leukapheresis /loo´kəfərē´-/, a process by which blood is withdrawn from a vein, white blood cells are selectively removed, and the remaining blood is recycled back into the donor. The white cells may be used for treating patients with blood deficiencies.

leukemia, a cancer of blood-forming tissues. Replacement of bone marrow with immature white blood cells (leukocytes) occurs, and abnormal numbers and forms of immature white cells appear in circulation. Leukemia is classified according to the kinds of abnormal cells, the course of the disease, and the duration of the disease. The two major types of leukemia are **acute lymphocytic leukemia (ALL)** and **acute myelocytic leukemia (AML).** ALL is usually a disease of children, whereas AML occurs in all age groups.

leukemia cutis, a condition affecting the skin of the face, in which yellowish, red, or purple lesions and large accumulations of white blood cells develop.

leukemoid reaction, a condition resembling leukemia in which the white blood cell count rises in response to an allergy, inflammatory disease, infection, poison, hemorrhage, burn, or other causes of severe physical stress.

leukocyte /loo´kəsīt/, a white blood cell. There are five types of leukocytes, classified by the presence or absence of small particles (granules) in the cytoplasm, the main substance of the cell. The agranulocytes, or those without granules, are lymphocytes and monocytes. The granulocytes, white cells with granules, are called neutrophils, basophils, and eosinophils. Leukocytes are larger than red blood cells (erythrocytes). A cubic millimeter of normal blood usually contains 5000 to 10,000 leukocytes. Among the most important functions of the leukocytes are the destruction of bacteria,

fungi, and viruses, and rendering harmless poisonous substances that may result from allergic reactions and cell injury.

leukocytosis /-sītō´-/, an abnormal increase in the number of circulating white blood cells. This often accompanies bacterial, but not usually viral, infections. Leukemia may be associated with a white blood cell count as high as 500,000 to 1 million per cubic millimeter of blood.

leukoderma /-dur´mə/, loss of skin pigment. Compare **vitiligo.**

leukonychia /-nik´ē·ə/, white patches under the nails.

leukopenia /-pē´nē·ə/, an abnormal decrease in the number of white blood cells.

leukoplakia /-plā´kē·ə/, a precancerous change in the normal tissue of a mucous membrane that causes raised white patches on the affected part.

leukotoxin /-tok´sin/, a substance that can inactivate or destroy white blood cells. –**leukotoxic,** *adj.*

leukotrienes, chemical compounds that occur naturally in leukocytes. They are able to produce allergic and inflammatory reactions, and may take part in the development of asthma and rheumatoid arthritis.

levator /ləvā´tər/, *pl.* **levatores** /lev´ətôr´ēz/, a muscle that raises a structure of the body. The **levator ani** is one of a pair of muscles of the pelvis that stretches across the bottom of the pelvic cavity like a hammock, supporting the pelvic organs. The **levator palpebrae superioris** is a muscle of the upper eyelid that raises the eyelid. The **levator scapulae** is a muscle of the back and sides of the neck that raises the scapula of the shoulder.

level of consciousness, the degree of awareness present in human functioning. Common descriptions include awake/oriented with appropriate behavior; awake but not oriented; unconscious—responds appropriately to noxious (painful) stimuli; unconscious—responds inappropriately to noxious stimuli; unconscious. *See also mental status exam.*

lever, any bone and associated joint of the body that act together so that force applied to one end of the bone will lift a weight at another point. An example is the action of muscles that move the forearm at the elbow joint.

levitation, a hallucination that one is floating or rising in the air. The sensation may also occur in dreams. –**levitate,** *v.*

Leydig cells /lī´dig/, cells of the testes that secrete testosterone, a male sex hormone.

liability, direct or indirect legal responsibility.

libel, written publication of statements known to be false, with malicious intent or reckless disregard.

liberation, **1.** the process of drug release into a body organ or system from the dosage given. **2.** the activation of an enzyme or chemical reaction.

libido /libē´dō, libī´dō/, the psychic energy or instinctual drive associated with sexual desire, pleasure, or creativity.

lice, small, wingless insects (order Anoplura) that live on the blood of their host. They are transmitters of systemic diseases, with three varieties (pubic, head, and body louse) preferring human hosts.

licensed practical nurse, a person trained in basic nursing techniques and direct patient care who practices under the supervision of a registered nurse. Also known as **Licensed Vocational Nurse, LPN, LVN.**

licensure, the process by which a recognized agency, usually governmental, gives permission to an individual to engage in a controlled profession.

lichenification /līken´ifikā´-/, a thickening and hardening of the skin, often resulting from irritation caused by repeated scratching. –**lichenified,** *adj.*

lichen nitidus /li´kən/, a skin disorder in which numerous small, flat, pale, glistening papules form. Also known as **Pinkus' disease.**

lichen planus, a skin disease with small, flat, purplish papules or patches. Common sites are wrists, forearms, ankles, abdomen, and lower back. On mucous membranes the lesions appear gray and lacy. Nails may have ridges running lengthwise.

lidocaine, an antidysrhythmic drug used in the presence of ventricular ectopics, ventricular tachycardia, and ventricular fibrillation. It decreases ventricular excitability and raises the threshold of ventricular fibrillation. Toxicity is the major side effect, causing anxiety, hypotension, numbness, nausea, seizures, and tinnitus. Not to be used in the presence of escape or pacemaker rhythms. Also known as **Xylocaine.**

lienal vein /lē·ē´nəl/, a large vein that is important in circulating blood from the spleen.

life belt, a personal flotation device worn around the waist. *See also personal flotation device.*

lifeboat, **1.** *(historical)* a land-based boat, launched when necessary to save overboard or shipwrecked victims. These boats were specially built and equipped for use in heavy seas. **2.** a small, rigid boat, carried by a ship for emergencies requiring off-loading of crew and passengers. Compare **life raft.**

life buoy. See **ring buoy.**

lifeguard, **1.** personnel trained in water rescue and emergency care who patrol swimming pools, lakes, and oceans. While the degree of training varies considerably, all categories are responsible for the safety of people around a water environment. **2.** call sign used by aircraft to indicate to air traffic control towers that an aircraft is engaged in a mission where a human life is in danger.

life island, a plastic bubble enclosing a bed, used to provide a germ-free environment for a patient.

life net, circular rescue device used to allow people to jump from the lower stories of a burning building. A round metal frame with fabric in the center, this tool has fallen into disuse because of the availability of tall ladders and other improved escape systems.

life raft, a small, usually inflatable boat used as refuge for victims of shipwreck. Several types of rafts are available, including **coastal** (basic, 4-50 persons), **lifefloat** (rigid plastic foam, 5-6 persons), **offshore** (inflatable, up to 50 persons for weeks), **rescue platform** (basic with cover, up to 50 persons), **SOLAS** (minimum of thirty days survival), and **USCG** (harsh or prolonged conditions). *See also lifeboat.*

life space, a term used by American psychologists to describe all of the influences existing at the same time that may affect individual behavior. The total of the influences make up the life space.

life-style-induced health problems, diseases with histories that include known exposure to certain health-threatening or risk factors, such as heart disease associated with cigarette smoking, poor eating habits, lack of exercise, and psychological stress.

lift, any of several techniques for raising a patient. These include the blanket lift, the three- four- or six-rescuer lift, and the chair lift. Utilization of any of these techniques should take into account the patient's injuries, the number of personnel available, and the distance to be lifted.

ligament /lig´əmənt/, **1.** a white, shiny, flexible band of fibrous tissue binding joints together and connecting various bones and cartilages. When part of a joint membrane, they are covered with fibrous tissue that blends with surrounding connective tissue. Yellow elastic ligaments connect certain parts of adjoining vertebrae. They help to hold the body erect. Compare **tendon. 2.** a layer of membrane with little or no stretching ability, extending from one abdominal organ to another. *See also broad ligament.*

ligamental tear, a tear of the fibers of a ligament connecting and surrounding the bones of a joint. An injury to the joint, such as from a sudden twisting motion, causes torn ligaments. This may occur at any joint but is most common in the knees and is often linked to sports injuries.

ligation /līgā´shən/, tying off a blood vessel or duct with a suture or wire to stop or prevent bleeding or to prevent passage of material through a duct, as in ligation of the fallopian tubes. *See also vein ligation and stripping.*

ligature /lig´əchər/, a suture or wire.

light, radiant energy of the wavelength and frequency that stimulate visual receptor cells in the retina of the eye to produce nerve impulses that are perceived in the brain as vision.

light accommodation, changes that occur in the eye in order that vision can occur at varying levels of light. Also known as **light adaptation.**

lightening, a sensation felt late in pregnancy as the fetus settles into the pelvis. The fetus is said to have "dropped."

lightning, an atmospheric electrical discharge caused by a difference in electrical charges between atmosphere and ground. These discharges can have an electrical current of 250,000 amperes. Multiple forms have been noted, including ball, bead, ribbon, streak, and sheet lightning.

light reflex, the mechanism by which the pupil of the eye reacts to changes in light and darkness. The **consensual reaction to light** is the narrowing of the pupil of one eye when the other eye is exposed to light.

limb, a body part, such as an arm or leg, or a branch of an internal organ.

limbic system, a group of related nervous system structures within the midbrain that are linked with various emotions and feelings, such as anger, fear, sexual arousal, pleasure, and sadness. The function of the system is poorly understood.

limited quantity, an amount of radioactive material that is exempted from specification packaging, marking, and labeling because of low radiological hazard. Includes small quantities and certain manufactured articles.

line, **1.** a stripe, streak, or narrow ridge, often imaginary, that connects areas of the body or that separates various parts of the body, as the hair line or nipple line. Also known as **linea. 2.** smaller diameter rope. **3.** the shortest distance between 2 points.

linea alba /lin´ē·ə/, a line that runs along the midline of the abdomen beneath the skin, formed by a tendon extending from the sternum to the pubic area. It contains the navel.

linea nigra, a dark line appearing on the abdomen of pregnant women during the latter part of the pregnancy. It usually extends from the pubic area to the navel.

linear fracture, a fracture that runs along the length of a bone.

lineman's gloves, nonconducting rubber gloves with leather exteriors that are used when working with downed or energized power lines.

line throwing gun, rescue device that shoots a length of line across a distance. A larger rope can then be pulled across and used to access and remove a trapped victim; generally used during water and mountain rescues.

lingual artery /ling´gwal/, one of a pair of arteries that branch along the sides of the neck and head to supply the tongue and surrounding muscles.

lingual frenum, a band of tissue that extends from the floor of the mouth to the underside of the tongue.

liniment /lin´imənt/, a remedy, usually containing an alcoholic, oily, or soapy substance, that is rubbed on the skin, producing an inflammatory reaction to reduce one elsewhere.

lip, any rimlike structure bordering a cavity or groove, such as that surrounding the opening of the mouth.

lipase /lī´pās/, any of several digestive system enzymes that increase the breakdown of lipids.

lipectomy /lipek´-/, surgical removal of fat beneath the skin, as from the abdominal wall.

lipid, any of the various fats or fatlike substances in plant or animal tissues. Lipids are insoluble in water but soluble in alcohol and other organic solvents. They are stored in the body and serve as an energy reserve, but may be elevated in certain diseases, such as atherosclerosis. Kinds of lipids include **cholesterol, fatty acids, phospholipids, triglycerides.**

lipidosis /lip´idō´-/, any disorder that involves the buildup of abnormal levels of certain fats in the body. Kinds of lipidoses are **Gaucher's disease, Krabbe's disease, Niemann-Pick disease, Tay-Sachs disease.**

lipodystrophy /lip´ōdis´trəfē/, any abnormality in the use of fats in the body, particularly one in which the fat deposits under the skin are affected.

lipoid /lip´oid/, any substance that resembles a fat.

lipoma /lipō´mə/, a tumor consisting of fat cells. A **lipoma arborescens** is a fatty tumor of a joint, with a treelike distribution of fat cells. A **lipoma capsulare** is in the capsule of an organ, such as the capsule or sheath covering the kidney. A **lipoma fibrosum** contains masses of fibrous tissue.

lipomatosis /-mətō´-/, abnormal tumorlike accumulations of fat in body tissues.

lipomatous myxoma /lipō´mətəs/, a tumor containing fatty tissue that begins in connective tissue.

lipoprotein /lip´ōprō´tēn/, a protein in which fats form a part of the molecule. Practically all of the lipids in human blood are present as lipoproteins. Lipoproteins are classified by their size or density. *See also cholesterol, triglyceride.*

liquefaction, 1. a physical process where soil, usually silts and sands, lose their holding strength temporarily and act as viscous fluids rather than solids. This process is most common in clay-deficient soil and is activated by ground movement, as during an earthquake. **2.** Conversion of solid tissue to a fluid state.

liquid, a state of matter between solid and gas, in which the substance flows freely and assumes the shape of the vessel in which it is contained.

liquid breathing, experimental concept that utilizes a liquid in place of air to add oxygen and remove carbon dioxide within the lungs. This concept would allow divers to descend to any depth, stay as long as necessary and surface immediately. Fluorocarbon liquids have been the most promising, but human use awaits further advances.

listeriosis, a disease caused by a germ that infects shellfish, birds, spiders, and mammals in all areas of the world. It is transmitted to humans by direct contact with infected animals, by breathing of dust, or by contact with contaminated sewage or soil. All secretions from an infected person may contain the organism. Signs include enlarged liver and spleen, and a dark, red rash over the trunk and legs.

listlessness, a state of apathy and decreased activity brought on by illness or depression.

lithiasis /lithī´əsis/, the formation of stones (calculi) from mineral salts in the hollow organs or ducts of the body. This occurs most commonly in the gallbladder, kidney, and lower urinary tract.

lithotomy /lithot´/, the surgical removal of a stone (calculus), especially one from the urinary tract.

litter, any device for carrying ill or injured victims. Most commonly, this term is used to mean a carrying device without wheels, such as a folding litter, Neil-Robertson litter, Stokes litter. Also known as **carrier, cot, stretcher.** *See also gurney.*

live birth, the birth of an infant that exhibits any sign of life, such as breathing, heart beat, umbilical cord pulsation, or movement of voluntary muscles. Length of pregnancy of the mother is not considered. A live birth is not always one in which the infant is viable.

livedo /livē´dō/, a blue or reddish blotching of the skin, usually caused by a spasm of arterioles.

live ice. See **water ice.**

liver, the largest gland of the body and one of its most complex organs. Located in the upper right portion of the abdominal cavity, the liver attaches to the diaphragm by two ligaments. It is completely covered by peritoneum except where it attaches to a ligament. The liver is divided into four lobes, with the right lobe much larger than the others. The hepatic artery conveys oxygenated blood from the heart to the liver. The hepatic portal vein conveys nutrient-filled blood from the stomach and the intestines. At any given moment the liver holds about 13% of the total blood supply of the body. Dark reddish-brown in color, it has a soft, solid consistency shaped like an irregular hemisphere. Its major functions are producing bile, processing glucose, proteins, vitamins, and fats, producing hemoglobin and converting ammonia to urea. It also renders harmless numerous substances, such as alcohol and nicotine. *See also gallbladder.*

liver disease, any of a group of liver disorders. The most important diseases in this group are cirrhosis, cholestasis, and hepatitis. Characteristics of liver disease are jaundice, loss of appetite, enlarged liver ascites, and altered level of consciousness. *See also cholestasis, cirrhosis, hepatitis.*

liver spot, (*informal*) a brown or black lesion seen on older persons. Also known as **Chloasma hepaticum.**

lividity, bluish discoloration of the skin. **Postmortem lividity** is discoloration of dependent parts of the body, which appears within one-half to two hours after cardiac arrest, due to gravitational movement of blood.

living will, a written agreement between a patient and physician to withhold heroic measures if the patient's condition is found to be terminal.

lizard bite, a bite of the large Gila monster of Arizona, New Mexico, and Utah, or the beaded lizard of Mexico. They are the only lizards known to be venomous. The symptoms of their bites and the recommended treatment are similar to those of the bites from moderately poisonous snakes.

load-bearing, primarily responsible for holding weight.

loaded bumper, a compressed energy-absorbing bumper, in which the piston that absorbs the energy of an accident remains compressed after the accident. There is a danger in that it may release while personnel are standing in front of it, causing serious injury or death.

loam, a soil type composed of clay and sand.

lobar pneumonia. See **pneumonia.**

lobe, a partly detached portion of any organ, outlined by clefts, furrows, or connective tissue, as in the lobes of the brain, liver, and lungs. **–lobar, lobular,** *adj.*

lobectomy /lōbek´-/, surgery in which a lobe of a lung is removed.

lobotomy /lōbot´-/, surgery in which nerve fibers in the frontal lobe of the brain are severed. The operation is rarely done because it has many unpredictable and undesirable effects, including loss of bladder and bowel control, personality change, and socially unacceptable behavior.

local, **1.** a small, defined area. **2.** a treatment or drug applied to a small area, such as a local anesthetic.

local anesthetic, a substance used to reduce or eliminate nerve sensation, specifically pain, in a limited area of the body.

local emergency, the situation that exists after a finding by the local chief executive that an immediate danger exists to the community such that the public safety is imperiled. Earthquake, rioting, and weather disasters that affect areas of cities, counties, towns, or villages can be deemed local emergencies. The local declaration of emergency is superseded if a state or federal emergency including the local area is declared.

lochia /lō´kē·ə/, the discharge that flows from the vagina following childbirth.

locked-in syndrome, state in which a patient blinks, breathes, has vertical eye movement, but no voluntary movement. Hemorrhage and/or infarction of the pons of the brain causes the patient to appear unresponsive, while remaining totally aware of surroundings.

lockjaw. See **tetanus.**

locus, a specific place or position, such as the locus of a particular gene on a chromosome, or the locus of infection, a site in the body where an infection originates.

logistics officer, staff person within the incident command system responsible for the section that obtains all of the personnel, equipment, and services required during any multiple-patient incident. At large incidents, this position may be subdivided into the support and service branch director positions. *See also incident command system, logistics section.*

logistics section, division within the incident command system that provides all personnel, equipment, and services required at a multiple-patient incident. This section may be subdivided into support (facilities, supplies, and equipment) and service (communications, food, and medical care for responding personnel). Once these resources are obtained, their management becomes the responsibility of planning and operations. *See also incident command system, logistics officer.*

logroll, technique for moving patients by rolling them onto their sides, inserting a lifting or immobilization device behind, and then rolling them back onto the device. This procedure requires at least three persons to be effective.

long-acting thyroid stimulator, a natural substance that causes prolonged stimulation of the thyroid gland. Rapid growth of the gland and excess activity of thyroid function results in hyperthyroidism. It is found in the blood of 50% of patients affected with Graves' disease.

longitudinal, referring to a measurement in the direction of the long axis of an organ, object, or body, such as an imaginary line from head to toe.

long line haul, helicopter rescue technique utilizing rope to retrieve and fly a victim to a relatively distant landing zone. This method of rescue is used when no suitable landing area for helicopter or victim is located close to the rescue site. A rescuer usually flies with the victim to provide care and reassurance en route. The helicopter generally lands to take the victim onboard for interior transport to another location. Also known as **long line.** *See also short haul.*

long-range navigation, electronic navigation device by which a ship or aircraft finds its position by noting the difference in time between two or more radio signals generated from fixed locations. Also known as **LORAN.**

long tract signs, signs of nervous system disorders, such as repeated involuntary muscle contractions or loss of bladder control. They usually indicate a lesion in the middle or upper portion of the spinal cord or in the brain, disrupting nerve impulses normally transmitted over long nerve tracts.

loose snow avalanche. See **avalanche.**

loosening, a psychologic disturbance in which the association of ideas become vague and unfocused. The condition is frequently a symptom of schizophrenia.

lotion, a liquid preparation applied to protect the skin or to treat a skin disorder.

Lou Gehrig's disease. See **amyotrophic lateral sclerosis.**

louse bite, a tiny puncture wound produced by a louse, a small, wingless insect. Diseases such as typhus and relapsing fever may be transmitted by lice. Head and body lice are common parasites and often found among school children. The bite may cause intense itching.

low birth weight infant, an infant whose weight at birth is less than 2500 grams (5.5 pounds).

low-density lipoprotein. See **lilpoprotein.**

lower explosive limit, the minimum amount of vapor necessary for a chemical to burn. Below this point there can be no chemical combustion. Also known as **LEL.**

lowering, the process of dropping a rescuer and/or a victim to a preferred location. This technique allows the use of gravity in the rescuer's favor, requiring less force than raising.

Lown-Ganong-Levine syndrome, a rare cardiac accessory pathway syndrome, associated with preexcitation. This causes a normal QRS complex, paroxysmal tachycardia, and a short PR interval. *See also preexcitation, Wolff-Parkinson-White syndrome.*

low-specific activity material, material containing uniformly distributed radioactive material in low concentrations. This type of material does not constitute a radiological safety hazard.

low velocity, **1.** low vehicular speed, generally below 25 miles per hour (about 40 kilometers/hour). **2.** weapons with projectile speed below 2000 feet per second (about 609 meters/second).

lucid /loo´sid/, clear, rational, and able to be understood. A **lucid interval** refers to a period of relative mental clarity between periods of irrationality, especially in organic brain disorders or seizures.

Ludwig's angina /lood´viks/, an acute streptococcal infection of the mouth and neck. It causes the tongue to become edematous, blocking the airway.

lumbago /lumbā´gō/, pain in the low back due to muscle strain, rheumatoid arthritis, osteoarthritis, or ruptured disk. **Ischemic lumbago** is pain in the lower back and buttocks, caused by poor blood circulation to the area.

lumbar /lum´bär/, pertaining to the lower back.

lumbar nerves, the five pairs of spinal nerves in the lumbar region. The **lumbar plexus** is a network of nerves formed by divisions of the lumbar nerves. It is located on the inside of the posterior abdominal wall.

lumbar puncture, placing a hollow needle into the lumbar portion of the spine to obtain samples of fluid for diagnostic and treatment purposes. Also known as **LP.**

lumbar veins, four pairs of veins that collect blood by dorsal tributaries from the flanks and by abdominal tributaries from the walls of the abdomen.

lumbar vertebra. See **vertebra.**

lumbosacral plexus /lum´bōsā´krəl/, a network of lumbar, sacral, and coccygeal nerves that supply the legs and pelvis.

lumen /loo´mən/, a cavity or channel.

lumpectomy /lumpek´-/, surgical removal of a breast tumor without removing large amounts of surrounding tissue or adjacent lymph nodes. *See also breast cancer, mastectomy.*

lunate bone /loo´nāt/, one of the bones of the wrist.

Lund and Browder method, procedure for most accurately determining percentage of body surface burns, based on age. This method utilizes body surface charts that factor age (growth) into the equation for calculating burn percentages. *See also rule of nines, rule of palms.*

lung, one of a pair of light, spongy organs in the chest. The lungs provide the mechanisms for inhaling air from which oxygen is extracted and for exhaling carbon dioxide. The pulmonary arteries transport blood to the lungs where oxygen is replaced. The bronchial arteries supply blood to the lung tissues. Most of this blood returns to the heart through the pulmonary veins. The apex of the lung extends into the base of the neck above the first rib. The base rests on and moves with the diaphragm. The lungs are composed of lobes that are smooth and shiny on their surface. The right lung contains three lobes; the left lung, two lobes. Each lung is covered with a thin, moist (pleural) membrane. An inner fibrous layer contains secondary small lobes (lobules) divided into primary lobules, each of which consists of blood vessels, lymph vessels, nerves, and a duct (alveolar) connecting with the alveoli.

lunula /loon´yələ/, *pl.* **lunulae,** the crescent-shaped pale area at the base of a fingernail or toenail.

lupus erythematosus, a chronic and usually fatal disease that causes changes in the vascular system, resulting in rashes, fever, and compromised function of the cardiac, pulmonary, and renal systems. Intense joint pain is a common symptom. Also known as **lupus.**

lupus vulgaris, a form of dermal tuberculosis in which areas of the skin become ulcerated and heal slowly, leaving deeply scarred tissue. The disease is not related to lupus erythematosus.

luteal /loo´tē·əl/, pertaining to the corpus luteum of the female ovary or its functions or effects.

luteinizing hormone /loo´tē·inī´zing/, a hormone produced by the pituitary gland. In men, it stimulates the secretion of testosterone by the testes. Testosterone, together with follicle stimulating hormone (FSH), stimulates the testes to produce sperm. In females, luteinizing hormone, working together with FSH, stimulates the follicles containing ova, or egg cells, in the ovary to secrete estrogen, the female sex hormone.

Lyme arthritis, an acute inflammatory disease, involving one or more joints, believed to be transmitted by a tick-borne disease organism. The condition was first noted in Lyme, Connecticut, but has since been reported in other parts of the United States. Symptoms include chills, fever, headache, and inflammation with joint edema. Knee and temperomandibular joints are most commonly involved.

lymph, a thin, clear, slightly yellow fluid originating in many organs and tissues of the body.

It circulates through the lymphatic vessels and is filtered by the lymph nodes. Its composition varies depending on the organ or tissue it is in, but generally contains about 95% water, a few red blood cells, and variable numbers of white blood cells. It is similar to blood plasma except for a lower amount of protein material. *See also chyle.*

lumphadenitis /limfad´ənī´-/, an inflammatory condition of the lymph nodes, usually the result of a bacterial infection or other inflammatory condition. The nodes may be swollen, hard, smooth or irregular, and may feel hot. The location of the affected node is usually related to the site or origin of disease.

lymphangioma /-jē·ō´mə/, a yellowish-tan tumor on the skin, composed of a mass of dilated lymph vessels.

lymphangitis /lim´fanjī´-/, an inflammation of one or more lymphatic vessels, often resulting from an acute streptococcal infection caused by an insect or animal bite in an arm or leg. Fine red streaks may extend from the infected area to the axilla or groin. Other signs are fever, headache, and muscle ache.

lymphatic /limfat´ik/, pertaining to the lymphatic system of the body.

lymphatic system, a complex network of capillaries, thin vessels, valves, ducts, nodes, and organs. It helps to protect and maintain the liquid environment of the body by producing, filtering, and conveying lymph and by producing various blood cells. The lymphatic network transports fats, proteins, and other substances to the blood system. It also restores 60% of the fluid that leaks out of cells into spaces between cells. Small valves help to control the flow of lymph and prevent blood from flowing into the lymphatic vessels. The lymph collected throughout the body drains into the blood through two ducts situated in the neck. Various body movements combine to move lymph through the lymphatic system. The thoracic duct on the left side of the neck is the major vessel of the lymphatic system and conveys lymph from the whole body, except for the upper right side, which is served by the right lymphatic duct. Lymphatic vessels resemble veins but have more valves, thinner walls, and contain lymph nodes. The lymphatic capillaries, which are the beginning of the system, form a continuous network over the entire body, except for the cornea of the eye. The system also includes specialized lymphatic organs, such as the tonsils, thymus, and spleen. The lymphatics of the intestine contain a special milky substance called chyle. *See also chyle, lymph, lymph node, spleen, thymus.*

lymphedema /lim´fədē´mə/, a disorder in which lymph accumulates in soft tissue with swelling caused by inflammation, obstruction, or removal of lymph vessels.

lymph node, one of many small oval structures that filter lymph, fight infection, and in which are formed white blood cells and blood plasma cells. Lymph nodes are of varying sizes. Each node is enclosed in a fibrous capsule, and consists of closely packed lymphocytes, connective tissue, and lymph pathways. Most lymph nodes are clustered in specific areas, such as the mouth, neck, lower arm, axilla, and groin. A **visceral lymph node** filters lymph circulating in the lymphatic vessels of the viscera of the chest, lower body, and pelvis. Also known as **lymph gland.**

lymphocyte /lim´fəsīt/, one of two kinds of small white blood cells (leukocytes). Lymphocytes normally include 25% of the total white blood cell count but increase in number in response to infection. They occur in two forms: **B cells** and **T cells.** Each has its own function. The function of the B cell is to search out, identify, and bind with specific intruders (allergens or antigens). B cells create antibodies for insertion into their own cell membranes. When exposed to a specific allergen or antigen, the B cell is activated. It travels to the spleen or to the lymph nodes, and rapidly produces large amounts of antibody. T cells are lymphocytes that have circulated through the thymus gland and have become thymocytes. When exposed to an antigen, they divide rapidly and produce large numbers of new T cells sensitized to that antigen. T cells are often called "killer cells" because they secrete special chemical compounds and assist B cells in destroying foreign protein.

lymphocytic choriomeningitis /-sit´ik/, a viral infection of the brain and spinal cord. Symptoms include fever, headache, and stiff neck. The infection occurs primarily in young adults, most often in the fall and winter months.

lymphocytopenia /-sī´təpē´nē·ə/, a smaller than normal number of lymphocytes in the blood. This may occur as a blood disorder or with nutritional deficiency, cancer, or infectious mononucleosis.

lymphogranuloma venereum /-gran´yəlō´mə/, a sexually transmitted disease caused by a strain of the germ *Chlamydia trachomatis*. Signs are genital lesions, headache, and fever. *See also Chlamydia.*

lymphoma /limfō´mə/, a tumor of lymphoid tissue. Lymphoid tissue is netlike and holds lymphocytes in its spaces. The various lymphomas differ in degree of structure and content, but their effects are similar. The appearance of one or more painless, enlarged lymph nodes in the neck is followed by weakness, fever, weight loss, and anemia. The spleen and liver may enlarge. Men are more likely than women to develop lymphoid tumors.

lysine /lī´sin/, an essential amino acid needed for proper growth in infants and for maintenance of nitrogen balance in adults. *See also amino acid, protein.*

lysinemia /-ē´mē·ə/, a congenital disorder that causes the inability of the body to use the essential amino acid lysine. This results in muscle weakness and mental retardation.

lysis /lī´sis/, destruction, as of a cell through the action of an enzyme or antibody.

lysosome /lī´səsōm/, a particle in a cell that contains enzymes capable of destroying the cell. It is believed that lysosomes may play an important role in certain self-destructive diseases in which the wasting of tissue occurs, such as muscular dystrophy.

lysozyme /-zīm/, an enzyme with antiseptic action that destroys some foreign organisms. It is found in white blood cells and is normally present in saliva, sweat, breast milk, and tears.

M

macerate /mas´ərāt/, to soften by soaking.
–**maceration,** *n.*

macrocephaly /mak´rōsef´əlē/, a birth defect marked by a head and brain that are too large in relation to the body.

macrocyte /mak´rəsīt/, an unusually large, mature red blood cell.

macrognathia /-nā´thē·ə/, an abnormally large jaw.

macronutrient /-noo´trē·ənt/, a chemical element needed in large amounts for the body. Macronutrients include carbon, hydrogen, oxygen, nitrogen, potassium, sodium, calcium, chloride, magnesium, phosphorus, and sulfur. Also known as **major element.** Compare **micronutrient.**

macrophage /mak´rəfāj/, any large cell that can surround and digest foreign substances in the body, such as protozoa or bacteria. They are found in the liver, spleen, and in the loose connective tissue.

macula /mak´yələ/, *pl.* **maculae,** a small colored area or a spot. It may be permanent.

Mae West, an inflatable personal flotation device worn by some pilots and crew while flying over large bodies of water. *See also personal flotation device.*

Magill forceps, an elongated pair of forceps used to advance an endotracheal tube during intubation or remove a foreign body during complete airway obstruction. Also known as **Magills.**

magma, molten rock located within a volcano. *See also lava.*

magnesium, a silver-white mineral needed for many chemical reactions in the body. About 50% of the body's magnesium is in the bones.

magnesium sulfate, a central nervous system depressant effective in the management of seizures, particularly those associated with toxemia of pregnancy (eclampsia). It is also being used in the management of torsades de pointes and dysrhythmias secondary to tricyclic overdose and digitalis toxicity. Side effects include bradycardia, hypotension, and respiratory/cardiac depression and/or arrest. Do not administer to any patient with heart block. Also known as **mag sulfate.**

magnetometer, instrument that detects deviations of magnetic field, used to locate metal or rock.

main rotor, the primary horizontal rotor(s) of a helicopter. This rotor provides the power to lift, move, and land. *See also tail rotor.*

major disaster, *(U.S. government)* any catastrophe, such as hurricane, flood, tidal wave, drought, fire, or mudslide that in the determination of the President causes damage of sufficient severity and magnitude to warrant assistance under the Federal Disaster Relief Act.

major medical incident, a level-II multiple casualty incident producing large numbers of casualties for which routinely available regional medical mutual aid is necessary and adequate.

major medical insurance, insurance coverage developed to offset the costs of lengthy or major illness and injury.

mal, 1. an illness or disease. **2.** bad.

malabsorption, a failure of the small intestine to absorb nutrients. It may result from a birth defect, malnutrition, or any abnormal condition of the digestive system that prevents needed food elements from being absorbed.

malabsorption syndrome, a group of symptoms resulting from disorders in the intestine's ability to absorb nutrients from food. Symptoms include anorexia, weight loss, arthralgias, and myalgias. Anemia and lethargy can occur due to inadequate absorption of iron, folic acid, and vitamin B$_{12}$.

malacia /məlā´shə/, a softening of any tissue of the body.

malaise /malāz´/, a vague feeling of body weakness or discomfort, often indicating the beginning of illness.

malalignment /mal´əlīn´mənt/, a failure of parts of the body to line up normally, as in teeth that do not conform to the dental arch.

malaria /məler´ē·ə/, an infection caused by one or more of at least four different species of the protozoan organism *Plasmodium,* transmitted by mosquito bite. Malaria can also be spread by blood transfusion or by the use of an infected needle. Symptoms include chills, fever, anemia, and enlarged spleen. Malaria is generally a chronic disease. Because the life cycle of the infecting parasite changes with the species, the patterns of chills and fever differ, as do the length and seriousness of the disease. The disease is mostly found in tropical areas. However, a number of new cases are brought to North America by refugees, military personnel, and travelers. Prevention with antimalarial drugs is important for those visiting areas where infection is possible. –**malarial,** *adj.*

male, 1. referring to the sex that produces sperm cells and fertilizes the female to have offspring; masculine. **2.** a male person.

malformation, an abnormal structure in the body. *See also birth defect.*

malignant, 1. relating to a lesion that is cancerous and spreading. **2.** tending to become worse, probably life-threatening, such as malignant hypertension.

malingering, a conscious faking of the symptoms of a disease or injury to gain some desired end.

malleable, 1. able to have its shape changed permanently by the application of stress, as can a metal. **2.** easily affected by external influences.

malleolus /məlē´ələs/, *pl.* **malleoli,** a rounded bony structure, as the protrusion on each side of the ankle.

malleus /mal´ē·əs/, one of the three ossicles in the middle ear, resembling a hammer or mallet. It is connected to the eardrum and carries sound vibrations to the anvil (incus). *See also ear.*

Mallory-Weiss syndrome, a tear in the lower esophagus resulting in hemorrhage, which is often caused by severe and prolonged vomiting.

malnutrition, any disorder concerning nutrition. It may result from an unbalanced diet or from eating too little or too much food. It may also result from improper body utilization of foods. Compare **deficiency disease.**

malocclusion /mal´əklo͞o´zhən/, abnormal contact of the teeth of the maxilla with the teeth of the mandible. *See also occlusion.*

malpractice, negligent treatment of a patient by medical personnel resulting in harm or injury to the patient. It may occur as a result of deviation from accepted standards of reasonable judgment and care.

mammalian diving reflex, bradycardia and peripheral vasoconstriction, initiated by facial submersion in cool or cold water. This reflex maintains arterial blood pressure and cerebral blood flow. Most active in the young, this may allow for successful resuscitation of prolonged cases of submersion without permanent central nervous system damage or deficit. Also known as **diving reflex.**

mammary gland, one of two half-sphere-shaped glands on the chest of mature females. It is also seen in simple form in children and in males. Glandular tissue forms a ring of lobes with small sacs (alveoli). Each lobe has a system of ducts for the passage of milk from the alveoli to the nipple. The inner portion of the breast is filled with gland tissue. The outer portion is composed of fatty tissue. Also known as **breast.**

mammogram, an x-ray film of the soft tissues of the breast made to identify various cysts or tumors.

mandible /man´dibəl/, large bone forming the lower jaw. It consists of a horizontal portion that has the lower teeth and two vertical portions that form a joint with the maxilla.

manhole, an access into sewer/storm drains used for maintenance and inspection.

mania, a mood disorder with excitement, elation, overactivity, nervousness, and flight of ideas. Violent or self-destructive behavior occurs at times. **Transitory mania** features a sudden onset of excessive reactions that only last a short time, usually from 1 hour to a few days. **Hysteric mania** has combined symptoms of hysteria and mania. **Puerperal mania** is a disorder that sometimes occurs in women after childbirth. –**maniac,** *n., adj.,* **maniacal,** *adj.*

manic depressive, a mental disorder presenting as alternating moods of hyperexcitability and severe depression. Also known as **bipolar disorder.**

manifold, a hose, tubing, or pipe fitted with several inlets and/or outlets.

mannitol, an osmotic diuretic used to decrease intracranial pressure and to increase the urinary excretion of toxic substances (rhabdomyolysis) from the body. Side effects include hypotension (excessive diuresis), pulmonary edema, and transient volume overload. Its use is contraindicated in severe hypotension and pulmonary edema. Also known as **Osmitrol.**

Mannkopf's sign (Emil Mannkopf, German physician, 1836-1918), acceleration of pulse after pressing a painful point; not present in feigned pain.

manubrium, superior bone of the sternum that articulates with the clavicle and first costal cartilages. Also known as **manubrium sterni.**

MAO inhibitor. See **monoamine oxidase inhibitor.**

maple bark disease, lung disease (pneumonitis) caused by a mold *Cryptostroma corticale,* found in the bark of maple trees. In a sensitive patient the condition may be acute with fever, cough, and vomiting. It also may be chronic with weakness, weight loss, and coughing up sputum.

maple syrup urine disease, an inherited disorder in which an enzyme needed for the breakdown of three amino acids (valine, leucine, and isoleucine) is lacking. The disease is recognized by the typical maple syrup odor of the urine and

by altered reflexes. Also known as **branched chain ketoaciduria.**

marasmus /məraz´məs/, malnutrition and wasting, resulting from a lack of calories and protein and seen in failure to thrive children and starvation. Less commonly, it occurs as a result of an inability to absorb or use protein. *See also failure to thrive, kwashiorkor.*

march foot, a condition of the foot caused by excess use, as in a long march. The foot is swollen and painful. One or more of the bones involved may be fractured. *See also stress fracture.*

Marchiafava-Micheli disease, recurring episodes of hemoglobin in the urine due to cold exposure (cold hemoglobinuria) or strenuous exercise (march hemoglobinuria). Also known as **paroxysmal hemoglobinuria.**

Marey's law, arterial blood pressure varies inversely with heart rate.

Marfan's syndrome (Bernard-Jean Antonin Marfan, French physician, 1858-1942), a hereditary connective tissue disorder that causes cardiovascular (aortic weakness), ocular (lens dislocation), and skeletal (tall and thin with sternum and joint deformities) abnormalities.

marijuana. See **cannabis.**

masculine, having the physical characteristics of a male. –**masculinize,** *v.*

mask, **1.** device that provides a sealed environment around the eyes, allowing them to focus properly, to protect the face and respiratory system from communicable disease and in toxic, hazardous, and foreign environments or to allow oxygen to be supplied to the body. **2.** to conceal or cover up.

masking, the unconscious display of a personality trait that hides a behavior disorder.

masochism /mas´əkizm/, allowing physical, mental, or emotional abuse. The abuse may be from another person or oneself. Compare **sadism.**

mass casualty incident, a situation creating large numbers of ill or injured casualties in excess of the local health care system's capability. The number of victims will alter the type and quality of care delivered. Adapting to the crisis will require the local system to call for outside help, institute care similar to that used by the military (battlefield medicine), simplify treatment, and ration the care given via triage. Nurses, paramedics, and physicians on-scene will share similar professional responsibilities and may be required to perform outside their usual scope of practice to accommodate more victims. *See also disaster, multiple casualty incident, triage.*

masseter /maseˉ´tər/, the thick, rectangular muscle in the cheek that closes the mandible. It is one of four muscles used in chewing.

mastectomy /mastek´-/, surgical removal of one or both breasts. *See also breast cancer.*

mastication, chewing, tearing, or grinding food with the teeth while it becomes mixed with saliva. *See also bolus, digestion, ptyalin.*

masticatory system /mas´tikətôr´ē/, the group of organs, structures, and nerves used in chewing. It includes the jaws, teeth and supporting structures, temporomandibular joints, tongue, lips, and cheeks. Also known as **masticatory apparatus.**

mastitis /mastīˉ´-/, an inflamed breast.

mastoidectomy /mas´toidek´-/, surgical removal of a portion of the mastoid bone.

mastoiditis /-dīˉ´-/, an infection of one of the mastoid bones, usually an extension of a middle ear infection.

mastoid process, a bulge of a portion of the temporal bone on the lateral skull where various muscles attach. *See also temporal bone.*

MAST. See **military antishock trousers, pneumatic antishock garment.**

MAST survey, technique advocated by the American College of Emergency Physicians for the rapid examination of the abdomen, pelvis, and legs when the primary survey identifies a critical trauma situation. This allows the placement of the antishock trousers (MAST) without missing serious injuries of the lower extremities.

masturbation, sexual activity in which the penis or clitoris is stimulated by means other than sexual intercourse.

materia medica, **1.** the study of drugs and other substances used in medicine, their origins, preparation, uses, and effects. **2.** a substance or a drug used in medicine.

maternal deprivation syndrome, a condition in which slowed growth occurs as a result of a lack of physical or emotional stimulation. It is seen most often in infants. Symptoms include a lack of physical growth, with weight abnormally low for age and size, malnutrition, withdrawal, and irritability. *See also failure to thrive.*

matrix, **1.** a substance found between tissue cells. **2.** a basic substance from which a specific organ or kind of tissue develops. **3.** problem solving using graphs or algorithms.

matter, **1.** anything that has mass and occupies space. **2.** any substance not otherwise identified as to its parts, as gray matter.

maturation, **1.** the process or condition of coming to complete development. **2.** the final stages in the formation of ova or spermatozoa in which the number of chromosomes in each cell is reduced to the number needed for reproduction.

mature, to become fully developed; to ripen.

maturity, **1.** a state of complete growth or development, usually the period of life between adolescence and old age. **2.** the stage at which an organism can reproduce.

Mauriceau's maneuver, technique for delivery of the head of the breech birth infant. This procedure involves the rotation of the trunk so that the infant's back faces the clinician. A downward traction is applied until the hairline is visible. Supporting the body with the hand and forearm, the infant's mouth and chin are held with the index and middle fingers. The opposite hand is then used to support the back and shoulders and the body is gently brought upward. A second caregiver then applies pressure to the mother's suprapubic area to assist in delivery of the head with a minimum of neck traction. Slow delivery of the head is the goal.

maxilla /maksil´ə/, *pl.* **maxillae,** one of a pair of large bones that form the upper jaw.

maxillary sinus /mak´siler´ē/. See **nasal sinus.**

maximal breathing capacity, the amount of oxygen and carbon dioxide that can be exchanged per minute at the greatest rate and depth of breathing by a person.

mayday, (M'aidez = Help me) the highest priority of all radio distress calls, indicating that persons onboard are threatened by imminent danger, requiring immediate assistance. The Morse code equivalent is SOS (code signal only, not an abbreviation). *See also pan, securite.*

maypole, a single power pole, usually in rural areas, with several individual distribution lines radiating from the primary line to other structures on the property.

McBurney's point (Charles McBurney, American surgeon, 1845-1913), point of abdominal tenderness in appendicitis, located on a line between the umbilicus and the right iliac crest.

McMurray's sign, a click heard when moving the tibia on the femur, indicating injury to cartilage in the knee.

mean arterial pressure, the average pressure of blood flow as measured in a major artery.

measles, an acute, highly contagious, viral disease that occurs foremost in young children who have not been vaccinated. Measles is carried by direct contact with droplets spread from the nose, throat, and mouth of infected patients, usually in the early stage of the disease. Symptoms include fever, cough, eye irritation, sensitivity to light, and loss of appetite. Diagnosis is based on laboratory tests or on identifying small red spots (Koplik spots) inside the cheeks, which appear 1 to 2 days before the appearance of the rash. Also known as **rubeola.**

meatus /mē·ā´təs/, an opening or tunnel through any part of the body, as the external acoustic meatus that leads from the outer ear to the tympanic membrane.

mechanical advantage, the degree of assistance given by a device or technique that can offset a lack of power or strength. It is the ratio between the working force derived to the force applied, as in 2:1.

mechanical stress, the result of a transfer of energy when one object physically contacts or collides with another. Indications are punctures, gouges, breaks, or tears in the container. A container may also be weakened but have no visible signs of potential release.

mechanism of entrapment, method or object that causes the confinement or trapping of a victim.

mechanism of injury, the method or force that causes a victim's injuries. Many of these mechanisms cause predictable patterns of injury.

meconium /mēkō´nē·əm/, a material that collects in the intestines of a fetus. It forms the first stool of a newborn. Thick and sticky, it is usually greenish to black in color. Meconium is composed of secretions of the intestinal glands, some amniotic fluid and debris, as bile dyes, fatty acids, skin cells, mucus, fine hair, and blood. Aspiration of meconium from the amniotic fluid can result in loss of surfactant and a failure of the lungs to expand or pneumonia.

media, the middle or muscular layer of an artery.

medial /mē´dē·əl/, located near the middle of the body.

medial cuneiform bone, the largest of the cuneiform bones of the foot.

median effective dose, the dose of a drug that causes a specific effect in one half of the patients to whom it is given.

median nerve, a nerve that extends along the forearm and the hand.

median plane, anatomical description for an imaginary line that divides the body vertically through the trunk and head into right and left halves. Also known as **midsagittal plane.**

mediastinal emphysema, air in the mediastinal space caused by trauma or overpressurization of the lungs. Although this can be accompanied by pneumothorax, it is not a requirement. Air dissecting into the mediastinum may be the sole cause, particularly during scuba diving. Symptoms include voice distortion, subcutaneous emphysema, and a fullness in the throat. *See also Hamman's sign.*

mediastinum /mē´dē·əstī´nəm/, the space in the center of the chest, between the lungs. It extends from the sternum to the spine. It contains all of the thoracic structures, except the lungs.

medic, **1.** a field medical person in the armed forces (in the United States, specifically the Army and Air Force). **2.** a general term describing a military combat medical person, a paramedic, or other field medical person.

medical antishock trousers. See **military antishock trousers, pneumatic antishock garment.**

medical center, **1.** a health care facility. **2.** a hospital, especially one staffed to care for many patients and for a large number of diseases and disorders, using modern technology.

medical control, the medical authority providing guidance to an emergency medical system, particularly related to advanced life support. Types of control include on-line, off-line, direct, and indirect. *See also specific entry.*

medical history, previous health states, illnesses, and injuries of a patient.

Medical Practices Act, laws requiring an individual to be licensed or certified to practice medicine or defining the scope of practice.

Medicare, federally paid national health insurance. The program is divided into two parts. Part A protects against costs of medical, surgical, and mental hospital care. Part B is a voluntary medical insurance program paid in part from federal funds and in part from premiums paid by persons enrolled in the program. Medicare enrollment is offered to persons who can receive Social Security or railroad retirement benefits.

medication, a substance that is used as a drug or remedy for illness.

medication abuse, a type of adult abuse (particularly elderly or dependent) that results in harm or potential harm by overadministering, underadministering, withholding, or otherwise inappropriately using medication.

medicine, 1. a drug or a remedy for illness. 2. the art and science of the diagnosis, treatment, and prevention of disease and keeping good health. 3. the art of treating disease without surgery.

medium, a substance through which something moves or through which it acts.

medulla /mədul´ə/, the most inner part of a structure or organ, such as the adrenal medulla, or inner part of the adrenal gland.

medulla oblongata. See **brain.**

medullary canal, hollow area within the shaft of a long bone, which contains yellow bone marrow.

megacaryocyte /me´gəker´ē·əsīt´/, a very large bone marrow cell. Megacaryocytes are needed to make the platelets in the marrow. They are normally not in the circulation. *See also platelet.* –**megacaryocytic,** *adj.*

megacolon /-kō´lən/, massive, abnormal widening of the large intestine (colon) that may be congenital or may develop later in life. *See also Hirschsprung's disease.*

megalomania, an abnormal mental state with delusions of grandeur in which one believes oneself to be a person of great power, fame, or wealth. *See also mania.*

meiosis /mī·ō´-/, dividing a sex cell, as it matures, into two, then four gametes. The nucleus of each gamete receives one half of the number of chromosomes in the body cells of the species. In humans, meiosis results in gametes each containing 23 chromosomes, including one sex chromosome. Compare **mitosis.**

melancholia /mel´angkō´lē·ə/, excess sadness; melancholy.

melanin /mel´ənin/, a black or dark brown color that occurs naturally in the hair, skin, and in the iris and choroid membrane of the eye. *See also melanocyte.*

melanocyte /mel´ənōsīt´/, a body cell able to produce melanin. Such cells are found throughout the basal cell layer of the skin. They form melanin color from an amino acid (tyrosine).

melanoma /mel´ənō´mə/, any of a group of skin tumors (benign or malignant) that are composed of melanocytes. Most melanomas form flat dark skin patches over several months or years. Compare **blue nevus.**

melena, black, tarry stools containing blood resulting from gastrointestinal bleeding.

melting point, the temperature at which a solid changes to a liquid. This temperature is also the freezing point, depending on the direction of the change. For mixtures, a melting point range may be given.

membrana tectoria, the broad, strong ligament that holds the spinal column to the skull.

membrane, a layer of tissue that covers a surface, lines or divides a space. *See also mucous membrane, serous membrane, skin, synovial membrane.*

membranous labyrinth /mem´brənəs/, a network of three fluid-filled, membrane-lined ducts in the bony half-circle canals of the inner ear. They are linked to the sense of balance. The ducts contain a fluid called endolymph.

memory, the recall, through unconscious means of association, of previous sensations, ideas, or information that has been consciously learned. **Anterograde memory** is the memory of events of long ago but not of those that happen recently. **Long-term memory** is the ability to recall sensations, events, ideas, and other information for long periods of time without apparent effort. **Short-term memory** is memory of recent events.

menarche /menär´kē/, the first menstruation and the beginning of the menstrual cycle in females. It usually occurs between 9 and 17 years of age. *See also pubarche.*

Mendelson's syndrome, a type of chemical pneumonia resulting from aspiration of gastric secretions into the lungs.

Meniere's disease /mānē·erz´/, a disease of the inner ear with periods of vertigo, nerve deafness, and tinnitus. The cause is not known.

meninges /minin´jēz/, *sing.* **meninx** /mē´ningks, men´-/, any one of the three membranes that cover the brain and the spinal cord: the outer layer (dura mater), an inner layer (pia mater), and a spiderweb-like middle layer (arachnoid). –**meningeal,** *adj.*

meningitis /men´injī´-/, any infection or inflammation of the membranes covering the brain and spinal cord. Symptoms vary depending on the cause. They may include fever, headache, stiff neck and back, nausea, and skin rash. The most common causes are bacterial infection with *Streptococcus pneumoniae, Neisseris meningitis,* or *Haemophilus influenzae.* **Aseptic meningitis** may be caused by other bacteria, chemical irritation, or viruses including coxsackieviruses, echoviruses, and mumps.

meningocele /mining´gōsēl´/, a bulge of meninges through a defect in the skull or spinal column. It forms a hernial cyst that is filled with fluid from the brain and spine. *See also neural tube defect.*

meningococcemia /-koksē´mē·ə/, a disease caused by bacteria (*Neissera meningitidis*) in the blood. Symptoms include chills, pain in the muscles and joints, headache, petechiae, sore throat, and weakness.

meningoencephalocele /-ensef´əlōsēl´/, a cyst that contains brain tissue, cerebrospinal fluid, and meninges. It pushes through a defect in the skull. The condition is often linked to other defects in the brain. *See also neural tube defect.*

meniscus /minis´kəs/, cartilage in the knees and other joints.

menometrorrhagia /men´ōmet´rôrā´jə/, excess menstrual and uterine bleeding that is not caused by menstruation. It may be a sign of cancer of the cervix.

menopause /men´əpōz/, the end of menstruation, generally meaning the period ending the female reproductive phase of life (climacteric). Menses stop naturally with the decline of monthly hormonal cycles between 45 and 60 years of age.

menorrhagia /men´ôrā´jə/, abnormally heavy or long menstrual periods.

menses /men´sēz/, the normal flow of blood and cast-off uterine cells that occurs during menstruation. The first day of the flow of the menses is the first day of the menstrual cycle.

menstrual age, the age of an embryo or fetus as counted from the first day of the last menstrual period.

menstrual cycle, the repeating cycle of change in the endometrium of the uterus. The temporary layer of the endometrium sheds during menstruation. It then regrows, thickens, is kept for several days through ovulation, and sheds again at the next menstruation. The average length of the cycle, from the first day of bleeding of one cycle to the first of another, is 28 days. However, the length and character vary greatly among individual women. Menstrual cycles begin at puberty. They end with the menopause.

menstruation, the periodic discharge through the vagina from the nonpregnant uterus. It is composed of a bloody mass containing cast-off tissue from the endometrium. The average length of menstruation is 4 to 5 days. *See also menstrual cycle.* –**menstruate,** *v.*

mental, relating to, or characteristic of, the mind.

mental derangement, a disorder of intellect, or mind. Mild derangement is known as **psychoneuroses.** More severe disorders are categorized as **psychoses.**

mental health, a state of mind in which a person who is healthy is able to cope with and adjust to the stresses of everyday living.

mental illness, any disorder of emotional balance, as shown in abnormal behavior or mental problems. It may be due to genetic, physical, chemical, biologic, mental, or social and cultural factors.

mental retardation, a disorder marked by less than average general intellectual function with difficulty in the ability to learn and to act socially. It may be classified according to the intelligence quotient as: borderline, IQ 71 to 84; mild, IQ 50 to 70; moderate, IQ 35 to 49; severe, IQ 20 to 34; and profound, IQ below 20.

mental status exam, evaluation of a patient's mental state, utilizing appearance and behavior, speech, mood, thought content, orientation, and perception as parameters for assessment. Failure to be appropriate for the situation in two or more areas constitutes failure of the exam. This may place the emergency medical provider in the position of invoking implied consent to treat or transport an otherwise unwilling patient.

meperidine hydrochloride, a synthetic narcotic used to treat moderate to severe pain and anxiety. Side effects include altered level of consciousness, dizziness, and respiratory depression. Not to be used in patients with undiagnosed abdominal pain, multiple trauma, head injury, or those taking monoamine oxidase (MAO) inhibitors, such as Eutron, Nardil, Parnate. Also known as **Demerol.**

Mercalli scale, subjective scale for measuring earthquake intensity. This intensity is derived from observations of the damage noted at a particular earthquake location. Also known as the **Modified Mercalli Intensity Scale of 1931.** See Appendix 3-20.

mercury, a metal element used in thermometers and blood pressure measuring instruments. It forms many poisonous compounds.

mercury poisoning, a toxicity caused by swallowing or breathing mercury or a mercury compound. A chronic form results from breathing the vapors or dust of mercury compounds or from repeated swallowing of small amounts. It leads to irritability, excess saliva, loosened teeth, slurred speech, trembling, and staggering. Symptoms of acute mercury poisoning include a metal taste in the mouth, thirst, nausea, vomiting, severe abdominal pain, bloody diarrhea, and kidney failure. Free mercury, as in thermometers, is not absorbed by the stomach or intestine. Mercury compounds are found in farming chemicals and in certain antiseptics and dyes. They are used heavily in industry.

mesa, a high, flat landform rising steeply above the surrounding terrain. This land area is smaller than a plateau and larger than a butte.

mescaline /mes´kəlēn/, a mind-altering, poisonous alkaline drug derived from the cactus. Closely related chemically to epinephrine, mescaline causes an irregular heart rate, diaphoresis, anxiety, and hallucinations. Also known as **peyote.**

mesencephalon /mes´ensef´əlon/. See **brain.**

mesenteric node /mes´enter´ik/, a lymph gland in one of three groups serving parts of the intestine. The mesenteric nodes receive lymph from the small and large intestine and the appendix.

mesentery proper /mes´enter¯e/, a broad, fanshaped fold of peritoneum. It connects the jejunum and ileum with the posterior wall of the abdomen. It holds the small intestine and various nerves and arteries of the abdomen.

mesothelium /-thē´lē·əm/, a layer of cells that lines the body cavities of the embryo. It becomes, after birth, a covering, such as the pleura of the chest and pericardium of the heart.

metabolic /met´əbol´ik/, referring to **metabolism.**

metabolic acidosis. See **acidosis.**

metabolic alkalosis. See **alkalosis.**

metabolic disorder, any disorder that interferes with normal digestion and use of food in the body.

metabolic equivalent, the amount of oxygen taken in per kilogram of body weight per minute when a person is at rest.

metabolic rate, the amount of energy released or used in a given unit of time. The metabolic rate is listed in calories as the amount of heat released during metabolism at the cell level.

metabolism /mətab´əlizm/, the sum of all chemical processes that take place in the body as they relate to the movement of nutrients in the blood after digestion, resulting in growth, energy, release of wastes, and other body functions. Metabolism takes place in two steps. The first step is the constructive phase (anabolism). Amino acids are converted to proteins. The second step is the destructive phase (catabolism).

Larger molecules (such as glycogen) are converted into smaller molecules (such as glucose). Exercise, body temperature, hormone activity, and digestion can increase the rate of metabolism. *See also acid-base metabolism, anabolism, basal metabolism, catabolism.* **–metabolic,** *adj.*

metabolite /-līt/, a substance made by metabolic action or one necessary for a metabolic process. An essential metabolite is one needed for an important metabolic process. For example, urea and ammonia are metabolites of proteins.

metacarpus /me´təkär´pəs/, the middle portion of the hand. It consists of five bones numbered from the thumb side, metacarpals I through V. **–metacarpal,** *adj., n.*

metamorphopsia /-môrfop´sē·ə/, a defect in seeing. Objects are seen as distorted in shape, resulting from a disease of the retina.

metaphase, stage of mitosis in which the nuclear membrane and nucleolus disappear and the chromosomes become aligned in an equatorial plane; occurs after prophase and before anaphase. Also known as **metakinesis.** *See also anaphase, prophase, telophase.*

metaproterenol sulfate, a bronchodilator used in the treatment of asthma. Side effects include tachycardia and hypertension. It should be used with caution in patients with a history of cardiac dysrhythmias. Also known as **Alupent, Metaprel.**

metastasis /mətas´təsis/, *pl.* **metastases,** the tumor or the process by which tumor cells are spread to distant parts of the body. **–metastatic,** *adj.,* **metastasize,** *v.*

metatarsus /-tär´səs/, a part of the foot, made up of five bones numbered I to V, from the large toe. Each bone connects with the first row of phalanges at the outer end. **–metatarsal,** *adj.*

meteorotropism /mē´tē·ərətrō´pizm/, a reaction to influences of climate shown by biologic occurrences, such as sudden death, arthritis, and angina during weather changes. **–meteorotropic,** *adj.*

meter, a metric unit of length equal to 39.37 inches.

metered dose inhaler, device, containing aerosolized medication, that distributes a specific dose each time the trigger is depressed.

methanol, a colorless, toxic liquid distilled from wood. It is commonly used as a solvent and as a component of gasoline, antifreeze, and washer fluid. Drinking methanol may cause blindness or death. Also known as **wood alcohol.**

methemoglobin /met·hē´məglō´bin/, a form of hemoglobin in which iron is oxidized so it cannot carry oxygen and thus causes cellular hypoxia. *See also hemoglobin.*

method, a technique or procedure for creating a desired effect, as in an intubation technique or method of patient assessment.

methylprednisolone, a corticosteroid used primarily in the treatment of cerebral/spinal cord edema and anaphylaxis. Side effects include headache and hypertension. It should be used with caution in patients with diabetes or gastrointestinal bleeding. Onset of action may be up to two hours after administration. Also known as **Solu-Medrol.**

metralgia /mətral´jə/, tenderness or pain in the uterus.

metric equivalent, any value in metric units of measurement that equals the same value in English units, as 2.54 centimeters equal 1 inch or 1 liter equals 1.0567 quarts.

metric system, a decimal system of measurement based on the meter (39.37 inches) as the unit of length. The gram (15.432 grains) is the unit of weight or mass. The liter (0.908 US dry quart or 1.0567 US liquid quart) is the unit of volume.

metritis /mətrī´-/, inflammation of the walls of the uterus. Kinds of metritis are **endometritis** and **parametritis.**

metrorrhagia /met´rôrā´jə/, uterine bleeding other than that caused by menstruation. It may be caused by tumors in the uterus or cervical cancer.

microangiopathy /mī´krō·an´jē·op´əthē/, a disease of the small blood vessels in which capillaries thicken (diabetic microangiopathy) or in which clots form in the arterioles and the capillaries (thrombotic microangiopathy).

microbe /mī´krōb/, a microorganism. **–microbial,** *adj.*

microcephaly /-sef´əlē/, a birth defect with an abnormally small head in relation to the rest of the body.

microcheiria /-kī´rē·ə/, a birth defect with abnormally small hands. The condition is often linked to bone and muscle disorders.

microcurie, one-millionth of a curie or 37,000 disintegrations per second. *See also curie.*

microcyte /mī´krəsīt/, an abnormally small red blood cell. It occurs in iron deficiency and other anemias.

microdactyly /-dak´tilē/, a birth defect with abnormally small fingers and toes. The condition is usually linked to bone and muscle disorders.

micrognathia /-nā´thē·ə/, slowed growth of the mandible.

micromelic dwarf /-mel´ik/, a dwarf whose arms and legs are abnormally short.

micronutrient /-noo͞´trē·ənt/, an organic compound, such as a vitamin, or a chemical element, such as zinc or iodine. Micronutrients are needed only in small amounts for the normal processes of the body. Also known as **trace element.**

microorganism, a microscopic animal or plant able to carry on living processes. It may or may not be a cause of disease. Kinds of microorganisms include **bacteria, fungi, protozoa, viruses.**

microphage /mī´krəfāj/, a white blood cell able to ingest microorganisms, such as bacteria.

micropodia /-pō´dē·ə/, a birth defect with small feet. The condition is often linked to other defects or to bone disorders.

micropsia /mīkrop´sē·ə/, an abnormal condition of sight, in which objects are seen as smaller than they really are. It often occurs during hallucinations. –**microptic,** *adj.*

microscopic, referring to very small objects, visible only when seen with a microscope.

microsomia /-sō´mē·ə/, a condition of an abnormally small and underdeveloped, yet otherwise perfectly formed body with normal relationships of the various parts.

micturate, urinate; to pass urine.

midazolam hydrochloride, a benzodiazepine central nervous system depressant used during grand mal seizures and to provide sedation in conscious or combative patients prior to tracheal intubation. Side effects include nausea or vomiting, hypotension, and respiratory depression. It should not be used in patients exhibiting signs of shock or toxic drug ingestion. Also known as **Versed.**

midbrain, the part of the brain stem that connects the pons and cerebellum with the hemispheres of the cerebrum. It is the superior portion of the brainstem located above the pons, consisting of white matter with small bits of gray matter. Also known as **mesencephalon.**

middle cardiac vein, one of five veins of the heart muscle.

middle ear. See **ear.**

middle lobe syndrome, collapse of the middle lobe of the right lung, linked to chronic infection, cough, wheezing, or inflammation. Blockage of the bronchus may occur.

midwife, a person who assists women in childbirth.

migraine /mī´grān/, a throbbing headache, usually occurring on only one side of the head with severe pain, sensitivity to light, and other disturbances. Attacks may last for hours or days. The disorder occurs more often in women than in men. The exact cause is not known.

Migrainous cranial neuralgia, also called **cluster headache,** a variation of migraine. Its significant symptom is painful, throbbing headaches. The headaches usually occur in groups within a few days or weeks.

miliaria /mil´ē·er´ē·ə/. See **heat rash.**

military antishock trousers, inflatable device used around the abdomen and legs that assists in shunting blood from the lower extremities back into the central circulation. Developed in the 1960s and used extensively in the Vietnam War, this device is currently used in cases of hypovolemia and low resistance shock and for stabilization of lower extremity fractures. Also known as **MAST, medical antishock trousers, PASG, pneumatic antishock garment.** *See also pneumatic antishock garment.*

mind, the part of the brain that is the seat of mental action. It allows one to know, reason, understand, remember, think, feel, react, and adapt to all external and internal stimulations or surroundings.

mine drift, a horizontal mine passageway.

mineral, **1.** an inorganic substance occurring naturally in the earth's crust. It has a particular chemical makeup and, usually, a crystal-like structure. **2.** a nutrient that is eaten in food as a compound, such as table salt (sodium chloride), rather than as a free element. Minerals are important in regulating body functions.

mineral deficiency,   the inability to use one or more of the mineral elements needed for human nutrition. Minerals are part of all body tissue and fluids. They act in muscle contractions, regulate electrolyte balance, and strengthen skeletal structures. *See also electrolyte and specific minerals.*

mineralocorticoid,   a hormone, released by the adrenal glands, that keeps blood volume normal. An excess of mineralocorticoid causes high blood pressure, decreased potassium, and a slight increase in sodium. A lack of the hormone results in low blood pressure, excess potassium, and heavy salt loss. Without this hormone an adult may lose as much of 25 g of salt a day. Injury and stress increase mineralocorticoid release.

minor surgery,   any surgical procedure that does not require general anesthetia.

miosis /mī·ō´-/,   **1.** narrowing of the muscle of the iris, causing the pupil of the eye to become smaller. Certain drugs or an increase in light on the eye cause miosis. **2.** an abnormal condition in which excess narrowing of the iris results in pin-point pupils. Compare **mydriasis.**

miotic /mī·ot´ik/,   any substance or drug, as pilocarpine, that causes narrowing of the pupil of the eye. Such drugs are used to treat glaucoma.

miscarriage,   an end of pregnancy before the twentieth week occurring naturally because of defects of the fetus or womb. More than 10% of pregnancies end as spontaneous abortions, almost all caused by defective eggs. *See also abortion.*

missile fracture,   a fracture caused by a fast-moving object, such as a bullet or a piece of shrapnel.

mist,   liquid droplets dispersed in air.

mite,   insects of the class Arachnida responsible for various allergy and disease outbreaks. They have a body consisting of a head/chest section and an abdominal section. About 35,000 species exist, with scabies and chiggers being the best known. Some female mites burrow into the skin and lay eggs that hatch into larvae. *See also scabies.*

mitigation,   action taken to prevent or reduce harm.

mitochondrion /mī´təkon´drē·on/, *pl.* **mitochondria,**   a component of the cytoplasm of a cell that regulates cell activity. Mitochondria are the main source of cell energy.

mitosis /mītō´-/,   a type of cell division. It occurs in body cells and results in forming two identical cells, or daughter cells. Mitosis is the process by which the body makes new cells for both growth and repair of injured tissue. Compare **meiosis.**

mitral regurgitation,   a partial reversal of blood flow back into the left atrium from the left ventricle due to an incompetent mitral valve. Symptoms include dyspnea, fatigue, and irregular heart rate. The condition may result from congenital deformity, rheumatic fever, or cardiac tissue inflammation. Congestive heart failure may eventually occur. Also known as **mitral insufficiency.** *See also mitral valve prolapse, valvular heart disease.*

mitral valve.   See **heart valve.**

mitral valve prolapse,   a failure of the mitral valve to close properly, causing a flow of blood back into the left atrium. It is caused by one or both cusps of the mitral valve pushing back into the atrium during contraction of the ventricle. Most patients feel no symptoms. *See also valvular heart disease.*

mittelschmerz,   abdominal pain at the time of ovulation due to peritoneal irritation from bleeding at the ovulation site.

mixed connective tissue disease,   a disorder with the combined symptoms of two or more diseases that affect connective tissue such as synovitis, myositis, and systemic lupus erythematosus. This condition may cause joint pain, inflammation of the muscles, arthritis, and dyspnea.

mixed gas diving,   scuba diving utilizing mixtures of breathing gases (besides compressed air) to offset the effects of pressure and work effort. Generally this involves gas combinations, such as helium/oxygen/nitrogen or compressed air/nitrogen.

mixture,   **1.** a substance composed of portions not chemically combined. **2.** a liquid drug containing more than one drug. Compare **compound, solution.**

mobile repeater,   a mobile radio unit capable of automatically retransmitting any radio traffic received. This extends the range of radios with inadequate transmitting power. Also known as **extender, repeater, vehicular repeater.**

mobilization center, an off-incident location at which emergency service personnel and equipment are temporarily located, pending assignment, release, or reassignment. Also known as **staging area.**

Mobitz type I, second-degree AV block (Woldemar Mobitz, German physician, 1889-?), a cardiac rhythm, characterized on EKG by a progressively lengthening PR interval until a QRS complex is dropped, with the cycle then repeating. The ratio of conducted beats may be variable, usually 3:1, 4:1, or 5:1. Patients with this condition may show signs of low cardiac output, depending on the number of conducted beats. Also known as **Wenchebach.** *See also Mobitz type II, second-degree AV block.*

Mobitz type II, second-degree AV block, a cardiac rhythm, characterized by either consistently normal or lengthened PR interval (but not both) with an occasional dropped QRS complex. The ratio of conducted beats may be variable, but is usually 3:1, 4:1, or 5:1. Patients with this condition may show signs of low cardiac output, depending on the number of dropped beats. *See also Mobitz type I, second-degree AV block.*

modem, communications device that allows computer information to be transmitted over a telephone line by converting digital signals into analog. The process is reversed at the receiving end.

modified chest lead, EKG electrode positions that utilize modifications of precordial (chest) leads to better view the cardiac rhythm during continuous monitoring. Modified chest lead 1 (MCL1) is the most commonly utilized of the modified chest leads.

modified jaw thrust. See **jaw thrust.**

modulation, intermittently changing the frequency or amplitude of a sound wave.

modulator, device that converts electrical energy into sound waves.

moisture regain, the ability of a material to absorb moisture and still retain heat; the amount of moisture a material can absorb before it feels cold.

molar, any of the 12 molar teeth, 6 in both the upper and lower dental arch. Each of the upper molars has three roots. The lower molars are larger than the upper and each has two roots.

molar pregnancy, pregnancy in which a mass of cysts (called **hydatid mole**) instead of an embryo grows from the tissue of the early stage of the fertilized egg. The cause of the disorder is not known.

mold, a fungus.

molding, the natural process by which a baby's head is shaped during labor as it is squeezed into and through the birth canal by the forces of labor. The head often becomes quite long. The bones of the skull may be caused to overlap slightly, without damage. Most of the changes caused by molding return to normal during the first few days of life.

molecule, the smallest unit of a substance that has the properties of an element or compound. *See also compound, element.*

molluscum /məlus´kəm/, any skin disease marked by soft, rounded masses. **Molluscum contagiosum** is a disease of the skin and mucous membranes caused by a virus. It appears as scattered white masses and occurs most often in children.

Monash method /mənash´/, immobilization and compression technique of first aid for Elapidae (cobras, kraits, coral snakes) snakebite. This technique uses a thick pad, tied in place over the snakebite with a tight bandage, to collapse superficial veins and lymph vessels, impending the spread of venom. A similar method **[Commonwealth Serum Laboratory technique]** uses an elastic bandage or air splint to perform the same function. Both procedures (developed in Australia) have been shown to be effective in the prehospital care of venomous Elapidae bites but have not yet been evaluated for other types of venomous snakebite.

Mongolian spot, a harmless, bluish-black spot, occurring over the sacrum between the hipbones or the buttocks of some newborns. It is especially common in blacks, Native Americans, Southern Europeans, and Orientals. It usually disappears during early childhood.

monitor, 1. to watch a situation or condition for change. 2. equipment used to watch for change, such as EKG monitor, security (TV) monitor, vital sign monitor.

monitoring survey, periodic or continuous determination of the amount of ionizing radiation or radioactive contamination present for purposes of health protection. Also known as **monitoring.**

monoamine oxidase /mon´ō·am´in/, an enzyme that deactivates nervous system hormones, such as epinephrine. Also known as **MAO.**

monoamine oxidase inhibitor, any of a group of drugs used to treat depression, attention deficit, and obsessive compulsive disorder. They are especially useful for anxiety linked to phobias. MAO inhibitors are sometimes used to treat migraine headache and high blood pressure. Side effects include drowsiness, dry mouth, orthostatic hypotension, and constipation, Patients taking MAO inhibitors also should avoid foods such as cheeses, red wine, smoked or pickled herring, beer, and yogurt. Also known as **MAO inhibitor.**

monoblast /mon´əblast/, a large, immature white blood cell. Some leukemias are diagnosed by an excess amount of these cells in the marrow and their presence in the circulation.

monocyte /-sīt/, the largest of the white blood cells. They have two to four times the diameter of a red blood cell.

monocytic leukemia /-sit´ik/, a cancer of blood-forming tissues in which the major cells are monocytes. Symptoms include weakness, fever, loss of appetite, weight loss, a large spleen, skin disorders, and anemia. There are two forms: **Schilling's leukemia** and the more common **Naegeli's leukemia.**

monocytosis /-sītō´-/, increased numbers of monocytes in the circulation.

mononeuropathy, a medical or traumatic disorder affecting a single nerve. Common causes are accidental injection of drugs into a nerve, electric shock, displaced fractures or improper application of splints or casts, and diabetes mellitus. *See also sciatica.*

mononuclear cell /-nōō´klē·ər/, a white blood cell, including lymphocytes and monocytes, with a round or oval nucleus.

mononucleosis /-nōō´klē·ō´-/, an abnormal increase in the number of mononuclear cells in the circulation. *See also infectious mononucleosis.*

monosaccharide /-sak´ərid/, a carbohydrate composed of one basic sugar unit.

monozygotic /-zīgot´ik/, referring to offspring grown from one fertilized egg (zygote), as occurs in identical twins.

mons pubis, a pad of fatty tissue and rough skin that lies over the anterior portion of the female pelvis.

moon face, a condition in which a rounded, puffy face occurs in patients given large doses of steroid drugs, as those with rheumatoid arthritis or acute childhood leukemia. Features return to normal when the drug is discontinued.

morbidity, an illness or an abnormal condition or quality.

morning sickness, a common condition of early pregnancy. There may be frequent and long-lasting nausea, often in the morning, with vomiting, weight and appetite loss, general weakness, and discomfort. The cause is not known. It usually does not begin before the sixth week after the last menstrual period and ends by the twelfth to the fourteenth week of pregnancy.

morphea /môr´fē·ə/, local hardening of the skin, with yellowish or ivory-colored, rigid, dry, smooth patches. It may lead to sclerosis elsewhere in the body. It is more common in women than men.

morphine sulfate, a narcotic used for the treatment of pain, including that of cardiac origin. Side effects include respiratory depression and/or arrest, hypotension, decreased level of consciousness, nausea, and vomiting. Should be avoided in patients with multiple trauma, shock, head injury, undiagnosed abdominal pain, and compromised respirations. Also known as **morphine, MS, MSO4.**

mortality, **1.** the condition of being subject to death. **2.** the death rate, noted as the number of deaths per unit of population for a specific region, age group, disease, or other grouping.

mosquito bite, a bite of a bloodsucking insect of the subfamily Culicidae. It may result in an allergic reaction, an infection, or pruritic sores. Mosquitoes are carriers of many infectious diseases and are attracted by moisture, carbon dioxide, estrogens, sweat, or warmth.

motion sickness, a condition caused by uneven or rhythmic motions, as in a car, boat, or airplane. Severe cases include nausea, vomiting, dizziness, and headache. With mild cases, there is headache and general discomfort.

motor, 1. referring to motion, as the body involved in movement, or the brain functions that direct body movements. **2.** referring to a muscle, nerve, or brain center that makes or takes part in motion.

motor apraxia, the inability to carry out certain planned movements or to handle small objects, although one knows the use of the object. The cause is a lesion in the brain on the opposite side of the arm that cannot move. *See also apraxia.*

motor area, the cerebral cortex. Removing the motor area from one of the brain's hemispheres causes paralysis of voluntary muscles, especially to the opposite side of the body. Various areas of the motor area are linked to different body structures, such as the lower arm, face, and hand.

motor neuron, one of various nerve cells that carry nerve impulses from the brain or spinal cord to muscle or glandular tissue. *See also nervous system.*

motor neuron paralysis, an injury to the spinal cord that causes damage to motor neurons. It results in various degrees of loss of movement, depending on the damage. **Lower motor neuron paralysis** involves an injury or lesion in the spinal cord. There is decreased muscle tone, weak or absent reflexes, and progressive wasting of the muscles. **Upper motor neuron paralysis** involves an injury or lesion in the brain or spinal cord. Signs include increased muscle tone and spasticity of the muscles involved, hyperactive deep tendon reflexes, and weak or absent superficial reflexes.

motor nerve, nerve pathway that transmits impulses from the brain to the body. *See also sensory nerve.*

mouth, 1. *(anatomy)* the opening of any cavity, such as the opening at the upper end of the digestive tract. **2.** *(special operations)* the point

where a small body of water empties into a larger body of water.

mucin /myōō´sin/, a carbohydrate that is the primary component of mucus. It is present in most glands that release mucus. Mucin is the oily material that protects body surfaces from rubbing or wearing.

mucking, shoveling of ore in a mine.

mucocutaneous, referring to the mucous membrane and the skin.

mucocutaneous lymph node syndrome, a sudden illness with fever, primarily of young children. Symptoms include inflamed mouth membranes, "strawberry tongue," swollen lymph nodes in the neck, and redness and shedding of the skin on the arms and legs. Joint pain, diarrhea, pneumonia, and cardiac rhythm changes may also occur. The cause is unknown. Also known as **Kawasaki syndrome.**

mucolytic /-lit´ik/, anything that dissolves, thins, or destroys mucus.

mucopolysaccharidosis /-pol´ēsak´əridō´-/, one of a group of inherited disorders of carbohydrate metabolism that cause higher than normal amounts of sugars and mucins in the tissues. Symptoms include skeletal deformity, mental retardation, and slowed growth. There is a lowered life expectancy. **Hunter's syndrome (II)** affects only males. Males born of women who have the trait have a 50% chance of having the disorder. **Hurler's syndrome (I)** causes severe mental retardation. Hurler's syndrome usually results in death during childhood from heart or lung failure. **Morquio's disease (IV)** results in abnormal muscle and bone growth in childhood. Dwarfism may occur.

mucoprotein /-prō´tēn/, a chemical compound present in all connective and supporting tissue that contains carbohydrates combined with protein.

mucopurulent /-pyōōr´yələnt/, referring to a combination of mucus and pus.

mucosa, mucous membrane, such as that lining the nose, mouth, stomach, intestine.

mucous /myōō´kəs/. See **mucus.**

mucous membrane, any of the four major kinds of thin sheets of tissue cells that cover or line various parts of the body. Examples include linings of the mouth, digestive tube, breathing passage, genital and urinary tracts. It releases mucus and absorbs water, salts, and other substances. Compare **serous membrane, skin, synovial membrane.**

mucous plug, a collection of thick mucus, usually in the cervix of the uterus or in the respiratory tract. The plug may be dry and firm or moist and streaked with blood.

mucus /myoōˊkəs/, the sticky, slippery material released by mucous membranes and glands. It has mucin, white blood cells, water, and cast-off tissue cells. –**mucoid,** *adj.,* **mucous,** *adj.*

Müllerian duct, one of a pair of tubes in the human embryo that become the fallopian tubes, uterus, and vagina in females.

multiagency coordination system, the combination of facilities, equipment, personnel, procedures, and communications integrated into a common system with responsibility for coordination or assisting agency emergency operations. Also known as **MACS.**

multifactorial, referring to any condition or disease caused by two or more factors. Examples are diseases that involve inherited and environmental factors, such as spina bifida, asthma, and Hirschsprung's disease.

multifocal, originating at more than one site.

multigravida /mulˊtigravˊidə/, a woman who has been pregnant more than once.

multipara /multipˊərə/, *pl.* **multiparae,** a woman who has given birth to more than one living child.

multiple casualty incident, a situation with more ill or injured victims than normally encountered in a response. This situation alters the methods of patient assessment, treatment, and transport. The degree of alteration will depend on the number of victims and local protocol. Also known as **MCI.** *See also disaster, mass casualty incident, triage.*

multiple personality, an abnormal condition in which two or more personalities exist within the same individual. Awareness of the others among the various personalities may not occur. Change from one to another is usually sudden and linked to stress.

multiple sclerosis, a disease marked by loss of the protective myelin covering of the nerve fibers of the brain and spinal cord. There are cycles in which symptoms worsen. Initial signs are numbness, or abnormal sensations in the arms and legs or on one side of the face, muscle weakness, dizziness, and sight disturbances, such as double vision and partial blindness. Later, there may be loss of muscle control, abnormal reflexes and dysuria.

multiplex, type of radio system that allows two or more different types of signal (simultaneous voice and/or telemetry transmissions) to be sent over the same frequency at the same time. *See also duplex, simplex.*

multiplexer, device that combines several signals into one for transmission over a single channel.

multitrauma dressing, large gauze dressing (36 × 36 × 10 in.) used for covering large wounds, such as an evisceration, amputation, or large laceration.

mumps, a viral disease with enlargement of the salivary glands near the neck. It is most likely to affect children between 5 and 15 years of age. Antibodies from the mother usually prevent this disease in children under 1 year of age. Mumps is most contagious during the late winter and early spring. The mumps virus is carried in droplets or by direct contact. Symptoms include loss of appetite, headache, discomfort, and fever. Complications include arthritis, inflammation of the pancreas, heart muscle, ovary, testicles, and kidney. Also known as **infectious parotitis.**

Munchausen's syndrome, repeated fabrication of disease for the purpose of gaining attention, medical treatment, and/or hospitalization.

Munchausen's syndrome by proxy, any condition fabricated or induced in a child by a parent for purposes of gaining attention, medical treatment, and/or hospitalization. Although harm to the patient may occur, it is not intended. The goal is to attract attention for the benefit of the involved parent. Also known as **Polle's syndrome.**

murmur, a low pitched fluttering or humming sound in the body. *See also heart murmur.*

Murray-Jones splint. See **splint.**

muscle, a tissue composed of fibers that contract, allowing movement within the body. There are two basic types, striated and smooth. **Striated muscle,** also called voluntary muscle, includes all the muscles of the skeleton. It is composed of bundles of parallel, streaklike fibers under conscious control. It responds quickly to stimulation but is paralyzed by any pause in nerve signal. **Smooth muscle** is found in internal organs, such as the stomach and intestine. This kind of muscle is involuntary and reacts slowly to stimulation. It does not entirely lose its ability to contract if the nerves are damaged. The myocardium is sometimes referred to as cardiac muscle.

muscular dystrophy, a group of diseases that feature weakness and wasting of skeletal muscles without the breakdown of nerve tissue. The cause is unknown. **Duchenne's muscular dystrophy** occurs with progressive wasting of the muscles in the legs and pelvis and affects mostly males. **Fascioscapulohumeral dystrophy** causes wasting of the muscles of the face, shoulders, and upper arms. This form usually occurs before 10 years of age. **Becker's muscular dystrophy** is a milder form and occurs in childhood between 8 and 20 years of age. **Distal muscular dystrophy** is a rare form that most often affects adults. It causes weakness and muscle wasting that begins in the arms and legs and then moves to the trunk and face. With **limb-girdle muscular dystrophy,** weakness and atrophy of the muscles begins in the shoulder or in the pelvis. The condition is progressive, spreading to other body areas, regardless of the area in which it begins. **Myotonic muscular dystrophy** occurs first in the hands and feet, and later in the shoulders and hips, drooping eyelids, facial weakness, and speaking difficulties. **Pelvifemoral muscular dystrophy** is a form that begins in the hip. **Scapulohumeral muscular dystrophy** first affects the shoulder muscles and later often involves the pelvic muscles.

muscular system, all of the muscles of the body, namely, the smooth, cardiac, and striated muscles, considered as one structural group.

musculoskeletal /mus´kyəlōskel´ətəl/ , referring to the muscles and the skeleton.

musculoskeletal system, all of the muscles, bones, joints, and related structures, such as the tendons and connective tissue, that function in the movement of the parts and organs of the body.

mushroom poisoning, a condition caused by eating certain mushrooms, particularly two species of the genus *Amanita.* Muscarine, a substance in *Amanita muscaria,* causes poisoning in a few minutes to 2 hours. Symptoms include diaphoresis, vomiting, dyspnea, and diarrhea. In severe cases, seizures, coma, and shock may occur. The more deadly but slower acting phalloidine, a substance in *A. phalloides* and *A. verna,* causes similar symptoms. It also causes liver damage, kidney failure, and death in 30% to 50% of the cases.

mutagen /myōō´təjən/, any chemical or physical agent that causes a mutation or speeds up the rate of mutation. –**mutagenic,** *adj.,* **mutagenicity,** *n.*

mutation, change in a person's genes that occurs by itself with or without the influence of a mutagen, such as x-rays: The alteration changes the physical trait carried by the gene. Genes are stable units, but a mutation often is passed on to future generations.

mute, 1. a person without the ability to speak. **2.** silent.

mutism /myōō´tizm/, the inability or refusal to speak. The condition often results from an emotional conflict. It is most commonly seen in patients who are psychotic, neurotic, apathetic, or depressed. **Akinetic mutism** is a state in which a person is not able to or will not move or make sounds.

myalgia /mī·al´jə/, muscle pain. It may be linked to infectious diseases, as influenza, measles, and rheumatic fever. Muscle pain occurs in many disorders, as inflammation of connective and muscle tissue, low blood sugar, and muscle tumors. –**myalgic,** *adj.*

myasthenia /mī´əsthē´nē·ə/, weakness of a muscle or a group of muscles. –**myasthenic,** *adj.*

myasthenia gravis, chronic weakness of muscles, especially in the face and throat. It results from a defect in nerve transmissions between nerve fibers to muscles. Occurs most often in young women and in men over 60 years of age. Symptoms include dyspnea, muscular weakness, dysphagia, and fever.

mycetoma /mī´sētō´mə/, a fungal infection involving skin, connective tissue, and bone. One type, **Madura foot,** is a tropical fungal infection of the foot.

Mycoplasma /-plaz´mə/, microscopic organisms without rigid cell walls. They are considered to be the smallest of all free-living organisms.

mycosis /mīkō´-/, any disease caused by a fungus. Some kinds of mycoses are tinea pedis and candidiasis. –**mycotic,** *adj.*

mydriasis /midrī´əsis/, widening of the pupil of the eye.

myelin /mī´əlin/, a fatty substance found in the coverings of various nerve fibers. The fat gives the normally gray fibers a white color. –**myelinic,** *adj.*

myelinolysis /-ol´-/, a disorder that dissolves the myelin sheaths around certain nerve fibers. It occurs in alcoholic and undernourished patients.

myelin sheath, a fatty layer of myelin that wraps the axons. Some diseases, such as multiple sclerosis, can destroy the myelin wrappings.

myelitis /mī´elī´-/, inflammation of the spinal cord with motor or sensory nerve deficits. *See also poliomyelitis.*

myelocele /mī´əlōsēl´/, a saclike bulge of the spinal cord through a defect in the spinal column, seen at birth. *See also myelomeningocele.*

myeloclast /-klast´/, a cell that breaks down the myelin sheaths of nerves of the central nervous system.

myelocyte /-sīt´/, an immature white blood cell. It is normally found in the bone marrow. These cells appear in the circulating blood only in certain forms of leukemia. –**myelocytic,** *adj.*

myelogram /-gram´/, **1.** an x-ray film of the spinal cord taken after the injection of a dye. It shows any distortions of the spinal cord, spinal nerve roots, or surrounding space. **2.** a count of the different kinds of cells in a sample of bone marrow.

myeloid /mī´əloid/, **1.** referring to the bone marrow. **2.** referring to the spinal cord.

myeloma /mī´əlō´mə/, a tumor of the bone marrow.

myelomeningocele /-məning´gōsēl´/, a central nervous system hernia. A sac containing the spinal cord, meninges, and cerebrospinal fluid extends out through a weakened area in the vertebral column. The hernia may be located at any point along the spine, but usually occurs in the lower back. *See also neural tube defect, spina bifida.*

myelopathy /mī´əlop´əthē/, any disease of the spinal cord.

myelopoiesis /-pō·ē´sis/, the formation and growth of the bone marrow.

myiasis /mī´yəsis/, infection or infestation of the body by the larvae of flies. They usually enter through a wound or an ulcer.

mylohyoideus /mī´lōhī·oi´dē·əs/, one of a pair of flat triangular muscles that form the floor of the mouth. It acts to raise the tongue.

myocardial infarction, death of cardiac tissue usually resulting from myocardial ischemia following occlusion of a coronary artery.

myocardial rupture, any laceration or perforation of the atria, ventricles, or other cardiac structure. Damage usually occurs acutely due to trauma to the chest or heart but may be delayed for weeks and occur due to necrosis of a contused or infarcted myocardium.

myocardiopathy /-kär´dē·op´əthē/, any disease of the heart muscle. Also known as **cardiomyopathy.**

myocarditis /-kärdī´-/, inflammation of the cardiac muscle. It most often occurs as a viral disease, but may also be caused by bacteria, fungus, or a chemical agent.

myocardium /-kär´dē·əm/, a thick layer of muscle cells that forms most of the heart wall. The myocardium contains few other tissues, except for blood vessels. It is covered inside by endocardium. The tissue of the myocardium that causes it to contract is made up of fibers like skeletal muscle tissue, but contains less connective tissue. Special fibers of myocardial muscle include the sinoatrial node, the atrioventricular node, the atrioventricular bundle, and the Purkinje fibers. Most of the myocardial fibers contract the heart. The heart uses free fatty acids as its main fuel, as well as important amounts of sugar and a small amount of amino acids. Oxygen, which affects the ability of muscle tissue to contract, is an important food for the myocardium. Without an oxygen supply, myocardial contractions decrease in a few minutes. The heart normally takes in about 70% of the oxygen reaching it by the coronary arteries. *See also epicardium, heart.* **–myocardial,** *adj.*

myoclonus /mī·ok´lənəs, mī´ōklō´nəs/, a spasm of a muscle or a group of muscles. **–myoclonic,** *adj.*

myoglobin, an oxygen-binding protein found in muscle cells, similar in structure and function to hemoglobin.

myoma /mī·ō´mə/, a tumor of muscle. *See also fibroids, leiomyoma, rhabdomyoma.*

myometritis /-mətrī´-/, inflammation of the myometrium.

myometrium /-mē´trē·əm/, the muscular layer of the wall of the uterus.

myoneural /-nŏŏr´əl/, referring to a muscle and its nearby nerve, especially to nerve endings in muscles.

myopathy /mī·op´əthē/, a disorder of skeletal muscle that causes weakness, wasting, and changes within muscle cells. Examples include any of the muscular dystrophies. A myopathy is different from a muscle disorder caused by nerve dysfunction. *See also muscular dystrophy.* **–myopathic,** *adj.*

myopia /mī·ō´pē·ə/, a condition of nearsightedness. Causes include lengthening of the eyeball or an error in deflecting rays so that parallel rays of light are focused in front of instead of on the retina. Also known as **nearsightedness.**

myorrhexis /mi´ôrek´sis/, a tearing or break in a muscle. **–myorrhectic,** *adj.*

myosin /mī´əsin/, a protein that makes up nearly one half of the proteins in muscle tissue.

An interaction between myosin and another protein, actin, makes muscle contraction possible.

myositis /-si´-/, inflammation of muscle tissue, usually of the voluntary muscles. Causes of myositis include injury, infection, and invasion by parasites.

myotome /-tōm/, **1.** a group of muscles stimulated by a single spinal nerve segment. **2.** an instrument for cutting or dissecting a muscle.

myotonia /-tō´nē·ə/, any condition in which muscles do not relax after contracting.

myotonic myopathy /-ton´ik/, any of a group of disorders with increased skeletal muscle contractions and decreased relaxation of muscles after contraction.

myringectomy /mir´injek´-/, surgical removal of the tympanic membrane.

myringitis /-jī´-/, inflammation or infection of the tympanic membrane.

mysophobia /mī´sə-/, an anxiety disorder with an abnormal fear of dirt, contamination, or getting dirty.

myxedema /mik´sədē´mə/, the most severe form of hypothyroidism. Signs include edema of the hands, face, feet, and tissues around the eye.

myxoma /miksō´mə/, a tumor of connective tissue.

myxovirus, any of a group of viruses usually carried by mucus. Some kinds of myxoviruses are the viruses that cause influenza, mumps, and croup.

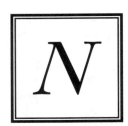

nacelle /näsel´/, streamlined housing for an aircraft engine, generally attached to a wing.

nail, **1.** a structure with a horny surface at the end of a finger or toe. Each nail has a root, body, and edge. The root is embedded in the skin. **2.** any of many metal nails used in bone and joint surgery to join bones or pieces of bone.

nalbuphine, an analgesic used in the relief of pain, particularly that of cardiac origin. Side effects include altered level of consciousness, bradycardia, hypotension, and respiratory depression. It is contraindicated in the presence of head injury, multiple trauma, shock, undiagnosed abdominal pain, and compromised respirations. Also known as **Nubain.**

naloxone, a narcotic antagonist used to reverse the central nervous system and respiratory effects of natural and synthetic narcotic overdoses. Side effects include diaphoresis, nausea or vomiting, precipitation of withdrawal syndrome, and tachycardia. Use with caution in suspected narcotic addicts. Also known as **Narcan.**

nanism /nä´nizm/, an abnormal smallness or stunted growth; dwarfism.

nanomelia /-mē´lyə/, abnormally small arms and legs in relation to the head and body.

nape, the back of the neck.

naphthalene poisoning, a toxic condition caused by swallowing naphthalene. Symptoms include nausea, vomiting, headache, abdominal pain, and seizures. Naphthalene is used in mothballs and moth crystals.

narcissism /när´sisizm/, an abnormal interest in oneself, especially in one's own body and sexual characteristics; self-love. Compare **egotism.**

narcissistic personality /-sis´-/, a personality with behavior and attitudes that show an abnormal love of self. Such a person is self-centered and self-absorbed, is very unrealistic concerning abilities and goals, and, in general, assumes the right to more than is reasonable in relationships with others.

narcolepsy /när´kōlep´sē/, a disorder with sudden sleep, sleep paralysis, and sight or hearing hallucinations at the onset of sleep. It begins in adolescence or young adulthood and lasts throughout life. Sleep periods may last from a few minutes to several hours. **—narcoleptic,** *adj.*

narcoleptic /-lep´-/, **1.** referring to a condition or substance that causes an uncontrollable desire for sleep. **2.** a patient with narcolepsy.

narcosis /närkō´-/, a state of stupor caused by narcotic drugs.

narcotic, **1.** a substance that produces stupor. **2.** a narcotic drug. Narcotics (synthetic or opium-derived analgesics) change one's sense of pain, cause a heightened sense of well-being, mental confusion, and deep sleep. They may slow breathing, cause nausea and vomiting, and reduce motility. Repeated use of narcotics may result in physical and psychologic addiction.

narcotic antagonist, a drug that prevents or reverses the effects of narcotics.

nares /ner´ēz/, *sing.* **naris,** the openings in the nose that allow the passage of air to the pharynx and lungs during respiration.

nasal, referring to the nose and nasal cavity.

nasal cannula, oxygen supply device that is placed in the nose of a patient when low (1–6 liters per minute) flows of oxygen are desired. Consists of a supply tubing that ends in a two-pronged tip and a head strap. Also known as **nasal prongs.**

nasal cavity, the open area inside the nose that is divided into two chambers by the nasal wall (septum). Each chamber, called a **nasal fossa,** opens externally through the nostrils, and internally into the pharynx.

nasal flaring, widening of the nostrils during respirations, usually a sign of air hunger or respiratory distress.

nasal prongs. See **nasal cannula.**

nasal sinus, any one of the many cavities in various bones of the skull. A sinus is lined with mucous membrane which lines the nasal cavity and is very sensitive. When irritated, the membrane may swell and block the sinuses. **Ethmoidal air cells** are many small, thin-walled cavities in the ethmoid bone of the skull. The **frontal sinuses** are two small cavities in the frontal bone of the skull. They connect to the nasal cavity. The **maxillary sinuses** are a pair of large air cells forming a hole in the body of the maxilla. The **sphenoidal sinuses** are a pair of cavities lateral to the nose.

nasogastric intubation, the placement of a tube through the nose into the stomach to remove air and gastric contents or to irrigate the stomach. Also known as **NG intubation.**

nasolabial reflex /-lā´bē·əl/, an infant's quick backward movement of the head, arching of the back, and stretching of the limbs in response to a light touch to the tip of the nose with an upward sweeping motion. The reflex disappears by about 5 months of age.

nasolacrimal /-lak´riməl/, referring to the nasal cavity and nearby tear (lacrimal) ducts. The **nasolacrimal duct** is a channel that carries tears from the lacrimal sac to the nasal cavity.

nasopharyngeal airway, a basic airway that is inserted via the nose into the posterior oropharynx, behind the tongue. This prevents the tongue from blocking the airway in a patient with an altered level of consciousness. Types include Robertazzi (fixed flange) and Rüsch (adjustable flange). Also known as **nasal airway, nasal trumpet.**

nasotracheal intubation, procedure involving placement of an endotracheal tube in the trachea via the nose. This technique is useful only in a patient with spontaneous respirations. Also known as **NT intubation.**

natal, **1.** referring to birth. **2.** referring to the buttocks (nates).

nates /nā´tēz/. See **buttocks.**

National Interagency Incident Management System, consists of five major subsystems that collectively provide a total systems approach to all-risk incident management. The subsystems are: the incident command system; training; qualifications and certification; supporting technologies; and publications management. Also known as **NIIMS.**

National Search and Rescue Plan, a document that identifies federal (U.S.) responsibilities for assistance in situations of injured, lost, overdue, and stranded persons. It defines all inland federal search and rescue (SAR) responsibilities as belonging to the U.S. Air Force and all maritime or navigable waters SAR as U.S. Coast Guard responsibility. This document also forms the basis for the *National Search and Rescue Manual.*

natriuresis /nā´trēyŏŏrē´-/, the release of more than normal amounts of sodium in the urine. It may be caused by diuretics or from various disorders of chemical or physical processes.

natural childbirth, labor and childbirth with little or no medication.

natural hazard, a natural event with the potential to cause damage or death, such as a storm, earthquake, or drought.

nausea /nô´zē·ə, nô´zhə/, the sensation leading to the urge to vomit. Common causes are motion sickness, early pregnancy, intense pain, emotional stress, gallbladder disease, food poisoning, and various infections. **–nauseate,** *v.,* **nauseous,** *adj.*

navel, the point on the abdomen at which the umbilical cord joined the fetal abdomen. It is located about halfway between the breastbone and the genital area. Also known as **umbilicus.**

near-drowning, a submersion incident in which the victim survives at least 24 hours, possibly accompanied by alterations in body chemistry, cardiac function, core temperature, and/or level of consciousness. *See also drowning.*

nearsightedness. See **myopia.**

nebula /neb´yələ/, *pl.* **nebulae,** a corneal spot or scar that usually does not obstruct vision.

nebulizer, a device for creating a fine spray. Also known as **atomizer.**

neck, a narrowed section, as the part of the body that connects the head with the body, or the neck of the femur.

necrobiosis lipoidica /nek´rōbī·ō´-/, a skin disease with thin, shiny, yellow to red plaques on the legs or forearms. These plaques may form crusts or ulcers. Usually linked to diabetes mellitus, it occurs most often in women.

necropsy. See **autopsy.**

necrosis /nekrō´-/, local tissue death that occurs because of disease or injury. *See also gangrene.*

necrotizing, causing tissue death.

necrotizing enteritis. See **food poisoning.**

necrotizing enterocolitis, an acute inflammatory bowel disorder that occurs mainly in premature or low birth weight infants. The disease causes tissue death with bacterial invasion of the intestinal wall. The stomach and intestinal lining are destroyed, which leads to peritonitis. Its cause is unknown.

needle chest decompression. See **needle thoracostomy.**

needle cricothyrotomy, technique involving placement of a catheter-needle combination through the cricothyroid membrane, utilizing the catheter as a temporary airway in cases of foreign body obstruction or trauma to the trachea. Also known as **needle cric.** *See also surgical cricothyrotomy.*

needle thoracostomy, technique of relieving the pressure of a tension pneumothorax by insertion of a large-bore needle into the involved lateral (fourth or fifth costal interspace) or anterior (second or third costal interspace) chest wall. This will improve the patient's vital signs, so as to allow more time to prepare for insertion of a chest tube. Also known as **needle chest decompression, needle decompression.** *See also tube thoracostomy.*

negative feedback, a decrease in a body function in response to stimulation. For example, when the release of certain hormones reaches a certain level, a signal is given by another hormone to slow the release.

negative pressure, less than standard atmospheric pressure, as in a vacuum or at an altitude above sea level.

negativism, a behavior attitude of resistance or refusal to cooperate with reasonable requests. The response may be passive, as the stiff postures seen in catatonic schizophrenia, or active, as in a contrary act, like sitting down when asked to stand.

neglect, an act of omission that may result in harm to a dependent person by those on whom they depend. Confinement, failure to provide supervision, isolation, or the withholding of necessities may constitute neglect. *See also abuse, self-neglect.*

negligence, failure to follow accepted practice, as defined by that expected of a reasonable and prudent person. Proving negligence requires that four points of law be shown to exist: a duty to act, a breach of duty, existing damage, and that the damage was caused by the failure to act (proximate cause).

Neil-Robertson litter, semirigid, poleless litter consisting of a canvas or plastic sheet, reinforced with wood or plastic slats, that can be wrapped around the entire body and fastened. This transport device is used to evacuate victims from mountaineering and shipboard accidents and when helicopter hoisting may be necessary. Also known as **Neil-Robertson.** *See also rigid transport vehicles.*

Nelson's syndrome, a hormone disorder that may follow removal of the adrenal gland. There is an increase in the production of hormones by the pituitary gland.

nematocyst, stinging cell located on the outer surfaces of jellyfish, sea anemones, and corals. These venom-charged cells are used for defense and for paralyzing prey.

nematode /nem´ətōd/, a parasitic worm of the phylum Nematoda. All roundworms belong to this group.

neologism /nē·ol´əjizm/, a word made up by a psychiatric patient that has meaning only to the patient.

neonate, an infant from birth to one month of age.

neonatal death. See **perinatal death.**

neonatal period, the period from birth to 28 days of age, a time of the greatest risk to the infant. About 65% of all deaths that occur in the first year of life happen in this 4-week period.

neoplasm /-plazm/, any abnormal growth of new tissue. A **benign neoplasm** is a tumor that has a fiber capsule and a regular shape. It does not grow fast, become widespread, invade surrounding tissue, or spread to distant sites. It causes harm only by pressure and does not usually return after removal. A **malignant neoplasm** is a tumor that tends to grow, invade nearby tissues, and spread through the bloodstream. It usually has an irregular shape and is made up of imperfectly developed cells. Also known as **tumor.** See also cancer. –**neoplastic,** adj.

neoplastic fracture, a fracture resulting from bone tissue weakened by a tumor.

nephrectomy /nefrek´-/, the surgical removal of a kidney.

nephritis /nefrī´-/, any disease of the kidney with inflammation and abnormal function. See also glomerulonephritis.

nephroangiosclerosis /nef´rō·an´jēōsklerō´-/, destruction of the small renal arteries, linked to high blood pressure. This condition is present in some patients between 30 and 50 years of age with high blood pressure. Early signs are headaches, blurred vision, and a diastolic blood pressure greater than 120 mm Hg. Also known as **malignant hypertension.** See also hypertension, kidney failure.

nephrocalcinosis /-kal´sinō´-/, an abnormal condition of the kidneys in which deposits of calcium form in the filtering units. It usually occurs at the site of a previous inflammation or breakdown.

nephrogenic /-jen´ik/, beginning in the kidney.

nephrolith /-lith/, a stone (calculus) formed in a kidney. –**nephrolithic,** adj.

nephrolithiasis /-lithī´əsis/, the presence of calculi in the kidney. See also kidney stone.

nephron /nef´ron/, a filtering unit of the kidney. Each kidney contains about 1.25 million nephrons. See also kidney.

nephropathy /nefrop´əthē/, any inflammation or disorder of the kidney. See also kidney disease.

nephrotic syndrome /nefrot´ik/, a kidney disease marked by protein in the urine, decreased albumin, and edema. Also known as **nephrosis.**

nephrostomy /nefros´təmē/, a surgically created opening in which a catheter is inserted into the kidney for drainage.

nephrotoxic /-tok´sik/, anything poisonous or destructive to a kidney.

nephrotoxin /-tok´sin/, a poison specifically destructive to the kidneys.

nerve, one or more bundles of signal-carrying fibers that connect the brain and the spinal cord with other parts of the body. Nerves carry inward (afferent) signals from receiving organs toward the brain and spinal cord, and outward (efferent) signals to the various organs and tissues. Each nerve consists of an outer sheath enclosing a bundle of nerve fibers. The sheath is made up of joining tissue. Single nerve fibers are wrapped in a membrane (neurilemma) in which some nerve fibers are also enclosed in a fatty insulating substance (myelin). See also axon, dendrite, neuroglia, neuron.

nerve accommodation, the ability of nerve tissue to adjust to a constant source and strength of stimulation so that some change in either strength or length of stimulation is needed to alter its function.

nerve agent, toxic chemical agents that interfere with parasympathetic nerve transmission by inhibiting cholinesterase. These gases or liquids will produce alterations of consciousness, respiratory distress, salivation, and seizures. Initially created to produce casualties during war, they were later found to be effective insecticides, such as Malathion (organophosphate).

nerve compression, pressure on one or more nerve branches, resulting in nerve damage and muscle atrophy. The degree of damage depends on the amount and length of time of pressure and nerve location.

nerve impulse, the electric and chemical processes that generate and send messages through the nervous system.

nervous breakdown, (informal) any mental condition that disrupts normal functioning.

nervous emesis,   vomiting resulting from anemia, brain tumor, concussion, meningitis, Meniere's disease, migraine, motion sickness, or skull fracture.

nervous system,   the arrangement of nerve cells that controls all of the functions of the body. It is divided into the central nervous system, composed of the brain and spinal cord, and the peripheral nervous system, which includes the cranial nerves and spinal nerves. These nerves combine and communicate to interact with all organs and tissues of the body with inward (afferent) and outward (efferent) nerve fibers. Afferent fibers carry sense signals, as pain and cold, to the central nervous system. Efferent fibers carry motor signals and movement commands from the central nervous system to the muscles and other organs. Somatic nerve fibers are linked to bones, muscles, and skin. Visceral nerve fibers are linked to the internal organs, blood vessels, and mucous membranes. The many functions of the nervous system are linked through a vast system of tiny structures, as neurons, axons, dendrites, and ganglia. *See also autonomic nervous system, central nervous system, peripheral nervous system.*

nettle rash,   an eruption resulting from skin contact with the stinging nettle. This common weed has leaves containing histamine. The stinging and itching provoked lasts from a few minutes to several hours.

neural /nŏor´əl/,   referring to nerve cells and their fibers.

neuralgia /nŏoral´jə/,   a painful condition caused by a variety of disorders that affect the nervous system. The term is usually linked to an affected body area, as facial neuralgia.

neural tube,   the tube of tissue that lies along the central axis of the early embryo. It gives rise to the brain, the spinal cord, and other parts of the central nervous system.

neural tube defect,   any defect of the brain and spinal cord caused by failure of the neural tube to close during growth during pregnancy. The defect often results from an abnormal increase in spinal fluid pressure on the neural tube during the first 3 months of pregnancy. It may occur at any point along the spinal column. The most severe defect is absence of the skull and defective brain growth. Most neural tube defects involve incomplete joining of one or more parts of the spinal column. *See also meningocele, myelomeningocele, spina bifida.*

neurasthenia /nŏor´əsthē´nē·ə/,   **1.** a condition of mental and physical exhaustion that often follows depression. **2.** a stage in the recovery from schizophrenia in which the patient is listless and seems unable to cope with routine activities and relationships. –**neurasthenic,** *adj.*

neurinoma /nŏor´inō´mə/,   a tumor of the nerve sheath.

neuritis /nŏorī´-/, *pl.* **neuritides,**   inflammation of a nerve. Signs include neuralgia, loss of sensation, paralysis, muscular weakness, and slowed reflexes.

neuro check,   *(informal)* simplified examination of the neurological status of a patient. This assessment usually consists of level of consciousness, movement of extremities, and pupillary reaction. *See also mental status exam, neurologic assessment.*

neurocoele /-sēl/,   a system of cavities in the brain and the central canal of the spinal cord. Also known as **neural canal.**

neurodermatitis /-dur´mətī´-/,   a pruritic skin disorder seen in anxious, nervous patients. Scratches and skin thickening are found on exposed areas of the body, as the forearms and forehead.

neurofibroma /-fībrō´mə/,   a fiberlike growth of nerve tissue. Many growths of this type in the nervous system are often linked to defects in other tissues.

neurofibromatosis /-fī´brōmətō´-/,   a congenital condition with many fiberlike growths (neurofibromas) of the nerves, skin, and other organs, and light brown (café au lait) spots on the skin. There may also be defects of the muscles, bones, and abdominal organs. The disorder is sometimes linked to meningocele, spina bifida, or epilepsy. Also known as **multiple neuroma.**

neuroglia /nŏorog´lē·ə/,   the supporting or connective tissue cells of the central nervous system. Compare **neuron.**

neurohormonal regulation /-hôr´mōnəl/,   control of an organ or a gland by the combined effect of nervous system and hormone activity.

neurohypophyseal hormone /-hī´pōfiz´ē·əl/, a hormone released by the pituitary gland. Kinds of neurohypophyseal hormones are **oxytocin** and **vasopressin.** *See also pituitary gland.*

neurolepsis /-lep´-/, an altered state of consciousness with reduced physical movement, anxiety, and indifference to surroundings. Sleep may occur, but usually the person can wake up and can respond to commands. Antipsychotic drugs usually cause neurolepsis.

neuroleptic /-lep´tik/, a drug that causes neurolepsis, as droperidol.

neuroleptic malignant syndrome, a disorder induced by tranquilizers, such as haloperidol, and that is characterized by muscular rigidity, hyperthermia, tachycardia, dyspnea, and diaphoresis.

neurologic assessment, physical assessment of the nervous system, consisting of evaluation of respirations, mental status, pupillary reaction, and extremity movement. For patients displaying neurological symptoms, additional evaluation of eye movement, reflexes, and sensation may be necessary. Also known as **neuro exam.** *See also mental status exam, neuro check.*

neuroma /nŏŏrō´mə/, a tumor of nerve cells and fibers. It may vary in size up to 6 inches or more. Pain moves from the tumor to the ends of the affected nerve. It is not usually constant but may become continuous and severe.

neuromuscular /-mus´kyələr/, referring to nerves and muscles.

neuromuscular blocking agent, a drug that interferes with the signals from motor nerves to skeletal muscles. Neuromuscular blocking agents are used to induce muscle relaxation and paralysis and as an aid to facilitate endotracheal intubation.

neuromyelitis /-mī´əlī´-/, inflammation of the spinal cord and nearby nerves.

neuron /nŏŏr´on/, the nerve cell of the nervous system. It contains a nucleus within a cell body with one or more fibers (axons or dendrites) extending from it. Some fibers are insulated by a fatty substance (myelin) and some fibers are uninsulated (unmyelinated). Some myelinated fibers carry signals of pressure, temperature, touch, and sharp pain. Unmyelinated fibers carry impulses from the abdomen and outer body. Neurons are named according to the direction in which they carry impulses and to the number of fibers they extend. Sensory neurons carry nerve impulses toward the spinal cord and brain. Motor neurons carry nerve impulses from the brain and spinal cord to muscles and gland tissue. Usually multipolar neurons have one axon to carry impulses away from the cell body and several dendrites to carry impulses toward the cell body. Most of the neurons in the brain and spinal cord are multipolar. Bipolar neurons, which are fewer than the other types, have only one axon and one dendrite. All neurons have at least one axon and one or more dendrites and are slightly gray in color when clustered, as in the brain and spinal cord.

neuronitis /-nī´-/, an inflammation of a nerve or nerve cell, especially of spinal nerves.

neuropathic joint disease /-path´ik/, a wasting disease of one or more joints. There is instability of the joint, bleeding, and edema. Pain is usually less severe than would be expected for the damage to the joint. The disease results from an underlying disease, as syphilis, diabetes, leprosy, or a defect in pain sensation.

neuropathy /nŏŏrop´əthē/, inflammation and wasting of the nerves, as that linked to lead poisoning. **Autonomic neuropathy** refers to nerve damage to the autonomic nervous system, causing orthostatic hypotension. **Compression neuropathy** is any disorder in which nerves are damaged by pressure or injury. Symptoms are numbness, weakness, or paralysis. **—neuropathic,** *adj.*

neurosis, defective handling of worry or inner conflict. This usually involves using unconscious defense mechanisms that may lead to a neurotic disorder. This process, called **neurotic process,** in which an unconscious conflict, as a struggle between an idealized self-image and the real self, leads to feelings of anxiety. Defense mechanisms are used to avoid these uncomfortable feelings. Personality change and the symptoms of neurosis result. *See also neurotic disorder.*

neurosurgery, any surgery involving the brain, spinal cord, or nerves.

neurotic, 1. referring to neurosis or to a neurotic disorder. **2.** one who is afflicted with a neurosis. **3.** *(informal)* an emotionally unstable person.

neurotic disorder, any mental disorder with symptoms that are distressing, unacceptable, and foreign to one's personality. Examples include severe anxiety, obsessions, and compulsive acts. The ability to function may be affected, but behavior generally stays within acceptable norms and sense of reality is not changed. Kinds of neurotic disorders include **anxiety neurosis, obsessive-compulsive neurosis, psychosexual disorder, somatoform disorder.**

neurotoxic /-tok´sik/, anything having a poisonous effect on nerves and nerve cells, as the effect of lead on the brain and nervous system.

neurotoxin /-tok´sin/, a poison that acts directly on the tissues of the central nervous system, as the venom of certain snakes or the botulism toxin.

neurotransmitter, any chemical that changes or results in the transmission of nerve signals across the synapse separating nerve fibers. Kinds of neurotransmitters include **acetylcholine, epinephrine, norepinephrine.**

neutral, a state exactly between two opposing values, qualities, or properties, as when a substance is neither acid nor alkaline. *See also acid, base.*

neutralization, the interaction between an acid and a base that makes a solution that is neither acidic nor basic. The usual products of neutralization are a salt and water.

neutralize, to negate or render harmless.

neutralizing agents, those materials that can be used to neutralize the effects of a corrosive material.

neutral thermal environment, an artificial environment that keeps the body temperature normal.

neutron, an elementary nuclear particle with a mass approximately the same as that of a hydrogen atom and carrying no electrical charge.

neutropenia /nooˊtrəpēˊnē·ə/, a drop in white blood cells (neutrophils) in the blood. Neutropenia is linked to leukemia, infections, rheumatoid arthritis, vitamin B_{12} deficiency, and splenomegaly. Also known as **granulocytopenia.**

neutrophil /-fil/, a grainlike white blood cell (leukocyte). Neutrophils are the circulating white blood cells necessary for removing or destroying bacteria, cell debris, and solid particles in the blood.

nevus /nēˊvəs/, a colored area of skin that is usually harmless but can become cancerous. Also known as **birthmark, mole.**

newborn, an infant from birth to 24 hours.

Newton's laws (Sir Isaac Newton, English astronomer and philosopher, 1642-1727), three laws that define the relationship between motion and force. Newton's first law of motion states that an object, whether at rest or in uniform motion, remains in that state unless acted upon by an outside force. The second law states that force is equal to mass times acceleration or deceleration. The third law asserts that for every action there is an equal and opposite reaction.

Nezelof's syndrome /nezˊəlofs/, a lack of immune responses and little or no specific antibodies. The cause is not known. It affects brothers and sisters, pointing to a possible hereditary disorder. It causes increasingly severe and finally fatal infections. Signs that often are seen in children up to 4 years of age include frequent pneumonia, middle ear, nose, and throat infections, and splenomegaly.

niacin /nīˊəsin/, a vitamin of the B complex group that dissolves in water, found in various plant and animal tissues. It acts in the breakdown and use of all major foods. Also known as **nicotinic acid.**

niacinamide /-amˊīd/, a B complex vitamin. Also known as **nicotinamide.**

nickel, a silvery-white metal element. Nickel causes more cases of allergic dermatitis than all other metals combined.

nickel dermatitis, an allergic contact skin inflammation (dermatitis) caused by the metal, nickel. Exposure comes from jewelry, wristwatches, metal clasps, and coins.

nicotine, a colorless, quick-acting poison in tobacco. It is used as an insecticide in farming and an anti-parasitic agent in veterinary medicine. Swallowing large amounts of nicotine causes excessive salivation, nausea, vomiting, diarrhea, headache, dizziness, bradycardia, and respiratory paralysis.

nifedipine, a calcium channel blocker used in the treatment of angina pectoris. Side effects include headache, dizziness, nausea, and facial flushing. Should be avoided with patients receiving IV beta blockers or experiencing hypotension. Also known as **Procardia.**

night blindness, poor vision at night or in dim light due to a lack of vitamin A, a birth defect, or diseases. Temporary night blindness is caused by sudden exposure to bright light in a person with dark-adapted sight. *See also dark adaptation, night vision.*

nightmare, a dream occurring during rapid eye movement sleep that brings out feelings of strong, inescapable fear or extreme anxiety, usually awakening the sleeper. Compare **sleep terror disorder.**

night vision, an ability to see dimly lit objects. It stems from a condition linked to the rod cells of the retina. The rods contain a highly light-sensitive chemical, rhodopsin, or visual purple, which is necessary for being able to see in dim light. Light destroys rhodopsin, requiring at least 30 minutes of dark adaption before again developing effective night vision. Night vision may also be reduced by a lack of vitamin A, an important part of rhodopsin.

911, national (U.S.) emergency telephone system that utilizes trained operators from local public safety agencies to give advice and take phone requests for emergency assistance via the number 911. When computer processing allows the operator to ascertain the caller's address and phone number without speaking to the caller, the system is known as **enhanced 911.**

nipple, **1.** the conical protuberance of erectile tissue in the center of the areola of the breast, capable of secreting milk in the postpartum female. **2.** any small protuberance, particularly related to mechanical objects.

nit, the egg of a parasitic insect, as a louse. It may be found attached to human or animal hair or to clothing. *See also pediculosis.*

nitric acid /nī´trik/, a colorless, highly toxic acid that gives off fumes of nitrogen dioxide when exposed to air.

nitrite /nī´trīt/, a salt of nitrous acid used as a vasodilator and antispasmosdic. Among the nitrites used in medicine are amyl, ethyl, potassium, and sodium nitrite.

nitrobenzene poisoning /nī´trōben´zēn/, poisoning from the absorption into the body of ni-

trobenzene, a pale yellow, oily liquid used in shoe dyes, soap, perfume, and artificial flavors. Exposure in industry occurs from breathing the fumes or absorbing it through the skin. Symptoms include headache, drowsiness, nausea, cyanosis, and respiratory failure.

nitrogen, an element that is a gas at normal temperatures. Nitrogen makes up about 78% of the atmosphere and is a part of all proteins and most substances.

nitrogen narcosis, compressed air intoxication seen during scuba diving at depths below 100 feet. This phenomenon is seen as the partial pressure of nitrogen increases, creating euphoria, overconfidence, slowed reflexes, hallucination, and unconsciousness. Also known as **rapture of the deep.**

nitroglycerin, a vasodilator used in the treatment of suspected cardiac chest pain, hypertensive emergencies, and pulmonary edema resulting from congestive heart failure. Side effects include transient hypotension, pulsating headache, and facial flushing. Should not be used with hypotensive or pediatric patients. Also known as **nitro, NTG.**

nitrous oxide, a gaseous analgesic/anesthetic that, when mixed 50:50 with oxygen, is used to relieve anxiety and pain, particularly of cardiac origin. Side effects include dizziness and nausea or vomiting. It is contraindicated in cases of altered levels of consciousness, decompression sickness, head injury, multiple trauma, respiratory depression, shock, and undiagnosed abdominal pain. Also known as **Nitronox, N_2O.**

NOAA weather station, a mobile weather data collection and forecasting facility (including personnel) provided by the National Oceanic and Atmospheric Administration which can be used within the incident area.

no code, *(informal)* a patient suffering from a terminal condition for whom resuscitation would be inappropriate. Also known as **DNR.** *See also Do not resuscitate.*

nocturia /noktoor´ē-ə/, urination, especially excess urination, at night. It may be a symptom of prostate or kidney disease, or it may occur in persons who drink excess amounts of fluids, especially alcohol or coffee, before bedtime. Also known as **nycturia.** Compare **enuresis.**

nocturnal /noktur´nəl/, **1.** referring to or occurring at night. **2.** describing an individual or animal that is active at night and sleeps during the day.

nodal rhythm, atrioventricular junctional rhythm. Also known as **AV junctional rhythm, junctional rhythm.**

node, 1. a small, rounded mass. **2.** a lymph node.

nodular /nod´yələr/, referring to a small, firm structure or mass.

nodule /nod´yo͞ol/, a small node or nodelike structure.

noma /nō´mə/, an acute ulcerating disease of the mucous membranes of the mouth or genitals. The condition is most often seen in children with poor nutrition and cleanliness. There is rapid and painless breakdown of bone and soft tissue. Healing eventually occurs but often with disfiguring defects. Also known as **gangrenous stomatitis.**

nonaccidential trauma, physical (usually child) abuse. Also known as **NAT.** *See also physical abuse.*

non-bulk packaging, packaging that has an internal volume of 119 gallons (450 liters) or less for liquids, a capacity of 882 pounds (400 kg) or less for solids, or a water capacity of 1000 pounds (453.6 kg) or less for gases. It may consist of single packaging (e.g., drum, carboy, cylinder) or combination packaging, which is one or more inner packagings inside an outer packaging (e.g., glass bottles inside a fiberboard box). Non-bulk packaging may be palletized or placed in overpacks for transport in vehicles, vessels, and freight containers. Examples include carboys, cylinders, and drums.

noncompliance, the failure of a patient to follow medical advice. The patient may have a health belief, a cultural or spiritual value, an economic difficulty, or a problem with the physician that results in missing appointments or not using drugs as ordered.

nondirectional beacon, a ground-based radio transmitter that works in conjunction with an aircraft's automatic direction finder to provide a signal source that the aircraft can use for electronic navigation. The transmitter broadcasts in the 200 to 415 kilohertz range in all directions.

Aeronautical maps mark each beacon's location, name, frequency, and code letters. Also known as **NDB.**

noninvasive, a procedure or treatment that does not require the skin to be broken or a cavity or organ of the body to be entered, as taking a blood pressure with a stethoscope and sphygmomanometer.

nonprotein nitrogen, the nitrogen in the blood that is not a part of protein. Examples include the nitrogen linked to urea and uric acid.

non-rebreather oxygen mask, an oxygen administration device used to deliver high (greater than 60%) concentrations of oxygen. The mask has one-way valves attached that allow expired gas exhalation out of the mask without allowing room air in to dilute inspired oxygen. A reservoir (bag) is attached to allow buildup of oxygen concentration. Removal of one or both of the one-way valves converts the device to a **partial non-rebreather mask,** decreasing oxygen concentration. Also known as **non-rebreather, non-rebreather face mask, NRFM.**

nonspecific urethritis. See **urethritis.**

nontoxic, not poisonous.

Noonan's syndrome, a disorder in males, marked by short stature, low-set ears, webbing of the neck, and skeletal problems. The cause is unknown.

normal, 1. describing a usual, regular, or typical example of a set of objects or values. **2.** referring to persons in a nondiseased population.

normal-form radioactive materials, radionuclides in liquid, powder, gaseous, or other physical form, such that they might be dispersed if released from a shipping container.

normal human serum albumin, a colloid volume expander used to increase circulating blood volume in the presence of hypovolemia, particularly when due to burns and trauma. Also known as **Plasmanate.**

normal sinus rhythm, the predominant cardiac rhythm in healthy people, consisting of a regular rhythm, P wave, P-R interval (0.12-0.20 second in length), QRS complex (0.12 second or less in duration), T wave, Q-T interval (usually 0.4 second or less in duration), constant R-R interval, and a rate of 60-100 per minute. The electrical impulse creating this rhythm originates in the sinoatrial (SA) node in the right atrium. Also known as **NSR, sinus rhythm, SR.**

normoblast /nôr´məblast/, an immature red blood cell that still has a nucleus. After the nucleus is released, the young red blood cell (erythrocyte) becomes known as a reticulocyte. Compare **erythrocyte.** *See also reticulocyte.* **–normoblastic,** *adj.*

normochromic /-krō´mik/, referring to a red blood cell of normal color, usually because it contains the right amount of hemoglobin.

normotensive, referring to normal blood pressure. **–normotension,** *n.*

normothermic, normal temperature.

nose, a structure on the front of the skull that is a passageway for air to and from the lungs. The nose filters, warms, and moistens the air. The nose is the organ of smell and aids in speaking. The external portion, which grows out of the face, is much smaller than the internal portion, which lies over the roof of the mouth. The hollow interior portion is divided by a wall (septum) into a right and a left cavity. Each cavity is subdivided into a top, middle, and bottom opening by bony ridges (nasal conchae). The external nose has two nostrils, and the internal portion has two rear nostrils (posterior nares). Four pairs of sinuses drain into the nose. Mucous membrane with hairlike projections (cilia) lines the nose. *See also nasal cavity.*

nosebleed. See **epistaxis.**

nosecup, a device, inside a facepiece, that directs the wearer's exhalations away from the facepiece lens and thus prevents internal fogging (condensation) on the lens.

nosocomial infection /nō´sōkō´mē·əl/, an infection acquired during hospitalization. Also known as **hospital-acquired infection.**

notch, a gap or a depression in a bone or other organ.

notifiable, referring to conditions, diseases, and events that must, by law, be reported to a government agency. Examples include birth, death, smallpox, serious communicable diseases, and certain violations of public health regulations.

noxious, harmful; irritating.

nuchal cord /noo´kəl/, a condition in which the umbilical cord is wrapped around the neck of the fetus in the uterus or as it is being born. Usu-

ally the cord is slipped over the infant's head. The shoulders may come through a single loose loop. The condition is the most common complication of childbirth and occurs in more than 25% of births.

nuclear medicine, a branch of medicine that uses radioactive chemical elements (isotopes) in the diagnosis and treatment of disease.

nuclear radiation, particulate and electromagnetic radiation emitted from atomic nuclei in various nuclear processes. *See also alpha particle, beta particle, gamma ray, x ray, neutron.*

nuclear scanning, a method of medical diagnosis. The size, shape, location, and function of various body parts is seen using radioactive material and a device that senses the radioactivity in the body. Also known as **radionuclide organ imaging.**

nuclear weapon, a general term given to any weapon in which the explosion results from the energy released by reactions involving atomic nuclei—fission, fusion or both.

nucleic acid /nookle´ik/, a chemical compound involved in making and storing energy, and carrying hereditary characteristics. A capsule-like protein coat **(nucleocapsid)** surrounds nucleic acid. Some viruses are made only of bare nucleocapsids. Kinds of nucleic acid are **deoxyribonucleic acid** and **ribonucleic acid.**

nucleolus /nookle´ələs/, *pl.* **nucleoli,** any of the small, dense structures made up mostly of ribonucleic acid and located in the cytoplasm of cells. Nucleoli are needed to make cell proteins.

nucleon /noo´kle-on/, a term applied to protons and neutrons within the nucleus.

nucleoplasm /-plazm´/, the protoplasm of the nucleus, as opposed to the protoplasm of the cell outside of the nucleus. Compare **cytoplasm.**

nucleus /noo´kle·əs/, **1.** the main controlling body in a living cell, usually surrounded by a membrane. It contains genetic codes for continuing life systems of the organism and for controlling growth and reproduction. **2.** a group of nerve cells of the central nervous system that have the same function, as supporting the sense of hearing or smell.

nucleus pulposus, the gelatinous mass which provides cushioning within the intervertebral disk. *See also herniated disk.*

nuclide, a general term referring to any nuclear species of the chemical elements. There are about 270 stable nuclides and about 1250 radioactive nuclides.

null cell, a white blood cell (lymphocyte) that grows in bone marrow. Stimulated by an antibody, these cells can apparently attack certain cells directly and are known as "killer," or K, cells.

nullipara /nulip´ərə/, a woman who has not given birth to a living infant. The term "para 0" also means nullipara. Compare **multipara, primipara.**

numbness, a partial or total lack of sensation in part of the body, because of an interruption of signals from sensory nerve fibers. Numbness is often felt with tingling.

nurse. See **registered nurse.**

nurse's aide, a person who does basic nonmedical tasks in the care of a patient, as bathing and feeding, making beds, and moving patients.

nursing, **1.** acting as a nurse, giving care that encourages and promotes the health of the patient being served. **2.** breast feeding an infant.

nursing home. See **extended care facility.**

nut, climbing tool consisting of a large square nut with a cable or webbing attachment that provides an artificial anchoring point on rock that can be relied on to hold a climber who falls.

nutation, **1.** (ballistics) an aerodynamic force acting upon a projectile that causes a forward rotation in a rosette pattern. See also bullet tumble, bullet yaw, precession. **2.** nodding.

nutrient, a substance that provides nourishment and assists in the growth and development of the body. **Essential nutrient** refers to the carbohydrates, proteins, fats, minerals, and vitamins necessary for growth and normal function. These substances are supplied by food, since some are not produced in the body in large enough amounts for normal health. **Secondary nutrient** refers to a substance that helps to digest food in the intestine.

nutrient artery of the humerus, one of a pair of branches of the arteries near the middle of the arm.

nutrition, **1.** nourishment. **2.** the sum of the steps involved in taking in nutrients and in their use by the body for proper functioning and health. The stages are ingestion, digestion, absorption, assimilation, and excretion. **3.** the study of food and drink as related to the growth and health of living organisms. A **nutritionist** is one who studies and puts into practice the rules and science of nutrition.

nutritional anemia, a disorder with inadequate production of red blood cells caused by a lack of iron, folic acid, vitamin B_{12}, or other food disorders. **Iron deficiency anemia** may be caused by too little dietary iron, poor absorption of iron, or chronic bleeding. **Macrocytic anemia** features large, fragile, red blood cells (macrocytes). **Megaloblastic anemia** is a blood disorder in which abnormal red blood cells (megaloblasts) are produced. These red blood cells are usually linked to a form of anemia (pernicious) in which there is a lack of vitamin B_{12} or folic acid. **Pernicious anemia** affects mainly older patients. It results from a lack of intrinsic factor that is needed to process the vitamin B_{12} (cyanocobalamin) for red blood cells.

nyctophobia /nik´tō-/, an obsessive fear of darkness.

nymphomania, excessive sexual desire in women.

nystagmus /nistag´mus/, involuntary, cyclical movement of the eyes in any direction, usually seen as the result of neurologic disease or injury. The plane of movement is usually horizontal (lateral) or vertical. A direction of rapid movement is followed by slow movement in the other direction. The direction of rapid movement describes the type of nystagmus, as in left lateral nystagmus, upward nystagmus.

Nysten's law (Pierre H. Nysten, French physician, 1771-1818), rigor mortis begins in the muscles of mastication and progresses through the face, trunk, and arms, reaching the legs last.

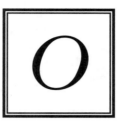

obese, extremely fat.

obesity, an abnormal increase in the amount of fat, mainly in the stomach and intestines, and in tissues beneath the skin. **Endogenous obesity** is caused by poor function of the endocrine or metabolic systems. **Exogenous obesity** is overweight caused by greater calorie intake than the body needs. The characteristics of obesity include excess weight, low activity level, and poor eating habits, as eating when not hungry.

objective, **1.** having a real, substantial existence apparent to an observer, such as objective symptoms. **2.** an aim or goal.

oblique, referring to a slanting angle or any point between vertical and horizontal. Some muscles have an oblique pattern. An **oblique fracture** is a fracture at a slanting angle.

obliquus externus abdominis /oblī´kwəs/, one of a pair of muscles of the abdomen, which assists in urination, defecation, vomiting, childbirth, and forced breathing. Both sides acting together flex the vertebral column. Also known as **descending oblique muscle.**

obliquus internus abdominis, one of pair of muscles of the abdomen, assisting in urination, defecation, vomiting, childbirth, and forced breathing. Both sides acting together flex the vertebral column. Also known as **ascending oblique muscle.**

observation, **1.** the act of watching carefully and closely. **2.** a report of what is seen or noticed.

obsession, a thought or idea with which the mind is always concerned and that usually deals with something irrational. The thought is not easily removed by thinking or talking it through. If often leads to a compulsion, as an uncontrollable urge to clean a room that is not dirty. *See also compulsion.*

obsessional personality, a type of personality in which continuous, abnormal, uncontrollable, and unwanted thoughts lead to compulsive actions.

obsessive-compulsive neurosis, a neurotic condition of being unable to resist or stop urges, thoughts, or fears that are different from the person's judgments.

obsessive-compulsive personality, a type of personality in which there is an uncontrollable need to do certain acts or rituals, as continuous washing of hands or changing of clothes. When the acts or rituals become abnormal and more obvious, they can become neurotic reactions.

obstetrics, the branch of medicine dealing with pregnancy and childbirth. An **obstetrician** is a physician who specializes in obstetrics.

obstipation, serious and continuing constipation caused by intestinal blockage. *See also constipation.*

obstruction, **1.** something that blocks or plugs an opening or passageway. **2.** the condition of being blocked.

obstructive lung disease, increased resistance to air movement due to narrowing of the bronchial tree. This resistance usually forms as the result of prolonged irritation or disease processes. *See also chronic obstructive pulmonary disease.*

obstructive uropathy,   any disease that blocks the flow of urine. The condition may lead to kidney disorders and a higher risk of urinary infection.

obturator /ob´tərā´tər/,   a device used to block a passage or a canal or to fill a space.

obturator externus,   the flat, triangle-shaped muscle covering the outer surface of the front wall of the pelvis. It rotates the femur laterally.

obturator internus,   a muscle that covers a large area of the lower part of the pelvis, where it surrounds the obturator foramen. It rotates the femur laterally and raises the thigh when it is flexed.

obvious death,   body condition where death is easily ascertained or assumed due to obvious incompatibilities with life. Signs of obvious death include decapitation, decomposition, evisceration of vital organs (i.e., brain or heart), incineration, and rigor mortis.

Occam's razor (William of Occam, 14th century),   the assumptions introduced to explain a thing must not be multiplied beyond necessity. Also known as the **law of scientific briefness.**

occipital artery /oksip´itəl/,   one of a pair of branched arteries from the external carotid arteries that supplies blood to parts of the head and scalp.

occipital bone,   the posterior portion of the skull where the foramen magnum links with the spinal canal.

occipital lobe.   See **brain.**

occipitofrontalis /oksip´itōfrontā´lis/,   one of a pair of thin, broad muscles covering the top of the skull. It is the muscle that pulls the scalp and raises the eyebrows and contains branches of the nerves for the face.

occiput /ok´sipət/,   the posterior part of the head.

occlude,   to close or obstruct.

occlusal trauma,   an injury to a tooth beneath the gum resulting from accidents, disorders of the temporomandibular joints, and teeth grinding.

occlusion,   **1.** a blockage in a canal, blood vessel, or passage of the body. **2.** any contact between the biting or chewing surfaces of the upper and lower teeth.

occlusive,   something that blocks or closes.

occult blood,   blood that comes from an unknown place, with unclear signs and symptoms. Occult blood is usually in the stools of patients with stomach and intestinal disorders.

occult fracture,   a fracture that cannot be seen on initial x-ray, but appears on films taken later.

occupational accident,   an injury caused by an accident to an employee in the workplace. Accidents account for more than 95% of workplace injuries.

occupational disability,   a condition in which a worker is unable to perform a job properly because of an occupational disease or a workplace accident.

occupational disease,   an illness due to performing a certain job, usually from contact with disease, or from performing certain actions repeatedly.

occupational health,   the state of a worker being able to work well enough and hard enough to do the job well, not to miss work because of illness, to have few claims for disability, and to be able to work for a significant portion of his or her life.

occupational medicine,   medicine that deals with the prevention, treatment, and diagnosis of medical problems relating to work and to the health of workers in different types of workplaces and jobs.

ochronosis /ō´krənō´-/,   deposits of brown-black color in connective tissue and cartilage. It is often caused by alkaptonuria or poisoning with phenol. Bluish spots may be seen on the whites of the eyes, fingers, ears, nose, genitals, mouth, and armpits. The urine may be dark colored.

ocular /ok´yələr/,   **1.** referring to the eye. **2.** an eyepiece or system of lenses, as in a microscope.

ocular myopathy,   slow weakening of the muscles that move the eye. There may be drooping of the upper lid. It may affect one or both eyes and may be caused by damage to the nerve necessary for eye movement, a brain tumor, or a disease that affects nerves and muscles.

oculocephalic reflex /ok´yəlōsefal´ik/,   a test of the brainstem. When the patient's head is quickly moved to one side and then to the other, the eyes will usually take a moment to catch up with the head movement and then slowly move to the middle position. Failure of the eyes to do this (doll's eyes) means damage or pressure on the opposite side of the brainstem.

oculomotor nerve, either of a pair of cranial nerves that control eye movements, supplying certain extrinsic and intrinsic eye muscles. Also known as **third cranial nerve.**

odontectomy /ō´dontek´-/, the removal of a tooth.

odontoid process, the protuberance on the upper surface of the second cervical vertebrae (axis). It is the place around which the first cervical vertebrae (atlas) turns, allowing the head to turn. Also known as **dens.**

odor, a scent or smell. The sense of smell is set off when molecules in the air carry the odor to the nerve (olfactory) located inside the nose. See Appendix 1-6.

odynophagia /od´inōfā´jə/, painful swallowing; a strong sensation of burning, squeezing pain while swallowing. It is caused by irritation of the mucous membranes or a disorder of the esophagus (gastroesophageal reflux).

Oedipus complex /ed´əpəs, ē´də-/, a sexual feeling by a child for the parent of the opposite sex, usually with strong negative feelings for the parent of the same sex.

Ohm's law (Georg S. Ohm, German physicist, 1787-1854), voltage equals amperage times resistance.

oil, any of a large number of fatty liquid substances from animal, vegetable, or mineral matter that will not mix with water.

ointment, a delivery vehicle for medication used on the skin. Various ointments are used as local anesthetics, antiinfectives, astringents, irritants, or keratolytic agents. Also known as **salve, unction, unguent.**

olecranon /ōlek´rənon/, a process on the ulna that forms the point of the elbow. It fits into the olecranon fossa of the humerus when the forearm is straightened.

oleic acid /ōlē´ik/, a colorless, liquid fatty acid found in vegetable and animal fats. In store products, oleic acid is found in lotions, soaps, ointments, and food additives.

olfactory /olfak´tərē/, referring to the sense of smell. **–olfaction,** *n.*

olfactory center, the part of the brain responsible for being aware of odors.

olfactory nerve, one of a pair of nerves linked to the sense of smell, composed of fibers that spread through the mucous membrane of the nasal cavity. Passing into the skull, the fibers form links with the fibers of the cells in the olfactory bulb, a relay center between the nose and the brain. Also known as **cranial nerve I.**

oligodactyly /ol´igōdak´tilē/, a birth defect causing the lack of one or more fingers or toes.

oliguria /ol´igo͞or´ē·ə/, a decreased ability to produce and excrete urine (usually less than 500 ml (1 pint) a day). The result is that waste products of metabolism cannot be released properly. Compare **anuria.**

omentum /ōmen´təm/, an extension of the peritoneum that surrounds one or more nearby organs in the abdomen. It divides into the greater omentum and lesser omentum. **–omental,** *adj.*

omphalitis /om´fəlī´-/, a disorder of the umbilicus with injection, edema, and purulant drainage.

omphalocele /om´fəlōsēl´/, a hernia of intestinal organ material through a hole in the abdominal wall at the navel. The hole is usually closed surgically soon after birth.

oncology /ongkol´-/, the branch of medicine that deals with the study of tumors.

oncotic pressure. See **blood colloid osmotic pressure.**

Ondine's curse, loss of respiratory drive in which the brainstem is unable to stimulate breathing in response to high carbon dioxide levels in the blood. Causes include drug overdose and polio. Also known as **hypothalamic alveolar hypoventilation syndrome.**

on-line medical control. See **direct medical control.**

onset of action, length of time necessary for a drug to begin exerting its effect.

ontogeny /ontoj´ənē/, the life history of one living thing from a single-celled egg to the time of birth, including all phases of cell division and growth. Compare **phylogeny.**

onychia /ōnik´ē·ə/, inflammation of the finger in the nail bed. Compare **paronychia.**

onychogryphosis /on´ikōgrifō´-/, a thickened, curved, clawlike overgrowth of fingernails or toenails.

ooblast /ō´əblast/, the female germ cell from which the egg grows.

oocyesis /ō´əsī·ē´sis/, a pregnancy with an embryo growing within the ovary instead of the uterus where it normally grows.

oogenesis /ō´əjen´əsis/, the growth of female eggs (ova).

oophorectomy /ō´əfôrek´-/, surgery to remove one or both ovaries. **Oophorosalpingectomy** is surgery to remove one or both ovaries and the fallopian tubes.

oophoritis /ō´əfôrī´-/, inflammation of one or both ovaries, usually occurring with inflammation of the fallopian tubes (salpingitis).

oosperm /ō´əspurm/, a fertilized egg; the cell caused by the joining of the sperm and the egg after fertilization occurs; a zygote.

opacity /ōpas´itē/, the condition of something that cannot be seen through (opaque or nontransparent), as a cataract opacity.

opaque /ōpāk´/, referring to a substance or surface that neither carries nor allows adequate light through.

open-circuit apparatus, breathing apparatus in which the wearer's exhalations are vented to the surrounding environment.

operation, **1.** surgery **2.** a single event, involving execution of a specified set of actions.

operational ceiling. See **service ceiling.**

operational period, the period of time scheduled for execution of a given set of operation actions.

Operations Coordination Center, the primary facility of the Multiagency Coordination System. It houses the staff and equipment necessary to its function. Also known as **OCC.**

operations section, the part of the incident command system responsible for all operations at an incident. This section may be divided into branches, divisions, groups, resources, strike teams, and/or task forces. *See also incident command system.*

operating radius, **1.** distance an agency or service is able to operate around their location. **2.** the horizontal distance from the certerline of rotation to a vertical line through a load's center of gravity (the radius of operation of a crane or similar machine).

operculum /ōpur´kyələm/, a covering.

ophthalmia /ofthal´mē·ə/, inflammation of the conjunctiva or more posterior parts of the eye. *See also conjunctivitis.*

ophthalmology /-mol´-/, the branch of medicine that deals with function, structure, and diseases of the eye. An **ophthalmologist** is the physician who practices this medicine.

ophthalmoplegia /-mōplē´jə/, the loss of movement of the eye muscles. It may occur acutely in both eyes with myasthenia gravis, thiamin deficiency, or botulism.

ophthalmoscope /ofthal´məskōp/, a device for looking into the eye.

opiate /ō´pē·āt/, a narcotic that contains opium, drugs made from opium or any of several semisynthetic drugs that behave like opium. These drugs are used to ease pain and have great potential for misuse and addiction.

opisthorchiasis /ō´pisthôrkī´əsis/, infection with a kind of *Opisthorchis* liver worm commonly found in Asia, the Pacific Islands, and parts of Europe. Cancer of the bile ducts may result. This infection is prevented by eating adequately cooked fish.

opisthotonos /ō´pisthot´ənəs/, a continuous severe spasm of the muscles causing the back to arch, the head to bend, and the arms and hands to flex rigidly at the joints.

opium alkaloid, any of several substances taken from the unripe seed pods of the opium poppy (*Papaver album* and *Papaver somniferum*). Three of the alkaloids, codeine, papaverine, and morphine, are used for pain relief. Morphine is the basic, most common drug of its kind against which the painkiller effect of newer drugs for pain relief are tested. The opium alkaloids and the drugs made from them, including heroin, act on the central nervous system, causing loss of pain. In usual doses, the relief from pain is achieved without loss of consciousness.

Oppenheim reflex, a sign of central nervous system disease. It is provoked by firmly stroking downward on the anterior and medial surfaces of the lower leg, causing the great toe to straighten out and fanning of other toes. *See also Babinski's reflex.*

opportunistic infection, an infection caused by a virus or other germ that is not usually harmful. The patient becomes infected because the ability to fight off disease has been reduced by a present disorder, such as diabetes mellitus.

optic, referring to the eyes or to sight.

optic atrophy, wasting away of the optic disc in the retina, caused by a breakdown of optic nerve fibers. Optic atrophy may be caused by a birth defect, inflammation, blockage of the central retinal artery or internal carotid artery, alcohol, or poisons. Breakdown of the disc may be seen with arteriosclerosis, diabetes, glaucoma, hydrocephalus, anemia, and different types of nervous system disorders.

optic disc, the small blind spot on the surface of the retina. It is the only part of the retina that is not sensitive to light. At its center is the entrance of the central artery of the retina. Also known as *(informal)* **blind spot.**

optic nerve, one of a pair of cranial nerves made up mainly of fibers that start in the retina, travel through the thalamus at the base of the brain, and join with the visual cortex at the back of the brain. At a structure in the front part of the brain, called the optic chiasm, there is a crossing over of fibers from the inner half of the retina of one eye to the fibers of the other eye. The fibers left over from the outer half of each retina are uncrossed and pass to the visual cortex on the same side. The visual cortex works to sense light and shade and to sense objects by decoding nerve signals from the retina. Also known as **cranial nerve II.**

optics, a field of study that deals with sight and the way that the eye and the brain are linked in order to sense shapes, patterns, movements, distance, and color. **–optic, optical,** *adj.*

optometry /optom´ətrē/, the practice of testing the eyes for the ability to focus and see, making corrective lenses, and suggesting eye exercises.

oral, relating to the mouth.

oral administration of medication, giving a tablet, capsule, or solution of a drug by mouth. Placing a tablet between the cheek and the teeth or gum is known as **buccal administration.** Placing it beneath the tongue until the tablet dissolves is **sublingual administration.**

oral contraceptive, an oral steroid for birth control. The two major steroids used are progestogen and a combination of progestogen and estrogen. *See also contraception.*

orbicularis oculi /ôrbik´yəler´is/, the muscular part of the eyelid composed of the palpebral, orbital, and lacrimal muscles. The palpebral muscle closes the eyelid gently; the orbital muscle closes tighter as in winking.

orbicularis oris, the muscle around the mouth, composed of fibers from facial muscle and fibers in the lips. It closes and purses the lips.

orbit, one of a pair of bony, cup-shaped openings in the skull that contain the eyes and various eye muscles, nerves, and blood vessels.

orchidectomy /ôr´kidek´-/, an operation to remove one or both testicles. Also known as **orchiectomy.**

orchitis /ôrkī´-/, inflammation of one or both testicles, often due to mumps, syphilis, or tuberculosis.

ordinate /ōr´dənət/, the vertical line that crosses the abscissa at a right angle, used to define a point in graphs.

oreximania /ôrek´sē-/, a condition of extreme appetite. It often results from an unusual or unnatural fear of becoming thin. Compare **anorexia.**

organ, any structural part of a system of the body composed of tissues and cells that allow it to perform a certain job, such as the liver, spleen, or heart. Each one of the organs that occur in pairs, such as the lungs, can function by itself. The liver, pancreas, spleen, and brain may continue normal or near normal function with over 30% of their tissue lost.

organelle, a specialized part of a single-celled organism that has a membrane and performs a specific function; a cell organ.

organic, **1.** referring to any chemical compound that has carbon in it. **2.** referring to an organ.

organic mental disorder, any mental or behavioral problem due to damage and/or impaired function of brain tissue. Causes may include cerebral arteriosclerosis, lead poisoning, or neurosyphilis. Also known as **OBS, organic brain syndrome.**

organoid, any structure that looks like an organ physically or functionally, especially a tumor mass.

organophosphate poisoning, toxicity due to inhalation or absorption of cholinergic insecticides such as **Parathion** or **Malathion.** Symptoms include bradycardia, altered levels of consciousness, confusion, increased secretions, muscle cramping, and vomiting.

orgasm, the sexual climax, a series of strong muscle contractions of the genitals over which there is no control.

orientation, being aware of where one is with regard to person, place, and time. *See also mental status exam.*

orifice /ôr´ifis/, the entrance or outlet of any opening.

origin, **1.** beginning of a nerve or the fixed attachment of a muscle. **2.** the starting point; source.

ornithine /ôr´nithin/, an amino acid that is not a part of protein, but is a substance made while food is being metabolized.

Ornithodoros /ôr´nithod´ərəs/, a type of tick, some kinds of which carry the sprirochetes of relapsing fevers.

oropharyngeal airway, basic airway that is inserted via the mouth into the posterior pharynx, behind the tongue. This prevents the tongue from blocking the airway during altered states of consciousness. It can also be used as a biteblock, to prevent the teeth from damaging the tongue or a tube inserted in the oropharynx. *See also nasopharyngeal airway.*

orphan drug, a medication that is not cost-effective to produce, usually because there are an inadequate number of patients needing it to justify the cost. The Orphan Drug Act of 1983 (U.S.) allows drug companies and research groups to obtain federal money to offset the cost of creating and producing these drugs.

orthopantogram /-pan´təgram/, an x-ray film showing all of the teeth, jaw, and nearby structures on a single film.

orthopedics, the medical science that studies the correction and prevention of disorders of the locomotor (movement) structures of the body, such as the joints, muscles, skeleton. The physician who specializes in this science is known as an **orthopedist** or **orthopod.** Also spelled **orthopaedics.**

orthophoto maps, aerial photographs corrected to scale such that geographic measurements may be taken directly from the prints. They may contain graphically emphasized geographic features and may be provided with overlays of such features as water systems and important facility locations.

orthopnea /-pnē´ə, ôrthop´nē·ə/, a condition in which a patient must sit or stand to breathe deeply or comfortably. It occurs in many disorders of the cardiac and respiratory systems, such as angina pectoris, asthma, emphysema, pneumonia. *See also dyspnea.*

orthoptic /ôrthop´tik/, referring to normal two-eyed (binocular) sight.

orthostatic, relating to or caused by an erect position.

orthostatic vital signs, taking blood pressure and pulse in supine, sitting, and, possibly, standing positions to determine if an absolute or relative hypovolemia exists. A systolic blood pressure drop of 15 mmHg or an increase in pulse rate of 15 beats per minute is considered a positive sign of at least 15% loss of blood volume. If the patient becomes symptomatic when sitting, do not proceed to the standing position. Also known as **orthostatics, tilt test.**

orthotonos /ôrthot´ənəs/, a straight, rigid posture of the body caused by muscle spasm, as after tetanus infection or strychnine poisoning.

os, **1.** an opening, commonly related to the cervix. **2.** relating to bone.

Osborn wave. See **J wave.**

oscilloscope /osil´əskōp/, a device that converts electrical impulses into a visual signal, such as an EKG monitor.

Osgood-Schlatter disease, inflammation or partial detachment of the patellar ligament from the tibia. Symptoms include swelling and tenderness near the proximal portion of the tibia. It is usually due to overuse of the quadriceps.

Osler's nodes, tender, red papules on the ends of fingers or toes. The condition is seen in bacterial endocarditis and usually lasts 1 or 2 days.

Osler-Weber-Rendu syndrome /-randōō´/, an inherited blood vessel disorder, bleeding from capillaries and mucous membranes. Small red-to-violet sores are found on the lips, mouth and nasal mucous membranes, tongue, and tips of fingers and toes. Bleeding from the sores may be heavy and may result in anemia.

osmolality, the osmotic concentration of solute per kilogram of solvent.

osmolarity, the osmotic concentration of a solution defined as osmoles of solute per liter of solution.

osmosis /ozmō´-, os-/, the movement of a fluid, such as water, through a semipermeable membrane from a solution that has a lower amount of a dissolved substance to one that has a higher amount. Movement through the tissue occurs until the levels of dissolved material in the solutions become equal.

osseous labyrinth /os´ē·əs/, the bony part of the inside of the ear. It is composed of three cavities: the vestibule, the semicircular canals, and the cochlea, carrying sound vibrations from the middle ear to the acoustic nerve. All three cavities hold a fluid called perilymph.

ossicle, any small bone, particularly the three bones of the inner ear (incus, malleus, stapes).

ossification, the growth of bone.

ostealgia /os´tē·al´jə/, pain that is linked to an abnormal condition within a bone, such as osteomyelitis.

osteitis /os´tē·ī´-/, an inflammation of bone, caused by infection or injury. Symptoms include swelling, tenderness, dull, aching pain, and redness in the skin over the affected bone.

osteoarthritis /os´tē·ō·ärthrī´-/, a common form of arthritis in which one or more joints have tissue changes. Symptoms include pain after exercise or use of the joint, stiffness, tenderness to touch, and crepitus. Its cause is unknown but may include chemical, mechanical, congenital, metabolic, and endocrine factors. Also known as **degenerative joint disease.** Compare **rheumatoid arthritis.**

osteoblast /-blast´-/, a cell that begins in the embryo and, during the early growth of the skeleton, works in forming bone tissue. Osteoblasts bring together the substances that form the bone and over time grow into osteocytes.

osteochondrosis /-kondrō´-/, a disease that affects the bone-forming centers in children. It begins by destroying and killing bone tissue, followed by regrowth of bone tissue. *See also Osgood-Schlatter disease.*

osteoclasia /-klā´zhə/, a condition in which bony tissue is destroyed and absorbed by large bone cells (osteoclasts). It may occur during growth or the healing of fractures.

osteocyte /-sīt´/, a bone cell; a fully grown osteoblast that has become buried in the bone material (matrix). It connects with other osteoblasts to form a system of tiny canals within the bone substance.

osteogenesis /-jen´əsis/, the beginning and growth of bone tissue.

osteogenesis imperfecta, an inherited condition that causes poor growth of connective tissue and brittle bones that are easily broken. In its worst form, the disease may be seen at birth (osteogenesis imperfecta congenita). Also known as **brittle bones.**

osteolysis /os´tē·ol´isis/, the destruction of bone tissue, caused by disease, infection, or poor blood supply. The condition often affects bones of the hands and feet. It is seen in disorders that affect blood vessels, as in Raynaud's disease and systemic lupus erythematosus.

osteoma /os´tē·o´mə/, a tumor of bone tissue.

osteomalacia /-məlā´shə/, softening of the bone. There is a loss of calcium in the bone material, along with weakness, fractures, pain, anorexia, and weight loss. The condition may be due to inadequate phosphorus and calcium.

osteomyelitis /-mī´əlī´-/, an infection of bone and marrow. Symptoms include bone pain, tenderness, local muscle spasm, and fever. It is usually caused by bacteria (often staphylococci) that enter the bone during an injury or surgery, from infection or via the bloodstream.

osteonecrosis /-nekrō´-/, the destruction and death of bone tissue, as caused by cancer, infection, injury, or ischemia.

osteopathy /os´tē·op´əthē/, the practice of medicine that uses all of the usual techniques of drugs, surgery, and radiation but assesses the relationship between the organs and the muscle and skeletal system. Osteopathic physicians may correct structural problems by changing the position of bones in the treatment of health problems.

osteoporosis /-pôrō´-/, a loss of normal bone density with thinning of bone tissue and the growth of small holes in the bone. The disorder may cause pain, fractures, loss of body height, and deformation of parts of the body. It occurs most often in women who have gone through menopause, patients who are inactive or paralyzed, and patients taking steroid hormones. Estrogen, a female sex hormone, is often used to prevent postmenopausal osteoporosis.

osteosarcoma /-särkō´mə/, a type of cancer composed of bone cells.

osteosclerosis /-sklerō´-/, an abnormal increase in bone density. The condition occurs in different kinds of diseases and is often linked to poor blood circulation in the bone tissue, infection, and tumors.

osteotomy /os´te·ot´əmē/, the sawing or cutting of a bone. Kinds of osteotomy include block osteotomy, in which a section of bone is removed; cuneiform osteotomy to remove a bone wedge; and displacement osteotomy, in which a bone is rebuilt to change the way that the skeleton carries most of the body's weight.

ostomy /os´təmē/, (informal) surgical opening in the body to allow the release of urine from the bladder or of feces from the bowel.

otic /ō´tik/, referring to the ear.

otitis /ōtī´-/, inflammation or infection of the ear. **Otitis externa** affects the outside canal of the ear. **Otitis media** affects the middle ear, a common disease of childhood. Symptoms include a sense of fullness in the ear, with impaired hearing, pain, and fever.

otolaryngology /ō´tōler´ing·gol´-/, a branch of medicine that deals with diseases and disorders of the ears, nose, and throat and nearby parts of the head and neck.

otorrhea /ō´tôrē´ə/, any substance discharged from the external ear. Otorrhea may contain blood, pus, or cerebrospinal fluid.

otoscope /-skōp/, a device used to examine the outer ear, the tympanic membrane, and the tiny bones (ossicles) of the middle ear.

ototoxic /-tok´sik/, having a toxic effect on the organs of hearing and balance or the eighth cranial (vestibulocochlear) nerve. Common ototoxic drugs include certain antibiotics, aspirin, and quinine.

ounce, a unit of weight equal to 1/16 of 1 pound avoirdupois.

outcome, the status of a patient or situation at the end of a procedure or disease.

outer perimeter, (special operations) the safe area surrounding a high-hazard area of operations; a buffer zone that limits and controls access to an incident area. See also inner perimeter.

outlet, an opening through which something can pass.

out-of-ground effect. See **ground effect.**

out-of-service resources, the assets assigned to an agency or incident that are unable to respond due to mechanical failure, lack of personnel, or physical (need for rest) reasons.

oupatient, 1. a patient, not in a hospital, who is being treated in an office, clinic, or other walk-in ambulatory care facility. 2. a health care facility for patients who do not need to be in a hospital. Compare **inpatient.**

outwash, downstream water flowing from a hydraulic.

ovarian artery /ōver´ē·ən/, a branch of the abdominal aorta that carries blood to an ovary.

ovarian cyst, a sac that grows in or on the ovary.

ovarian vein, one of a pair of veins that come out from the broad ligament near the ovaries and the fallopian tubes.

ovary, one of the pair of female sexual reproduction organs found on each side of the lower abdomen in a fold of the broad ligament, beside the uterus. Each ovary is normally firm, smooth, and almond in size and shape. At ovulation, an egg (ovum) is released from a small cavity (follicle) on the surface of the ovary. See also ovulation.

overcompensation, an extreme attempt to overcome a real or unreal physical or mental problem. The patient may or may not be aware of the problem. See also compensation.

overload, anything that pushes beyond normal limits.

over the counter, referring to a drug that the consumer can buy without a prescription. Also known as **OTC.**

overweight, more than normal in body weight after taking into account height, body build, and age. See also obesity.

ovoflavin /ō´vəflā´vin/, a riboflavin (vitamin B₂) taken from the yolk of eggs.

ovoglobulin /-glob´yəlin/, a protein (globulin) taken from the white of eggs.

ovulation /ov´yəlā´shən/, releasing an egg (ovum) from the ovary after the breaking of a mature small cavity (follicle). Ovulation is brought on by the gonadotrophic hormones, follicle stimulating hormone, and luteinizing hormone. Ovulation usually occurs on the fourteenth day following the first day of the last menstrual period and often causes brief, sharp pain on the side of the ovulating ovary. **–ovulate,** *v.*

ovum /ō´vəm/, *pl.* **ova, 1.** an egg. **2.** a female germ cell released from the ovary at ovulation.

oxalates, naturally occuring plant substances that are toxic due to their irritating and potentially corrosive nature. Dieffenbachia and caladium plants (insoluble oxalates) cause severe burning and edema in mucous membranes, and rhubarb leaves (soluble oxalate) cause hypotension, seizures, and muscle rigidity after ingestion.

oxidation, any process in which the amount of oxygen of a chemical compound is increased. **–oxidize,** *v.*

oxidizing agent, a chemical compound that easily gives up oxygen and attracts hydrogen from another compound. Also known as **oxidizer.**

oximeter, photoelectric device used to determine the oxygen content of the blood. *See also pulse oximeter.*

oxygen, a gas necessary for life processes that has no taste, odor, or color. Oxygen may be administered to increase the amount of oxygen and thus to lower the amount of other gases in the blood. *See also oxygen toxicity.*

oxygenation, the process of combining or treating with oxygen. **–oxygenate,** *v.*

oxygen consumption, the amount of oxygen in milliliters per minute necessary for normal body functions.

oxygen content, total amount of oxygen in the blood, expressed as milliliters per 100 milliliters of blood. Also known as **volumes per cent.**

oxygen mask. See **non-rebreather oxygen mask, simple oxygen mask.**

oxygen saturation, amount of oxygen bound to hemoglobin, expressed as a percentage.

oxygen therapy, any method used to administer oxygen to relieve hypoxia.

oxygen toxicity, toxic effects of breathing oxygen for prolonged periods of time or under pressures at or below 33 feet of seawater. **Central nervous system oxygen toxicity** is caused when 100% oxygen is breathed at more than 2 atmospheres absolute pressure. Manifestations of this condition include seizures and altered levels of consciousness. **Pulmonary oxygen toxicity** occurs when breathing low levels of oxygen over prolonged periods of time (>20 hours). Symptoms include pulmonary edema and hemorrhage. *See also Paul Bert effect, retrolental fibroplasia.*

oxygen transport, the method by which oxygen is absorbed in the lungs by the hemoglobin in red blood cells and carried to tissue cells all over the body. *See also hemoglobin.*

oxyopia /ok´sē·ō´pē·ə/, unusually good sight. A patient with normal (20/20) vision when standing 20 feet from the standard Snellen eye chart can read the seventh line of letters, each of which is 1/8 inch high. A patient with oxyopia can read smaller letters at that distance.

oxytocic, /-tō´sik/, any one of many drugs that cause the smooth muscle of the uterus to contract. They are also used to control post partum bleeding and correct uterine muscle tone after childbirth.

oxytocin, an oxytocic agent (pituitary hormone), effective in the management of postpartum hemorrhage. Side effects include uterine cramping. This medication should not be used prior to delivery of the infant due to increased risk of uterine rupture. Use with extreme caution in patients with previous cesarean section or uterine surgery. Also known as **Pitocin.**

ozone shield, the layer of ozone (a form of oxygen) in the atmosphere from 20 to 40 miles above the surface of the earth. It protects the earth from excess ultraviolet radiation.

P

pacemaker, **1.** specialized cardiac cells that generate impulses, stimulating the remaining cardiac cells to depolarize. In the normal heart, this depolarization creates a stimulus that causes mechanical contraction of the cardiac muscle. The normal pacemaker site of the heart is the sinoatrial (SA) node in the right atrium. There are many other pacemaker sites, but they are generally dominated by the SA node. *See also AV node, Bundle of His, Purkinje fibers.* **2.** an electrical device that can generate rhythmic electrical discharges, simulating the heart's natural pacemaker. It may be used when the heart fails to provide a satisfactory electrical stimulus for contraction, as in asystole, third-degree block. A pacemaker used outside the chest wall is known as a **transcutaneous,** or **external, pacemaker.** One used inside the chest wall is an **internal pacemaker.** These may function full-time (fixed pacemaker) or only as the rhythm requires it (demand pacemaker).

pacemaker cell, myocardial cell capable of initiating an electrical impulse.

pacemaker rhythm, the EKG rhythm created when an artificial cardiac pacemaker is originating the heart's electrical impulse.

pacer, *(informal)* a pacemaker.

pachyderma /pak´ēdur´mə/, thick skin.

Pacini's corpuscles /päsē´nēz/, sense organs joined to the end of one nerve fiber in the skin. They are found in the palm of the hand, sole of the foot, genitals, and joints.

pack, **1.** to cover with wet or dry heat or cold. This may be done to stimulate circulation, reduce swelling, or raise/lower the body temperature, as with an ice pack. **2.** to fill a cavity or wound with gauze or similar material. **3.** device for transporting equipment or supplies on a person's back.

packaging, those emergency care procedures necessary to properly transfer a patient from the scene to an ambulance, such as spinal immobilization.

packed cells, blood cells removed from plasma. They are given in severe anemia and post-fluid resuscitation in hypovolemia to restore normal levels of hemoglobin and red cells without overloading the cardiovascular system with excess fluid. *See also bank blood.*

pad, **1.** a mass of soft material used to cushion, prevent wear, or soak up fluids. **2.** a mass of adipose tissue that cushions many structures, as the fat pad of the patella.

padded dash syndrome, injuries resulting when the anterior neck strikes the steering wheel or dashboard during an accident. The compression of the larynx against the cervical spine may deform the arytenoid cartilages, dislocate the cricothyroid joint, and/or fracture the thyroid cartilage. Airway obstruction, dyspnea, pain, and subcutaneous emphysema may follow. Wearing a shoulder harness with a lap seat belt prevents many of these injuries.

pager, portable device using tone activation to receive a message.

Paget's disease /paj´əts/ (Sir James Paget, British surgeon, 1814-1899), skeletal disease of the elderly, causing chronic bone inflammation and deformities. The cause is unknown. Also known as **osteitis deformans.**

pagophagia /pā´gōfā´jə/, a craving to eat large amounts of ice due to a lack of iron in the diet.

pain, an unpleasant sense transmitted from sensory nerve endings. It is a symptom of inflammation and is an important clue to the cause of many disorders. Pain may be mild, severe, chronic, acute, cutting, burning, dull or sharp, exactly or poorly located, or referred. **Acute pain** is pain of sudden onset, generally not previously experienced. **Chronic pain** refers to pain that continues or returns over a long period. This is typically secondary to chronic illness or previous injury. **Referred pain** is felt at a place different from that of the actual injury or disorder. It is commonly seen with internal injuries.

pain receptors, sensory nerve endings that are sensitive to damage, irritation, or excess temperature and/or pressure. Receptors located on or near the skin surface are stimulated directly and are sensitive to minute changes. Receptors located in the body's interior (bone, muscle, organs) are less sensitive and require more profound stimulation. Referred pain can occur on activation of deeper receptors but not the superficial ones.

pain threshold, the point at which a stimulus activates one or more pain receptors.

paint, 1. to apply a solution to the skin. 2. a drug solution that is used in this way. Kinds of paint include **antiseptic, germicide,** and **sporicide drugs.**

paint sniffing, the practice of inhaling the vapor (toluene) contained in most spray paints to obtain a euphoric effect (high). Chronic inhalation damages cerebral tissue. Metallic spray paints (particularly gold and silver) contain the highest amounts of toluene and appear to cause the most intense effect. Also known as **huffing.**

palate /pal´it/, the roof of the mouth, anatomically divided into the hard palate and the soft palate. **–palatal, palatine,** *adj.*

palatine bone /pal´ətin/, one of a pair of bones of the skull, forming the posterior portion of the hard palate and part of the nasal cavity.

palatine tonsil, one of two oval masses of lymphoidal tissue located on the lateral wall of the oropharynx.

palladium /pəlā´dē·əm/, a hard, silvery metal element used in surgical instruments and dental devices.

pallet, portable platforms of wood or metal used to store and move material and packages.

palliate /pal´ē·āt/, to soothe or relieve.

pallor, paleness or lack of color in the skin.

palm, the anterior surface of the hand, between the wrist and fingers. **–palmar,** *adj.*

palmar aponeurosis /pä´mər/, connective tissue (fascia) that surrounds the muscles of the palm. Also known as **palmar fascia.**

palmar erythema, redness from inflammation of the palms of the hands.

palmaris longus /palmer´is/, a long, slender muscle of the forearm which flexes the hand.

palmar reflex, a reflex that causes flexion of the fingers when the palm of the hand is tickled.

palpation, technique used in a physical examination in which the examiner checks the texture, size, and location of parts of the body with the hands.

palpebra /pal´pəbrə/. See **eyelid.**

palpebral fissure /pal´pəbrəl/, the opening between the upper and lower eyelids.

palpitate, to flutter or throb rapidly, as in a tachycardia.

palpitation, a sensation of pounding or racing of the heart.

palsy /pôl´zē/, a loss of muscle control in an area of the body, usually due to an interruption of nerve impulses, as in **Bell's palsy, cerebral palsy, Erb's palsy.**

pan, a maritime distress code indicating an urgent message regarding the safety of an aircraft, person, or vessel. As the second highest priority distress call, it takes precedence over all other communications except Mayday. Reports of a vessel aground, an urgent medical condition, or a potential aircraft mechanical problem that is not yet critical are examples of pan messages. *See also Mayday, securité.*

pancarditis /-kärdī´-/, inflammation of the entire heart.

Pancoast's syndrome, 1. a lung tumor characterized by pain in the arm and weakening of the muscles of the arm and hand. This is caused by the damaging effects of the tumor on the brachial plexus. **2.** bone destruction in one or more ribs and the spine.

pancreas /pan′krē·əs/, a fish-shaped, grayish-pink gland about 5 inches long that stretches across the posterior portion of the abdomen, behind the stomach. It releases insulin, glucagon, somastatin, and enzymes of digestion. Small ducts empty into the main duct that runs the length of the organ. The main duct empties into the intestine at the same spot as the exit of the common bile duct. About 1 million cell units (islands of Langerhans) are in the pancreas. Beta cells release insulin, which helps control the body's use of carbohydrate. Alpha cells release glucagon, which counters the action of insulin. Other units of the pancreas release enzymes that help digest fats and proteins.

pancreatectomy /pan′krē·ətek′-/, surgical removal of all or part of the pancreas.

pancreatic dornase, an enzyme from beef pancreas, used to treat lung disease.

pancreatic duct, the main releasing channel of the pancreas. The **accessory pancreatic duct** is a small opening into the pancreatic duct or the first section of the duodenum.

pancreatic enzyme, any one of the several digestion enzymes released by the pancreas. *See also chymotrypsin, pancreatic juice.*

pancreatic hormone, any one of several hormones released by the pancreas. Major hormones are insulin and glucagon. *See also glucagon, insulin.*

pancreatic insufficiency, inadequate release of pancreatic hormones or enzymes. Loss of appetite, failure of the body to absorb food and heavy weight loss often occur. Alcohol-induced pancreatitis is the most common form of this condition.

pancreatic juice, the fluids released by the pancreas. They are made as a reaction to the arrival of food in the duodenum. Pancreatic juice contains water, protein, salts, and many enzymes. The juice is necessary to break down proteins into amino acids, turn fats in the diet to fatty acids, and to change starch to simple sugars.

pancreatitis /-tī′-/, inflammation of the pancreas. **Acute pancreatitis** is often the result of damage to the gallbladder by alcohol, injury, in-

fection, or drugs. Symptoms are severe abdominal pain radiating to the back, fever, anorexia, nausea, and vomiting. Jaundice may also be present. The causes of **chronic pancreatitis** are like those of the acute form. When the cause is alcohol abuse, there may be calcium deposits and scars in the smaller ducts of the pancreas. There is abdominal pain, nausea, and vomiting.

pancreatolith /pan′krē·at′ōlith/, a stone in the pancreas.

pancytopenia /pan′sītəpē′nē·ə/, a marked reduction in the number of red and white blood cells and platelets. *See also anemia.*

pandemic /pandem′ik/, a disease that occurs throughout a population, as a large influenza epidemic.

panel, 1. a group or series of laboratory tests. **2.** multilayered wood sheet used to support the walls of a trench.

panencephalitis /pan′ensef′əlī′-/, inflammation of the entire brain. It is often viral in origin.

panesthesia /pan′esthē′zhə/, the total of all feelings. Compare **cenesthesia.**

panic, a strong, sudden fear that causes terror that may result in being unable to move or in senseless, uncontrolled behavior.

panniculus /panik′yələs/, *pl.* **panniculi,** a membrane made of many sheets of fascia covering a structure in the body.

panophthalmitis /pan′ofthalmī′-/, inflammation of the entire eye, usually caused by a bacteria. Symptoms are pain, fever, headache, and edema. The iris may appear muddy and gray.

pantothenic acid /pan′təthen′ik/, a member of the vitamin B complex, and an important element in food.

paper bag syndrome, *(informal)* the occurrence of a pneumothorax when trauma occurs against an expanded chest and a closed glottis. The resultant large increase in intrathoracic and alveolar pressures causes rupture of alveoli without rib fracture necessarily occurring. *See also pneumothorax, pulmonary overpressurization syndrome.*

papilla /pəpil′ə/, *pl.* **papillae, 1.** a small papule, as the cone-shaped (conoid) papillae on the surface of the tongue. **2.** the optic papilla, a tiny white disc in the retina of the eye, known as the "blind spot."

papillary muscle, any of the muscles joined to the chordae tendineae in the ventricles of the heart. The papillary muscles help to open and close the valves.

papilledema /pap´iləde¯´mə/, swelling of the optic disc caused by increased intracranial pressure.

papillitis /pap´ilī´-/, inflammation of a papilla.

papule /pap´yo͞ol/, a small, solid, raised pimple-like bump, as of acne. Compare **macula. –papular,** *adj.*

-para, a combining form meaning a "woman who has given birth to children in a number of pregnancies." *See also parity.*

paracoccidioidomycosis /-koksid´e¯oi´do¯mīko¯´-/, a chronic, sometimes fatal, fungal infection. It causes ulcers of the mouth, larynx, and nose. The disease typically occurs in Mexico and South America.

paradoxic agitation, a period of unexpected excitement that sometimes follows the use of a tranquilizer.

paradoxical motion, the opposing movement to normal chest motion, of the detached section of ribs, seen in flail chest. *See also flail chest, paradoxic breathing.*

paradoxical pulse. See **pulsus paradoxus.**

paradoxical respirations. See **paradoxic breathing.**

paradoxic breathing, the respiratory situation induced when the fractured segment of a flail chest moves opposite that of the normal chest. This decreases effectiveness of pulmonary function and may lead to hypoxia. Also known as **paradoxical respirations.** *See also paradoxical motion.*

paragonimiasis /per´əgon´imī´əsis/, an infection with a lung fluke (*Paragonimus kellicotti*). It occurs most often in North American minks and can be carried to humans. The disease may also be caused by eating fluke cysts from infected freshwater crabs or crayfish.

parainfluenza virus /-in´flo͞o·en´zə/, a virus that causes respiratory infections in infants and young children and, less commonly, in adults. There are four types of the virus. Types 1 and 2 parainfluenza viruses may cause a form of bronchitis or croup. Type 3 may cause croup, bronchitis, and bronchopneumonia in children. Types 1, 3, and 4 are linked to pharyngitis and the common cold. Compare **influenza, rhinovirus.**

parallel trench, (*trench rescue*) a previously excavated and backfilled trench that is near and parallel to another trench being dug.

paralysis /pəral´əsis/, *pl.* **paralyses,** the loss of muscle use or sensation or both. It may be caused by injury or disease. Paralyses may be named for their cause, the effects on muscle tone and their spread, or the part of the body affected. **–paralytic,** *adj.*

paralysis agitans /aj´itəns/. See **Parkinson's disease.**

paralytic ileus, a decrease or absence of intestinal peristalsis due to illness, injury, or surgery; frequently, this condition results in intestinal obstruction. Signs/symptoms include absent bowel sounds, nausea or vomiting, and a tender abdomen. Also known as **adynamic ileus.**

paramedic, prehospital provider of advanced emergency medical care; a physician extender. Advanced skills usually include EKG interpretation, endotracheal intubation, intermediate-to-advanced pharmacology and intravenous therapy, and sophisticated physical assessment. Requirements for certification or licensure vary from state to state, with educational programs varying from 300 to 2500 hours in length. The emergency department physician is the person to whom the paramedic is responsible. Physician treatment decisions may be communicated via radio/phone, written protocols, or both. *See also EMT, off-line medical control, on-line medical control.*

parametritis, inflammation of the tissue of the structures near the uterus. *See also pelvic inflammatory disease.*

paramnesia /per´amne¯´zhə/, a memory defect in which one believes one remembers events that never happened. Compare **déjà vu.**

paramyxovirus /-mik´so¯-/, a member of a family of viruses that includes those that cause mumps.

paranasal /-nā´zəl/, near or alongside the nose.

paranasal sinus, one of the cavities in bones around the nose, such as the frontal sinus in the forehead.

paranoia, a mental disorder marked by a complex system of thinking. Delusions of persecution and grandeur usually center on one major theme, as a job situation or an unfaithful spouse.

Symptoms include resentment or hostility, severe anger, and demanding unrealistic things of others. **Acute hallucinatory paranoia** is a disorder in which one sees and hears things that are not there and believes things that are not true.

paranoid, 1. a person with a paranoid disorder. 2. (*informal*) a person who is too suspicious or who feels overly persecuted.

paranoid disorder, any of a large group of mental disorders marked by a damaged sense of reality and continuing delusions. An **acute paranoid disorder** is a condition that develops quickly, lasting usually less than 6 months. It is most commonly seen in persons who have had major changes in their environment, such as immigrants, refugees, prisoners, and military inductees. A **shared paranoid disorder** is one in which two close or related patients have exactly the same symptoms. *See also paranoia.*

paranoid reaction, a behavior associated with aging and with the gradual formation of delusions, usually of a persecution, and often accompanied by hallucinations. Other signs of senility, such as memory loss and confusion, do not usually accompany the reaction, and the person is aware of time, place, and self.

paranoid schizophrenia, a form of schizophrenia marked by preoccupation with absurd and changeable delusions, usually of persecution or jealousy, accompanied by hallucinations. Symptoms include extreme anxiety, exaggerated suspiciousness, anger, and violence. The condition occurs most often during middle age. *See also schizophrenia.*

parapertussis /-pərtus´is/, an acute bacterial infection with symptoms closely resembling those of whooping cough (pertussis). It is usually milder, although it can be fatal. It is possible to have both infections at the same time.

parapharyngeal abscess /-ferin´jē·əl/, an infection of tissues near the throat, usually as a complication of tonsillitis.

paraplegia /-plē´jə/, motor nerve or sensory loss in the legs, resulting from damage to the spinal cord. This condition usually occurs after trauma or in disease conditions, such as scoliosis and spina bifida. Signs of paraplegia often develop immediately after injury and include loss of sensation, motion, and reflexes below the nerve root damaged.

parapsychology, a branch of psychology concerned with the study of alleged psychic phenomena, such as clairvoyance, extrasensory perception, and telepathy.

paraquat /per´əkwət/, a toxic pesticide (paraquat dichloride).

parasagittal plane, an imaginary vertical plane passing through the body parallel to the medial plane, thereby dividing the body into right and left segments.

parasite /-sīt/, an organism which depends on a host for nourishment in order to survive. A **facultative parasite** may live on a host but is capable of living independently. An **obligate parasite** is one that depends entirely on its host for survival.

parasitemia /-ē´mē·ə/, the presence of parasites in the blood.

parasympathetic, referring to the properties of the parasympathetic nervous system.

parasympathetic nervous system, a division of the autonomic nervous system. Mediated by the action of the neurotransmitter acetylcholine, this system performs many functions, including increased intestinal activity during digestion and slowed heart rates. *See also autonomic nervous system, peripheral nervous system, central nervous system, sympathetic nervous system.*

parasympatholytic /-sim´pəthōlit´ik/. See **anticholinergic.**

parasympathomimetic /-mimet´ik/, a substance causing effects similar to those caused by acting on a parasympathetic nerve. Also known as **cholinergic.**

parasystole, an ectopic rhythm whose pacemaker cannot be discharged by the dominant rhythm because of depressed conduction in the area surrounding the parasystolic focus.

parathyroid hormone, a hormone released by the parathyroid glands that acts to control the absorption or release of calcium and phosphorus in the body.

paratyphoid fever /-tī´foid/, a bacterial infection, caused by *Salmonella*. Symptoms appear like typhoid fever, although milder. *See also salmonellosis, typhoid fever.*

parenchyma /pəreng´kimə/, the working tissue of an organ as opposed to supporting or connective tissue.

parent, a mother or father; one who has offspring. **–parental,** *adj.*

parenteral /pəren´tərəl/, a method of administration which allows medication to be absorbed across or through tissues that are not part of the gastrointestinal tract, as intravenous, intramuscular. **–parenterally,** *adv.*

parenteral absorption, taking up substances into the body other than by the digestive tract.

paresis /pərē´-, per´əsis/, less than total paralysis or muscular weakness.

paresthesia, heightened sensitivity; tingling or prickling sensations due to disease or body position.

parietal /pərī´ətəl/, **1.** the outer wall of a space or organ. **2.** referring to the parietal bones of the skull or the parietal lobe of the brain.

parietal lobe. See **brain.**

parietal pericardium, the portion of serous pericardium that lines the fibrous pericardium.

parietal peritoneum, the peritoneum that lines the abdominal walls.

parity, 1. a woman's condition with regard to the number of children she has borne. This is part of a description of a woman's childbearing history, which comprises three categories: gravid (number of pregnancies), parity (number of live births), and abort (number of abortions, miscarriages, and stillbirths). This information is charted as gravida/para/ab. A woman with a history of 3 pregnancies, 2 of which were born alive and 1 of which was a miscarriage, is noted as gravida 3, para 2, ab 1. **2.** similar; equal to.

parkinsonism, having symptoms characteristic of Parkinson's disease. Difficulty with daily activities, paralysis, shuffling gait, and tremors are hallmarks of this disorder. Precipitating factors include carbon monoxide poisoning, malaria, polio, and tranquilizer use.

Parkinson's disease (James Parkinson, British physician, 1755-1824), a chronic nervous system disease characterized by muscular weakness and rigidity, shuffling gait, and fine muscle tremors. Thinking and reasoning are generally not affected. Although the cause is unknown, imbalances of dopamine and acetylcholine are noted. Also known as **paralysis agitans.**

Parkland formula, formula for estimating fluid requirements in burn patients. This formula is equal to 4 ml/kg/% body surface area burned. One-half of the total amount is given over the first 8 hours from time of injury, and the remainder is given over the following 16 hours. Also known as **Baxter formula.** *See also Brooke formula, consensus formula, Shrine burn formula.*

paronychia /per´ənik´ē·ə/, an infection of the fold of skin at the edge of a nail.

parosmia /pəroz´mē·ə/, any disorder of the sense of smell.

parotitis /per´ətī´-/. See **mumps.**

paroxysm /per´əksizm/, **1.** a marked rise in symptoms. **2.** a seizure or spasm. **–paroxysmal,** *adj.*

paroxysmal atrial tachycardia, atrial tachycardia characterized by sudden onset and termination. Also known as **PAT.**

paroxysmal nocturnal dyspnea, sudden onset of shortness of breath while sleeping, usually due to positional pulmonary edema in cardiac patients. A patient with borderline congestive heart failure sleeps on several pillows at night to avoid this symptom. Slipping off this support may precipitate pulmonary edema, waking them with difficulty breathing. Although due to the same factors that cause orthopnea, this condition is not always relieved by sitting upright. Symptoms include coughing and wheezing. Also known as **PND.** *See also orthopnea.*

paroxysmal supraventricular tachycardia, any tachycardia with a pacemaker site above the level of the ventricles that begins and ends suddenly and otherwise cannot be more accurately identified. Also known as **PSVT, SVT.** *See also supraventricular tachycardia.*

Parrot's sign (Jules Marie Parrot, French physician, 1839-1883), in meningitis, the pupils dilate when the skin of the neck is pinched.

parthenogenesis /pär´thənōjen´əsis/, a type of reproduction in which an organism grows from an unfertilized egg (ovum).

partial non-rebreather oxygen mask. See **non-rebreather oxygen mask.**

partial pressure, the pressure that is exerted by a single gas in a mixture of gases. It can be denoted by the letter P preceding the gas symbol (PCO_2).

partial reabsorption, amount of a drug reabsorbed from the renal tubule by passive diffusion.

parturition /pär´tyərish´ən/, the process of giving birth.

Pascal's law, a pressure applied to any part of a fluid will be transmitted equally throughout the fluid.

passive-aggressive personality, a behavior in which strong actions or opinions are given in an indirect, nonviolent manner, as pouting, being difficult, or forgetful.

passive-dependent personality, a behavior marked by helplessness, being unable to make a decision, and often clinging to and seeking support from others.

passive glomerular filtration, fluid in the blood that is filtered across capillaries of the glomerulus and into Bowman's capsule.

passive smoking, the breathing in by nonsmokers of the smoke from other people's smoking.

Pasteurella /pas´tərel´ə/, a group of bacteria, including species that cause disease in humans. *Pasteurella* infections may be carried by animal bites.

patch, a small, flat spot on skin that differs in color or texture from skin in close proximity to it. Also known as **macule.**

patella, the sesamoid bone, located anterior to the knee joint. Also known as **kneecap, kneepan.**

patellar ligament, a ligament that stretches from the tendon above the knee across the patella. It joins with the tibia.

patellar reflex. See **deep tendon reflex.**

patent, accessible; intact; open; evident.

patent ductus arteriosus, an opening between the pulmonary artery and aorta caused by the fetal ductus arteriosus failing to close after birth. *See also congenital heart disease.*

-pathic, 1. a combining form referring to an illness or affected part of the body. **2.** a combining form referring to a form or system of treatment.

pathogen /path´əjən/, any microorganism able to cause a disease. **–pathogenic,** *adj.*

pathogenicity, capable of producing disease in a susceptible host.

pathognomonic, indicative of a disease.

pathology /pathol´-/, the study of the traits, etiology, and effects of disease, as seen in the structure and workings of the body. In **autopsy pathology,** a disease is studied in a body after death. **Clinical pathology** is the laboratory study of disease by a pathologist. It includes hematology, bacteriology, chemistry, and serology. **–pathologic,** *adj.*

pathway, a group of neurons that make a route for nerve signals between any part of the body and the spinal cord or the brain.

patient, one who requires health care assessment or who is ill or injured and receiving health care. Also known as **pt.** *See also victim.*

patient assessment. See **assessment.**

patient record, compiled documentation of patient care and treatment. For prehospital purposes, this is one form upon which all patient history, physical exam, and treatment information is recorded. For hospital purposes, this is a group of forms that combine laboratory, x-ray, and other diagnostic information with patient examination and treatment information. Also known as **chart, EMS form.**

Patient's Bill of Rights, a list of patient's rights drawn up by the American Hospital Association. It offers guidelines for patient and family treatment during a stay in the hospital.

Pauwel's fracture /pou´əlz/, a fracture of the proximal neck of the femur, near the socket.

peak plasma level, the highest circulating concentration achieved by a drug, gas, or toxin. Also known as **peak level.**

peak time, the time (usually minutes or hours) when a substance exerts its maximum effect.

pectin, a substance found in fruits and vegetables. It adds bulk to the diet. *See also dietary fiber.*

pectineus /pektin´ē·əs/, one of the femoral muscles. It moves the thigh and turns it toward the midline of the body.

pectoralis major /pek´tərā´lis/, a large fan-shaped muscle of the upper thoracic wall. It flexes and rotates the arm at the shoulder joint.

pectoralis minor, a thin, triangle-shaped muscle under the pectoralis major. It rotates the scapula, pulling it down and forward, and raises the upper ribs in forced inspiration.

pectus deformity, deformed chest wall.

pediatric dose /pē´dē·at´-/, the correct dose of a drug given to a child or infant based on the age, weight, body surface area, and the action of the drug in the child. **Cowling's rule:** (age at next birthday/24) × adult dose.

pediatrics, a branch of medicine focusing on the growth and care of children. Its special focus is on the diseases of children and their treatment and prevention. **–pediatric,** *adj.*

Pediatric Trauma Score, an injury severity scale for children that categorizes six elements of trauma. These elements are airway, systolic blood pressure, central nervous system function, wounds, weight, and skeletal injury. When combined together, the scores of each of these elements can accurately and objectively reflect a pediatric trauma patient's condition.

pediculosis, infestation with lice (pediculus). Lice are vectors for transmission of bubonic plague, trench fever, typhus, and relapsing fever. **Pediculosis capitis** is infestation with head lice (*Pediculus humanus*). **Pediculosis corporis** is infestation with body lice (*Pediculus humanus corporis*). **Pediculosis pubis** is infestation with crab lice (*Phthirus pubis*). Also known as **louse.**

pedophilia /ped´əfil´ə/, **1.** an abnormal interest in children. **2.** a disorder in which adults participate in sexual activity with children. **–pedophilic,** *adj.*

peduncle /pədung´kəl/, a stalk or stemlike connecting part of a growth or tissue.

peer review, process of review of documentation, manuscripts, procedures, or research for their professional and technical merit by others in the same field.

pellagra /pəlag´rə, pəlā´grə/, a disease resulting from a lack of niacin or tryptophan. Persons with diets made up of foods lacking in tryptophan, such as cornmeal and porkfat, are at risk. Symptoms include lesions, especially on skin exposed to the sun, inflammation of the mucous membranes, and diarrhea. **Pellagra sine pellagra** is a form in which skin symptoms are absent. **Typhoid pellagra** is a type in which the symptoms also include fever.

pelvic, referring to the pelvis.

pelvic cellulitis, a bacterial infection of the tissues around the cervix.

pelvic floor, the muscles and tissues surrounding the inferior portion of the pelvis.

pelvic inflammatory disease, a disease of the female pelvic organs, usually caused by bacteria. Symptoms include fever, vaginal discharge, pain in the lower abdomen, bleeding, and painful sexual intercourse. Also known as **PID.** *See also endometritis.*

pelvifemoral /pel´vifem´ərəl/, referring to the structures of the hip joint. Included are the muscles and the space around the bony pelvis and the head of the femur.

pelvis, *pl.* **pelves,** the lower portion of the trunk of the body. It is composed of four bones: the two hip (innominate) bones located anterio-laterally and the sacrum and coccyx. It divides into the greater (false) pelvis and the lesser (true) pelvis. The greater pelvis is the larger part of the space above a bony rim that divides the two parts. The lesser pelvis is inferior to the rim. Its bony walls are more complete than those of the greater pelvis.

pendulum maneuver, a helicopter technique for delivering supplies to rescuers located on a vertical or overhanging wall. A rope or hoist cable is set into a swinging motion by rocking the helicopter or directly pushing and pulling the rope. A rescuer tied into the wall grasps the rope and pulls the rope to the ledge.

penetrate, to pierce; to pass deeper into.

penetration, **1.** forcing into; spreading through. **2.** the passage of a hazardous chemical through pinholes, stitched seams, zippers, or imperfections in the material. Chemical protective clothing can be penetrated at several locations, including the face piece and exhalation valve, suit exhaust valves, and suit fasteners. The potential for penetration generally increases in excessively cold or hot temperatures.

penicillinase /-ās/, an enzyme produced by certain bacteria, including staphylococci, that stops the action of penicillin. This causes resistance to the antibiotic. Also known as **beta-lacta-mase.**

peninsula, a body of land nearly surrounded by water.

penis, the outer reproductive organ of a male. The penis is made up of three tubular masses of spongy tissue covered with skin. Two of these masses (corpora cavernosa) partially surround the third one (corpus spongiosum). The corpus spongiosum contains the urethra.

penniform,   referring to the shape of a feather, especially in muscle fibers.

pentose,   a five carbon sugar produced by the body and also found in some fruits, as plums and cherries.

pentosuria /pen´təsŏŏr´e·ə/,   sugar (pentose) in the urine.

pepper gas,   oleoresin capsicum; the riot control agent (harassing chemical) in most frequent use by law enforcement agencies. It causes a burning sensation on the skin, severe tearing, and increased mucous production for up to one hour after contact. *See also chemical agent.*

pep pills,   *(slang)* amphetamines.

pepsin,   an enzyme released in the stomach that speeds up the breakdown of protein. *See also enzyme.*

pepsinogen,   a primary component of the enzyme pepsin, secreted by cells of the gastric mucosa and used in protein digestion.

peptic,   1. relating to digestion. **2.** relating to pepsin.

peptic ulcer,   loss of mucous membrane in any part of the digestive system, which allows unprotected tissue to come in contact with gastric fluid. A **duodenal ulcer** is the most common type of peptic ulcer. A **channel ulcer** is a rare type of peptic ulcer found in the pyloric canal, which is between the stomach and the duodenum. Acute ulcers are almost always shallow and occur in groups. They may occur with or without symptoms and heal without scars. Chronic ulcers are true ulcers. They are deep, occur singly, and cause symptoms. The muscular wall of the tract is permanently damaged. A scar forms, and the mucous membrane may heal, but not the muscle under it. Also known as **gastric ulcer.** *See also ulcer.*

peptide /pep´tīd/,   a molecular chain of two or more amino acids. *See also amino acid, polypeptide, protein.*

peptide bond,   the chemical bond between amino acids.

percentage,   the number of parts in a hundred, denoted by the symbol %.

perception,   detecting and interpreting nerve impulses from the sense organs. The ability to judge depth or the distance between objects is called **depth perception.** Vision from both eyes is essential to this ability. **Facial perception** refers to the ability to judge the distance and direction of objects through feeling in the skin of the face. It is commonly felt by those who are blind. **Stereognostic perception** refers to the ability to recognize objects by the sense of touch.

perceptual defect,   any of a broad group of disorders of the nervous system which dampens the conscious sensing of nerve signals.

percussion,   a tapping of the body's surface used to ascertain the size and texture of thoracic and abdominal organs. It is also used to detect the presence of fluid or gas in a body space. **Immediate** or **direct percussion** refers to percussion done by striking the fingers on the surface of the chest or abdomen. **Indirect, mediate** or **finger percussion** is striking a finger of one hand on a finger of the other hand as it is placed over an organ. **Palpatory percussion** is done using light pressure with the flat of the hand.

percutaneous /pur´kyŏŏtā´ne·əs/,   a medical procedure performed through the skin, such as a biopsy or intravenous cannulation.

percutaneous transtracheal ventilation.   See **jet insufflation.**

perforate,   to make a hole. **–perforation,** *n.*

perforating fracture,   an open fracture caused by an object, such as a bullet.

perfusion,   1. fluid passing through an organ or a part of the body. **2.** supplying an organ or tissue with nutrients and oxygen via the circulatory system.

periapical /per´e·ap´ikəl/,   the tissues around the root of a tooth, including the gums and bones.

periapical abscess,   an infection around the root of a tooth, usually spread from tooth cavities. The abscess may penetrate nearby bone or soft tissues.

periappendiceal abscess,   a purulent and inflamed tissue sac near the vermiform appendix.

periarteritis /per´e·är´təri´-/,   an inflammation of the outer layer of an artery and the tissue around it.

periarteritis nodosa, a connective tissue disease with many nodules along arteries. This causes blockage of the vessel, resulting in ischemia, bleeding, and pain. Symptoms include tachycardia, fever, weight loss, and abdominal pain.

pericardial fluid, a lubricating fluid found between the visceral and parietal pericardium.

pericardial friction rub, a dry, grating sound heard during thoracic auscultation that may be indicative of pericarditis.

pericardial sac, a loose-fitting membrane that surrounds the heart. It is divided into an outer fibrous membrane and an inner serous layer. Also known as **pericardium.**

pericardial tamponade, compression of the heart due to increased pressure within the pericardial sac due to accumulated fluid or blood.

pericardiocentesis, withdrawing fluid from the pericardial sac to relieve pressure being exerted on the heart.

pericarditis, inflammation of the pericardium. Symptoms include chest pain, dry cough, dyspnea, fever, and palpitations.

pericardium /-kär´dē·əm/, *pl.* **pericardia,** a double-layered membrane around the heart. **–pericardial,** *adj.*

pericholangitis /-kō´lanjī´-/, inflammation of the tissues around bile ducts in the liver due to ulcerative colitis. Symptoms include fever, chills, and jaundice. *See also colitis.*

perilymph /-limf/, a clear fluid in the inner ear.

perimeter, a boundary that restricts movement into areas of interest or danger. *See also inner perimeter, kill zone, outer perimeter.*

perinatal /-nā´təl/, referring to the time and process of giving birth or being born.

perinatology /-tol´-/, a branch of medicine that studies the anatomy and physiology of the mother and her infant during pregnancy, childbirth, and the 28 days after birth.

perineum, the area comprising the pelvic floor, medial to the thighs. The penis, rectum, vagina, and supporting structures are located here.

period, *(nontechnical)* menses.

periodic, rhythmic repetition.

periodontal /per´ē·ōdon´təl/, the space and tissues surrounding the teeth.

periodontal disease, disease of the tissues around the teeth.

periodontitis /-ōdontī´-/, inflammation of the tissue that joins the teeth and gums.

periosteum /per´ē·os´tē·əm/, a fiberlike covering of the bones, except at their ends. There is an outer layer of connective tissue with fat cells and an inner layer of fine elastic fibers. Periosteum contains the nerves and blood vessels that supply the bones.

periostitis /-ostī´-/, inflammation of the elastic periosteum. Infection or injury causes tenderness and swelling around the bone with pain, fever, and chills.

peripheral, referring to the outer portions or surface of a body, organ, or structure; the periphery.

peripheral nervous system, the motor and sensory nerves excluding the brain and spinal cord. The system has 12 pairs of cranial nerves, 31 pairs of spinal nerves, and their many branches in body organs. Sensory nerves carry signals to the brain and spinal cord. Motor nerves carry signals from the brain to other parts of the body. Somatic nerves act on the body wall; visceral nerves supply internal organs. *See also autonomic nervous system.*

peripheral neuropathy, any disorder of the peripheral nervous system.

peripheral thermoreceptors, heat-sensitive nerve endings located in skin and some mucous membranes. These receptors provide an awareness of both hot and cold.

peripheral vascular disease, any condition that affects the blood vessels outside of the heart and the major vessels. Symptoms include numbness, pain, high blood pressure, and pulse deficits. Causes include being overweight, cigarette smoking, stress, and lack of activity. When linked to an infection of the heart (bacterial endocarditis), blood clots may form in arterioles causing necrosis in many parts of the body, such as the tip of the nose, fingers, or toes. Some forms of peripheral vascular disease include **arteriosclerosis** and **atherosclerosis.**

peripheral vascular resistance, the total resistance against which blood is pumped. This resistance is determined by blood vessel size and blood viscosity. Also known as **afterload, systemic vascular resistance.**

peripheral vision, sight that occurs at the outer edges of perceptible vision. Objects that move into our field of vision are first perceived in the periphery. The ability to see these objects requires that sight be focused not on one object but on the area as a whole. Normal is approximately 180°. *See also photopic vision, purkinje shift, scotopic vision.*

peristalsis /per´istôl-/, the wavelike, rhythmic contraction of smooth muscle. It forces food through the digestive tract, bile through the bile duct, and urine through the ureters.

peritoneal cavity /per´itōnē´əl/, a space between the parietal and visceral layers of the peritoneum.

peritoneal dialysis. See **dialysis.**

peritoneum /-tōnē´əm/, membrane that covers the entire wall of the abdomen and is folded over the inner organs (viscera). It is divided into outer (parietal) and inner (visceral) membranes. The **parietal peritoneum** is the layer that lines the wall of the abdomen. The **visceral peritoneum** is the largest membrane in the body that covers the viscera. The free surface of the peritoneum permits the organs to glide against the wall and against one another. **–peritoneal,** *adj.*

peritonitis /-tōnī´-/, inflammation of the peritoneum, caused by bacteria or substances from a wound or perforation of an organ. Peritonitis is caused most often by a ruptured appendix. When the condition is caused by scar tissue between two surfaces, it is known as **adhesive peritonitis.** Symptoms of peritonitis include ascites, pain, nausea, vomiting, and fever. *See also appendectomy, appendicitis.*

peritubular capillary, a network of capillaries located in the cortex of the kidney.

permanent tooth. See **dentition, tooth.**

permeable /pur´mē·əbəl/, allowing fluids and/or other substances to pass through. *See also osmosis.*

permeation, the process by which a liquid moves through a given material on the molecular level. This process is significant in personal protective equipment contamination and decontamination.

Permissible Exposure Limit, the maximum time-weighted concentration at which 95% of exposed, healthy adults suffer no adverse effects over a 40-hour work week. It is an 8-hour, time-weighted average concentration, unless otherwise noted, expressed in either ppm or mg/cu meter. They are commonly used by OSHA in evaluating work place exposures and can be found in the NIOSH *Pocket Guide to Chemical Hazards.* Also known as **recommended exposure limit.**

pernicious anemia /pərnish´əs/. See **nutritional anemia.**

pernio. See **chilblains.**

peroneal, referring to the lateral portion of the lower leg or the fibula.

persistent generalized lymphadenopathy, lymph node enlargement found in at least two sites other than the groin. HIV infections show this symptom at an early stage in the disease.

persona, *pl.* **personae,** the role that a person takes and presents to the world to satisfy the demands of society or as part of some mental conflict. The persona masks the person's inner being.

personal flotation device, flotation equipment, approved by the U.S. Coast Guard for use while around water. These devices, used for boating, swimming, and scuba diving, may provide full-time flotation or require inflation prior to use. They may be wearable, such as buoyant vests, life preservers, and special-purpose vests, or throwable, such as ring buoys and throwable cushions. Also known as **life preserver, PFD.** *See also life belt, ring buoy.*

personality, pattern of behavior each person develops as a means of dealing with the surroundings and their cultural, ethnic, and other standards.

perspiration. See **diaphoresis.**

pertinent negative, a physical finding that is within normal limits, but pertains to the patient's chief complaint. These are usually discussed with other medical caregivers to provide an accurate picture of a patient's condition.

pertussis, an acute, contagious illness with severe coughing that ends in a loud whooping sound. Seen primarily in unimmunized children under four years old, it is spread directly by airborne droplets via coughing or sneezing and indirectly by contact with patient belongings.

Signs/symptoms include cough, dyspnea, fever, lack of appetite, and sneezing. Also known as **whooping cough.**

perversion, any variation from what is considered normal or natural behavior.

pes /pēz/, the foot or a footlike structure.

pes planus, flatfoot.

petechiae small purple or red spots that appear on the skin because of isolated areas of hemorrhage under the skin. Petechiae range from pinpoint to pinhead size and are flat with the surface. Compare **ecchymosis. –petechial,** *adj.*

petit mal seizure /pətē´mäl´, pet´emal´/. See **seizure.**

petrolatum, a soft, purified substance obtained from petroleum and used in ointments. Also known as **petroleum jelly.**

petroleum distillate poisoning, a toxic condition caused by swallowing or breathing a petroleum product, such as gasoline, kerosene, fuel oil, model airplane cement, and some solvents. Nausea, vomiting, chest pain, dizziness, and altered levels of consciousness are symptoms.

peyote /pā·ō´tē/, a cactus from which a hallucinogenic drug, mescaline, is made.

pH, symbol for the negative logarithm of hydrogen ion concentration of a substance (moles per liter). A value of 7.0 is neutral (at 71.6° F, or 22° C); greater than 7.0 is alkaline; less than 7.0 is acidic. Normal blood pH is 7.4 (range of 7.36-7.44).

phagocyte /fag´əsīt/, a cell that is able to surround, engulf, and digest small living things, as bacteria. **Fixed phagocytes** do not move in the blood. They include fixed cells and some connective tissue cells. **Free phagocytes** move in the blood and include white blood cells (leukocytes) and free cells.

phagocytosis /-sītō´-/, the process by which some cells of the body engulf and digest bacteria and cell wastes.

phakomatosis /fak´ōmətō´-/, *pl.* **phakomatoses,** a group of congenital diseases characterized by nodules of the eye, skin, and brain.

phalanx /fālan´gks/, *pl.* **phalanges** /fālan´jēz/, any one of the bones making up the fingers of each hand and the toes of each foot. Each hand or foot has 14 phalanges.

phantom limb syndrome, a sensation common after the removal of a limb. The patient has the impression of sensation in the missing limb.

pharmaceutic /fär´məsoō´-/, referring to pharmacy or medical drugs.

pharmacodynamics, the study of a drug's action on a living organism; the biochemical response of the cells to a drug.

pharmacokinetics /fär´məkōkinet´-/, the study of the movement of drugs in the body.

pharmacology /-kol´-/, the study of the production ingredients, uses, and actions of drugs.

pharyngeal reflex /ferin´jē·əl/. See **gag reflex.**

pharyngeal tonsil. See **adenoid.**

pharyngitis /fer´injī´-/, inflammation or infection of the pharynx, usually causing a sore throat. *See also strep throat.*

pharynx /fer´ingks/, the throat, a tubelike structure that is a passage for both the respiratory and digestive systems. The pharynx is made of muscle and is lined with mucous membrane. It contains openings for the eustachian tubes, posterior nares, larynx, esophagus, and tonsils. It is divided into three regions. The **nasopharynx** is posterior to the nasal cavity. It originates posterior to the internal nare and extends to the level of the uvula. The **oropharynx** extends inferiorly from the soft palate in the posterior oral cavity to the level of the hyoid bone below the mandible. The **laryngopharynx** extends from the hyoid bone at the base of the tongue to the esophagus. Also known as **throat.** *See also larynx.*

phencyclidine psychosis, a psychiatric emergency with behaviors ranging from unresponsive to violent. The illicit drug phencyclidine precipitates this crisis, and an occurrence may last days to weeks. Also known as **PCP.**

phenocopy /fē´nōkop´ē/, a physical trait or condition that one is not born with, but appears as a trait that is congenital. Conditions as deafness, mental retardation, and cataracts can be inherited, but they can also result from infections or other causes.

phenol /fē´nôl/, a highly poisonous, harsh chemical taken from coal or plant tar or made in a laboratory. It has a strong odor and is a potent cleaning fluid (carbolic acid).

phenol poisoning, poisoning caused by swallowing compounds with phenol, such as carbolic acid, creosote, and naphthol. Phenol poisoning causes burns of the mouth, seizures, and major organ failure.

phenomenon /finom´ənon/, a sign that is often connected to a particular illness or condition and is important in diagnosing.

phenothiazine, the organic compound that is the primary component of a class of tranquilizers. Also used to produce dyes, insecticides, and veterinary antihelmintics. *See also extrapyramidal reaction.*

phenotype /fē´nōtīp/, **1.** the traits of an individual or group one can see. They are caused by the interactions of heredity and the environment. **2.** a group of organisms that look like each other. Compare **genotype. –phenotypic,** *adj.*

phenylalanine, an amino acid needed for the normal growth of infants and children. It is also needed for normal protein utilization throughout life. It is found in large amounts in milk, eggs, and other foods. *See also amino acid, phenylketonuria, protein.*

phenylketonuria /fe´nəlkē´tōno̅o̅r´ē·ə/, a birth defect in which an enzyme needed to change an amino acid (phenylalanine) into tyrosine is lacking.

phenytoin, an anticonvulsant, effective in the field management of status epilepticus. Central nervous system depression and hypotension are potential side effects of this medication. Although there are no contraindications for field use, it is generally used for status epilepticus only when the patient is allergic and/or unresponsive to diazepam or midazolam. Also known as **Dilantin.**

pheochromocytoma /fē´ōkrō´mōsītō´mə/, a tumor of the adrenal gland that increases the release of epinephrine and norepinephrine. Symptoms include high blood pressure, headache, excess blood glucose, nausea, vomiting, and syncope.

phimosis vaginalis /vaj´inā´lis/, a congenital narrowing of the opening of the vagina.

phi phenomenon /fī/, a feeling of motion that is caused by lights that flash on and off at a certain rate. Also known as **stroboscopic illusion.**

phlebitis /flebī´-/, inflammation of a vein, often along with formation of a clot. It occurs most commonly as the result of injury to the vessel wall, infection, and chemical irritation. Also known as **thrombophlebitis.**

phlebotomus fever /flēbot´əmas/, a mild inflection, due to a virus transmitted to humans by the bite of an infected sandfly. Symptoms include fever, headache, eye pain and inflammation, muscle pain, and a rash.

phlebotomy /flebot´-/, venous blood removal to treat an excess of red blood cells (polycythemia vera). Also known as **venesection.**

phlegm /flem/, thick mucus released by tissues lining the respiratory passages.

phobia, an anxiety problem with an overwhelming and irrational fear.

phonetic alphabet, a word system, utilizing easily spoken words, to represent letters of the alphabet, such as Tango for the letter T. This system is frequently used in radio communications to clarify pronunciation. See Appendix 4-6.

phonic /fon´ik, fō´-/, referring to voice, sounds, or speech.

phosgene, toxic, colorless gas causing severe pulmonary edema by destruction of alveolar tissue. Generally seen as a chemical war gas, it has an odor like new-mown hay. It is categorized as a choking or lung agent.

phosphatase /fos´fətāz/, an enzyme that accelerates chemical reactions with phosphorus. *See also catalyst, enzyme, phosphorus.*

phosphate /fos´fāt/, a substance used in cells for storing and using energy. It also helps transport genetic data within a cell and from one cell to another.

phosphorus /fos´fərəs/, a nonmetal chemical element. It is needed to digest protein, calcium compounds, and glucose. The body uses phosphorus from milk, cheese, meat, egg yolk, whole grains, peas, and nuts. A lack of phosphorus can cause weight loss, anemia, and abnormal growth.

phosphorus poisoning, a condition caused by swallowing white or yellow phosphorus, sometimes found in rat poisons, fertilizers, and fireworks. Symptoms include nausea, throat and stomach pain, vomiting, diarrhea, and an odor of garlic on the breath.

photoallergic contact dermatitis, a skin reaction that occurs 24 to 48 hours after being exposed to light in a person who is put at risk by a substance (photosensitizer) that builds up in the skin. It is changed to active allergic material by light. *See also photosensitizer.*

photodermatoses, skin conditions due to sensitivity to light.

photophobia, 1. abnormal reaction to light, as by the eyes. It occurs in many diseases that affect the conjunctiva and cornea, such as measles. **2.** an anxiety disorder caused by a fear of light.

photopic vision, normal daytime sight; vision primarily utilizing the color-sensitive cones of the eye. *See also peripheral vision, purkinje shift, scotopic vision.*

photosensitive, referring to a reaction of skin to sunlight often caused by certain drugs. A brief exposure to sunlight or to an ultraviolet lamp may cause edema, hives, or burns in patients who are photosensitive. *See also photosensitizer, phototoxic.*

photosensitizer, any substance that may cause an allergic reaction when combined with light. Common photosensitizers are antibiotics (sulfanilamide), antiseptics (hexachlorophene), some birth control pills, tranquilizers (phenothiazene), and a substance (psoralen) found in many plants, as carrots and mustard.

photosynthesis /-sin´thəsis/, a process by which plants with chlorophyll make carbohydrates from carbon dioxide and water. They use sunlight for energy and release oxygen.

phototherapy, treatment of disorders by using light. Ultraviolet light may be used to treat acne, decubitus ulcers, and other skin disorders.

phototoxic, a rapid reaction of the skin to light when exposed to a photosensitizer and light. *See also photosensitive, photosensitizer.*

phrenic nerve /fren´ik/, one of a pair of branches of the fourth cervical nerve. It is a motor nerve to the diaphragm. The **accessory phrenic nerve** joins the phrenic nerve at the base of the neck or in the chest.

phycomycosis /fī´kōmīkō´-/, a fungal infection. Respiratory infection sometimes occurs with late diabetes mellitus that is untreated or out of control. *See also zygomycosis.*

phylogeny /filoj´ənē/, the growth of the structure of a species as it changed from simpler forms of life. Compare **ontogeny.**

physical abuse, physical injury, generally caused by another with whom the injured party has a legal or social relationship, under circumstances that indicate that the injured party's health or welfare is being harmed or threatened. Also known as **nonaccidental trauma.**

physical diagnosis, diagnosis made by external examination only. *See also diagnosis.*

physical or **chemical hazard statement,** a statement displayed on a side panel, as necessary. It will list special flammability, explosion, or chemical hazards posed by the product.

physical examination, examining the body by auscultation, inspection, palpation, percussion, and scent. Although the depth of a prehospital examination is limited by the examiner's proficiency and the patient's chief complaint, much information is gained from a thorough examination. Also known as **physical exam, secondary survey.**

physical fitness, the ability to carry out daily tasks with alertness and vigor with enough energy left to meet emergencies or to enjoy leisure activities.

physician, 1. a person who has earned a degree Doctor of Medicine (MD) after a course of study at an approved medical school. To practice medicine, an MD has to be licensed in the state in which services will be performed. **2.** a person who has earned a degree of Doctor of Osteopathy (D.O.) by completing a course of study at an approved college of osteopathy. Osteopathic physicians and medical physicians follow nearly the same courses of training and practice. Osteopathic medicine places special emphasis on the physical defects of tissues as a cause of illness.

physician extender, a health care provider who is not a physician but who performs certain medical functions done by physicians.

physician's assistant, a person trained to assist a physician. A physician directs and oversees the physician's assistant. Also known as **PA.**

physiologic dead space, those portions of the airway that do not participate in oxygen–carbon dioxide exchange; the anatomic dead space plus nonfunctional alveoli.

physiologic retraction ring, a ridge around the inside of the uterus that forms during the second stage of normal labor. Compare **constriction ring, pathologic retraction ring.**

physiology /fiz´ē·ol´-/, study of the function of the human body.

phytotoxicology, the study of plant poisons.

phytotoxin, the most toxic substances originating in plants. These poisons are grouped into the families Euphorbiaceae (castor bean) and Fabaceae (jequirity bean). They can cause burning of the mouth, nausea, vomiting, altered levels of consciousness, tachydysrhythmias, seizures, and liver failure.

pia mater /pī´ə mā´tər, pē´ə/, the innermost of the meninges covering the brain and the spinal cord. It carries a rich supply of blood vessels, which serve the nervous tissue. Compare **arachnoid, dura mater.**

pica /pī´kə/, a craving to eat things that are not foods, such as dirt, clay, chalk, glue, ice, starch, or hair. It may occur with poor diet, with pregnancy, and in some forms of mental illness.

Pick's disease, a mental disorder that occurs in middle age. Affecting the anterior portion of the brain, it causes neurotic behavior, slow changes in personality, emotions, reasoning, and judgment. *See also dementia.*

Pickwickian syndrome, *(from a morbidly obese character in the works of Charles Dickens)* decreased pulmonary function, grotesque obesity, somnolence, and general debility; theoretically resulting from the hypoventilation induced by obesity. Cor pulmonale, hypercapnia, and pulmonary hypertension can result.

picrotoxin, a nervous system stimulant taken from the seeds of a Southeast Asian fruit *(Anamirta cocculus).*

piebald /pī´bôld/, patches of white hair or skin due to a lack of pigment cells (melanocytes) in those areas. It is inherited. Compare **albinism, vitiligo.**

Pierre Robin syndrome /pē·er´ rōbaN´/, congenital defect involving a smaller than normal jaw. Due to the small size of the mandible, the tongue is easily forced back against the posterior pharynx, causing airway obstruction. These infants may require an oral/nasal airway or endotracheal intubation to maintain airway patency.

pig, *(informal)* a lead container, used for shielding radioactive materials.

pigeon breast, a congenital defect with a sternum that protrudes outward. Also known as **pectus carinatum.**

piggyback, 1. to introduce a second container of intravenous fluid into the line of one already established. This is usually done to administer a medication over a period of time. **2.** one object added to another.

pigment, any organic coloring material made by body tissues, as melanin. **–pigmentary, pigmented,** *adj.,* **pigmentation,** *n.*

piles /pīlz/. See **hemorrhoids.**

pill, a rounded or oval-shaped drug to be swallowed whole.

pillow, phenomenon observed in a body of water when water flows over a rock or obstruction.

pilomotor reflex /pī´lō-/, erection of the hairs of the skin in response to cold, emotion, or irritation of the skin. Also known as **gooseflesh.**

pilonidal cyst /-nī´dəl/, a cyst that grows in the skin of the lower back.

pilonidal fistula, a channel close to the tip of the coccyx. Also known as **pilonidal sinus.**

pilosebaceous /-sibā´shəs/, referring to a hair follicle and its oil gland.

pilus /pē´ləs/, *pl.* **pili,** a hairlike structure.

pin, 1. a small metal peg or rod. **2.** to join fragments of bone together surgically with metal rods or screws. **3.** *(informal)* an entrapping situation with the victim being physically held by an object. *See also extrication, rescue.*

pineal gland /pin´ī·əl/, a cone-shaped structure in the brain with unknown function. It may release a hormone (melatonin), which appears to halt the release of another (luteinizing) hormone. Also known as **pineal body.**

pinealoma /pin´ē·əlō´mə/, a tumor of the pineal gland in the brain.

ping-ponging, an illegal practice in which a patient is passed from one physician to another so that a health program or service can charge for unnecessary tests.

pinocytosis /pī´nōsītō´-/, the process by which fluid is taken into a cell. The cell membrane envelopes fluid from outside the cell, forming a tiny reservoir of fluid in the cell.

pinta /pēn´tə/, a skin infection carried by flies or other insects in Latin America.

pin track infection, a condition in which infections may develop at the sites where traction pins are inserted into a body part. Signs of infection include irritation, purulent drainage, and pain.

pinworm infection, an infection by the common pinworm *(Enterobius vermicularis),* which looks like a small white thread. The worms infect the large intestine and deposits eggs in the anal area, causing itching and insomnia.

pipe, a tube for fluid, gas, or divided solids.

piriformis /pir´ifôr´mis/, a flat, triangular muscle that moves and helps to extend the thigh.

pitch, **1.** the horizontal (nose up or down) axis of three-dimensional movement, usually related to aircraft and ship motion. *See also roll, yaw.* **2.** a steep grade. **3.** the frequency of vibration that allows its sound to be classified on a scale from high to low. **4.** dark, sticky resin that is liquid when heated, hard when cold; an oil or tar.

piton /pē´tän, pētōN´/, a metal spike used for an anchor point to provide security for a rope. This device is designed to hold a falling climber by anchoring the rope and slowing or stopping the fall. Designed to be hammered into cracks in the rock, they are quick to insert and very strong when placed correctly. *See also anchor point, bolt, nut.*

pitting, **1.** small, puncturelike indentations in fingernails or toenails, often a result of psoriasis. **2.** an indentation that briefly remains after applying pressure to edematous skin.

pituitary gland, the small gland joined to the hypothalamus at the base of the brain. It supplies hormones that control many processes of the body. The pituitary is divided into two lobes. The **adenohypophysis** is the anterior lobe. It secretes many hormones, including growth hormone. These hormones control the thyroid, gonads, adrenal cortex, breast, and other endocrine glands. Hormones from the hypothalamus gland control the adenohypophysis. The **neurohypophysis** is the posterior lobe of the pituitary gland. It is the source of antidiuretic hormone (ADH) and oxytocin. ADH hormone causes cells in the kidney to reabsorb more water, thereby reducing the amount of urine. Oxytocin causes strong contractions of the pregnant uterus and causes milk to flow from breasts. The pituitary gland is larger in a woman than in a man and becomes larger during pregnancy. Also known as **hypophysis cerebri.**

pityriasis alba /pit´ərī´əsis/, a common skin disease marked by round or oval, finely scaling patches without pigmentation, usually on the cheeks.

pityriasis rosea, a skin disease in which a scaling, pink rash spreads over unexposed parts of the body. The **herald patch,** a large area of irritation, appears before the pink rash by several days. The rash tends to follow the normal crease lines of the skin.

pivot joint, a joint in which movement is limited to motion in one plane. The elbow is a pivot joint. *See also synovial joint.*

placard. See **vehicle warning placard.**

placebo, an inactive substance given as if it were a medication. Studies have shown them to be as effective as physiologically active drugs when both the patient and physician believe in the treatment.

placenta /pləsen´tə/, a temporary blood-rich structure in the uterus through which the fetus exchanges oxygen, nutrients, and other substances. The fetus also eliminates carbon dioxide and metabolic wastes through the placental structure. The placenta begins to form on about the eighth day of pregnancy when the forming embryo (blastocyst) implants into the wall of the uterus and becomes joined to it. **Placenta accreta** refers to a placenta that invades the uterine muscle, making separation from the muscle difficult. **Placenta battledore** is a condition in which the umbilical cord is in the margin or edge of the placenta, instead of near the center.

placental insufficiency, an abnormal condition of pregnancy, marked by slowed growth of the fetus and uterus. Also known as **placental dysfunction.**

placenta previa /prē´vē·ə/, a condition in which the placenta is placed abnormally in the uterus so that it partly or completely covers the opening of the cervix. It is the most common cause of painless bleeding in the third trimester of pregnancy. Its cause is unknown. As the cervix opens during labor, the placenta is slowly separated from the blood vessels of the uterus. This results in bleeding that begins slowly, is painless, but may continue until the mother and fetus are hypovolemic.

plague /plāg/, an infectious disease transmitted by the bite of a flea from a rodent infected with the bacillus *Yersinia pestis*. Plague is primarily an infectious disease of rats or other rodents. The fleas feed on humans when their normal hosts have been killed by the plague. Widespread human infections may follow. **Bubonic plague** is the most common form of plague. **Black Death** usually refers to the epidemic of bubonic plague in the fourteenth century that killed over 25,000,000 people in Europe. Symptoms include painful swollen lymph nodes (buboes) in the neck, axillae, and groin, fever as high as 106° F, exhaustion, tachycardia, hypotension, petechue, and altered level of consciousness. *See also bubo.*

plain, a large area of flat or nearly flat land.

planning section, the part of the incident command system that collects, evaluates, disseminates, and uses information about an incident's development and the status of incident resources.

plantar, the sole of the foot. Also known as **volar.**

plantaris /plantär´is/, one of the muscles located on the posterior aspect of the lower leg. It flexes the foot and the leg. Compare **gastrocnemius, soleus.**

plantar reflex, the normal response of flexing the toes when the outer surface of the sole is firmly stroked from the heel to the toes. Compare **Babinski's reflex.**

plantigrade /plan´tigrād/, referring to the human pattern of walking on the sole of the foot with the heel touching the ground.

plaque /plak/, **1.** a flat, often raised patch on the skin or any other organ of the body. **2.** a deposit of atherosclerosis on the lining of an artery.

plasma /plaz´mə/, the colorless fluid in lymph and blood containing white and red blood cells and platelets. It is composed of water, electrolytes, proteins, glucose, fats, bilirubin, and gases. Plasma makes up about 50% of the total volume of blood. Compare **serum.**

plasma cell, a cell found in bone marrow, connective tissue, and blood, used to fight disease.

plasmapheresis /-fərē´-/, separating plasma from the blood and returning the remaining cells to the patient. Compare **leukapheresis, plateletpharesis.**

plasma protein, any of the proteins in blood plasma. These substances (such as albumin, fibrinogen, prothrombin, and the gammaglobulins) help to maintain fluid balance and blood pressure. Fibrinogen and prothrombin are needed for proper blood clotting.

plasma protein binding, a process in which drugs attach to proteins in the blood and form a drug-protein combination. The most commonly bound protein is albumin, whose molecules are too large to diffuse through the blood vessel membrane. This traps the attached drug in the bloodstream while it is bound.

plaster, 1. any material made of a liquid and a powder that hardens when it dries. **2.** a home treatment made of a semisolid mixture placed on a part of the body, as a mustard plaster.

plastic surgery, the surgical change, replacement, or rebuilding of outer surfaces of the body. It is done to correct a structural or cosmetic defect.

plate, a flat structure or layer, such as a thin bone.

plateau, a large, flat landform rising steeply above the surrounding land.

plateau phase, prolongation of the cardiac muscle cell depolarization phase. This results in a prolonged refractory period.

platelet /plāt´lit/, the smallest of the cells in the blood. Platelets are disk-shaped, have no hemoglobin, and affect blood clotting. Compare **erythrocyte, leucocyte.** *See also hemoglobin.*

plateletpheresis /-fərē´-/, the removal of platelets from blood with the remainder being infused back into the patient. Compare **leukapheresis, plasmapheresis.**

platinum, a silvery-white, soft metallic element, used in the manufacture of chemicals able to withstand high temperatures.

Platyhelminthes, a group of parasitic flatworms that includes tapeworms and flukes.

platypnea, dyspnea occurring only when in the upright position. This may be seen in conditions causing severe abdominal muscle weakness, advanced obstructive lung disease, and some congenital cardiac diseases.

platysma /plətiz´mə/, one of a pair of wide muscles of the lateral neck. The platysma draws down the lower lip and the corner of the mouth.

pledget /plej´ət/, a small, flat compress of gauze or cotton, used to wipe skin, soak up fluids, or clean a small surface.

–plegia, a combining form meaning paralysis of a certain area.

pleura /plo͞or´ə/, *pl.* **pleurae,** a two-layered membrane surrounding the lung. The visceral pleura adheres to the surface of the lung. The parietal pleura lines the chest wall. The two pleura are separated from each other by a serous fluid.

pleural, relating to the membrane enveloping the lungs and lining the thoracic cavity.

pleural cavity, the space within the thorax that contains the lungs.

pleural effusion, fluid between the parietal and visceral pleurae that remains unabsorbed. Symptoms include chest pain, dyspnea, dry cough, fever.

pleural space, the potential space that exists between the surface of the lung and the internal chest wall.

pleurisy /plo͞or´əsē/, inflammation of the pleura. Symptoms include dyspnea and sharp, localized pain when breathing or moving. Causes include cancer, pneumonia, pulmonary embolus, and tuberculosis.

pleurodynia, sharp chest pain due to inflammation of the costal muscles.

pleuropneumonia, a combination of pleurisy and pneumonia.

pleurothotonos /-thot´ənəs/, a severe, chronic contraction of the muscles of one side of the body, usually connected to tetanus or strychnine poisoning. **–pleurothotonic,** *adj.*

plexus, *pl.* **plexuses,** a group of nerves, blood, or lymph vessels. The body has many plexuses, such as the cardiac plexus and the solar plexus.

plica /plī´kə/, *pl.* **plicae** /plī´sē/, a fold of tissue in the body, as the circular folds (plicae circulares) of the small intestine. **–plical,** *adj.*

plug, a mass of tissue cells, mucus, or other matter that blocks a normal opening or passage of the body, such as a cervical plug.

pneumatic antishock garment, an inflatable device, fastening around the abdomen and lower extremities, used in the management of hypovolemia and for splinting. Its action was thought to increase peripheral vascular resistance of the abdomen and lower extremities, but this effect has been shown to be only theoretical. The amount of blood actually shunted into the upper portion of the body remains controversial. Also known as **MAST, medical antishock trousers, military antishock trousers, PASG.**

pneumatic shoring, *(trench rescue)* shoring or jacks with moveable parts operated by compressed air. Also known as **speedshore.**

pneumococcus /-kok´əs/, *pl.* **pneumococci** /-kok´sī/, a bacterium (*Diplococcus pneumoniae*), the most common cause of bacterial pneumonia. More than 85 subtypes are known. *See also pneumonia.*

pneumoconiosis /-kō´ne·ō-/, any disease of the lung caused by chronic inhalation of dust, most often mineral dusts. *See also anthracosis, asbestosis, silicosis.*

pneumocystosis /-sistō´-/, a respiratory infection from a parasite (*Pneumocystis carinii*) commonly seen in patients who are at high risk because of loss of resistance to infections. Symptoms include fever, cough, tachypnea, and cyanosis. The death rate is near 100% in untreated patients. Also known as **interstitial plasma cell pneumonia,** *Pneumocystis carinii* **pneumonia.** *See also acquired immune deficiency syndrome (AIDS).*

pneumomediastinum /-mē´de·əstī´nəm/, the presence of air or gas in the thoracic cavity medial to the lungs, where the heart and great vessels are located.

pneumonectomy /-nek´-/, the removal of all or part of a lung.

pneumonia /no͞omō´ne·ə/, inflammation of the lungs, commonly caused by bacteria (*Diplococcus pneumoniae*). Symptoms include fever (which may reach 105° F/40.5° C), headache, cough, and chest pain. Red blood cells leaking into the alveoli cause a rust-colored sputum. **Aspiration pneumonia** is caused by the presence of foreign material or emesis in the lungs. It occurs when a patient has an unprotected airway and regurgitates gastric contents into the lungs. **Hypostatic pneumonia** occurs in elderly or weak persons who remain in the same position for long periods. **Lobar pneumonia** is a bacterial infection of one or more of the lobes of the lungs. **Mycoplasma pneumonia,** also called walking pneumonia, is a contagious disease of children and young adults. Symptoms include dry cough and fever. *See also bronchopneumonia.*

pneumonitis /-ni´-/, *pl* **pneumonitides,** inflammation of the lung, caused by a virus or a reaction to chemicals or organic dusts. Dry cough is a common symptom.

pneumotaxic center, a group of neurons in the pons that inhibits the inspiratory (respirations) center of the brain.

pneumothorax, air or gas in the pleural cavity, causing collapse of the lung on the affected side. This may be due to infection or trauma. If there is no penetration of the chest wall, this condition is known as **closed,** or **spontaneous, pneumothorax.** Symptoms include sudden dyspnea and lateral chest pain. Lung sounds may be absent on the affected side. An **open pneumothorax** has a wound that penetrates the chest wall and, generally, allows the escape of air from the thoracic cavity (sucking chest wound). *See also hemothorax, paradoxic breathing, tension pneumothorax.*

pocket dosimeter, portable radiation detection device utilizing an electrically charged crosshair within an ionization chamber. The amount of electric charge dissipated is passively recorded on a scale within the chamber. Total accumulated gamma radiation exposure is recorded. Also known as **pencil dosimeter, pocket chamber.**

pocket mask, a basic life support ventilation device, used to protect a rescuer from potential infection during artificial ventilation. An oxygen inlet valve allows the use of supplemental oxygen when available.

podalic /pōdal´ik/, referring to the feet.

podiatry /pōdī´ətrē/, the diagnosis and treatment of diseases and disorders of the feet.

poikilothermy /poi´kəlōthur´mē/, the varying of body temperature in response to external temperature This state occurs with the sympathetic block that can be caused from spinal injury. With the loss of the ability to vasodilate (sweat) and vasoconstrict (shiver), the patient's core temperature moves toward the environmental temperature.

point of maximum impulse, the area over the left thorax where the heart's action is most noticeably palpated or visualized. It is generally found in the fifth intercostal space, just to the left of the midclavicular line. This parameter may be of use in determining a shift in the heart's position during pneumothorax or cardiac enlargement. Also known as **apex beat, PMI.**

Poisenuille's law /pwäzwēz´/ (Jean Marie Poisenuille, French physiologist, 1799-1869), a law of physiology that states that blood flow through a vessel is directly proportional to the diameter of the vessel to the fourth power.

poison, any substance that damages health or destroys life when ingested, injected, inhaled, or absorbed. Depending on the size of the dose, any substance can be harmful. Harmful effects may be divided into local and systemic. Local effects, such as those from swallowing harmful substances, involve the site of the first contact between the body and the poison. Systemic effects depend on the spread of the poison but affect the entire body. *See also specific types of poisoning.* **–poisonous,** *adj.*

poison control center, one of a nearly worldwide group of services that offer data about all aspects of poisoning, keep epidemiologic records, and refer patients to treatment centers.

poison ivy, any of several species of climbing vine (*Rhus*), with shiny, three-pointed leaves. Common in North America, it causes pruritic lesions in many people. Also common in North America, and of the *Rhus* group, are **poison oak,** a vine, and **poison sumac,** a shrub. Symptoms of contact with these plants are like those for poison ivy. *See also rhus dermatitis, urushiol.*

polarity /pōler´itə/, the existence or display of opposing qualities, or emotions, such as pleasure and pain, love and hate, or strength and weakness. It is important for psychological stability.

polio /pō´lē·ō/, *(informal)* poliomyelitis.

polioencephalitis /-ensef´əlī´-/, inflammation of the gray matter of the brain caused by poliovirus. **Polioencephalomyelitis** includes the spinal cord.

poliomyelitis /-mī´əlī´-/, a disease caused by poliovirus. There are mild forms and others that are more serious. The disease is contagious. The mild form lasts only a few hours with fever, headache, nausea, and vomiting. The more severe form may include irritation of the meninges or paralysis. *See also poliovirus.*

poliosis /pō´lē·ō´-/, loss of hair coloring. It may be inherited and can occur over the whole body or only in patches.

poliovirus, the virus that causes poliomyelitis. There are three different types of this virus.

Polle's syndrome. See **Munchausen's syndrome by proxy.**

pollutant, an undesired substance in the environment, usually with unhealthy effects. Pollutants can be in the atmosphere as gases or dust that irritate lungs, eyes, and skin, or as substances in water, foods, or beverages.

polyarteritis nodosa /pol´ē·är´təri´-/, a vascular disease in which small and medium-sized arteries become damaged. This causes the death of the tissues they supply with blood. Any organ or organ system may be affected. The disease attacks men and women between 20 and 50 years of age. Symptoms are elevated temperatures, abdominal pain, weight loss, and neurological damage.

polychlorinated biphenyls, a group of chemical compounds used to make plastics, insulation, and chemicals to slow the spread of flames. All can be poisonous. Also known as **PCB.**

polyclonal /-klō´nəl/, referring to a group of cells or organisms that are exactly alike and come from cells that are exactly alike.

polycythemia /-sīthē´mē·ə/, an abnormal increase in the number of red blood cells. It may occur in cardiac or respiratory diseases, or in prolonged exposure to high altitudes. Also known as **Osler's disease.** *See also acute mountain sickness, erythrocytosis.*

polydactyly /-dak´-tile/, a birth defect resulting in the newborn having more than the normal number of fingers or toes. Also known as **hyperdactyly, polydactylism.**

polydipsia /-dip´sē·ə/, increased thirst. Some conditions increase urination, which leads to dehydration and thirst. These include diabetes and some kidney disorders.

polygene /-jēn/, any of a group of genes that together form a trait. Examples include genes that affect size, weight, or intelligence.

polyleptic /-lep´-/, any disease or condition with varying levels of seriousness of symptoms.

polymer /-mər/, a chemical compound formed by linking a number of smaller molecular units (monomers).

polymerization, a reaction during which monomers are induced to bond and form chains, often by the addition of a catalyst or other unintentional influences, such as excessive heat, friction, contamination.

polymorphous /-môr´fəs/, referring to things that exist in many different forms, possibly changing in structure at different stages.

polymorphous light eruption, a common reaction to sunlight or ultraviolet light in patients who are sensitive to sunlight. Small, red papules and blisters appear on otherwise normal skin.

polymyalgia rheumatica /-mī·al´jə/, a disease of the large arteries. One form (polymyalgia rheumatica) affects the muscles, with pain of the back, shoulder, or neck. The other form (cranial arteritis) affects the cerebral arteries, causing a severe headache. *See also temporal arteritis.*

polyopia /-ō´pē·ə/, a vision disorder, resulting in multiple images; multiple vision. The condition can occur in one or both eyes. *See also diplopia.*

polyp, a small growth that comes from a mucous membrane surface.

polypeptide /-pep´tīd/, a chain of amino acids that is usually smaller than a protein. *See also amino acid, peptide.*

polyposis /-po´-/, a condition with many tumors or growths (polyps) on an organ or tissue.

polysaccharide /-sak´ərīd/, a carbohydrate that contains three or more molecules of simple carbohydrates. Starch is an example.

polyuria /-yŏŏr´ē·ə/, excretion of large amounts of urine. Some causes are diabetes, diuretics, and increased fluid intake.

polyvinyl chloride, a common plastic material that releases hydrochloric acid when burned. Also known as **PVC.**

Pompe's disease. See **glycogen storage disease.**

ponophobia, 1. dread of pain. **2.** distaste for exerting oneself.

pons /ponz/, *pl.* **pontes** /pon´tēz/, any bridge of tissue that connects two parts of a structure or an organ of the body. *See also brain.*

popliteal, the posterior surface of the knee.

popliteal artery, the portion of the femoral artery that is inferior to the knee.

population, any group that is marked by a certain trait or situation.

population at risk, a group of people who share a trait that causes each member to be at risk to a disease, such as cigarette smokers who work with asbestos.

porphyria /pôrfir´ē·ə/, an abnormal increase of porphyrins. There are two major kinds of porphyria: **erythropoietic porphyria,** in which large amounts of porphyrins are made in bone marrow, and **hepatic porphyria,** in which large amounts are made in the liver. Signs common to both are photopobia and abdominal pain. Other effects can include seizures, hallucinations, and dyspnea.

port, 1. an outlet through which fluid or medications are injected. **2.** the left side of a boat or ship when looking forward. **3.** a place where ships load and unload goods. **4.** a location for input-output data exchange.

portable, 1. designed to be moveable; easily moveable. **2.** a handheld radio; a walkie-talkie.

portal hypertension, increased blood pressure of the hepatic vasculature caused by an increase in vascular resistance in the liver and associated blood vessels. This condition generally decreases hepatic blood flow. Also known as **renovascular hypertension.**

portal system, the network of veins that drains blood from the stomach, intestine, spleen, pancreas, and gallbladder and carries blood from these organs to the liver.

portal vein, a large vein that collects blood from capillaries of the gallbladder, intestine, pancreas, spleen, and stomach and sends it to the capillaries of the liver. After passing through the liver, this blood is sent to the inferior vena cava via the hepatic vein. This route of blood flow is termed **hepatic portal circulation.**

Porto-power. See **hydraulic jack tool.**

port-wine stain. See **hemangioma.**

positive, 1. referring to a test or exam result indicating the presence of a substance or a reaction. **2.** referring to physical examination showing that there is a disease change.

positive end-expiratory pressure, maintaining mechanical ventilation airway pressures above atmospheric at the end of exhalation. This creates a positive airway pressure throughout the ventilatory cycle and serves to increase the amount of air left in the lungs at the end of expiration (functional residual capacity) in patients who are unable to maintain spontaneous respirations with adequate tidal volume. The technique is indicated when a patient is mechanically ventilated through an endotracheal tube and is unable to maintain adequate tissue oxygenation. Also known as **PEEP.** Compare **continuous positive airway pressure.**

positive-pressure ventilation, delivering gases to the hypoventilating patient using a gas-powered, manually triggered ventilating device.

posterior, dorsal to or toward the back. Compare **anterior.**

posterior cerebral artery, the artery supplying the posterior portion of the cerebrum.

posterior chamber of the eye, the space between the iris and the lens.

posterior communicating artery, the artery, branching off each internal carotid artery, that connects to the posterior cerebral artery on that side of the body.

posterior costotransverse ligament, one of the five ligaments for each joint in the spine.

posterior longitudinal ligament, a ligament attached to the back of each vertebra and extending from the base of the skull to the coccyx.

posterior superior iliac spine, one of the two bony segments that form the iliac crest.

posterior tibial artery, one of the parts of the popliteal artery of the leg.

postictal /pōstik´təl/, **1.** the time immediately following a seizure. **2.** referring to the appearance and demeanor of one who has had a seizure, characterized by combativeness, confusion, incontinence, and sleepiness.

postinfectious, period of time when the patient or organism is no longer able to cause infection.

postmature, overly developed or matured. *See also dysmaturity.* **–postmaturity,** *n.*

postmature infant, an infant born after the end of the forty-second week of pregnancy.

postmenopausal, referring to the period of life following menopause.

postmortem, examination after death. Also known as **autopsy, necropsy, postmortem examination.**

postoperative, the period of time following surgery.

postpartal care /-pär´təl/, care of the mother and her newborn baby during the first few days after childbirth.

postpartum /-pär´təm/, after childbirth.

postpartum depression, mental dysfunction of the mother following childbirth. This condition can range from mild depression to psychosis and occurs approximately once every 3000 pregnancies.

postprandial /-pran´dē·əl/, after a meal.

postsynaptic /-sinap´-/, **1.** located after the synapse. **2.** occurring after a synapse has been crossed by an impulse. *See also synapse.*

posttraumatic stress disorder. See **stress reaction.**

posture, the position of the body with respect to the space around it. Posture is created by the muscles that move the limbs, by the sensation of muscles and joints (proprioception), and by the sense of balance.

potassium, an alkali-metal element needed by all plants and animals to live. Potassium helps to control nerves and muscles. Foods that have potassium are whole grains, meat, beans (legumes), fruit, and vegetables. Loss of potassium can occur through vomiting, diarrhea, or the long-term use of laxatives. Also known as **K.**

potassium-sparing agent, a group of medications that allow the body to retain potassium while increasing the excretion of sodium and water.

potential difference, the difference in electrical potential, measured as the difference in charge across a cell membrane.

potentiation /pōten´shē·ā´shən/, activation or enhancement of one substance, such as a drug, by the addition or presence of another substance.

poultice /pōl´tis/, a soft, moist substance spread between layers of gauze or cloth and placed hot onto a body surface.

pox, **1.** any of several skin disorders marked by a rash of small blisters or purulent sores. **2.** the scars of smallpox.

PQRST, a mnemonic representing a patient assessment format, used with conditions from which subjective information can be obtained (difficulty breathing, dizziness, pain, weakness). This format allows most special questions to be answered about a particular medical condition in an orderly fashion. P—what **p**rovoked the condition, what makes it better (**p**alliates); Q—the **q**uality of the condition (aching chest pain, difficulty getting air in, room spinning around the patient); R—**r**ecurrence, **r**egion, or **r**adiation; S—**s**everity (usually subjectively determined by the patient on a 1 to 10 scale or objectively by the examiner on a +1 to +4 scale, with +1—complains only when asked; no outward signs of pain; +2—complains spontaneously that pain is serious; no physical sign of pain; +3—visible signs of distress (grimacing, guarding, pallor, splinting, tachycardia); and +4—altered level of consciousness, crying, writhing); and T—**t**ime since the condition began.

practitioner, one with the education and skills to practice in the medical field.

Prader-Willi syndrome, a disorder with a congenital lack of muscle tone, excessive appetite, overweight, and retardation. When diabetes mellitus occurs with these other symptoms, the condition is known as **Royer's syndrome.**

prandial /pran´dē·əl/, referring to a meal; used in relation to timing, as after eating (postprandial) or before eating (preprandial). **–prandiality,** *n.*

prayer of Maimonides /mīmon´ədēz´/ (Rabbi Moses ben Maimon, Jewish physician (Egypt), 1135-1204), a pledge or prayer given during graduation ceremonies at some medical schools, committing oneself to certain standards in the practice of medicine. *See also Declaration of Geneva, Hippocratic oath.*

precapillary sphincter, the smooth muscle sphincter regulating blood flow into a capillary.

precession, *(ballistics)* the motion, related to spin, that is a circular yaw around a projectile's center of mass, in a spiral fashion. This motion can describe any object but is most often used in relation to bullet or missile motion. *See also bullet tumble, bullet yaw, nutation.*

precipitate /prəsip´itāt/, **1.** to cause a substance to separate or to settle out of a liquid in which it is dissolved. **2.** an event that occurs quickly or without being expected. **3.** an event which causes another event to happen.

precipitous delivery, birth of an infant via spontaneous delivery, where the time of onset of labor until birth is less than 3 hours.

precordial, referring to the precordium, which is the area of the chest anterior to the heart.

precordial movement, any motion of the front wall of the chest in the area over the heart.

precordial thump, a sudden strike to the chest, delivered with the fist. This is done in cases of witnessed, monitored cardiac arrest. The technique may convert a heart in ventricular tachycardia or ventricular fibrillation to a perfusing rhythm. *See also fist pacing.*

preeclampsia /prē´əklamp´sē·ə/, a toxemia of pregnancy with headache, increasing hypertension, and pedal edema. Although the condition resolves once the pregnancy is completed, it can deteriorate to eclampsia during the pregnancy. *See also eclampsia.*

preexcitation, depolarization of the ventricles earlier than they are normally depolarized via the atrioventricular node. An accessory pathway is thought to exist that allows more rapid conduction from the atria to the ventricles. This pathway shortens conduction time, causing ta-

chycardia at rates greater than 200 beats per minute. *See also accelerated A-V conduction, delta wave, Lown-Ganong-Levine syndrome, Wolff-Parkinson-White syndrome.*

pregnancy, the process of growth and development of a fetus within a female's reproductive organs. It occurs from the time of conception through birth. Pregnancy lasts about 266 days (38 weeks) from the day the egg is fertilized by the sperm, but it may last 280 days (40 weeks; 10 lunar months; 9⅓ calendar months) from the first day of the last menstrual period. An **ectopic pregnancy** is one in which the fetus develops outside of the uterus. This can occur because of a defect in the fallopian tube or uterus. A **cornual pregnancy** is a type of ectopic pregnancy. An **ovarian pregnancy** is one in which the embryo grows in or attaches to the ovary rather than in the womb. *See also molar pregnancy, tubal pregnancy.*

pregravid, before pregnancy.

prehospital care report, any document used to record patient care and circumstances related to a prehospital response. Also known as **EMS form, patient care report, response report, run report.**

Prehospital Index, a system for categorizing trauma severity by scoring blood pressure, level of consciousness, presence/absence of penetrating chest or abdominal injuries, pulse, and respirations. The higher the score, the more severely injured the patient.

preinfarction syndrome, sudden development of angina pectoris or a worsening of existing angina by an increase in its frequency or severity; may be indicative of an impending myocardial infarction.

preload, the load to which a muscle is subjected when shortening. In the heart, the greater the amount of blood flow, the more the cardiac muscle fibers will be stretched. This will increase the velocity of the next contraction. *See also Starling's law.*

premature, 1. not fully grown or mature. **2.** occurring before the usual time. **–prematurity,** *n.*

premature atrial contraction, an ectopic beat originating in the atria from an irritable focus. Also known as **PAC.**

premature infant, any infant born before 37 weeks of pregnancy. Also called **preterm infant.**

premature junctional contraction, an ectopic beat originating in an irritable focus in the atrioventricular (AV) node. Also known as **PJC.**

premature labor. See **labor.**

premature rupture of membranes, amniotic sac rupture, prior to the onset of labor, at any gestational age.

premature ventricular contraction, an ectopic beat originating from an irritable focus in the ventricles; characterized as an early, wide QRS complex without a related P wave on the EKG. Also known as **PVC, ventricular ectopic.**

premenopausal, referring to the time of life prior to menopause.

prenatal /prēnā´təl/, occurring before birth.

preprandial /prēpran´dē·əl/, before a meal.

presacral edema, fluid accumulation in the sacral area of a recumbent patient, usually related to congestive heart failure.

presbycardia, decreased function of the cardiac muscle, caused by aging.

presbyopia, farsightedness, in the normal aging process, as a result of loss of elasticity in the lens.

prescribe, **1.** to write an order for a drug, treatment, or process. **2.** to suggest a certain way to treat a patient for a disorder.

prescribed fire, intentional ignition of vegetation for purposes of land management. These practices include improving habitat, reducing fire hazards, and insect control. Also known as **controlled burn.**

prescription drug, a drug that can be dispensed only with a physician's prescription.

presenile dementia /prēsē´nīl/. See **Alzheimer's disease.**

presenting part, the portion of the fetus that is closest to the cervix or appearing at the vaginal entrance.

pressor, **1.** a substance that causes elevation of the blood. **2.** increasing or stimulating the activity of a nerve.

pressure, a force or stress, placed against a surface by a fluid or an object; Force/Area = Pressure.

pressure bandage, a covering used to apply pressure to a dressing and/or wound to control blood flow. Elastic material is most often used as bandaging, since its tension can be adjusted, depending on the need for pressure.

pressure dressing, a dressing held with pressure to control blood flow. This dressing can be held by hand or with a pressure bandage. *See also direct pressure, pressure bandage, pressure point, tourniquet.*

pressure edema, **1.** edema of the legs caused by a pregnant uterus pushing against the large veins of the lower abdomen. **2.** edema of the scalp of the fetus after delivery.

pressure point, any area where an artery passes over bone that is used for applying pressure to control bleeding. Any location at which a pulse is felt provides such an area. Pressure at that location can control all bleeding distal to that point. *See also direct pressure, pressure dressing, tourniquet.*

pressure regulator, a device connected to a gas cylinder to reduce the cylinder pressure to a safer working level.

presumed consent, consent that is implied. *See also consent.*

presynaptic /prē´sinap´-/, **1.** located near a nerve synapse. **2.** occurring in a nerve before the synapse is crossed.

presynaptic neuron, the nerve ending that contains neurotransmitter vesicles.

presynaptic terminal, the enlarged axon terminal.

pretibial fever /prētib´ē·əl/, an infection with erythema on the lower legs, headache, fever, and muscle pain. Also known as **Fort Bragg fever.**

priapism, continual and painful erection of the penis due to disease or trauma. This is a reliable sign of damage to the spinal cord.

priapitis /prī´əpī´-/, inflammation of the penis.

prickly heat. See **heat rash.**

primary, first in order of time, place, development, or importance.

primary bronchus, one of two passages arising at the inferior end of the trachea and each leading into a lung.

primary epilepsy, epilepsy for which the cause is unknown. Also known as **idiopathic epilepsy.**

primary follicle, the ovarian follicle containing the primary oocyte.

primary injury, those injuries due to the initial air blast of an explosion. The most frequent damage occurs to the air-filled organs of the auditory, gastrointestinal, and pulmonary systems. *See also blast injury, secondary injury, tertiary injury.*

primary oocyte /ō´əsīt´/, the oocyte as it exists prior to the first meiotic division.

primary survey, the initial, rapid examination of a patient or scene for life-threatening conditions.

prime mover, a muscle or force that acts directly to bring about a movement. Most body movements need the combined action of several muscles.

primigravida /prim´igrav´idə/, first-time pregnancy. Compare **multigravida, primapara.** **–primigravid,** *adj.*

primipara /primip´ərə/, *pl.* **primiparae,** first time childbirth. Compare **multipara, nullipara, primagravida.**

primitive, formed early in the course of growing; existing in an early or simple form.

primum non nocere /prē´mō̄m nōn´ nōker´ā/, *(Latin)* "First, do no harm". As a basic principle of medicine, it is a treatment consideration for every patient.

PR interval, the time that elapses between the beginning of the P wave and the beginning of the QRS complex. Including both the P wave and the PR segment, this is indicative of the time necessary for atrial depolarization and conduction through the atrioventricular (AV) junction. Normal PR interval is 0.12 to 0.20 second.

Prinzmetal's angina, a form of angina, due to coronary artery spasm, that occurs at rest, rather than with effort. During an episode, the EKG may show noticeable ST elevation that disappears as the pain subsides. *See also angina.*

private line tone. See **channel guard.**

probing, manual method for searching for victims buried in avalanche debris. This method utilizes a probe line made of up to a dozen rescuers, each with avalanche probes 10 to 14 feet (about 3 to 4 meters) long. Probing may be coarse or fine, depending on whether the mode is rescue or body recovery. Coarse probing (one probe every 30 inches [about 75 cm]) can be very rapid, allowing for rescue of multiple victims in a short time. Fine probing (three probes every 12 inches [about 30 cm]) is very time consuming and, generally, useful only for body recovery.

procainamide, an antidysrhythmic agent, used to abolish ventricular ectopy refractory to lidocaine. Side effects include anxiety, hypotension, nausea, seizures, and a widened QRS complex. This drug is contraindicated in second- and third-degree heart blocks, premature ventricular contractions in the presence of bradycardia, and tricyclic drug overdose. Also known as **Pronestyl.**

procerus /prōsir´əs/, one of three muscles of the nose, that moves the eyebrows and the nose.

process, **1.** a series of connected events that follow one after another from a given state or condition. **2.** a natural growth from a bone or other body part.

procidentia /prō´siden´shə/, the falling or dropping of an organ, such as the uterus.

procreation, the process of producing offspring. **–procreate,** *v.,* **procreative,** *adj.*

proctitis /proktī´-/, inflammation of the rectum and anus. Symptoms include minor pain and the urge to defecate without being able to do so. Also known as **rectitis.**

proctology /proktol´-/, the branch of medicine that deals with treating disorders of the colon, rectum, and anus.

prodromal stage, early period of labor before uterine contractions become forceful and frequent enough to begin dilation of the cervix.

prodrome /prō´drōm/, an early sign of a health disorder or disease. **–prodromal,** *adj.*

product name, brand or trade name printed on front panel of a hazardous material container. If the product name includes the term "technical," as in Parathion-Technical, it generally indicates a highly concentrated pesticide with 70% to 99% active ingredients.

products of combustion, the end products of burning. The four major products are heat, fire gases, flame, and smoke. Fire gases include acrolein, ammonia, carbon dioxide, carbon monoxide, hydrogen chloride, hydrogen cyanide, hydrogen sulfide, phosgene, and/or sulfur dioxide.

progeny /proj´ənē/, **1.** offspring; an individual that comes from a mating. **2.** the descendants of a known or common ancestor.

progeria /prōjir´ē·ə/, disease process characterized by early aging. It commonly begins with the appearance in childhood of gray hair, wrinkled skin, and small size. There may be posture deformities and a lack of hair. Death usually occurs before 20 years of age. Compare **infantilism.**

progestin /projes´tin/, **1.** progesterone. **2.** any of a group of hormones, natural or synthetic, released by the corpus luteum, placenta, or adrenal cortex with progesterone-like effects on the uterus.

progestogen /projes´təjən/, a natural or synthetic female hormone. Also known as **progestin.**

prognathism /prog´nəthizm/, a condition in which the face appears abnormal because of abnormal projection of the jaw.

prognosis /prognō´-/, predicting the likely outcome of a disease based on the condition of the patient and the usual action of the disease.

progressive, the process of a disease or condition becoming more obvious and severe as it develops.

projection, **1.** anything that protrudes outward, as from a bone. **2.** a subconscious way to defend oneself by attributing traits, ideas, or actions that one cannot accept in oneself on another person.

projectile vomiting, vomiting that is very forceful.

prolactin /prōlak´tin/, a hormone that is secreted by the pituitary gland, which controls the growth of the mammary glands and the production of breast milk. Also known as **lactogenic hormone, luteotropin.**

prolapse /prō´laps/, the sinking or sliding of an organ away from its normal position or place in the body, as in a prolapsed uterus.

prolapsed umbilical cord, an umbilical cord that presents prior to or beside the presenting part of the fetus.

proliferation, spreading.

proliferative phase, time between the end of menses and ovulation in a 28-day menstrual cycle.

proline /prō´lin/, an important amino acid found in many proteins of the body, especially collagen. *See also amino acid, protein.*

prolonged release, the trait or quality of a drug that is released over a long period of time. The most common form is a soft capsule with tiny pellets of drug which dissolve at different rates in the intestine.

promethazine, an antiemetic/antihistamine, used to potentiate analgesics and in the treatment of nausea or vomiting. The primary side effect is drowsiness. Do not use in patients with altered levels of consciousness, toxic drug ingestion, or poisoning. Also known as **Phenergan.**

pronation /prōnā´shən/, **1.** lying-flat position, with the body facing downward. **2.** the turning of the forearm so that the palm of the hand faces downward and backward. **–pronate,** *v.,* **prone,** *adj.*

pronator teres, a muscle of the forearm, which pronates the hand.

prone, referring to the position of the body when lying face downward. Compare **supine.**

prophase, the first stage of cell division of germ cells (meiosis) and tissue cells (mitosis). The chromosomes initially appear in this stage. *See also anaphase, metaphase, telophase.*

prophylactic /prō´filak´-/, something that prevents, particularly related to disease. *See also condom.*

prophylaxis /prō´filak´sis/, prevention of or protection against disease.

Propionibacterium, a form of bacteria found on the skin of humans, in the gut of humans and animals, and in dairy products. One species (*P. acne*) is common in acne blisters.

propionicacidemia /prō´pē·on´ikas´idē´mē·ə/, a congenital defect in which the body is not able to use certain amino acids (threonine, isoleucine, and methionone). It causes mental and physical retardation.

proportion, an expression of the equality of two ratios (*a:b = c:d,* or *a* is to *b* as *c* is to *d*).

proprietary, referring to an institution or a product, operated or sold for profit.

proprietary medicine, any drug that is protected from competition because the chemicals it is made out of or the way it is made are protected by trademark or copyright.

proprietary name. See **trade name.**

proprioception /prō´prē·əsep´shən/, the ability to sense the positions of body parts and the motions of the muscles and joints.

proptosis /proptō´-/, bulging of a body organ or area.

propwash. See **slipstream.**

proscribe, to forbid. **–proscriptive,** *adj.*

prosencephalon /pros´ensef´əlon/, the part of the brain that has the thalamus and hypothalamus. It controls important body functions and affects thinking, appetite, and emotion. Also known as **forebrain.** Compare **mesencephalon. –prosencephalic,** *adj.*

prostacyclin /pros´təsī´klin/, a prostaglandin. It is formed mainly in human blood vessel walls and slows blood platelet clumping.

prostate /pros´tāt/, a male gland that surrounds the neck of the bladder and the urethra. It secretes a substance composed of alkaline phosphatase, citric acid, and various enzymes, which liquefies semen. **–prostatic,** *adj.*

prostatectomy /pros´tətek´-/, surgical removal of part or all of the prostate gland.

prostatic /prostat´ik/, referring to the prostate gland.

prostatitis /pros´tətī´-/, inflammation of the prostate gland. Characteristically the patient feels the need to urinate frequently and has a burning sensation during urination.

prosthesis /prosthē´-/, *pl.* **prostheses,** **1.** a device designed to replace a missing part of the body, as an artificial limb. **2.** a device designed and applied to make a part of the body work better, such as a hearing aid or denture.

prostration, a condition of being physically exhausted and unable to exert oneself further, as from heat or stress.

protease /prō´tē·ās/, an enzyme that helps the breakdown of protein. *See also proteolytic.*

protection factor, the ratio of contaminants in the atmosphere outside the facepiece to the contaminants inside the facepiece.

protein /prō´tēn, -tē·in/, any of a large group of complex, organic nitrogen compounds. Each is made up of linked amino acids that contain carbon, hydrogen, nitrogen, and oxygen. Some proteins also have sulfur, phosphorus, iron, iodine, or other necessary elements of living cells. Twenty-two amino acids are necessary for body growth, development, and health. The body can make 14 of these amino acids, called nonessential, while the other eight must be obtained from food.

protein metabolism, the method by which protein in foods is used by the body for energy and protein production.

proteinuria /-ōōr´ē·ə/, having large amounts of protein secreted in the urine, such as albumin. Proteinuria is often a sign of kidney disease, but it can also be caused by heavy exercise or fever. Also known as **albuminuria.**

Proteus /prō´tē·əs/, a type of bacteria often linked to hospital (nosocomial) infections. It is normally found in feces, water, and soil. It may cause wound infections and septicemia.

prothrombin /prōthrom´bin/, a blood plasma protein that forms thrombin in the liver, the first step in blood clotting. Also known as **factor II.**

proton, an elementary nuclear particle with a positive electric charge equal numerically to the charge of the electron and having a mass about equal to that of a hydrogen atom.

protoplasm /prō´tōplazm/, the living substance of a cell, usually made up of water, minerals, and animal and vegetable compounds.

protoporphyria /-pôrfir´ē·ə/, increased levels of protoporphyrin in the blood and feces.

protoporphyrin /-pôr´firin/, a coloring (porphyrin) that combines with iron and protein to make many important body chemicals, such as hemoglobin and myoglobin. *See also heme.*

protozoa /-zō´ə/, *sing.* **protozoon,** single-celled living organisms that are the lowest form of animal life. About 30 kinds of protozoa cause diseases in humans.

protozoal infection /-zō´əl/, any disease caused by protozoa. Some kinds of protozoal infections are **amebic dysentery, malaria, trichomonas vaginitis.**

protraction, movement in the anterior direction.

provider, a hospital, clinic, service, or health care professional, who provides a service to patients.

provitamin, a substance found in certain foods that the body may convert into a vitamin. Also known as **previtamin.**

proximal, referring to a body part that is closer to the center of the body, when compared to other parts of the body.

proximity suit, aluminized protective clothing for firefighters, which enables them to effectively fight fire and perform rescue with maximum safety from flames and heat. Also known as **approach suit, fire entry suit.**

prurigo /prŏŏrī´gō/, an inflammation of the skin with pruritus and weeping papules.

pruritus /prŏŏrī´təs/, itching.

prusik /prus´ik/, **1.** knot used when climbing a rope without mechanical devices. The design of the knot is such that it holds securely when weight is applied but moves easily when the weight is removed. This knot also works well as a safety device when rapelling and as a safety tie-off for the raising or lowering of rope. **2.** the climbing or safety device formed when the prusik knot is used to tie a sling to a rope. **3.** the climbing activity performed when ascending with a prusik.

pseudoaneurysm, condition resembling an aneurysm caused by blood vessel enlargement.

pseudocyst /-sist/, a cavity without a lining filled with gas or fluid.

pseudojaundice /-jôn´dis/, yellowish discoloration of the skin caused by eating too much carotene-rich food.

pseudomembranous colitis, inflammation of the colon caused by *Clostridium difficile*. This bacteria precipitates a life-threatening form of diarrhea.

Pseudomonas /sŏŏdom´ənas/, a kind of bacteria often found in wounds, burns, and infections of the urinary tract.

pseudotumor, a false tumor.

psittacosis /sit´əkō´-/, a respiratory illness caused by the bacterium *Chlamydia psittachi*. It is transmitted to humans by infected birds, especially parrots. The symptoms include fever, cough, and headache. Also known as **parrot fever.**

psoas major /sō´əs/, a long muscle in the lumbar area of the back. It moves the thigh and flexes the spine.

psoas minor, a long, slim muscle of the pelvis. It flexes the spine.

psoralen, a natural chemical that makes skin photosensitive. After being exposed to ultraviolet light, psoralens react to increase melanin in the skin. Natural psoralens are found in buttercups, carrot greens, celery, clover, dill, figs, limes, and parsley. Some psoralen-type chemicals are used

to help skin tanning and in the treatment of skin diseases, such as psoriasis and vitiligo.

psoriasis /sərī´əsis/, an inherited skin disorder in which there are red patches with thick, dry, silvery scales. It is caused by the body making too many skin cells. Sores are more common on arms, ears, pubis, and scalp.

psychedelic /sī´kədel´ik/, describing a state of altered senses in which a person may hallucinate.

psychiatry /sīkī´ətrē/, the branch of medical science that deals with the causes, treatment, and prevention of mental, emotional, and behavioral disorders. **–psychiatric,** *adj.*

psychic trauma, an emotional injury that leaves a lasting effect on the subconscious mind. Causes of psychic trauma are abuse in childhood, rape, and loss of a loved one.

psychobiology, the study of behavior in terms of the way the body and the mind work together.

psychogenic /-jen´ik/, originating in the mind. *See also psychosomatic.*

psychologic dependence, emotional dependence on an external stimulus, such as drugs, excitement, relationships.

psychologist, a person who specializes in the study of the structure and function of the brain and related mental processes.

psychology, the study of behavior and the functions and processes of the mind. **Applied psychology** is a practical use of psychology. *See also psychologist.*

psychomotor, self-controlled muscle movements linked with the nervous system.

psychomotor seizure. See **seizure.**

psychopath /-path/, a person with a personality disorder whose behavior is considered antisocial. Also known as **sociopath.**

psychopharmacology /-fär´məkol´-/, the study of the effects of drugs on behavior and mental functions.

psychophysiologic disorder /-fiz´ē·əloj´ik/, any of a large group of mental disorders that involve an organ or organ system controlled by the autonomic nervous system. For example, a peptic ulcer may be caused or made worse by stress. Also known as **psychosomatic illness, psychosomatic reaction.**

psychosexual, referring to the mental and emotional aspects of sex. *See also psychosexual development, psychosexual disorder.* **–psychosexuality,** *n.*

psychosis /sīkō´-/, *pl.* **psychoses,** any major mental disorder with a physical or emotional source. There may be severe depression, excitement, and illusions. These disturbances may prevent the patient from functioning normally. With **functional psychosis,** there are personality changes and the loss of ability to function in reality. *See also bipolar disorder, organic mental disorder, paranoia, schizophrenia.*

psychosomatic /-sōmat´ik/, the display of an emotional problem through physical disorders. *See also psychogenic.*

psychotic /sīkot´ik/, **1.** referring to psychosis. **2.** a patient who shows the symptoms of a psychosis.

psychotropic drugs /-trop´ik/, drugs that affect the mental function or behavior of a person.

pterygoideus lateralis /ter´igoi´dē·əs/, one of the mandibular muscles used to chew food.

ptomaine /tō´mān/, a group of nitrogen compounds found in decaying proteins.

ptosis /tō´sis/, the prolapse of an organ or part.

ptotic kidney /tō´tik/, a kidney that is abnormally located in the pelvis.

ptyalin /tī´əlin/, an enzyme in saliva that helps to digest starch. Also known as **amylase.**

pubarche /pyōō´bär´kē/, the beginning of puberty. It is marked by the first signs of adult sexual traits.

puberty /pyōō´bərtē/, the period of life at which both males and females are first able to reproduce.

pubic symphysis /pyōō´bik sim´fi-/, the slightly flexible joint of the anterior pelvis.

pubis /pyōō´bis/, *pl.* **pubes,** one of the bones that form the hip. Compare **ilium, ischium.**

public health, a field of medicine that deals with the health of the community. It is active in such areas as epidemiology, water supply, waste disposal, air pollution, and food safety.

pudendal nerve /pyōōden´dəl/, a branch of the nervous system that carries nerve impulses to the genitals and rectum.

puerperal /pyōō·ur´pərəl/, referring to the time after childbirth or to a woman who has just given birth.

puerperal fever, a bacterial infection that may follow childbirth. Symptoms include fever, bloody vaginal discharge, and diminished urine output. Also known as **childbed fever, puerperal sepsis.**

puerperal sepsis. See **puerperal fever.**

puerperium /pyōō´ərpir´ē·əm/, the period of 6 weeks following childbirth.

Pulex /pyōō´leks/, a type of flea that carries certain infections, such as plague and typhus.

pulmonary /pool´məner´ē/, referring to the lungs or the respiratory system. Also known as **pulmonic.**

pulmonary artery, one of two blood vessels that carry deoxygenated blood to the lungs from the right ventricle.

pulmonary capacity, the total of two or more pulmonary volumes.

pulmonary embolism, pulmonary artery blockage due to air, fat, thrombus, or tissue. This condition often causes sudden, unexplained shortness of breath and chest pain.

pulmonary hypertension, abnormally high pressure within the pulmonary circulation.

pulmonary overpressurization syndrome, overexpansion of trapped air in the lungs. This condition ruptures alveoli, forcing air into other lung tissue. Also known as **paper bag syndrome, POPS.** *See also hemothorax, pneumothorax, pulmonary embolism.*

pulmonary stenosis. See **stenosis.**

pulmonary surfactant, a phospholipid substance that reduces the surface tension of alveolar surfaces, allowing gas exchange and improving elasticity of pulmonary tissue.

pulmonary trunk, the large artery that carries blood from the right ventricle and branches into the right and left pulmonary arteries.

pulmonary valve. See **heart valve.**

pulmonary vein, one of a pair of blood vessels that return blood from the lungs to the left atrium. Compare **pulmonary trunk.**

pulmonary ventilation, air movement in and out of the lungs, replacing carbon dioxide with oxygen.

pulmonic pressure, right-sided pressure within the heart.

pulp, any soft, spongy tissue, such as that in the spleen or teeth.

pulp canal. See **root canal.**

pulp cavity, the space in a tooth that contains dental pulp.

pulpitis /pulpī´-/, infection of the dental pulp.

pulsatile /pul´sətīl/, referring to a rhythmic pulsing.

pulse, the palpable sensation felt over an artery which signifies the movement of blood from the heart. The pulse matches each beat of the heart. The normal pulse rate in the average adult is from 60 to 100 per minute. The average pulse rate for a newborn is 120 beats per minute. It slows throughout childhood and adolescence.

pulseless electrical activity, cardiac electrical activity without corresponding mechanical activity; no pulses. Previously known as **electromechanical dissociation, EMD.** Also known as **PEA.**

pulse oximeter, device used for the noninvasive monitoring of the oxygen level in the blood. The sampling technique of this device measures the intensity of color (colormetric) of blood to determine hemoglobin oxygen saturation. Also known as **oximeter, pulse ox.**

pulse point, any location on the surface of the body where the pulse can be easily felt. The most commonly used point is over the radial artery on the thumb side of the anterior wrist. An **apical pulse** is auscultated over the apex of the heart. A **brachial pulse** can be palpated on the medial upper arm, near the antecubital fossa. A **carotid pulse** can be felt by gently palpating the groove between the larynx and the sternocleidomastoid muscle. A **dorsalis pedis pulse** is felt between the first and second metatarsal of the foot. A **femoral pulse** is felt in the groin from the femoral artery. The **popliteal pulse** can be felt posterior to the knee. A **posterior tibialis pulse** is palpated near the ankle, posterior to the medial malleolus.

pulse pressure, difference between systolic and diastolic blood pressure. The number expressed relates to the vascular smooth muscle tone of arterial blood vessel walls. Pulse pressure is obtained by subtracting the diastolic pressure from the systolic. A pulse pressure under 30 or over 50 mmHg is considered abnormal.

pulsus alternans, alternating strong and weak palpated beats.

pulsus paradoxus, a pulse that becomes weaker during inspiration, due to changes in intrathoracic pressure, inhibiting cardiac return. This phenomenon may also be noted by a decrease in systolic blood pressure of more than 10 mmHg during inspiration and may be seen during cardiac tamponade. This is also the first phase of Beck's triad. Also known as **paradoxical pulse.**

pulvule /pul´vyo͞ol/, a gelatin capsule that has a dose of a drug in powder form.

pump, a device used to move liquids or gases by suction or pressure.

punctate, puncture marks; spotted. Marked with dots.

punctum lacrimale /lak´rimā´lē/, a tiny opening in the edge of each eyelid that is linked to the tear (lacrimal) duct.

puncture wound, an injury caused by the penetration of a narrow object, such as a knife, nail, glass, into the body.

pupil, an opening in the iris of the eye. It lies behind the cornea and in front of the lens. The pupil is the window through which light passes to the lens and the retina. Its size changes as the eye responds to changes in light intensity or body function. *See also dilatator pupillae.*

purge, to make free of an unwanted substance or problem.

purine /pyo͞or´ēn/, any one of a large group of nitrogen compounds. They may be the end products in the digestion of proteins in the diet.

Purkinje fibers, muscle tissue forming the terminal portion of the cardiac conduction system, which transmits electrical impulses from the bundle branches to the cells of the ventricles. Also known as the **Purkinje system.**

Purkinje shift, a phenomenon of vision that allows dark colors to be easily seen during the day, but to be almost totally indiscernible at night. The shifting of vision from color-sensitive cones to gray-sensitive rods creates this shift.

purpura /pur´pyərə/, minute hemorrhage beneath the skin or mucous membranes, causing ecchymoses or petechiae.

purulent /pyŏŏr´ŏŏlənt/, containing pus.

pus, fluid that comes from dead tissue, composed primarily of white blood cells. Its most common cause is bacterial infection.

pustule /pus´chŏŏl/, a small blister typically containing pus. **–pustular,** *adj.*

putrefaction /pyŏŏ´trəfak´shən/, the decay of animal or plant tissue, especially proteins. It makes foul-smelling compounds, such as ammonia.

putromaine /pyŏŏtrō´mān/, any poisonous substance made by the decay of food within a living body.

P wave, the first deflection in a normal cardiac cycle, representing atrial depolarization.

pyelonephritis /-nəfrī´-/, infection of the kidney.

pygmy /pig´mē/, a very small person with normal body shape; an undeveloped dwarf. Also spelled **pigmy.**

pyknic /pik´nik/. See **somatotype.**

pyloric sphincter /pīlôr´ik/, a thick muscular ring in the pylorus, separating the stomach from the duodenum. Also known as **pyloric valve.**

pyloric stenosis. See **stenosis.**

pylorospasm /-spazm/, a spasm of the pyloric sphincter of the stomach.

pylorus /pīlôr´əs/, a tube-shaped portion of the stomach that angles toward the duodenum.

pyoderma /pī´ōdur´mə/, any purulent skin disease, such as impetigo.

pyogenic /-jen´ik/, pus-forming.

pyorrhea /pi´ôrē´ə/, **1.** a releasing of pus. **2.** a purulent inflammation of the gums. **–pyorrheal,** *adj.*

pyramidal tract /pīram´idəl/, a nervous system pathway composed of nerve fibers that transmit voluntary muscle nerve impulses.

pyridoxine /pir´idox´sin/, a vitamin that is part of the B complex group of vitamins. It helps to build and break down amino acids. Also known as **vitamin B$_6$.**

pyrogen /pī´rəjən/, any drug or substance that causes an increase in body temperature See also *fever.* **–pyrogenic,** *adj.*

pyrolysis, the chemical phenomenon that occurs in fires, which causes the decomposition of the fuel involved.

pyromania /pīrō´-/, an uncontrollable urge to set fires. The condition is found primarily in men.

pyrophoric materials, materials that ignite spontaneously in air without an ignition source.

pyrosis /pīrō´-/. See **heartburn.**

pyruvate /pīrŏŏ´vāt/ the end product of glycolysis.

pyuria /pīyŏŏr´ē·ə/, white blood cells in the urine, typically a sign of infection in the urinary tract. See also *bacteriuria.*

Q

Q fever, a sudden illness, typically involving the respiratory system, caused by the *Rickettsia burnetii.* The disease is spread through contact with infected animals. This occurs by breathing in the rickettsiae from animal hides or drinking infected raw milk. A headache and fever may persist for 3 weeks or more. The name of the illness is derived from its unknown etiology (Q—query). Also known as **nine-mile fever, quadrilateral fever.**

Q law, as temperature decreases, so does chemical activity.

QRS complex, EKG waveform composed of the Q, R, and S waves. Representing ventricular depolarization, a normal complex is 0.12 second or less in duration.

QT interval, the time period of an EKG from the beginning of the QRS complex to the end of the T wave. This period varies with the duration of the QRS and T.

QT syndrome, prolongation of the time of ventricular repolarization. This condition increases a patient's susceptibility to dysrhythmias due to cardiac irritability. These dysrhythmias generally take the form of ventricular tachycardia (particularly torsades de pointes) and ventricular fibrillation. This syndrome is divided into pause-dependent and adrenergic-dependent conditions. Although this condition can be acquired or congenital, it is most often caused by drug therapy. Other than EKG abnormalities, the most common symptom is syncope.

quack, an incompetent practitioner.

quadrant, **1.** one of four regions of an area, divided for descriptive or diagnostic purposes. **2.** one-fourth of a circle.

quadriceps femoris /kwod´riseps fem´əris/, a group of four muscles of the anterior thigh that function to extend the leg.

quadrigeminal /-jem´inəl/, **1.** in four parts. **2.** a fourfold increase in size or frequency.

quadriplegia /-plē´jə/, paralysis of the extremities and trunk below the level of spinal cord injury. This disorder is often the result of injury in the cervical vertebrae. Automobile accidents and sporting mishaps are common causes. Compare **hemiplegia, paraplegia.**

quadruplet /kwod´rooplit, kwodrup´lit/, any one of four offspring born at the same time during a single pregnancy.

qualified, referring to a professional or facility that is recognized by an appropriate agency or organization as meeting established standards of performance.

qualitative test /kwol´itā´tiv/, a test that shows the presence or lack of a substance, typically described in subjective terms.

quality factor, the biologic damage that radiation can produce. Equal doses of different types of radiation cause varying levels of damage. *See also roentgen equivalent, man.*

quantitative test /kwon´titā´tiv/, a test that determines the amount of a substance per unit volume or unit weight. This can usually be described in objective terms.

quarantine /kwôr´əntēn/, **1.** the isolation of patients with a communicable disease or of those exposed to a communicable disease during the contagious period. The purpose is to prevent spread of the illness. **2.** the practice of holding travelers, ships, trucks, or airplanes coming from places of epidemic disease for the purpose of inspection or disinfection.

quartan /kwôr´tən/, happening again on the fourth day, or at about 72-hour intervals.

quick connect, a coupling that is rapidly engaged or disengaged. This device is used for changing pieces of equipment where time is critical, such as with hoses, hydraulic powered tools, masks, tanks.

Quick Look, trademark of Physio-Control Corp. describing the ability to monitor an EKG through paddles instead of patient cable/electrode configuration. This technique is thought to speed time to defibrillation. This term is occasionally used to describe the procedure.

quickening, the first feeling by a pregnant woman of movement of the baby in her uterus. It usually occurs between 16 and 20 weeks of gestation.

Quincke's pulse /kwing´kēz/, an abnormal alternate paleness and reddening of the skin seen by pressing the front edge of the fingernail and watching the blood in the nail bed disappear and return. This pulsation may be seen with disorders of the aorta and in otherwise healthy individuals. Also known as **capillary pulse.**

quinsy, *(historical)* peritonsillar abscess due to bacterial infection. *See also tonsillitis.*

quintan /kwin´tən/, happening again on the fifth day, or at about 96-hour intervals.

quintuplet /kwin´tō͞oplit, kwintup´lit/, any one of five offspring born at the same time during the same pregnancy.

Q wave, the first negative deflection following the P wave, but before the R wave. These deflections may be indicative of an old myocardial infraction, depending on the lead in which they are viewed. They may not be present on a normal EKG.

R

rabbit fever. See **tularemia.**

rabies /rā´bēz/, an often fatal viral disease of the nervous system. The virus is found primarily in wild animals, such as skunks and raccoons. Contact with an infected animal carries the virus to an unvaccinated dog or cat. Humans most often get the virus from a bite or exposure of a mucous membrane or break in the skin to the saliva of an infected animal. The virus travels along nerves to the brain, and then to other organs. A dormant period ranges from 10 days to 1 year. Symptoms include fever, headache, and paraesthias. Seizures, paralysis, coma, and death may result. There have been few nonfatal cases. Also known as **hydrophobia.**

raccoon's eyes, *(informal)* ecchymosis of the orbit(s) of the eye(s) due to sphenoid sinus fracture.

race, *(informal)* a group of genetically related people.

racemose /ras´əmōs´/, describing a structure in which many branches end in bunches, such as the alveoli of the lungs.

rachitic /rəkit´ik/, referring to rickets.

rachitis /rəkī´tis/, **1.** rickets. **2.** an inflammatory disease of the spine.

radial artery /rā´dē·əl/, an artery in the forearm. It divides into 12 branches in the forearm, wrist, and hand.

radial keratotomy, an operation in which a series of tiny incisions are made on the cornea of the eye. The incisions cause the cornea to bulge slightly. This most often corrects the eye for mild to moderate nearsightedness (myopia).

radial nerve, the largest branch of the brachial plexus that supplies the skin and musculature of the arm.

radial tuberosity, an oblong elevation of the distal end of the radius.

radiant energy, the energy given off by radiation, such as radio waves, visible light, and x-rays.

radiate, to move or spread from a common point.

radiate ligament, the ligament that connects each rib with a vertebra.

radiation, 1. the giving off of energy. **Electromagnetic radiation** refers to every kind of electrical and magnetic radiation. It includes energy with the shortest wavelength, such as gamma rays, to that with the longest wavelength, such as long radio waves. **Gamma radiation** refers to energy from radioactive elements that come from nuclear decay or nuclear reactions. **Ionizing radiation** refers to electromagnetic energy, such as x-rays, that break substances in their paths into ions. **Nonionizing radiation** does not change the electric charge of atoms in tissue. **Natural (background) radiation** is radioactivity in the soil and rocks or that reaches the earth from space, such as radiation from the sun. **2.** the use of a radioactive substance to diagnose or treat a disease.

radiation absorbed dose, the basic unit of an absorbed dose of ionizing radiation. It is approximately equal to the absorbed dose in tissue when the exposure in air is 1 roentgen of medium-voltage x-radiation. Also known as **rad.** *See also gray.*

radiation detector, a device used to detect presence and amount of radiation, which cannot be otherwise noted by human senses, such as a Geiger counter (Geiger-Müller detector).

radiation hazard, a condition under which persons might receive radiation in excess of the maximum permissible dose. There are both internal and external radiation hazards. *See also external exposure, internal exposure.*

radiation meter, device that detects and measures the presence of radiation emitted by the decay of radioactive substances. Also known as **radiation detector.** *See also Geiger counter, pocket dosimeter, radiation detector.*

radiation oncology, treatment of cancer with radiation.

radiation sickness, illness resulting from exposure to radiation. The seriousness of the condition depends on the amount, length of exposure, and the part of the body affected. Moderate exposure may cause headache, nausea, vomiting, loss of appetite, and diarrhea. Long-term exposure may cause sterility, cancer, and cataracts.

radical therapy, 1. a treatment meant to cure, not only relieve symptoms. **2.** an extreme treatment; not conservative, as radical mastectomy rather than simple or partial mastectomy.

radio cache, a cache may consist of a number of portable radios, a base station, and in some cases, a repeater stored in a predetermined location for dispatch to incidents.

radioactive element, a chemical element whose nucleus is subject to decay, releasing alpha or beta particles or gamma rays. All elements with atomic numbers greater than 83 are radioactive, such as radium, uranium.

radioactive isotope. See **isotope.**

radioactivity, the spontaneous emission of radiation (generally alpha or beta particles, accompanied by gamma rays) from the nucleus of an unstable atom. *See also alpha particle, beta particle, decay (radioactive), gamma radiation.*

radiobiology, the branch of science dealing with the effects of radiation on body systems.

radio frequency. See **amplitude modulation, frequency, frequency modulation.**

radiograph, an x-ray.

radiography /rā′dē·og′rəfē/, the use of radiation, as x-rays, to make images on photographic film. **Digital radiography** is an x-ray that uses a computer to create the image.

radiological survey. See **monitoring.**

radiology /-ol′-/, the branch of medicine that deals with radioactive substances used in diagnosing and treating a disease. A **radiologist** is a physician who studies and practices radiology.

radionuclide /-nōō′klīd/, any of the radioactive isotopes of cobalt, iodine, and other elements, used in nuclear medicine to treat tumors and cancers. They are also used for images of inner parts of the body. *See also nuclear scanning.*

radiopaque /-pāk′/, anything that stops the passage of x-rays or other radiant energy.

radioresistance, the ability of cells, tissues, or organs to resist the effects of radiation. **–radioresistant,** *adj.*

radiosensitivity, the lack of ability of cells, tissues, or organs to resist the effects of radiation. Cells of the intestine are the most radiosensitive of the body.

radioulnar syndesmosis, the complete articulation between the radius and ulna at both the proximal and distal locations.

radium (Ra), a radioactive metal element.

radius /rā′dē·əs/, *pl.* **radii,** one of the bones of the forearm. Its proximal end is small and forms a part of the elbow. The distal end is large and forms a part of the wrist.

radon, a radioactive, gaseous element. Radon is a decay product of radium and is used in radiation cancer therapy. A **radon seed** is a small sealed tube of glass or gold with a decay product of radium (radon) put into body tissues to treat cancers.

railroad jack. See **hydraulic jack tool.**

rales /rälz/. See **breath sounds.**

ram, 1. hydraulic rescue tool that pushes or pulls via a plunger(s) that extends from its end. It can be direct or remote controlled and of various size and capacity. Also known as **hydraulic rescue ram, power ram. 2.** forcible entry tool used in special operations when gaining entry by force is required. Made as a single-piece unit, it is primarily designed for forcing doors. Also known as a **battering ram.**

ramjet, a jet engine with no moving parts. Thrust is produced by taking air directly into the front and compressing it through a narrowed intake. Injected fuel is burned within the intake and gasses are forced out as exhaust. *See also turbojet.*

ramp, **1.** paved loading or parking area for aircraft. **2.** stairway from ground to aircraft door.

Ramsay Hunt's syndrome. See **herpes zoster oticus.**

ramus /rā′məs/, *pl.* **rami,** a small structure extending from a larger one, such as a branch of a nerve or artery.

random access memory, temporary computer data storage space; the area in which computer software uses the processor to manipulate data. All programs used by personal computer must first be moved from disk to random access memory (RAM). When a personal computer is turned off, all data in the RAM is lost, necessitating the saving of new data at periodic intervals. *See also read-only memory.*

range, **1.** a general coverage area, usually measured in miles. **2.** an area for practicing with firearms with targets located within the perimeter.

Rankine (William J. Rankine, Scottish physicist, 1820-1872), scale used for measuring temperature where zero degrees Rankine is −459.67° Fahrenheit (°F = °R + 459.67). A Rankine degree (°R) is the same size as a Fahrenheit degree. Also known as **Fahrenheit-absolute.**

ranula /ran′yələ/, *pl.* **ranulae,** a swelling to the floor of the mouth, most often caused by a blockage of the ducts of the salivary glands.

rape, a sexual attack that is a crime of violence or done under the threat of violence.

raphe /rā′fē/, a line that marks the halves of similar parts of the body.

rapid eye movement. See **sleep.**

rapid relief, *(hazardous materials)* ranges from several seconds to several minutes, depending on the size of the opening, type of container, and the nature of its contents. This behavior is associated with releases from containers under pressure, through relief valve actuations, broken or damaged valves, punctures, tears, or broken piping.

rapids, a narrowed portion of a river with rough, turbulent water flow.

rapid sequence induction, an anesthesia technique, used in emergency department and field situations, to sedate and paralyze patients who are hypoxic and/or combative. This will have the effect of decreasing oxygen consumption and facilitating endotracheal intubation. The procedure involves the intravenous use of a sedative, such as midazolam, and a respiratory paralytic, such as vecuronium. Atropine and lidocaine may also be used as adjuncts. This technique is especially valuable with increases in intracranial pressure (may prevent further increases) or patients having recently eaten (danger of regurgitation/aspiration).

rappel /rəpel′/, descending while attached to an anchored rope. This descent may involve a helicopter, a mountain face, or a structure.

rappel-extract. See **short haul.**

rappel rack, U-shaped rappelling device that supports a series of brake bars, designed to slow a descent by creating friction on the rope.

rapport /rapôr′/, a sense of understanding, harmony, and respect in relation between two persons.

raptus, having a sudden or violent onset or attack. **Raptus haemorrhagicus** is sudden, heavy bleeding. **Raptus maniacus** is sudden, violent mania.

rash, a skin irritation.

ratbite fever, an infection carried to humans by the bite of a rat or mouse. Symptoms include fever, headache, vomiting, a rash on palms and soles, and painful joints.

ratio, the relation of one quantity to another. It is shown as a relation of one to the other and written either as a fraction (8/3) or linearly (8:3).

rational, **1.** treatment based on an understanding of the cause and processes of a specific disease and the possible effects of the drugs or methods used in treating the disorder. **2.** sane; able to reason or act normally.

rationale /rash′ənal′/, a system of reasoning or a statement of the reasons used in explaining data or happenings.

rationalization, creating believable reasons to explain a behavior.

rattlesnake bite. See **snakebite.**

Raynaud's phenomenon /rānōz´/, arterial spasm of the fingers, usually precipitated by cold exposure or emotional stimulation. Fingers develop paresthesia (or pain) and become cold and pale. It is known as **Raynaud's disease** when symptoms have occurred for a minimum of two years without evidence of other cause.

Raynaud's sign. See **acrocyanosis.**

reaction, a response to an antigen substance or treatment.

reaction time, the elapsed time from initiation of a situation to initial execution of an action plan.

reactive hyperemia, the increase in blood flow that occurs with states of increased metabolism.

reactivity, the ability of a material to undergo a chemical reaction with the release of energy.

read-only memory, computer memory chip that permanently stores data and instructions. Created at the time of manufacture, its contents cannot be altered. Also known as **ROM.**

reagent /rē·ā´jənt/, a chemical substance known to react in a specific way. A reagent is used to find or make another substance in a chemical reaction.

reanimatology, the preparation and delivery of disaster search and rescue, including the early resuscitation of the severely injured who become accessible through detection and/or extrication.

rebound tenderness, a sign of peritoneal inflammation that is caused by the sudden release of pressure applied to the abdomen by the hand. See also appendicitis, peritonitis.

rebreather, closed-circuit scuba apparatus from which oxygen-enriched gas is inhaled and exhaled air is recycled for removal of carbon dioxide. Generally used above 33 feet (due to danger of oxygen toxicity), it leaves no bubble trail. This characteristic makes it useful for research and special operations. Also known as **oxygen rebreather.**

receptor, a sensory nerve ending that responds to specific stimuli.

receptor site, a chemical group on or within a cell that is partial to a specific drug or chemical.

recessive gene. See **gene.**

reciprocity, granting certification or licensure in one location, based on an equivalent from another location.

reclining, leaning backward. –**recline,** v.

recrudescence /rē´krōōdes´əns/, return of symptoms of a disease; a relapse.

rectal, referring to the rectum.

rectosigmoid /-sig´moid/, the sigmoid colon and the proximal end of the rectum.

rectum, lower part of the large intestine between the sigmoid colon and the anal canal.

rectus muscle, any muscle of the body with a straight form. The **rectus abdominis** is one of a pair of muscles of the abdomen. It flexes the spine and helps to contain the stomach and intestine. The **rectus femoris** is a muscle of the thigh and one of the components of the quadriceps femoris muscle. It flexes the leg.

recumbent /rikum´bənt/, lying down or leaning backward. See also reclining. –**recumbency,** n.

recurvatum /rē´kərva´təm/, backward-bending, as of the knee when caused by weakness of a leg muscle or a joint disorder.

red blood cell, red cell. See **erythrocyte.**

Red Cross, international symbol used to identify facilities and personnel that care for the ill and wounded, particularly during time of war. It is a simple red cross on a white background, also the symbol for the American Red Cross.

red marrow. See **bone marrow.**

reduce, **1.** to restore a body part to its usual position. **2.** to decrease.

reeve /rēv/, to pass the end of a rope through a hole; to thread.

referred pain /rifurd´/. See **pain.**

reflex, a response to stimulus that occurs without conscious thought.

reflex action, the involuntary function of any organ or part of the body in response to a specific action. An **attitudinal reflex** is any reflex triggered by a change in position of the head. A **chain reflex** is a series of reflexes, each stimulated by the preceding one. A **conditional reflex** is one that is developed by linking a behavior with a specific, repeated stimulus. A **coordinated reflex** is a series of muscular actions with a purposeful, set progression, as in swallowing.

reflex arc, the shortest portion of the nervous system that can receive a stimulus and produce a response.

reflex emesis, vomiting due to irritation of the mouth and/or throat. This may occur after airway insertion, anxiety, coughing, exposure to unpleasant sights/smells, hiccup, hypoperfusion, or suctioning.

reflux /rē´fluks/, backward or return flow of a fluid, such as **gastroesophageal reflux.** *See also hepatojugular reflux, vesicoureteral reflux.*

refraction, a change in direction of the path followed by energy-bearing waves, as light rays into water.

refractory /rifrak´tərē/, a disorder that resists treatment.

refractory shock, reversible shock that is resistant to treatment.

regimen /rej´əmen/, a strictly controlled treatment, such as a diet or exercise schedule.

registered nurse, a professional nurse who has completed a course of study at an approved school of nursing and passed the examination required by the state in which he or she will function. Also known as **RN.**

regression, **1.** a retreat in conditions, signs, or symptoms. **2.** a return to an early form of behavior.

regulator, a device that reduces or controls pressure from a higher pressure source.

regurgitation /rigur´jitā´shən/, **1.** the return of swallowed food into the mouth. **2.** the backward flow of blood through a defect in a heart valve, named for the affected valve. *See also reflux.*

rehabilitation, **1.** the process of restoring useful life or function to one who has suffered illness or injury. **2.** the procedure of physically assessing emergency services personnel after a prolonged or strenuous operation. Also known as **rehab.**

rehydration, the replacement or return of water to a system.

reinforced attack, *(firefighting)* those resources requested in addition to the initial attack.

reinforcement, a mental process in which a response is made stronger by the fear of punishment or the hope of reward.

Reiter's syndrome /rī´tərz/, an arthritic disorder of adult males that may result from a viral or fungal infection. It affects the ankles, feet, and lower back. Symptoms include diarrhea, fever, conjunctivitis, and ulcers on the hands and feet. Arthritis often continues after resolution of the other symptoms.

rejection, **1.** an immune system response to substances that body tissues see as foreign, such as grafts or transplants. **2.** the act of denying affection or recognition to another person.

relapse, the return of disease symptoms after apparent recovery.

relapsing fever, any of many infections marked by recurrent fever and caused by *Borrelia* bacteria. The disease is carried by lice and ticks and has occurred in the western United States, but is more common in South America, Asia, and Africa. Initial symptoms include sudden fever chills, headache, muscle pain, nausea, and rash. Jaundice is common during later stages. Victims often relapse after 7 to 10 days of normal temperature.

relapsing polychondritis, inflammation and breakdown of cartilage. Most often the ears and nose are affected. The disease results in hearing loss and airway damage to the larynx and trachea.

relative biologic effectiveness, a measure of ability of a specific radiation to kill cells, as for cancer. It is compared with a specific level of x-rays.

relative hypovolemia, inadequate circulating blood volume due to vasodilation.

relative refractory period, period of the cardiac electrical cycle where a greater than normal electrical stimulus could produce depolarization. This period follows the absolute refractory period and is the time of maximum vulnerability for ventricular irritablility causing fibrillation.

relative urgency assessment, *(search and rescue)* an evaluation of the urgency of a given situation, based on assessing the subject and equipment carried, terrain, and weather.

release, the entry of hazardous materials into the atmosphere or environment.

releasing hormone, one of many hormones made by the hypothalamus and released into the pituitary gland. Each of the releasing hormones acts on the pituitary to release a certain hormone. Also known as **releasing factor.**

reliability, 1. dependability. **2.** the number of false-positive test results in a given test. When a test locates every positive without giving any positives that are actually negative (false-positives), it is 100% reliable. *See also sensitivity.*

remission, the partial or complete lack of symptoms of a long-term disease. Remission may be natural or the result of treatment. If the remission lasts for years, the disease is said to be cured. Compare **cure.**

remittent fever /rimit´ənt/, daily changes of a fever with increases and decreases but never a return to normal.

renal /rē´nəl/, referring to the kidney.

renal artery, one of a pair of arterial branches of the abdominal aorta, serving the kidneys, adrenal glands, and ureters.

renal calculus, kidney stone.

renal calyx, the entry points (ducts) for urine from the interior of the kidney that lead to the ureter. They form the body of the renal pelvis. Also known as **renal calix.**

renal capsule, the cortical substance separating the renal pyramids.

renal corpuscle, Bowman's capsule and the glomerulus it contains.

renal cortex, the soft, outer layer of the kidney, containing approximately 1.25 million tubes. These remove wastes from the blood in the form of urine. A **renal corpuscle** is one of the small red bodies in the cortex of the kidney. The corpuscles are thought to be part of a filter system through which nonprotein substances in blood plasma enter tubules in the kidney for urination.

renal failure. See **kidney failure.**

renal medulla, the inner layer of the kidney.

renal osteodystrophy, uneven bone growth and loss of minerals caused by long-term kidney failure.

renal papilla, the apex of the renal pyramid.

renal pelvis, the funnel-shaped upper end of the ureter.

renal pyramid, one of several masses within the kidney that contains a portion of the loop of Henle and the collecting tubules.

renal tubule, one of the collecting ducts of the kidney.

renin, the enzyme that converts angiotensinogen to angiotensin I.

renin-angiotensin-aldosterone mechanism, an increase in blood pressure due to a release of renin from the kidneys. This hormone is released in response to low blood pressure and converts angiotensinogen to angiotensin I. Angiotensin I is converted by enzymes to angiotensin II. This causes vasoconstriction and increases secretion of aldosterone, which increases pressure by increasing blood volume through fluid retention.

repeater, a device designed to amplify and/or regenerate data signals and retransmit them in order to increase a signal's range.

reperfusion dysrhythmias, cardiac rhythm disturbances occurring after reestablishment of myocardial circulation, particularly following administration of a thrombolytic, such as streptokinase.

reperfusion injury, myocardial impairment after reestablishment of coronary artery blood flow.

replacement, the substitution of a missing part or substance with a like part or substance, as to replace blood.

replication, 1. reproducing; copying. **2.** the process by which chromosome material is doubled in the cell.

repolarization, the period of the cardiac action potential during which the heart recovers from depolarization. The end of this phase returns the heart to its resting membrane potential, ready for depolarization again. This phase is represented on the EKG by the T wave. Also known as **phase 4.**

reporting locations, any one of six facilities/locations where incident assigned resources may check in. The locations are: incident command–resources unit, base camp, staging area, helibase, or division supervisor for direct line assignments.

reposition, to move to an alternative position.

repression, 1. holding back or down. **2.** a defense mechanism in which unwanted thoughts, feelings, or desires are pushed from the conscious into the unconscious mind.

reprisal, an injury inflicted in return for one suffered; an act of revenge.

reproduction, **1.** the way animals and plants procreate. **2.** creating a like structure, situation, or factor.

reproductive system, the male and female sex glands, associated ducts and glands, and the outer sex organs. In women these include the ovaries, fallopian tubes, uterus, vagina, clitoris, and vulva. In men these include the testicles, epididymis, vas deferens, seminal vesicles, ejaculatory duct, prostate, and penis. Also known as **genital tract.**

rescue, **1.** finding and removing a victim who is passively restrained by environment, such as in an elevator, on a mountain, or in water. **2.** to free from confinement or danger. *See also extrication.*

rescue basket, helicopter hoisting device, shaped like a rectangular basket, used for the retrieval of uninjured or lightly injured victims. It is generally used by marine rescue services, to retrieve victims at sea.

rescue breathing. See **artificial respiration.**

rescue can, a buoyant cylinder with a towline that can be towed to a swimmer in distress and used to support him or her to safety.

rescue company, a tactical unit that utilizes a rescue vehicle and several (2-4) personnel, possibly with a company officer. These units are classified as light, medium, or heavy depending on the company's capability for rescue. A light or medium rescue company would be utilized at a vehicle accident. A heavy rescue company would be needed at a building collapse.

rescue eight. See **figure-eight descender.**

rescue net, helicopter hoisting device with a rigid floor panel and sides of flexible plastic or rope mesh netting. Although capable of lifting 2–3 lightly injured victims, it has generally been replaced by the rescue basket. Also known as **Billy Pugh net.** *See also rescue basket.*

rescue throw bag, a rope bag, held at one end while being thrown, used as a swimmer rescue device.

rescue tube, a buoyant, cylindrical device, that can be formed into a horsecollar shape. When towed to a swimmer in distress, it is attached around them or otherwise used to pull/support them. *See also rescue can.*

resect /risekt´/, to remove tissue or an organ from the body by surgery. Resection of an organ may be partial or complete.

reservoir of infection, a source of infectious disease. People, animals, and plants may be reservoirs of infection.

resident, a doctor in training after internship.

resident bacteria, bacteria living in a certain area of the body.

residential care facility, a health care center, such as a nursing home. It gives nonmedical care to patients who, because of physical, mental, or emotional disorders, are not able to care for themselves.

residual volume, the air that stays in the lungs after exhaling as much as possible.

resin, **1.** a nonvolatile solid or semisolid substance that has no nitrogen and is insoluble in water. It occurs as a natural residue from plants, with many of these residues being highly toxic, such as those from chinaberry, water hemlock **2.** any organic compound of natural or synthetic origin used to form plastics, such as polyethylene, polyvinyl.

res ipsa loquitur /räs´ip´sə lō´kwitoor/, *(Latin)* "the thing speaks for itself." This legal term defines an event that is so self-explanatory that it requires no further explanation or evidence, such as a postsurgical patient with an instrument left inside the surgical site.

resistance, the ability to oppose. When related to electrical energy flow, this would describe the amount of opposition to electron flow. When related to the immune system of the body, it would describe the ability to resist infection.

resonance, a sound made in the body by percussing the area over an organ or space to determine the integrity of underlying structures.

resorption, the loss of tissue, such as bone, by the intrinsic or extrinsic breakdown of the tissue.

resources, all personnel and major items of equipment available, or potentially available, for assignment.

resource tracking, the accounting of frequency of use, location, and status of those personnel and/or pieces of equipment assigned to an agency, area, or incident.

respiration,   1. breathing. **2.** the exchange of carbon dioxide and oxygen between an organism and the environment in which it lives. **Metabolic respiration** is this exchange between cellular and mitochondrial membranes. *See also alveolar ventilation, ventilation.*

respiratory /res´pərətôr´ē, rispī´rə-/,   referring to breathing or respiration.

respiratory acidosis.   See **acidosis.**

respiratory alkalosis.   See **alkalosis.**

respiratory bronchiole,   the smallest connector between the terminal bronchiole and the alveolar duct.

respiratory center,   a specialized group of neurons in the brain that control breathing in response to changes in levels of oxygen and carbon dioxide

respiratory exchange ratio,   the amount of carbon dioxide exhaled compared to the amount of oxygen inhaled.

respiratory membrane,   the membrane in the lungs through which gas exchange with the blood occurs.

respiratory syncytial virus /sin´sish´əl, sin´sish´ē·əl/,   a virus that is a common cause of epidemics of respiratory illness in adults and young children. Symptoms include cough, fever, and malaise. Also known as **RSV.**

respiratory tract,   the system of organs and structures that transfers oxygen and carbon dioxide between the alveolar capillary beds of the lungs. The respiratory tract is divided into two parts. The **lower respiratory tract** includes the left and the right bronchi and the alveoli where the exchange of oxygen and carbon dioxide occurs during the breathing cycle. The bronchi, which are branches of the trachea, divide into smaller bronchioles in the lung tissue; the bronchioles divide into alveolar ducts; the ducts into alveolar sacs; and the sacs into alveoli. The **upper respiratory tract** consists of the nose, nasal cavity, larynx, and the trachea. The upper tract moves air to and from the lungs and filters, moistens, and warms the air. *See also larynx, lung, nose, trachea.*

respondeat superior /rāspōndā´ät soōperə·ōr´/, *(Latin)* "Let the master answer." This doctrine of indirect legal responsibility holds that the employer is responsible for the actions of the employees. Additionally, this may be applied to an EMS physician's responsibility for medical acts performed by field personnel for whom the physician is responsible. Also known as **vicarious liability.**

resting membrane potential,   the difference in electrical charge between the inside and outside of the cell membrane, when no electrical activity is taking place.

restraint,   1. hindering or restricting from physical or mental action. **2.** a device that restricts patient movement. This term is most often used to refer to straps placed around the extremities, which prevent a combative or uncooperative patient from injuring themselves or others.

resuscitator,   1. person(s) responsible for resuscitation. **2.** *(historical)* oxygen-powered devices used to support breathing for a patient with dyspnea or respiratory arrest. Their principle of operation revolved around pressure-cycling. With the advent of closed-chest cardiopulmonary resuscitation, these devices proved ineffective in maintaining sufficient ventilation due to the pressure changes that chest compression develops. These devices were previously known by various trade names, such as **E&J, Emerson.** *See also demand valve.* **3.** *(informal)* any mechanical ventilation device, particularly those used in acute respiratory situations in the emergency department or prehospital setting, such as **bag-valve-mask devices.**

retarded,   slow.

retention,   1. resisting movement or being moved. **2.** holding in place; keeping. **3.** temporary containment of the material in an area where it can be absorbed, neutralized, or vacuumed for proper disposal.

reticular /ritik´yələr/,   having a netlike pattern or structure of veins.

reticular activating system,   a system of the brain essential for consciousness. Nerve fibers in the thalamus, hypothalamus, brainstem, and cerebral cortex are components of the system and are responsible for attention, concentration, and introspection.

reticular formation,   a cluster of nerve cells in the medulla, midbrain, pons, and spinal cord.

They control breathing, heart rate, blood pressure, and other vital functions. Also known as **formatio reticularis.**

reticulocyte /ritik´yələsīt´/, immature red blood cells that usually make up less than 1% of red blood cells.

reticuloendothelial system /-en´dōthē´lē·əl/, a system used to defend against infection and to dispose of the products of the breakdown of cells. It is composed of macrophages, the cells of the liver and cells of the lungs, bone marrow, spleen, and lymph nodes.

reticuloendotheliosis /-lē·ō´-/, increased growth and spread of cells of the reticuloendothelial system.

retina /ret´inə/, a 10-layered, nervous tissue membrane of the eye, continuous with the optic nerve. It receives images of objects outside the eye and carries signals through the optic nerve to the brain. The retina contains visual purple (rhodopsin), a substance that adapts the eye to changes in light. The retina becomes clouded if exposed to direct sunlight. The outer surface of the retina is in contact with the choroid; the inner surface with the vitreous body. *See also eye.*

retinaculum /ret´inak´yələm/, *pl.* **retinacula,** a structure that holds an organ or tissue in place.

retinal /ret´inəl/, **1.** the active form of vitamin A needed for night, day, and color vision. *See also retinene, vitamin A.* **2.** referring to the retina of the eye.

retinal detachment, a separation of the retina of the eye from the covering (choroid) in the posterior eye. Symptoms include the appearance of spots floating loosely in the affected eye and flashing lights seen as the eye is moved.

retinene /ret´inin/, either of the two yellow pigments (carotenoid pigments) found in the rods of the retina that are sources of vitamin A and are set into motion by light. *See also retinal, retinol.*

retinol /ret´inôl/, a form of vitamin A, found in the retinas of the eyes of mammals. Also known as **vitamin A$_1$.**

retinopathy, disease or disorder of the retina.

retraction, drawing backward or shortening.

retraction of the chest, visible depression of the soft tissues of the chest between the ribs, as occurs with increased breathing effort. In infants, sternal retraction also occurs with only a mild increase in breathing effort.

retroflexion, an abnormal placement of an organ in which the organ is tilted posteriorly and folded over on itself.

retrograde, 1. moving backward; moving in the opposite direction to that which is thought to be normal. **2.** breaking down; returning to an earlier state.

retrograde amnesia, memory loss for events occurring prior to the incident that caused the amnesia.

retrolental fibroplasia, development of an opaque membrane on the posterior surface of the lens. This condition primarily occurs in premature infants exposed to high concentrations of oxygen for 10 hours or more.

retroperitoneal, behind the peritoneum, referring to the space or organs located there.

retroperitoneal fibrosis, chronic inflammation in which fiberlike tissue surrounds the large blood vessels of the lower back. It often causes narrowing of the ureters. Symptoms include back and abdominal pain, weakness, fever, and frequency of urination. It may spread to involve the duodenum, bile ducts, and the superior vena cava.

retropharyngeal abscess /-ferin´jē·əl/, a buildup of pus in the tissues of the posterior pharynx causing dysphagia, fever, and pain.

retrouterine /ret´rōyōō´tərin/, behind the uterus.

retroversion /-vur´zhən/, **1.** a condition in which an organ is tilted back, often without bending or other twisting. The uterus may be retroverted in as many as 25% of women. **2.** a condition in which the teeth or mandible are posterior of their normal location.

retrovirus, a family of viruses whose specialty is converting RNA to DNA, as does the human immunodeficiency virus (HIV).

revascularization, surgically restoring blood flow to an organ or a tissue being replaced, as in bypass surgery.

reversal. See **hydraulic.**

reverse squeeze. See **squeeze.**

revised trauma score, a modified indicator of injury severity that combines the Glasgow coma scale with respiratory rate and systolic blood pressure. *See also Glasgow coma scale, trauma score.*

Reye's syndrome,   an acute, noninfectious, life-threatening condition primarily affecting children and adolescents. This syndrome is known to be associated with many viruses, especially influenza B and varicella. There is also a strong association between the development of Reye's syndrome and the ingestion of salicylate-containing medications during viral illness. Symptoms include altered level of consciousness, abdominal tenderness, dysrhythmias, and tachypnea.

rewarming,   the process of raising body core temperature following hypothermia. This process can be a combination of active and passive treatment. **Active rewarming** is the direct transfer of heat to the patient, which is done externally (with heating blanket, hot-water bottle) or internally (with warmed oxygen, intravenous fluids, peritoneal lavage). **Passive warming** is an external procedure in which the patient is covered with dry insulating materials in a warm environment. This allows the patient's body heat to rebuild the lowered core temperature.

rhabdomyolysis /rab´dōmī·ol´əsis/,   syndrome caused by injury of skeletal muscle, with a release of muscle contents into the circulation. The muscle injury may be due to direct injury, drugs, genetic disorders, infection, or metabolic dysfunction. Whereas the underlying process causes most of the early symptoms, the lethal complication is renal failure. Also known as **Meyer-Betz disease.**

rhabdovirus,   a member of a family of viruses that includes rabies.

rhagades /rag´ədēz/,   tears in skin that has lost its ability to stretch. It is very common around the mouth.

rheumatic aortitis /rōōmat´ik/,   an inflammatory condition of the aorta. It occurs in rheumatic fever and results in damage to the aortic wall. A similar condition connected to rheumatic fever, called **rheumatic arteritis,** may occur in arteries and arterioles.

rheumatic fever,   a systemic, febrile, inflammatory disease that is variable in duration, se-

quelae, and severity. Although the etiology is unknown, this disorder follows an infection with group A beta-hemolytic streptococci. Symptoms may include fever, cardiac involvement (endocarditis, pericarditis), and migratory polyarthritis.

rheumatic heart disease, dysfunction of the heart attributed to complications caused by rheumatic fever. These patients may develop cardiomegaly and pericardial effusion, but disruption of mitral valve function is the most common pathophysiology.

rheumatism,   *(nontechnical)* any of the many conditions with inflammation of the bursae, joints, ligaments, or muscles. Symptoms include pain, limited movement, and tissue damage. –**rheumatic, rheumatoid,** *adj.*

rheumatoid arthritis,   a chronic connective tissue disease that results from an autoimmune reaction. There is inflammation of the synovial lining of the joints and increased release of synovial fluid. This leads to thickening of the synovial membrane and swelling of the joint. First symptoms include fatigue, weakness, anemia, and joint pain or tenderness.

rheumatoid lungs, pulmonary dysfunction caused by rheumatoid arthritis, such as pleural effusion, pulmonary interstitial fibrosis.

Rh factor,   an antigen in the red blood cells of most people. A person with the factor is Rh+ (Rh positive). A person lacking the factor is Rh– (Rh negative). If an Rh– person receives Rh+ blood, red blood cells are destroyed and anemia occurs. Transfusion, blood typing, and crossmatching depend on Rh and ABO blood group labeling. The Rh factor was first found in the blood of a species of rhesus (Rh) monkey and is in the red cells of 85% of humans.

rhinencephalon, /rī´nensef´əlon/, *pl.* **rhinencephala,**   a portion of each cerebral hemisphere that contains the limbic system, which is linked to the emotions. *See also limbic system.*

rhinitis /rīnī´-/,   inflammation of the mucous membranes of the nose, with a nasal discharge. It may be seen with a sinus infection or common cold.

rhinopathy /rinōp´əthē/,   any disease or defect of the nose.

rhinorrhea /rī´nôrē´ə/, **1.** the free flow of mucus from the nose. **2.** spinal fluid from the nose following an injury to the head.

rhinosporidiosis /rī´nōspərid´ē·ō´-/, a fungal infection with polyps on the mucous membranes of nose, the conjunctiva, nasopharynx, and the soft palate.

rhinovirus, any of about 100 distinct, small RNA viruses that cause about 40% of respiratory illness. *See also cold.*

rhitidosis /rit´idō´-/, a wrinkling, as of the cornea of the eye.

Rh negative. See **Rh factor.**

rhodopsin /rōdop´sin/. See **rod.**

rhomboideus major /romboi´dē·əs/, a muscle of the upper back. It pulls the scapula toward the spine.

rhonchi. See **breath sounds.**

rhotacism /rō´təsizm/, a speech disorder marked by defective pronunciation of words with the sound /r/, by the excess use of the sound /r/, or by using another sound for /r/.

Rh positive. See **Rh factor.**

rhus dermatitis /rōōs/, a skin rash resulting from contact with a plant of the genus *Rhus,* such as poison ivy, poison oak, or poison sumac. *See also contact dermatitis.*

rhythm, **1.** repetitive sounds or motions that follow a particular pattern. **2.** *(informal)* the pattern of an EKG; the cardiac rhythm, such as sinus tachycardia.

rib, one of the 12 pairs of elastic arches of bone forming the largest portion of the thoracic skeleton. The first seven ribs on each side are called **true ribs** because they join to the sternum and the vertebrae. The other five ribs are called **false ribs.** The first three join with the ribs above. The last two are free anteriorly and are known as **floating ribs.**

riboflavin /rī´bōflā´vin/, a B vitamin, important in preventing sight disorders, such as cataracts. Small amounts of riboflavin are found in the liver and kidneys. Common sources are organ meats, milk, cheese, eggs, green leafy vegetables, meat, whole grains, and peas. Also known as **vitamin B₂.**

ribonucleic acid (RNA) /-nōōklē´ik/, a nucleic acid, found in both the nucleus and cytoplasm of cells. It carries gene data from the nucleus to the cytoplasm. In the cytoplasm, RNA binds proteins. **Messenger RNA** is a part of RNA that sends information from DNA (deoxyribonucleic acid) to the protein-making ribosomes of cells. *See also deoxyribonucleic acid.*

ribosome /-sōm/, an organelle in the cytoplasm of cells. Ribosomes act with messenger RNA and transfer RNA to join together amino acid units into a larger protein molecule according to a series of reactions by a genetic code.

Richter scale, measurement scale for determining the magnitude of an earthquake. This scale uses seismograph measurement of the amplitude of ground activity to determine intensity of an earthquake. An increase of one on the scale indicates ten times greater ground motion than the number before it. Although the scale is open-ended, magnitudes greater than 8 are rare. Magnitudes up to 6 are mild, 6-7 is moderate, and above 7 is great. *See also Mercalli scale.*

rickets, a condition caused by the lack of vitamin D, calcium, and phosphorus causing abnormal bone growth. Symptoms include soft bones, muscle pain, enlarged liver and spleen, diophoresis, and general tenderness.

rickettsia /riket´sē·ə/, *pl.* **rickettsiae,** any organism of the genus *Rickettsia.* Rickettsiae are rod-shaped bacteria. They live inside lice, fleas, ticks, and mites. They are carried to humans by bites from these insects. Rickettsial diseases have caused many of history's worst epidemics, including typhus and the spotted fevers.

right lymphatic duct, a vessel that carries lymph from the right superior area of the body to the blood stream. The duct dumps into the right internal jugular and right subclavian veins. *See also lymphatic system.*

rigidity, a condition of hardness or stiffness.

rigid transport vehicle, a specialized victim transport device with a rigid spine. Types include **Akja, cascade, forest/jungle penetrator, Jake's litter, Neil-Robertson litter, Stokes's litter,** and **Thompson litter.** While these devices offer excellent victim protection in rugged terrain, they are generally bulky and heavy. See specific entry. *See also soft transport vehicle.*

rigor /rig´ər, rī´gər/, **1.** a rigid condition of the tissues of the body, as in rigor mortis. **2.** a violent attack of shivering that may come with chills and fever.

rigor mortis /môr´tis/, the rigid stiffening of the muscles shortly after death. *See also Nystan's law.*

ring buoy, a circular personal flotation device, used as rescue equipment at pools and beaches. This device is approximately 18 inches in diameter, constructed of rigid, buoyant material with a grab line encircling the buoy and a 50-foot retrieving line attached. It is classified as a throwable personal floatation device by the U.S. Coast Guard.

Ringer's lactate (Sydney Ringer, British physiologist, 1835-1910), an intravenous solution generally used for volume replacement in the field. This solution consists of sterile distilled water, sodium chloride, sodium lactate, calcium chloride, and potassium chloride. Also known as **lactated Ringer's solution, LR, Ringer's, RL.**

ringworm, a contagious fungal disease with circular patches of erythema, scaling, and crusting. Also known as **tinea capitis.** *See also tinea.*

riot control agent. See **chemical agent, lacrimator, sternutator.**

rip, a seaward flow of water from a depression on the beach. The depression creates a funnel effect, which increases the pull (speed) of the water. This pull can carry a person from shallow water to beyond the breaker line. Swimming parallel to the shore or riding out the current are two means of escape. Also known as **riptide.** *See also runout.*

riprap, large pieces of rock placed along the shoreline of a body of water to prevent erosion. This material is also placed downstream of low-head dams to break up hydraulic backwash. Also known as **ripp-rapp.**

risk factor, a factor that causes a person or a group of people to be at risk for an unwanted or unhealthful event. **Relative risk** is the chance that a disease or side effect will occur given certain conditions or factors, such as the relative risk of lung cancer in someone who smokes cigarettes as compared with the risk in someone who does not smoke.

risorius /risôr´ē·əs/, one of the 12 muscles of the mouth. It retracts the angles of the mouth, as in a smile.

Rocky Mountain spotted fever, an infectious disease carried by ticks in the warm zones of North and South America. It is caused by bacteria *Rickettsia.* Symptoms include chills, fever, headache, muscle pain, confusion, and rash. *See also typhus.*

rod, one of the tiny nerve cells shaped like a cylinder on the surface of the retina of the eye. Rods have a chemical (rhodopsin) that allows the eye to detect dim light. It breaks down when exposed to bright light. Compare **cone.** *See also dark adaption.*

rodenticide poisoning, condition caused by swallowing a substance used to kill rats, mice, or other rodents. *See also phosphorus poisoning, warfarin poisoning.*

roentgen /rent´gən/ (Wilhelm Konrad Roentgen, German physicist, 1845-1923), a unit of x-ray or gamma radiation. One unit will produce ions that carry 1 electrostatic unit of charge (in 1 cubic centimeter of dry air at standard temperature and pressure).

roentgen equivalent, man, a unit-dose of biological radiation, calculated so that the number of roentgen equivalents, man (rems) is equal to the number of radiation absorbed doses (rads), multiplied by the quality factor of the given radiation, the distribution factor, and any modifying factors. *See also quality factor, radiation absorbed dose, sievert.*

roll, the longitudinal axis of movement, such as one wing dropping lower than the other; one of the axes of three-dimensional movement.

roller. See **hydraulic.**

roller bandage, a strip of soft, thick cotton material used to cover or hold a dressing in place. In addition, its thickness serves to absorb drainage. Commercially prepared material is rolled on its short axis (length 2-5 yards [1.8-4.6 meters]; width ½ to 6 inches [1.3-15.2 centimeters]). Also known as **Kerlix**™. *See also roller gauze.*

roller gauze, a strip of soft, thin cotton material used to cover or hold a dressing in place. Its dimensions are as those for roller bandage. Also known as **Kling**™. *See also roller bandage.*

Romberg sign, a loss of the sense of position in which the patient loses balance when standing erect, feet together, and eyes closed. Also known as **Romberg test.**

R-on-T phenomenon, a premature ventricular ectopic occurring during the relative refractory period of the T wave of the cardiac electrical cycle. A ventricular ectopic occurring at this time indicates an increase in cardiac irritability and places the patient at maximum risk for lethal ventricular rhythms.

roof bolt, a long metal bar that is driven into the overhead rock of an underground mine to stabilize the ceiling.

root, **1.** the proximal end of a nerve. **2.** the portion of an organ implanted in tissue, such as of a tooth. **3.** portion of the aircraft fuselage where the wing attaches.

rope climbers, small-diameter rope wrapped around the bottom of skis to create friction, easing ascents or descents for injured or tired skiers.

rosacea /rōzā´shē·ə/, a chronic form of acne seen in adults. Also known as **acne rosacea.**

roseola infantum /rōzē´ələ/, an illness of infants and young children with fever, sore throat, and enlarged lymph nodes.

rotation, **1.** turning around an axis. **External rotation** is a turning outward or away from the midline of the body. For example, a leg is turned out when the toes point away from the body's midline. **Lateral rotation** is turning away from the midline of the body, as when twisting to the left or right. **Medial rotation** is a turning toward the midline. **Neutral rotation** is turned neither toward nor away from the body's midline. **2.** one of the basic kinds of motion allowed by many joints, such as the rotation of the head on neck. **3.** the turning of a baby's head to go through the pelvis.

rotating tourniquets, constricting bands placed around the arms and legs to decrease blood return to the right side of the heart, by trapping blood in the extremities. The procedure has generally fallen into disuse due to concern regarding its effectiveness.

rouleaux formation /rōōlō´/, a collection of red blood cells that appears as a stack of coins and is seen microscopically in blood samples drawn during the final stages of irreversible shock.

round ligament, **1.** a ligament that attaches to the head of the femur on the articular surface. **2.** the remains of the umbilical vein.

roundworm, any worm of the class Nematoda, which includes the hookworm and the pinworm.

route of administration, any one of the ways in which a drug may be given, such as intramuscularly, intranasally, intravenously, orally, rectally, subcutaneously, sublingually, topically, and vaginally.

route of entry, one of four pathways through which a substance (toxic or otherwise) can enter the body; absorption, ingestion, inhalation, and/or injection, Also known as **portal of entry.**

roving gaze, slow, horizontal motions of the eye(s). This motion indicates integrity of the brainstem, thereby ruling out brainstem damage as a reason for unconsciousness.

R prime, a second positive deflection (**R'**) in the QRS complex of the EKG that extends above the baseline and is taller than the initial R wave.

R-R interval, EKG time interval measured from the beginning of an R wave to the next R wave. The measurement of several of these intervals indicates whether a rhythm is regular or irregular.

rubefacient /rōō´bəfā´shənt/, something that increases the reddish color of the skin.

rubella /rōōbel´ə/, the contagious viral disease German measles. Symptoms include fever, enlarged lymph nodes, joint pain, and rash. The virus is spread by respiratory droplets from coughs or sneezes.

rubeola /rōōbē´ələ/. See **measles.**

rubescent /rōōbes´ənt/, reddening.

rubivirus /rōō´bē-/, a member of the virus family, such as rubella virus.

rubor /rōō´bôr/, redness, especially when there is swelling.

rudder, **1.** a broad, flat steering device attached to the stern of a vessel. **2.** the upright moveable portion of the tail assembly, which controls the direction of an aircraft.

rudiment /rōō´dəmənt/, an organ or tissue that is incompletely developed or does not work. **–rudimentary,** *adj.*

ruga /rōō´gə/, *pl.* **rugae,** a ridge or fold, such as the rugae of the stomach, which form large folds in the mucous membrane of that organ.

rule of nines, method of estimating percentage of body surface area useful in determining the amount of skin damaged by burn injury. Using this method for adults, the head and upper extremities represent 9% of body surface; the trunk, front, and back each 18%; each lower extremity 18%; and the perineum 1%. *See also Appendix 3-11, rule of palms.*

rule of palms,   an estimate of body surface area with the palm of the patient's hand equaling 1%; generally used to estimate the amount of body surface area burned. *See also rule of nines.*

rumination /roō´minā´shən/,   the regurgitation of small amounts of undigested food after every feeding. It is commonly seen in infants and may be a symptom of overfeeding, eating too fast, or swallowing air.

runner,   **1.** a person used during periods of communications failure to carry messages between locations. **2.** a moving line (rope).

running soil,   loose, freely flowing soil, such as sandy soil, sugar sand.

runout,   seaward water flow through a hole in a sandbar, with the hole acting as a funnel. This funnel accelerates the water's speed, creating a hazardous current. This current can tire the strongest swimmer, although it dissipates about 25 yards beyond the sandbar. *See also rip.*

runout zone.   See **avalanche path.**

rupture /rup´chər/,   a tear in an organ or tissue. *See also hernia.*

R wave,   the first upward deflection of the QRS complex; the first positive deflection following the P wave.

S

sac, a pouch or a baglike organ.

saccharide /sak´ərīd/, any of a large group of carbohydrates, including all sugars and starches. Almost all carbohydrates are saccharides. *See also carbohydrate, sugar.*

saccharin /sak´ərin/, a white, crystal-like artificial sweetener, sweeter than table sugar (sucrose). Saccharin is often used as a substitute for sugar.

Saccharomyces /sak´ərōmī´sēz/, a genus of yeast fungi, including brewer's and baker's yeast, as well as some harmful fungi, that cause such diseases as bronchitis, candidiasis, and pharyngitis.

saccharomycosis /-mīkō´-/, infection with yeast fungi, as the genera *Candida* or *Cryptococcus.*

saccule /sak´yōol/, a small bag or sac, such as the air saccules of the lungs. **–saccular,** *adj.*

sacral /sā´krəl, sak´rəl/, referring to the sacrum.

sacral bone, the five fused segments of the vertebral column that form the sacrum, known as **S1-S5.**

sacral foramen, one of a number of openings between the vertebrae in the pelvic area through which nerves pass.

sacral plexus, a network of nerves that lie against the posterior wall of the pelvis. It becomes the sciatic nerve.

sacral promontory, the prominent portion of the pelvis at the base of the sacrum.

sacral sparing, the partial or complete preservation, after spinal injury, of nerve function of the anus, buttocks, perineum, and/or scrotum.

sacroiliac /sak´rō·il´ē·ak/, referring to the part of the skeleton that includes the sacrum and the ilium of the pelvis.

sacrospinalis /-spīnā´lis/, a large muscle of the back. It straightens and supports the vertebral column and the head, and it retracts the ribs inferiorly.

sacrum /sā´krəm/. See **vertebra.**

saddle joint, a type of joint, as the wrist and thumb. Compare **pivot joint.**

sadism /sā´dizm, sad´izm/, **1.** pleasure from causing physical or mental pain or abuse to others; cruelty. **2.** a disorder marked by a wish to hurt another person, willing or unwilling, for sexual satisfaction. Compare **masochism. –sadistic,** *adj.*

sadist, a person who suffers from or practices sadism.

safety line, a line or rope used as a backup to allow retrieval or prevent falls in the event of emergency.

safety officer, that person(s), in an incident command operation, who is responsible for assessing and monitoring safety hazards and developing contingency plans for personnel protection.

Safety of Life at Sea, an international organization, sponsored by the United Nations, that establishes maritime regulations. Under the

International Maritime Organization, 67 nations meet periodically to set standards for cargo, communications, fire protection, lifesaving, navigation, ship construction, and surveys at sea. Also known as **SOLAS.**

Saffir/Simpson Hurricane Scale, rating system for determining the severity of tropical cyclones. Parameters assessed include wind speed, damage sustained, and protective measures required. *See also tropical cyclone.* See Appendix 3-21.

safing, removing danger from an unsafe situation. While dealing with explosive ordnance disposal, this would entail rendering the device incapable of detonation. In trench rescue, this would be accomplished by the installation of sheeting and shoring. Vehicle rescue mandates that battery cables are removed to prevent the possibility of electrical fire.

sagittal plane /saj´itəl/, an anatomical view that divides the body vertically into right and left sections. This provides a side view of body structures, but does not necessarily divide the body into two equal halves. When the two sections are equal, this is termed a **midsagittal plane.**

sagittal suture, the saw-toothed line in the top of the skull that is formed where the parietal bones of the skull join.

Saint Bernard Hospice, traveler's stop on the Great Saint Bernard pass of the Pennine Alps (linking Switzerland and Italy), known for the large dogs used there for rescuing travelers in distress. The hospice and monastery located there were founded in the 11th century by St. Bernard de Menthon.

salicylate /səlis´ilāt/, any of several widely used drugs that are made from salicylic acid.

salicylate poisoning, a condition caused by ingesting salicylate, most often aspirin or oil of wintergreen. It manifests as tachypnea, vomiting, headache, seizures, and respiratory arrest.

saliva, the clear, viscous fluid secreted by glands in the mouth. Saliva contains water, mucin, organic salts, and the enzyme ptyalin that helps digest food. It aids in keeping the mouth wet, initiates the digestion of starches, and facilitates chewing and swallowing food.

salivary /sal´iver´ē/, relating to saliva or to the forming of saliva.

salivary amylase, a digestive enzyme excreted orally, that initiates the chemical conversion of carbohydrates for metabolism.

salivary duct, any of the tubes that carry saliva.

salivary fistula, a hole between a salivary gland or duct and the mouth or skin of the face or neck.

salivary gland, one of the three pairs of glands that aids in the digestion of food. The **parotid glands** are the largest pair of salivary glands. They lie near the tempromandibular joint. The **sublingual glands** are found inferior to the mucous membrane of the floor of the mouth beneath the tongue. The **submandibular glands** are a pair of walnut-sized salivary glands found inferior to the mandible in the anterior neck.

salivation, the secretion of saliva by the salivary glands.

Salmonella /sal´mənel´ə/, a genus of rod-shaped bacteria that includes species causing typhoid fever, paratyphoid fever, and some forms of gastroenteritis.

salmonellosis /sal´mənelō´-/, infection of the digestive tract caused by eating food contaminated with a species of *Salmonella*. Symptoms include sudden pain in the abdomen, fever, and watery diarrhea that occur 6 to 48 hours after eating. Nausea and vomiting are common. *See also food poisoning.*

salpingectomy /sal´pinjek´-/, surgical removal of one or both fallopian tubes.

salpingitis /-jī´-/, inflammation or infection of the fallopian tube. *See also pelvic inflammatory disease.*

salt, **1.** a substance made by mixing together an acid and a base. **2.** sodium chloride (common table salt).

saltatory conduction, irregular nerve conduction from one myelinated neuron to another.

salt depletion, the loss of salt from the body through increased diophoresis, diarrhea, vomiting, or urination.

salvage, to recover from an accident or fire for reuse.

salvo, two ectopic cardiac beats in a row. They may originate in the atria, atrioventricular junction, or ventricles. Also known as **couplets.**

SAM™ splint. See **splint.**

sandbags, burlap, cloth, or plastic bags, filled with sand, used to protect against flooding or as protection against explosions.

sanguineous /sang·gwin´ē·əs/, relating to blood.

sanitary sewer, a pipeline carrying sewage.

saphenous nerve /səfē´nəs/, the longest branch of the femoral nerve, located along the medial lower leg. One branch extends to the ankle. Another branch extends to the medial foot.

sarcoidosis /sär´koidō´-/, a chronic disease causing growths to form in the tissue around many organs of the body, including the lungs, spleen, liver, and skin. They lead to widespread inflammation and fibrous tissue. With **sarcoidosis cordis,** grainy growths develop in the heart.

sarcolemma, a portion of myofibril between adjacent Z lines.

sarcoma /särkō´mə/, a cancer of the soft tissues usually appearing as a painless swelling. About 40% of sarcomas occur in the legs and feet, 20% in the hands and arms, 20% in the trunk, with the remainder in the head or neck. The growth tends to spread very quickly.

sarcomere, the portion of skeletal muscle that contracts.

sarcoplasmic reticulum /sär´kōplaz´mik/, a network of canals and sacs in muscles attached to the skeleton that play an important part in muscle function.

sartorius /särtôr´ē·əs/, the longest muscle in the body, stretching from the pelvis to the inferior knee. It is a narrow muscle that extends across the anterior thigh, laterally to medially in relation to the knee. It causes the thigh to move up and out and the lower leg to move in.

saturated, having absorbed or dissolved the largest possible amount of a given substance; unable to absorb any further.

saturated fatty acid. See **fatty acid.**

saturated soil, soil containing a high quantity of water.

saturation diving, underwater diving of sufficient duration and depth that the tissues are saturated with inert gas. Breathing mixtures involve multiple gases (helium/oxygen) and depth may reach 500 meters (about 1500 feet). The saturation diver remains at depth for days at a time.

Also known as **long-duration diving, mixed-gas diving.**

satyriasis /sat´irī´əsis/, excessive or uncontrollable sexual desire in the male. Also known as **satyromania.** Compare **nymphomania.**

savanna, a grassy plain with high (about 3 m or 12 ft), thick grass and occasional shrubs and trees. Located in the earth's tropical zone, this terrain has dry and wet seasons, but moderate to heavy rainfall.

saw, a cutting tool with a toothed edge, such as **chain saw, circular saw, hacksaw.**

scabicide /skab´isīd/, any one of a large group of drugs that destroy the itch mite, *Sarcoptes scabiei.*

scabies /skā´bēz/, a contagious disease caused by the itch mite. There is intense pruritus and urticaria which often occurs on the fingers, wrists, and thighs. The mite, passed by close contact with infected humans or domestic animals, burrows into the layers of the skin where the female lays eggs. Two to 4 months later, the eggs hatch.

scalp, the skin that covers the top of the head. The face and ears are not included.

scaphocephaly /skaf´ōsef´əlē/, a defect of the skull present at birth in which the skull has an unusually long narrow shape.

scaphoid, hollowed; boat-shaped, as in the scaphoid bone (navicular) or a scaphoid abdomen.

scapulohumeral /skap´yəlōhyo͞o´mərəl/, referring to the muscles and the area around the scapula and humerus.

scapulohumeral reflex, a normal response to tapping the medial side of the scapula, causing arm jerk. If the arm does not move, it may be a sign of damage to the spine.

scarify /sker´əfī/, to make a number of light cuts into the skin; to scratch. Vaccination for smallpox is done by scarifying the skin under a drop of vaccine.

scarlet fever, a contagious disease of childhood caused by a type of *Streptococcus*. The infection causes sore throat, fever, enlarged lymph nodes in the neck, and a widespread bright red rash. Also known as **scarlatina.**

scene safety, evaluation of hazards and protection against them at the scene. Those protected include (in order of importance): emergency responders, bystanders, and victims. This phrase is most often used to refer to vehicle accidents, but it applies equally to any critical incident scene. Although risk cannot generally be eliminated, it can be minimized.

scent dog, a type of search dog that works without a leash to follow a person's scent to its source. The initial scent may be taken from clothing articles. This type of dog can detect scents that are buried in snow or water; winds affect this dog greatly. Also known as **air-scenting dog.** *See also tracking dog, trailing dog.*

Schäfer prone pressure method (Sir Edward Sharpey Schäfer, British physiologist, 1850-1935), *(historical)* technique of artificial respiration, advocated in 1903, which utilized a single rescuer positioned over a prone victim. The rescuer would straddle a victim's legs, placing both hands over the lower rib cage and, rocking forward, use the weight of the rescuer to force the diaphragm upward (forced expiration). Releasing pressure allowed relaxation of the diaphragm (return airflow into the chest). This method was eventually replaced by the back-pressure arm-lift and the chest-pressure arm-lift. *See also back-pressure arm-lift, chest-pressure arm-lift.*

schistosomiasis /shis´tōsōmī´əsis/, infection caused by the parasite *Schistosoma* due to contact with freshwater fouled with feces. Symptoms depend on the part of the body infected. *Schistosoma* may be found in the bladder, rectum, liver, lungs, spleen, intestine, and veins. It may cause pain, damage to the organ, and anemia. Schistosomiasis most often occurs in the tropics and in the Orient.

schizoid /skit´soid, skiz´oid/, **1.** typical of or resembling schizophrenia; schizophrenic. **2.** a person, not necessarily a schizophrenic, who shows the traits of a schizoid personality.

schizoid personality disorder, a state marked by the lack of the ability to make friends, a lack of feelings, the wish to be alone all the time and no concern for the opinions and feelings of others. The person is not able to show anger or any hostile feelings and does not seem to react to disturbing experiences. It may lead to schizophrenia.

schizophasia /skit´səfā´zhə, skiz´ə-/, the rambling babble typical of some types of schizophrenia.

schizophrenia /-frē´nē·ə/, any of a large group of mental disorders in which the patient loses touch with reality and is no longer able to think or act normally. **Acute schizophrenia** is the sudden onset of identity crisis. Symptoms include confusion, fear, depression, and inappropriate social behavior.

schizophrenic /-fren´ik/, **1.** relating to schizophrenia. **2.** a person with schizophrenia.

Schwann cell, the basic component that forms the myelin sheath around each peripheral nerve fiber.

sciatic /sī·at´ik/, near the hip, as is the sciatic nerve or the sciatic vein.

sciatica /sī·at´ikə/, inflammation of the sciatic nerve, usually with pain along the thigh and leg. It may cause muscle atrophy to the affected side.

sciatic nerve, a nerve which innervates the muscles of the thigh, leg, and foot.

science, an objective system for study or research that organizes facts and observations, controls variables, and provides the reproducibility necessary to explain how the world and everything in it works. **Pure science** is concerned with learning new facts for the sake of gaining new knowledge. **Applied science** is the practical use of scientific theory and laws.

scientific method, a system of obtaining knowledge by observing, hypothesizing, experimenting, and, when possible, reaching a conclusion.

sclera /sklir´ə/, the tough, white membrane covering most of the posterior eye. It helps the eye hold its shape. The muscles that move the eye are attached to the sclera.

sclerose /sklerōz´/, to harden or to cause hardening. **—sclerotic,** *adj.*

sclerosis /sklerō´-/, hardening of tissue resulting from any of several causes, including inflammation, the deposit of mineral salts, and damaged connective tissue fibers. **—sclerotic,** *adj.*

scoliosis /skō´lē·ō´-/, lateral curvature of the spine, resulting in an S shape to the spine.

scombroid poisoning, toxicity caused by eating inadequately preserved fish of the families

Scomberesocidae (saury) and *Scombridae* (bonito, mackerel, tuna). Symptoms include abdominal cramps, bronchospasm, diarrhea, hypotension, nausea, palpitations, pruritus, upper-body erythema, urticaria, and vomiting. Onset of symptoms occurs in 60 minutes or less.

scoop stretcher, patient-lifting device that can be separated longitudinally into halves. Although originally designed as a device that would separate, scoop under a patient, and then be reconnected, it is also used as a complete unit onto which a patient is logrolled. Effective for use with patients having a mechanism of injury (potential) for fractures and spinal injury, it is also used for lifting and moving patients found on the floor or in dwellings with restricted space. Originally known as **Greene splint, Robinson, Sarole.** *See also Greene splint.*

scopophilia /skō´pəfil´yə/, **1.** sexual pleasure from looking at sexually exciting scenes or at another person's genitals; voyeurism. **2.** a desire to be seen; exhibitionism.

scopophobia, fear of being seen or stared at by others. The condition is common in schizophrenia. *See also phobia.*

scorpion sting, the painful wound of a scorpion, a member of the spider family with a hollow stinger in its tail. The sting of certain scorpions may be lethal, especially in small children. Pain is followed within hours by numbness, nausea, muscle spasm, dyspnea, and seizures.

scotopic vision, human night vision. *See also peripheral vision, photopic vision, purkinje shift.*

scramble, 1. to code a transmission electronically so that it can be read only by a receiver with the proper decoding equipment. **2.** *(military aviation)* term that initiates an aircrew's response to their aircraft upon notification of an emergency.

scratch test, physical exam technique for determining the presence of a pneumothorax by scratching each side of the anterior chest, while listening with a stethoscope. If a finger is used to scratch an equal distance from the sternum, one side at a time, the louder sound will be found on the side with the pneumothorax.

screamer suit. See **soft transport vehicle.**

screening, 1. an initial evaluation, as an examination to determine fitness for a job. **2.** the testing of a large number of persons to locate disease, such as high blood pressure.

screw jack, a jack or trench shore with threaded parts, allowing lengthening or shortening.

scrotum /skrō´təm/, the pouch of skin that encapsulates the testicles. *See also testis.*

sculling, moving a paddle or oar from side to side, so that the boat or body is moved toward the side.

scurvy, a disease process due to a lack of vitamin C in the diet. Symptoms include weakness, anemia, edema, spongy gums, often with open sores in the mouth and loosening of the teeth, and bleeding of the mucous membranes. A **scorbutic pose** is the typical posture of a child with scurvy, with thighs and legs half-bent and hips turned laterally. The child usually lies still without moving the hands or feet because of the pain that movement causes.

Scyphozoa, group of sea animals that include the larger jellyfish and medusae. These animals possess the most potent venom in the world and range in size from millimeters (less than an inch) to meters (feet) and include the box jellyfish, giant jellyfish, and sea wasps. The man-of-war is not included in this group.

sealed source, a radioactive source sealed in an impervious container that has sufficient mechanical strength to prevent contact with and dispersion of the radioactive material under the conditions of use and wear for which it was designed.

search area determination, procedure for establishing an area of probability in which to conduct a search for person(s) lost. The four basic methods are Mattson, statistical, subjective, and theoretical. All these methods develop a zone around the point last seen. The Mattson method uses a large-group consensus to decide the search area. The statistical method uses predetermined lost-person statistics to calculate the area for search concentration. The subjective method uses the experiences of several searchers, combined with reasoning and speculation, to develop an area. The theoretical process uses known data, such as data on humans' speed, calculated from the point last seen, and variables of terrain and physical condition to narrow the region in which the subject of the search may be found.

search management,   the strategy and tactics of finding lost persons. This concept centers around analysis of lost-person behaviors and proper utilization of resources.

search pattern,   a specified method of physical search for lost persons, generally classified into three types. Type I is investigation of drainage areas, structures, trails, and ridges. This is the type used on initial or hasty team searches. Type II is a rapid, open-grid search, and type III calls for saturation of an area with a close-grid search.

search tactics,   methods of conducting time-dependent searches. Types I, II, and III may all be used, depending on length and type of search. Type I is the most rapid mode, happening early in a search. It utilizes hasty ground teams to check areas of highest probability. Type II methods are moderately fast, using dogs, aircraft, and rapid, open-grid ground searches. Type III is the slowest method, utilizing all resources to search exact areas of terrain (close-grid search) and covering those areas completely. *See also* Appendix 3-12.

seasickness.   See **motion sickness.**

seat harness,   a climbing device formed from tubular webbing wrapped around the waist and legs. Types include the diaper sling, double, figure of eight, and swami. Commercial models made of webbing are also available. Also known as **sit harness.**

sea urchin sting,   an injury from any sea urchin in which the skin is pierced and, in some species, venom released. A poisonous sting causes pain, paresis, numbness around the mouth, and dyspnea. *See also stingray.*

sebaceous   /sibā´shəs/, fatty, oily, or greasy, usually referring to the oil-secreting glands of the skin or to their secretions.

sebaceous cyst,   a closed sac filled with material from a sebaceous gland. Often due to blockage of sebaceous glands, they may grow to a large size. Also known as **wen.**

sebaceous gland,   one of the many small saclike organs in the skin. They are found all through the body, but especially in the scalp, face, anus, nose, mouth, and external ear. They are absent in the palms of the hands and the soles of the feet.

seborrhea   /seb´ôrē´ə/, any skin condition which causes increased sebum production.

seborrheic dermatitis   /-rē´ik/, a chronic inflammatory skin disease with dry or moist scales and yellowish crusts. Common sites are the scalp, eyelids, face, ears, breasts, and groin. **Seborrheic blepharitis** is a type in which the eyelids are red and the edges are covered with a grainy crust. *See also dandruff.*

sebum   /sē´bəm/, the oily secretion of the sebaceous glands of the skin, composed of keratin, fat, and cellular debris. Mixed with sweat, sebum forms a moist, oily, acidic film that is mildly harmful to bacteria and fungus and protects the skin against drying.

secondary,   **1.** less important; second in order. **2.** *(informal)* secondary assessment; physical exam.

secondary bronchus,   the air passage that leads to each lobe of the lungs; a branch of the primary bronchus.

secondary epilepsy,   epilepsy caused by illness or trauma.

secondary follicle,   container enclosing the secondary oocyte and surrounded by granulosa cells.

secondary injury,   the injuries sustained after being struck by material propelled from a blast. *See also blast injury, primary injury, tertiary injury.*

secondary sex characteristic,   any of the visible bodily features of sexual maturity that develop as a person grows older. These features include the growth of body hair and the development of the penis or breasts.

secondary survey,   the complete physical exam following the primary (or emergent, initial, rapid) survey. Generally, this exam consists of vital signs, medical history, and a head-to-toe evaluation of patient condition. This will be performed on stable patients at scene. Unstable patients will have it performed enroute to the medical facility. Also known as **head-to-toe survey, secondary.**

second-degree AV block,   heart block with intermittent conduction disturbances at the atrioventricular (AV) node. The two types are Mobitz I (Wenckebach) and Mobitz II (classic second-degree heart block). Also known as **second degree, Mobitz I or II.** *See also Mobitz I, second-degree AV block; Mobitz II, second-degree AV block.*

second opinion, an assessment and recommendation provided by a second practitioner, who will not participate in the patient's care or treatment. This opinion is often sought when the patient and/or clinician has unanswered questions about care or treatment.

second stage of labor, the period of time during labor occurring from the full dilation of the cervix until delivery.

secrete, to release a substance into a cavity, vessel, or organ or onto the surface of the skin, as does a gland.

secretin /sikrē´tin/, a hormone made by the lining of the intestine that helps digest food and produce bile.

secretory phase, that time of the menstrual cycle from formation of the corpus luteum to the beginning of the menstrual flow.

section, the level of organization within the incident command system that has functional responsibility for primary segments of an operation, such as finance, logistics, medical. The responsibilities of this level lie between the incident commander and branch level.

sector, a specific area of responsibility created as a subdivision of the incident command system.

sector officers, those individuals assigned by the incident commander to manage specific geographical areas or specific functions, hazard sector officer, safety officer.

securité, an urgent maritime safety signal that, when broadcast, is indicative of a forthcoming report regarding important weather or safety of navigation information. It is the lowest in priority of the three maritime distress signals. *See also Mayday, pan.*

security seal, a seal or device, provided on a hazardous materials package, that enables one to determine whether the package has been opened.

sedation, a drug-induced state of quiet, calmness, or sleep.

sedative, a drug that slows or calms the patient, such as barbiturates. *See also sedative-hypnotic.*

sedative-hypnotic, a drug that slows central nervous system function, used in the field to control seizure activity and to sedate patients, such as diazepam.

seizure, **1.** *(informal)* a sudden onset of a disease, pain, or symptoms. **2.** taking possession of. **3.** a sudden electrical dysfunction of the brain, manifesting as any combination of altered levels of consciousness and/or disruption of autonomic, motor, or sensory functions. Seizures are of two major categories: **generalized** and **partial.** Generalized seizures include **absence** seizures—of which **petit mal** (nonconvulsive suppression of awareness with immobility and blank stare) is a type and **tonic-clonic** (or **grand mal**) seizures. Grand mal seizures are characterized by unconsciousness and various involuntary, skeletal muscle activities, followed by a period (postictal) of urinary incontinence and unresponsiveness, then confusion, and increasing awareness. Partial seizures include **jacksonian** (or **focal-motor**) seizures (activity restricted to certain muscle groups or one side of the body with minimal alteration of consciousness) and **psychomotor** seizures. Psychomotor (or **temporal lobe**) seizures begin with an aura (an awareness or sensation), followed by autonomic changes (tachycardia, transient apnea, salivation, urinary/fecal urgency), and then impairment of consciousness with chewing, lip smacking, or a mechanical continuation of activity that preceded the episode. An **early** seizure is one that occurs within one week of head trauma. **Epilepsy** is a condition where seizures (generally of unknown cause) recur spontaneously for years. **Febrile** seizures are those that occur in children under age six, when associated with a fever in excess of 100.4° F (38° C) (while not under the influence of alcohol or drugs or having an intracranial infection). **Late** seizures happen more than a week after head injury. A prolonged/continuous (more than one hour) seizure or intermittent seizures with no lucid interval (awakening) between episodes is known as **status epilepticus.** Alcohol or drug abuse, degenerative disease, head trauma, hypoglycemia, and tumors are but a few of the known causes of seizures. Also known as *(informal)* **convulsion.** *See also jacksonian progression.*

seizure threshold,   the degree of stimulus necessary to cause a seizure. All humans can have seizures if the stimulus is strong enough. Those who have a seizure for no apparent reason have a low seizure threshold.

select fill,   soil chosen to replace previously excavated soil.

selenium,   a metal-like element related to sulfur, found in very small amounts in food.

self-contained breathing apparatus,   a portable environment, used in hazardous atmospheres, to allow safe completion of work. Such equipment usually consists of compressed air tank(s), facemask, and regulator. Also known as **airpack, BA, OBA, SCBA.**

self-contained underwater breathing apparatus,   life support equipment for use underwater. This equipment is of the open-circuit type and consists of high-pressure air tanks and a regulator. The regulator is of the pressure-demand type, originally being of double hose design and now designed with a single hose. Also known as **scuba.**

self-limited,   *(of a disease or condition)* tending to resolve without treatment.

self-rescue position,   lying on back with feet downstream, utilizing the arms in a sculling motion in order to move out of the current. This position is used in moving water to prevent injury to the head and allow removal of oneself from dangerous current.

Sellick's maneuver (Brian A. Selleck, British anesthetist, first described in 1961),   the application of gentle pressure anteriorly against the thyroid (cricoid) cartilage, thereby displacing the glottic opening posteriorly. This procedure is used during endotracheal intubation to improve visualization of the vocal cords and to decrease the risk of passive aspiration of material from the esophagus. Also known as **cricoid pressure.**

semen /sē´mən/,   the thick, whitish fluid released by the male sex organs that carries the sperm. Also known as **seminal fluid, sperm.**

semicircular canal,   any of three bony, fluid-filled loops inside the inner ear, involved in the sense of balance. *See also ear.*

semilunar valve,   1. a valve with half-moon-shaped cusps, such as the aortic valve and the pulmonary valve. **2.** any one of the cusps forming such a valve. *See also heart valve.*

semimembranosus   /sem´ēmem´brənō´səs/, one of three muscles on the posterior medial thigh. It helps to flex the leg.

seminal duct /sem´inəl/,   any tube through which semen passes, such as the vas deferens or the ejaculatory duct.

seminal vesicle,   either of the paired, saclike glands that lie posterior to the bladder in the male and function as part of the reproductive system. The seminal vesicles release a fluid that forms part of semen.

semination,   the introduction of semen into the female genital tract.

seminiferous /sem´inif´ərəs/,   carrying or releasing semen, as do the tubules of the testicles.

semipermeable membrane /-pur´mē·əbəl/,   a membrane that selectively allows substances to pass through, depending on the size of the molecule.

semitendinosus /-ten´dinō´səs/,   one of three muscles on the posterior thigh that help to flex the leg.

senescent /sines´ənt/,   aging or growing old. *See also senile.*

senile,   relating to or characteristic of old age, or the process of aging, especially the degeneration of the mind and body. *See also aging.*

senile involution,   a pattern of steady shrinking and breakdown in tissues and organs that occurs in old age.

senopia /senō´pē·ə/,   an eye condition in which hardening of the lenses causes the eyes to focus better on things nearby. It is linked with a disorder (lenticular nuclear sclerosis) that commonly leads to the development of cataracts.

sensation,   1. a feeling, impression, or awareness of a bodily state or condition that occurs whenever a nerve is stimulated and sends a signal to the brain. A **deep sensation** is the awareness of pain, pressure, or tension in the deep layers of the skin, muscles, or joints. A **primary sensation** comes directly from a stimulus that causes the sensation. A **referred sensation** is felt at a place other than where the stimulus occurs. **2.** a feeling of a mental or emotional state, which may or may not be caused by something outside of the body.

sense, **1.** the ability or structure that allows events both inside and outside of the body to be perceived and understood. The major senses are sight, hearing, smell, taste, touch, and pressure. Other senses include hunger, thirst, pain, temperature, space, and time. **2.** the ability to feel; a sensation. **3.** normal mental ability. **4.** to perceive through a sense organ.

sensitivity, **1.** the ability to feel or react to a stimulus. **2.** increased tendency to respond to a particular situation or substance as though allergic. *See also allergy, hypersensitivity.* **3.** the number of false negatives in the results of a given test. If a test indicates positive results in only 50% of the actual cases where positive exists, then the test has a sensitivity of 50%. *See also reliability.*

sensitization, an acquired reaction in which specific antibodies develop in response to an antigen. Allergic reactions are sensitization reactions that result from excess sensitization to a foreign protein.

sensitized, referring to tissues that have been made susceptible to antigenic substances. *See also allergy.*

sensory layer, the portion of the retina that contains the cones and rods. Also known as **sensory retina.**

sensory nerve, a nerve that transmits signals from the body to the brain or spinal cord. Compare **motor nerve.**

sensory-perceptual overload, a state in which the loudness and strength of numerous sensations go beyond the ability of the patient to sort them out.

sensory retina. See **sensory layer.**

sentinel headache, the slight headache and mild neck stiffness that may accompany subarachnoid or subdural hemorrhage in its early stages. *See also subarachnoid hemorrhage, subdural hemorrhage.*

sepsis /sep´sis/, infection.

septal defect /sep´təl/, a defect present at birth in the septum separating two chambers of the heart. **Atrial septal defect** is a defect with a hole in the septum between the two atria. A **ventricular septal defect** is a hole in the sep-tum separating the ventricles, permitting blood to flow from the left ventricle to the right ventricle and to recirculate through the pulmonary artery and lungs.

septate /sep´tāt/, relating to a structure divided by a septum.

septicemia, presence of pathogens, usually bacteria, in the bloodstream. This term is generally used to describe overwhelming infection, precipitating septic shock.

septic shock. See **shock.**

septum /sep´təm/, *pl.* **septa,** a dividing wall, as found separating the chambers of the heart.

sequester /sikwes´tər/, to keep apart, or away from others.

sequestration, **1.** an increase in the amount of blood inside and outside of the vascular system. **2.** loss of fluid from the capillaries into the lung.

sequestrum /sikwes´trəm/, *pl.* **sequestra,** a fragment of dead bone that is partially or completely broken free from the nearby healthy bone.

serine, an amino acid found in many proteins in the body.

serotonin /ser´ətō´nin, sir´-/, a substance found naturally in the brain and intestines. Serotonin is released from certain cells when the blood vessel walls are damaged. It acts as a vasodilator.

serous fluid /sir´əs/, a thin, watery liquid.

serous membrane, one of the many thin sheets of tissue that line certain areas inside the body, such as the sac that surrounds the heart. Between the inner layer of serous membrane covering various organs and the outer layer of the organ itself is a space kept wet by serous fluid. Compare **mucous membrane, skin, synovial membrane.**

serous pericardium, the inner layer of the pericardium that adheres to and surrounds the heart.

serratus anterior /serā´təs/, a thin muscle of the thoracic wall extending from the ribs inferior to the arm to the scapula. It moves to raise the shoulder and arm.

serum, **1.** any thin, watery fluid produced by the body. **2.** any clear, watery fluid that has been separated from its more solid elements. **3.** a vaccine made from the serum of a patient who has had disease and used to protect another patient against that same disease.

serum albumin, a protein substance in the blood, needed to help control blood pressure.

serum sickness, a sickness that may occur 2 to 3 weeks after being given an antiserum. It is caused by a reaction to the donor serum. Symptoms include fever, enlarged spleen, enlarged lymph nodes, rash, and joint pain. *See also antiserum.*

service ceiling, the maximum altitude that an aircraft can maintain a rate of climb of 100 feet per minute. Also known as **operational ceiling.**

sesamoid bone /ses´əmoid/, any of the round bones embedded in certain tendons, the largest being the patella.

severe local storm, a category of weather phenomena that includes hailstorms, thunderstorms, and tornadoes.

sex, **1.** a division of male or female based on many features, such as body parts and genetic differences. Compare **gender. 2.** sexual intercourse.

sex chromosome, a chromosome that is responsible for the sex determination of offspring; it carries genes that transmit sex-linked traits and conditions. In humans and mammals there are two distinct sex chromosomes, the X and the Y chromosomes, which are unequally paired and appear in females in the XX combination and in males as XY. Compare **autosome.**

sexual abuse, sexual exploitation of another individual, by coercion and/or threats, to satisfy the abuser's personal needs.

sexual assault, a forcible act of sexual contact without consent.

sexual harassment, any harassing act of a sexual nature, including speech.

sexual intercourse. See **coitus.**

sexuality, all of the functional, mental, and physical behaviors related to sexual conduct; may be overt or subtle.

sexually transmitted disease, a contagious disease usually transmitted by sexual intercourse or genital contact, such as acquired immune deficiency syndrome, gonorrhea, syphilis, trichomoniasis. Also known as **STD, venereal disease.** *See also specific entry.*

shackle, a U-shaped metal connector with a bolt or pin used to close the open end.

shaken baby syndrome, injuries sustained by a child who has been vigorously shaken. Children subject to this form of child abuse may present with bulging fontanelles, failure to thrive, lethargy, respiratory difficulty, or seizures. Injuries include concussion, neck injuries, retinal hemorrhage, and spinal hematomas.

shallow water blackout, unconsciousness occurring underwater, while breath-holding, after hyperventilation on the surface. This hyperventilation blows off carbon dioxide without appreciable increase in oxygen saturation. Because carbon dioxide is the normal stimulus to breathe, exercise-induced hypoxia can cause unconsciousness before the stimulus to breathe is felt.

shear, deformation caused by a force or pressure, which moves the same direction in two adjacent planes. **Ground shear** during an earthquake reshapes the terrain. **Trench shear** causes a portion of wall to separate, causing wall collapse. **Wind shear** can remove the lift from under an aircraft's wings.

sheath, a tubelike structure that surrounds any part of the body, as the sheath of the rectus abdominis muscle, the sheath of Schwann, which covers various nerve fibers.

sheeting, wood planks and panels that support trench walls when held with shoring. *See also shoring.*

self-neglect, failure to care for one's own personal needs and/or self-inflicted harm. Patients with decreased mental or physical capacities are typically involved. *See also neglect.*

shellfish poisoning, an illness caused by eating clams, oysters, or mussels that are tainted with the parasite red tide. The symptoms appear rapidly and include nausea, lightheadedness, vomiting, and tingling or numbness around the mouth, followed by paralysis of the hands and feet and, possibly, respiratory arrest. **Vibrio parahaemolyticus** is a microorganism linked to food poisoning caused by eating uncooked or under-cooked shellfish, especially crabs and shrimp. Symptoms include diarrhea, abdominal cramps, vomiting, headache, chills, and fever.

shell shock. See **shock, stress reaction.**

Shepherd's crook, a rescue device consisting of a long aluminum pole with a circular blunted hook at one end. The hook is large enough to encircle a victim, allowing reaching rescues at pools to be accomplished with minimal danger to the rescuer.

sickle cell anemia, a congenital disease in which red blood cells deform (sickle) in a patient with low hemoglobin and/or red blood cell count. These deformed cells may obstruct capillary flow. Signs/symptoms of the acute phase of this chronic disease include abdominal and/or joint pain, edema, fever, and malaise.

shield, any device or material used for protection against another force, as lead against radiation.

shigellosis /shig´əlō´-/, infection of the bowel marked by diarrhea, abdominal pain, and fever, that is carried by hand-to-mouth contact with the feces of infected individuals. The disease occurs only rarely in the United States, but is native to underdeveloped areas of the world. Also known as **bacillary dysentery.**

shingles. See **herpes zoster.**

shin splints, tenderness and pain with swelling of pretibial muscles, following athletic exertion. It is thought to be a mild form of anterior tibial compartment syndrome, and is more common in those with decreased foot arch (pes planus).

shipping name, the proper shipping name or other common name for a hazardous material; also any synonyms for the hazardous material.

shipping package warning label, a special label affixed to a package of hazardous material to identify the package contents. DOT regulation **shipping papers** or **documents** must accompany all shipments of hazardous material.

shipping paper (U.S. Department of Transportation), the document that describes materials being transported, particularly hazardous materials. This paper can be found on board the transporting vehicle.

shoaling, shallow water in navigable bodies of water; a sudden rise of the bottom.

shock, 1. a sudden mental or physical disturbance. Types include the following. **Chronic** (peripheral circulatory insufficiency in older patients with debilitating disease), **cultural** (stress associated with a change to a new culture very different from the one previously known), **delayed** (occurring a considerable time after an injury), **electric** (caused by electric current passing through the body), **insulin** (hypoglycemia due to increased circulating insulin and/or decreased circulating glucose), **primary** (that occurring from anxiety or pain after a mental or physical injury), and **shell** (battle fatigue). **2.** a clinical syndrome exhibiting varying degrees of inadequate tissue perfusion to the body. Types include **anaphylactic** (systemic allergic reaction, characterized by smooth muscle contraction and capillary dilation due to histamine release, causing reduced blood pressure), **cardiogenic** (poor tissue perfusion as a result of decreased cardiac output, usually as a result of heart disease), **hypovolemic** (decreased circulation from a reduction in blood volume, as from bleeding, dehydration), **metabolic** (a buildup of toxic waste products in the body due to organ failure, such as kidney, liver), **neurogenic** (vasodilation below a level of disruption of the spinal cord), **psychogenic** (fainting), and **septic** (vasodilation associated with the bacterial toxins of overwhelming infection). Anaphylactic, metabolic, neurogenic, and septic types of shock may also be known as **low resistance** types of shock (due to vasodilation). Shock may be **compensated** (the body is able to deal with the decreased perfusion by maintaining cardiac output and normal blood pressure), **uncompensated** (the body is no longer able to maintain systolic blood pressure), or **irreversible** (progressive cellular ischemia and necrosis, causing organ death).

shock index, a value indicative of the severity of low perfusion states, calculated by dividing the cardiac rate by the systolic blood pressure. When normal, it is around 0.5 but will be elevated in shock.

shock-loaded, an energy-absorbing vehicle bumper with pistons compressed into a retracted (loaded) position. These bumpers represent a risk at accident scenes, as they may release under pressure, striking those in their path. Also known as **loaded.** *See also bumper strike zone.*

shock lung. See **adult respiratory distress syndrome.**

shoring, timber or mechanical devices used to hold sheeting against trench walls or to support tunnels in mines. Also known as **crossbraces, shores, struts.** *See also sheeting.*

short-acting, referring to a drug that begins to take effect very soon after being administered.

short bones, bones as long as they are wide, such as the carpal bones, of the wrist.

short haul, technique of moving a victim via helicopter-mounted rope from a rescue location to any clear or accessible area a short distance away. The victim can then be transported by air or ground. Also known as **extract, fixed-line flyaway, rappel-extract.** *See also long line haul.*

shotgun. See **clampstick.**

shoulder, the place where the clavicle and scapula meet and where the arm attaches to the trunk of the body.

shoulder blade. See **scapula.**

shoulder dystocia, a complication of delivery caused when the fetal shoulders are obstructed in their movement by the mother's symphysis pubis.

shoulder girdle, term describing the combination of the clavicle and scapula. Also known as **pectoral girdle.**

shoulder joint, the ball and socket joint of the humerus and the scapula. Also known as **humeral articulation.**

shoulder presentation, the position of the fetus when its length lies perpendicular to the mother, exposing the shoulder. Also known as **transverse presentation.**

shreds, shiny threads of mucus in the urine, showing an infection in the urinary tract. Also known as **mucous shreds.**

Shrine burn formula, an equation for calculating fluid resuscitation requirements in pediatric patients, that also includes evaporative water loss in the calculation. The formula is 2000 milliliters times the total body surface area burned plus 5000 milliliters times the total body surface area burned to be infused over the first 24 hours following the injury ([2000 ml × BSA] + [5000 ml × BSA] = milliliters infused first 24 hours). That is followed by one-half the total amount given in the first 24 hours given over the next 16 hours (first-24-hour amount × 0.5 = milliliters given from hours 25 to 40 postinjury). *See also Brooke formula, consensus formula, Parkland formula.*

shrinkage, procedure in underground room-and-pillar mining where upward cuts are made in the roof (back) of a stope. These cuts continue upward, widening the stope, until all ore is removed from that area. *See also stope.*

shunt, 1. to reroute the flow of a body fluid from one place to another. **2.** a tube or device put into the body to redirect a body fluid from one place to another. An **external shunt** is a tube on the surface of the body.

sialogogue /sī·al´əgog/, anything that causes saliva to be released.

sialolith /sī·al´əlith/, a small stone formed in a salivary gland or duct.

sialorrhea /sī·al·ôrē´ə/, hypersalivation that may occur with a number of conditions, such as acute inflammation of the mouth, mercury poisoning, pregnancy, alcoholism, malnutrition, or a cholinergic overdose. Also known as **hypersalivation, ptyalism.**

sickle cell, an abnormal, crescent-shaped red blood cell, typical of sickle cell anemia.

sickle cell anemia, a chronic incurable blood disease that attacks red blood cells, causing pain, fever, splenomegaly, anemia, and paresis.

sick sinus syndrome, altered levels of consciousness or dizziness due to the irregular cardiac rhythm caused by an inability of the sinoatrial (SA) node to maintain an appropriate rate. Precipitated by electrolyte imbalance, hypoxia, or myocardial infarction, this syndrome is characterized by rapidly changing periods of sinus arrest, bradycardia/tachycardia and/or recurring ectopic beats.

side effect, an effect of a drug other than the effect(s) desired. The effect can be either beneficial or detrimental.

siderosis /sid´ərō´-/, **1.** a lung disease caused by the inhalation of iron dust or particles. **2.** an increase in iron in the blood.

sideways rolling, self-rescue technique when threatened by an avalanche. Removing packs and skis, the skier lies on the slope and rolls downhill, but toward the side of an avalanche flow. The object is to increase body speed above that of the snow and roll out of the path of the avalanche. Keeping the head uphill and rolling toward the side of the slope are critical points of the maneuver.

Siebe, Augustus (German coppersmith), *(historical)* invented the first practical deep-sea diving suit in London in 1837, based on his earlier design of 1817. His design was so successful, that the U.S. Navy's Mark 5 diving suit is an almost exact copy of the 1837 design.

sievert, a radiation measurement in the International System of Units (the SI) that equals 100 roentgen equivalents, man (rem). This unit is replacing the rem in scientific nomenclature. *See also gray.*

sigh, a deep inspiration followed by a slow exhalation.

sight, 1. the sense of vision. 2. that which is seen.

sigmoid /sig´moid/, 1. relating to an **S** shape. 2. the sigmoid colon. *See also colon.*

sigmoid mesocolon, a fold of membrane that connects the sigmoid colon to the pelvic wall.

sign, 1. an abbreviation or symbol. 2. an indication of the passage of an animal or person. 3. any objective abnormality indicative of disease or injury. See Appendix 1-5. *See also symptom.*

sign cutting, the process of searching for the initial evidence of a passing animal or person in a specific area. Also known as **cutting sign.** *See also tracking.*

silicosis /sil´ikō´-/, a lung disorder caused by inhaling silicon dioxide over a long period of time. Silicon dioxide is found in sands, quartzes, flints, and many other stones. Small fiberlike growths develop in the lungs.

silver, a whitish precious metal used in certain medications and, blended together with other metals, to fill teeth.

Silvester method. See **chest-pressure arm-lift method.**

silver salts poisoning, a condition caused by ingesting silver nitrate. Symptoms include discoloration of the lips, vomiting, abdominal pain, dizziness, and seizures.

simple oxygen mask, an oxygen administration device consisting of a mask, covering the mouth and nose. Oxygen concentration of 35-60% can be achieved at flow rates of 6 to 15 liters per minute. *See also non-rebreather oxygen mask, oxygen.*

simplex, a type of communications configuration where transmitting or receiving can occur in only one direction at a time on a given frequency. *See also duplex, multiplex.*

sinciput /sin´sipət/, the superior portion of the head.

sine wave, undulating EKG complex without the PQRST complex being apparent. The pattern is a rhythmically undulating baseline and occurs in patients with serious hyperkalemia. The pattern is formed from an extremely widened QRS complex, which may still be organized enough to cause cardiac depolarization and contraction. The patient will be symptomatic, generally requiring dialysis.

sinew, the tendon of a muscle. *See also tendon.*

sinoatrial node, site of the primary electrical impulse formation for the heart. Located at the junction of the right atrium and the superior vena cava, all normal cardiac activity originates from this site. Intrinsic electrical impulses at this location occur at a rate of approximately 60 to 100 per minute. Also known as **SA node, sinuatrial node, sinus node.**

sinus /sī´nəs/. See **nasal sinus.**

sinus arrest, periods of asystole due to intermittent or complete failure of the SA node and its lower pacemaker sites.

sinus arrhythmia, irregular sinus rhythm, with rate often varying with respirations. This is generally an asymptomatic variance of normal sinus rhythm, often seen in the physically fit and the young. Rate is usually 60-100 beats per minute.

sinus bradycardia, a sinus rhythm with rates below 60 beats per minute.

sinus exit block, cardiac dysrhythmia caused when the sinus-formed electrical impulse (P wave) does not leave the AV node. This will be seen on the EKG as a P wave without a QRS complex. There must be, at least, occasional conduction of the impulse (formation of a QRS complex) in order to differentiate this rhythm from ventricular standstill. *See also ventricular standstill.*

sinusitis /sī´nəsī´-/, inflammation of one or more nasal sinuses. It may be a complication of upper respiratory infection, dental infection, allergy, a change in atmosphere, as in air travel or underwater swimming, or a defect of the nose. With swelling of nasal mucous membranes the openings from sinuses to the nose may be blocked, causing pressure, pain, headache, fever, and local tenderness.

sinusoid, 1. a blood vessel, slightly larger than a capillary with a lining of reticuloendothelium. **2.** like a sinus.

sinus tachycardia, sinus rhythm with rate above 100 and, usually, below 150 beats per minute.

sirenomelia /sī´rənomē´lyə/, a birth defect in which both legs have grown together and there are no feet.

sit harness. See **seat harness.**

situs /sī´təs/, the normal position or location of an organ or part of the body.

SI units, the international units of physical amounts. Examples of these units are the volume of a liter, the length of a meter, or the precise amount of time in a minute. Comité International des Poids et Mesures meets regularly to define the units.

size-up, assessment for the purpose of determining situation and required resources. This procedure is generally divided into prearrival, initial, and sustained size-up.

skeletal fixation, any method of holding together fragments of broken bone by the attaching of wires, screws, plates, or nails.

skeletal muscle, muscle that attaches to the skeleton and is used in movement of the body. Also known as **striated muscle, voluntary muscle.**

skeletal system, all of the bones and cartilage of the body that provide the framework for the muscles and organs.

skeleton, the supporting frame for the body. It has 206 bones that protect delicate structures, provide attachments for muscles, allow body movement, serve as major reservoirs of blood, and produce red blood cells. *See also bone.*

Skene's glands /skēnz/, the largest of the glands that open into the urethra of women. Also known as **paraurethral glands.**

skilled nursing facility, an institution that provides skilled nursing care, including rehabilitation, for those unable to care for themselves.

skin, 1. the multilayered membrane that covers the entire surface of the body. It is the largest organ of the body and is composed of five layers of cells. The deepest layer is the **stratum basale.** It anchors the more superficial layers to the underlying tissues and provides new cells to replace cells lost. Above the stratum basale lies the **stratum spinosum.** The cells in this layer have tiny spines on their surfaces. As the cells move to the next layer, the **stratum granulosum,** they become flat, lying parallel with the surface of the skin. Over this layer lies a clear, thin band of tissue called the **stratum lucidum.** The outermost layer, the **stratum corneum,** is made up of dead cells that contain keratin. This layer is thick over areas of the body subject to abrasion, such as the palms of the hands, and thin over other more protected areas. The color of the skin varies according to the amount of melanin in the epidermis. Genetic differences determine the amount of melanin. The skin helps to cool the body when the temperature rises by radiating the heat flow in dilated blood vessels and by providing a surface for the evaporation of sweat. When the temperature drops, the blood vessels constrict and production of sweat decreases. Also known as **cutaneous membrane, integument. 2.** the outer covering of an aircraft.

skin absorption, the introduction of a chemical or toxic product into the body by way of the skin. Absorption is enhanced by abrasions, cuts, heat, and moisture.

skin graft, a portion of skin implanted to cover areas where skin has been lost due to burns, injury, or disease. To prevent tissue rejection of permanent grafts, the graft is taken from the patient's body or from an identical twin. Skin from another person or animal can be used temporarily for large burned areas to lessen fluid loss.

skip shoring, technique for supporting mine or trench walls with uprights and/or shores at spaced intervals. Also known as **spot bracing.**

skull, the bony structure of the head, consisting of the cranium and the facial skeleton. The cranium, which holds and protects the brain, consists of eight bones. The skeleton of the face has 14 bones. The base of the skull is the portion to which the spine attaches.

slander, knowingly speaking false statements about another with the intent of causing harm.

sleep, a state marked by decreased consciousness, diminished movement of the skeletal muscles, and slowed metabolism. People normally sleep in patterns that follow four definite, gradual stages. These four stages make up three-fourths of a period of typical sleep and are called, as a group, **non-rapid eye movement** sleep. The remaining time is usually occupied with **rapid eye movement (REM)** sleep. The REM sleep periods last from a few minutes to half an hour at a time. Dreaming occurs during REM time.

sleep apnea, periods of breathing cessation during sleep. Patients with cardiovascular compromise are at risk for sudden death during periods of apnea.

sleep deprivation, the state of inadequate sleep. This phenomenon is a quite common but generally unrecognized state, which is thought to be a factor in many accidents and complications at home and work.

sliding choker, a steel collar or hook attached to a wire rope sling. This enables the sling to adjust to different size loads.

sling, **1.** webbing of various lengths, tied together and used as an attachment device for climbers and equipment. **2.** a cloth securing device for immobilizing arm injuries, usually made from a triangular bandage, or cravat. **3.** the cable used under helicopters to secure and carry an external load.

sling load, cargo carried suspended under a helicopter. Also known as **external load.**

slipped disk. See **herniated disk.**

slipstream, wind around an aircraft caused by an operating propeller. Also known as **propwash.**

slough /sluf/, **1.** to shed or cast off dead tissue cells. **2.** the tissue that has been shed.

slough-in, collapse of a section of trench wall with an overhang remaining.

sloughing, the loss of necrotic tissue from the viable tissue to which it was attached.

slow reactive substance of anaphylaxis, a chemical mediator released from mast cells that causes bronchoconstriction and an increase in prostaglandin production.

slow ventricular tachycardia, ventricular tachycardia at rates up to 150 beats per minute. *See also ventricular tachycardia.*

sluff. See **avalanche.**

small cardiac vein, one of five veins within the heart. Also known as **right coronary vein.**

small intestine. See **intestine.**

smallpox, a highly contagious viral disease marked by fever and rash. It is caused by one of two species of poxvirus, variola major or variola minor **(alastrim).** Alastrim is a mild form of smallpox. Because human beings are the only carrier for the virus, worldwide vaccination with vaccinia, a related poxvirus, has been effective in wiping out smallpox. For several years no natural case of the disease has been known to occur. Also known as **variola.**

smegma /smeg´mə/, a substance released by sebaceous glands.

smell, 1. the sense that allows odors to be perceived. **2.** any odor, pleasant or unpleasant.

smoke diver, highly trained user of a self contained breathing apparatus.

smoke inhalation, the breathing in of noxious fumes. Symptoms include irritation of the throat and lungs, dyspnea, wheezing, restlessness, cough, and hoarseness. Pulmonary edema may develop up to 48 hours after exposure.

smooth muscle. See **muscle.**

snakebite, the puncture wound resulting from the fangs of a snake. Venomous snakes are found in five of the fourteen families that exist. Those five are the Colubridae (bird snake, boomslang), Crotalidae (rattlesnakes, fer-de-lance), Elapidae (cobras, coral snakes), Hydrophidae (sea snakes), and Viperidae (Russell's viper, puff adder). The toxic properties of the particular venom and the victim's response to those toxins are the primary determinants of the severity of a venomous bite. See Appendix 3-16. *See also Monash method.*

snatch block, a single pulley that opens on one side to permit placement of cable or rope.

sneeze, a sudden, forceful, involuntary burst of air through the nose and mouth occurring as a result of irritation to the mucous membranes of the throat, as by dust or pollen.

sniffing position, flexion of the patient's neck (at C5-6) while extending the head (at C1-2), in order to place the natural airway in the optimal position for endotracheal intubation.

sniperscope, a telescopic device that may be used in low light conditions, which focuses infrared light on a light-sensitive cathode and converts and enlarges the image.

snorkel, a J-shaped tube used by divers for breathing while swimming near the surface. This device allows divers prolonged surface swims with minimal exertion or visualization of the bottom from the surface.

snow anchor, any device or technique that provides an anchor point for climbers in the snow. Types include bollards, deadman, ice ax, snow fluke, and snow picket. A **bollard** is a horseshoe or teardrop-shaped trench cut into the snow, with the trench serving as a wrapping point for a rope or sling. A **deadman** is any flat, broad object that can be buried in the snow with a rope tied to it, such as a branch, ice axe, rock, or snow fluke. A **snow fluke** is an aluminum square with a cable tie-in that can be buried in the snow. A **snow picket** is a metal piton, made with holes along its length, whose size measures near 1 meter (about 3 feet). This is driven into the snow as an attachment point for carabiners/rope.

snow blindness, irritation of the eyes provoked by reflected sunlight (ultraviolet) from snow. Symptoms include a gritty sensation in the eyes, edema, pain, photophobia, and tearing. Also known as **ultraviolet keratitis.**

snow bridge, connection between two glacier edges made of snow. These bridges are very unstable, and the crevasses over which they form tend to be deep.

snow fluke. See **snow anchor.**

snow picket. See **snow anchor.**

snow shelter, any makeshift shelter made of snow, such as an igloo, snow cave or snow trench.

snub, wrapping rope or line around a stationary object in order to slow or stop movement.

Social Security Act, the federal law that provides for a national system of old age assistance, survivors' and old age insurance benefits, unemployment insurance and payments, and other public welfare programs, including Medicare and Medicaid.

socioeconomic strata, the various economic and social levels of a society. Persons are rated by amount of income, type of work, or family or personal history.

soda, a compound of sodium, particularly sodium bicarbonate, sodium carbonate, or sodium hydroxide.

sodium, a soft, grayish, highly reactive metallic element. In its ionized state, it is consumed as table salt and is the prevalent ion in all foods. It is the principal extracellular osmotic cation of the body.

sodium bicarbonate, an alkaline agent used in the treatment of metabolic acidosis, particularly during cardiac arrest, hyperkalemia, and tricyclic antidepressant intoxication. It should be used with caution in the poorly ventilated patient. Because it decreases the effectiveness of catecholamines upon contact, flush intravenous tubing before and after its administration. Also known as $NaHCO_3$.

sodium chloride, common table salt. See also *normal saline.*

sodium ion, electrically charged atom of sodium, critical to acid-base balance, kidney function, muscle contraction, and nerve conduction.

sodium-potassium exchange pump, biochemical process that actively moves potassium into a cell, while pushing sodium out of the cell. Using adenosine triphosphate (ATP) for energy, this process occurs in the impulse conduction systems of cardiac and nerve tissues. In cardiac tissue, this creates the electrical flow that allows repolarization of the heart in phase four of the depolarization cycle. Also known as **active transport.** See also *active transport.*

sodomy /sod′əmē/, **1.** anal intercourse. **2.** intercourse with an animal. **3.** a vague term for "unnatural" sexual intercourse.

soft ascender, any of several simple knots used as a nonmechanical ascending device, directly on a rope or in conjunction with a carabiner. Types include Bachmann, Headon, Kreuzklem, and Prusik. In addition to ascending, they are used as safeties in lowering-raising systems. These knots are useful in that they can be formed as needed from standard climbing equipment, can be cut under load if jammed, and can be used around more than one rope simultaneously. See also *ascender.*

soft collar, a soft foam device used to remind neck injury patients to limit the movement of their neck. Although previously used in immobilization of potential spinal injury victims, they are now obsolete for field use. The collar's lack of rigid support now limits its use to hospitalization and rehabilitation, for those patients with muscular injury of the neck.

soft palate, the structure composed of mucous membrane, muscular fibers, and mucous glands, forming the posterior portion of the roof of the mouth. The uvula is the round piece of flesh hanging from the posterior soft palate. Compare **hard palate.**

soft slab avalanche. See **avalanche.**

soft tissue, 1. the cells composing the surface and subsurface layers of the skin and muscle. **2.** any body tissue except dense connective (bone-cartilage) tissue.

soft transport vehicle, a specialized victim transport device that does not incorporate rigidity into its construction. These devices are easily carried, packed, or stored. Types may be as simple as a seat harness or as specific as a Tragsitz or screamer suit. The Tragsitz is a canvas or nylon sling that allows a rescuer to carry a victim with minor injuries on his or her back during mountain descent. A screamer or fishnet suit is a nylon coverall with positive closures and a sewn-in chest–seat harness. This device allows lowering-raising via rope or hoist, in a seated or horizontal position. *See also rigid transport device.*

software, instructions that make a computer perform tasks, such as for applications, device drivers, operating systems, and programs.

soil typing, testing soil to determine its critical properties, such as compressibility, permeability, and strength.

solar plexus, a network of nerves located posterior to the stomach.

solar radiation, the ultraviolet rays from the sun. Overexposure may result in sunburn, skin cancer, or sores linked with a sensitivity to light.

solar retinitis, retinal irritation or burns occurring after intense direct exposure to a laser or the sun, as when looking at an eclipse of the sun. Symptoms include pain, edema, and vision impairment. The lens of the eye focuses ultraviolet radiation on the retina to produce the syndrome. Also known as **eclipse retinopathy, foveomacular retinitis.**

solar still, survival device for producing drinkable water in arid and semiarid climates. Consisting of a piece of plastic covering a hole in the ground, this device can distill up to 3 liters (about 3 quarts) of water in 24 hours.

solar urticaria, hives or rash associated with exposure to sunlight.

soleus /sō´lē·əs/, one of three muscles found in the posterior calf. It is a broad flat muscle that moves the foot.

solid, material with a greater density than gases or liquids and a minimal tendency to disperse.

solid sheeting, placing sections of sheeting together (butting) to provide support of trench walls.

solubility, the ability of one material to blend uniformly with another; the ability of a material to dissolve in a solvent.

solution, two or more substances combined in a single homogenous gas, liquid, or solid.

solution cave. See **speleogenesis.**

solvent, a liquid capable of dissolving another substance.

somatic, related to the body.

somatic nervous system, the portion of the peripheral nervous system that conducts impulses from the central nervous system to skeletal muscle.

somatoform disorder /sō´mətōfôrm´, sōmat´ō-/, any of a group of nervous disorders with symptoms that look like a physical illness or disease, for which there is no disease. The symptoms are usually caused by conflict within the patient's mind. Kinds of somatoform disorders are **conversion disorder, hypochondria, psychogenic pain disorder.**

somatomegaly /-meg´əlē/, a condition in which the body is abnormally large because of hormonal imbalances.

somatomotor nerves, nerves that transmit motor impulses to skeletal muscle.

somatosplanchnic /sōmat´ōsplangk´nik/, relating to the trunk of the body and the internal organs of the lower body, such as the stomach or intestine.

somatostatin /-stat´in/, hormone that controls growth and helps to control the release of other hormones.

somatotype /-tīp/, **1.** body build or physique. **2.** the classification of body types based on certain physical traits.

somnolent /som´nələnt/, **1.** the state of sleepiness or drowsiness. **2.** tending to cause sleepiness. **—somnolence,** *n.*

soot, ash produced by the incomplete combustion of organic materials.

soporific /sop´ərif´ik/, referring to a substance, condition, or method that causes sleep. *See also hypnotic, sedative.*

sore, **1.** a wound, ulcer, or lesion. **2.** tender or painful.

sorting. See **triage.**

sound, **1.** healthy; without disease. **2.** a diagnostic instrument used for gaining access and/or probing into a canal or cavity; an introducer. **3.** auditory sensations produced by vibration. See Appendix 1-9.

source, referring to the origin, particularly of a body of water or a hazardous material spill.

souse hole, the hydraulic-like backflow that may be found behind a large obstruction in a flowing body of water.

space intrusion, structural movement into the passenger space of a vehicle during an accident. As a result of the body of the vehicle striking an object, deformation occurs to the vehicle's structure. The amount of intrusion can be indicative of the potential seriousness of a victim's injuries.

spalling, process that causes the primary injuries seen after exposure to a shock (blast) wave. The change in velocity of the shock wave as it moves between liquid-gas interfaces and tissues of different densities, disrupts the tissue. *See also blast injury, primary injury.*

spanish windlass, *(historical)* securing device used to create tension or traction. This device was usually constructed from a cravat or other cloth material and tightened by winding a rod or stick within the material until adequate tension was achieved. This technique was originally used to tighten a tourniquet. Later, it became the primary method of developing traction with the Thomas traction splint.

span-of-control, the supervisory ratio of from three to seven individuals with five being established as a general rule of thumb.

spasm, **1.** a sudden muscle tightening. **2.** a seizure. **3.** a sudden constriction of a blood vessel, bronchus, esophagus, pylorus, ureter, or other hollow organ. Compare **stricture.**

spastic, of or relating to spasms of the skeletal muscles. *See also cerebral palsy.*

spastic bladder. See **neurogenic bladder.**

spastic colon. See **irritable bowel syndrome.**

spatial zones, the areas of personal space in which most people function. Four basic spatial zones are the intimate zone, in which distance between individuals is less than 18 inches; the personal zone, between 18 inches and 4 feet; the social zone, extending between 4 and 12 feet; and the public zone, beyond 12 feet.

special emergency radio service, a group of radio frequencies designated for use by emergency agencies.

special-form radioactive materials, materials that are encapsulated or are in a solid form or matrix such that, if released from a package, they would maintain their integrity. Such materials might present a direct radiation exposure problem, but there would be little possibility of loose contamination and/or dispersal.

special operations, operations in hostile environments or those with the possibility of prolonged treatment or transport times that require fitness or skills beyond those normally needed during the standard emergency medical response. These would include advanced-level interhospital transport, aeromedical, mass-gathering emergency services, rescue (dive, mine, urban, water, wilderness), special weapons and tactics, and executive protection. Although first-responder and basic-level emergency medical technicians participate in these operations, a capacity for rapid, advanced assessment under adverse conditions and prolonged treatment with minimal equipment may be necessary. *See also combat austerity.*

species /spē´sēz, spē´shēz/, *pl.* **species** /spē´sēz, spē´shēz/, the category of living things below genus in rank. A species includes individuals of the same genus who are similar in structure and chemical composition and who can interbreed. *See also genus.*

specific activity, the total activity of a given radionuclide per unit mass. Units are generally curies per gram.

specific gravity, the weight of a material as compared with the weight of an equal volume of water. If the specific gravity is less than one, the material is lighter than water and will float. If the specific gravity is greater than one, the material is heavier than water and will sink.

specification packages, shipping packages meeting the design and construction standards prescribed in the Code of Federal Regulations, 49 CFR Part 178.

specimen /spes´imən/, a small sample, representing the nature of the whole, such as a blood specimen.

speculum /spek´yələm/, a tool used to hold open a body space to make examination possible, such as an ear speculum.

speech, sounds that form words to express one's thoughts or ideas.

speech dysfunction, a condition which affects the ability to speak. It may be caused by diminished blood flow to the brain, tumors, or certain medical procedures. **Anarthria** results from the loss of control of the muscles of speech. The patient is unable to say words. **Aphonic speech** is a defect in which everything is whispered. With **ataxic speech,** there is faulty formation of the sounds. **Mirror speech** has the order of syllables in a word reversed. With **slurred speech,** words are not spoken clearly or completely but are run together.

speech pathology, 1. the study of defects of speech or of the organs of speech. **2.** the diagnosis and treatment of defects of speech.

speleogenesis /spē´lē·ōjen´əsis/, the geological process by which a cave is formed. There are three major types of caves: lava, solution, and talus caves. Lava caves are formed when molten magma cools near the surface, but continues to flow underneath. Solution caves are the most common and are formed when groundwater dissolves carbonate rock. Talus caves form where rock debris piles up, due to glacier movement or rockfall at the base of mountains.

speleology, the study of caves.

sperm. See **semen, spermatozoon.**

spermatic cord /spərmat´ik/, a structure by which each testicle is attached to the body. The left spermatic cord is usually longer than the right, thus the left testis usually hangs lower than the right. Each cord is made up of arteries, veins, lymphatics, nerves, and the excretory duct of the testicles.

spermatic duct. See **vas deferens.**

spermatocele /spur´mətōsēl´/, a cystlike swelling that contains sperm. It lies posterior to the testis.

spermatocide /-sīd´/, a chemical substance that kills spermatozoa. Also known as **spermicide.**

spermatogenesis, the formation of spermatozoa.

spermatozoon /-zō´ən/, *pl.* **spermatozoa** /-zō´ə/, the male seed, contained in semen, that fertilizes the female egg to create a fetus.

sphenoid bone /sfē´noid/, the bone at the base of the skull.

sphenoid sinus, one of two mucous-lined cavities in the sphenoid bone, joined to the nasal cavity.

sphenomandibular ligament /sfē´nōmandib´yələr/, one of a pair of flat, thin ligaments that connect the mandible to the skull.

spherocytosis /-sītō´-/, the presence of diseased red blood cells in the blood.

sphincter /sfingk´tər/, a circular band of muscle fiber that narrows a passage or closes a natural opening in the body, such as the outer anal sphincter, which closes the anus.

spineboard, a rigid immobilization device used for securing a patient with actual or suspected spinal injury. Composed of wood, metal, or plastic, the **long spineboard** is used to immobilize the supine patient. It is usually 72L × 18 W inches with handholds along the sides and two runners on the underside. An extrication collar, straps and a lateral head immobilizer are used in conjunction with this device to properly secure the patient. The **short spineboard** (32L × 18W inches) is used to immobilize patients who are found seated or in a confined space until they can be moved to a supine position. While most often used during vehicle extrication, this device has generally been replaced by the newer flexible-vest type of immobilizers. These vest immobilizers also protect the spine but wrap around the victim to make application simpler and more secure. Also known as **board, long board, short board.**

sphygmomanometer /-mənom´ətər/, a device for measuring the blood pressure. It consists of an arm or leg cuff with an air bag attached to a tube and a bulb for pumping air into the bag, and a gauge for showing the amount of air pressure being pressed against the artery. *See also blood pressure.*

spiderbite, puncture wound caused by the bite of a spider. Of 30,000 species of spider, less than 100 are considered harmful to humans. Although most spiders have venom glands, few have sufficient amounts of venom or the length of fang necessary to penetrate skin. Venomous spiders in the western hemisphere include the banana spider, black widow, brown recluse, Chilean brown spider, Peruvian brown spider, pruning spider (Peruvian tarantula), and the red-legged widow.

spider strap, a net of webbing used to strap a patient into a litter or stretcher. Also known as **litter spider.**

spina bifida /spī´nə bif´ədə, bī´fədə/, a neural tube defect present at birth that results in a gap in the vertebrae that surround the spinal cord.

spinal canal /spī´nəl/, the canal within the vertebrae of the spinal column, which accommodates the spinal cord.

spinal column, the flexible group of vertebrae made up of 33 vertebrae separated by spongy disks. It protects the spinal cord inside. Also known as **spine, vertebral column.** *See also vertebra.*

spinal cord, a long, round structure found in the spinal canal and reaching from the base of the skull to the lumbar spine. A major part of the central nervous system, the adult cord is about 1 cm in diameter with an average length of 42 to 45 cm and a weight of 30 g. The cord carries sensory and motor signals to and from the brain and controls many reflexes. The **central canal** of the spinal cord is a tunnel that runs the entire length of the spinal cord. It contains cerebrospinal fluid and the spinal cord. *See also spinal nerves.*

spinal cord compression, a condition caused by pressure on the spinal cord. Symptoms range from temporary numbness of an arm or leg to permanent paralysis, depending on the cause and location of the pressure. Causes include spinal fracture, vertebral dislocation, tumor, bleeding, and edema secondary to an injury. *See also herniated disk.*

spinal fluid. See **cerebrospinal fluid.**

spinal ganglia, structures of the nervous system that contain the cell bodies of sensory neurons. Also known as **dorsal root ganglia.**

spinal hit, neurologic decompression sickness. *See also decompression sickness.*

spinal nerves, the 31 pairs of nerves that originate from the spinal cord. They are numbered according to the level where they exit the cord. *See also spinal cord.*

spinal puncture. See **lumbar puncture.**

spinal shock, neurogenic shock. *See also shock.*

spinal tract, any one of the pathways for nerve signals that are found in the white matter of the spinal cord.

spine. See **spinal column.**

spinocerebellar disorder /spī´nōser´əbel´ər/, a genetic disorder with a gradual degeneration of the spinal cord and brain. Some kinds of spinocerebellar wasting are **ataxia telangiectasia, Charcot-Marie-Tooth atrophy, Dejerine-Sottas disease, Friedreich's ataxia, Refsum's syndrome.**

spinous process, the portion of the spinal vertebrae that projects posteriorly from the vertebral arch. This process serves to attach muscles of the back.

splanchnocele /splangk´nōsēl/, hernia of any internal organ of the lower body.

spleen, an egg-shaped organ of the lymphatic system, located in the upper-left quadrant of the abdomen. It removes old red blood cells from the circulation and produces various globulin proteins for the immune system. Enlarging during digestion and illness, it is easily ruptured during blunt abdominal trauma. *See also lymphatic system.*

splenectomy /splēnek´-/, the removal by surgery of the spleen.

splenic flexure syndrome, bloating, fullness, gas, and pain in the upper-left quadrant of the abdomen as a result of air trapped in the splenic flexure of the large intestine. The symptoms may occasionally radiate upward and cause anterior–left chest discomfort.

splenomegaly /splē´nōmeg´əlē/, enlargement of the spleen.

splint, **1.** a device or the materials used to prevent the movement of the ends of a broken bone. An **air** splint consists of a plastic sleeve that is inflated with air to create rigidity. The **cardboard** splint is a three-sided piece of cardboard taped or tied to an injured extremity. A **pillow** splint is effective for use around an injured ankle. The **Thomas full-ring** or **half-ring**

splint was the first traction splinting device developed for immobilizing femur fractures. The leg splint extended from a ring at the hip to beyond the foot via two parallel bars joined at the end. This provided a platform from which to tie an ankle hitch (Collin's hitch) that was tightened (a Spanish windlass) to create traction. Later traction splints, though improved, imitated the technique developed by Sir Hugh Owen Thomas (British surgeon, 1834-1891). Other traction splints include Kendrick™, Klippel™, and Sager™. **Wire ladder** or **ladder** splints use wire mesh or braces (shaped like a ladder) that provide rigidity when folded or shaped around a potential fracture site. A variation of this splint is the **SAM**™ splint, which uses a flexible metal and foam structure to create a rigid structure. A **vacuum** splint envelops the injured extremity and, when the air inside is removed, develops enough rigidity to immobilize a fracture. *See also Spanish windlass, ladder splint.* **2.** the technique of immobilizing a fracture. **3.** stiffening of a portion of the body to avoid movement pain in an infected or injured part.

splinter hemorrhage, bleeding that looks like a splinter under a finger- or toenail. It is seen after injury and in patients with bacterial endocarditis.

spoil pile, a mound of excavated material created when digging a hole or trench.

spondylitis /spon´dilī´-/, inflammation of the spinal vertebrae, usually marked by stiffness and pain. The condition may follow injury to the spine or be the result of infection or rheumatoid disease. *See also ankylosing spondylitis.*

spondylosis /spon´dilō´-/, a condition of the spine marked by stiffness of a vertebral joint.

spontaneous abortion, an unplanned termination of pregnancy occurring before the twelfth week. Also known as **miscarriage.**

spontaneous combustion, the heating of materials to ignition temperature, without the deliberate application of heat, due to atmospheric conditions and composition of the materials.

sporadic, *(of a number of events)* occurring at scattered, interrupted, and seemingly random intervals.

spore, a form taken by some bacteria that is resistant to heat, drying, and chemicals. Under proper conditions the spore may change back into the active form of the bacterium. Diseases caused by spore-forming bacteria include anthrax, botulism, and tetanus.

sporicide /spôr´isīd/, any substance used to kill spores.

spot bracing. See **skip shoring.**

spotter, 1. person(s) outside the rear of a vehicle who assists the driver in safe backing maneuvers. **2.** the second person of a sniper-countersniper team, who observes targets and protects the sniper.

sprain, an injury to the tendons, muscles, or ligaments of a joint, with pain, swelling, and discoloration over the joint.

S prime, a second negative deflection (S′) occurring after the positive R wave in the QRS complex.

sprue, a chronic disorder caused by poor absorption of nutrients in the small intestine. Symptoms include diarrhea, weakness, weight loss, and cramps. It occurs in both tropic and nontropic forms and affects both children and adults. **Nontropical sprue** is a condition due to an inherited inability to digest foods that contain gluten. **Tropical sprue** is of unknown cause and occurs in the tropics and subtropics. *See also celiac disease, malabsorption syndrome.*

sputum /spyōō´təm/, material coughed up from the lungs. It contains mucus, cellular debris, and may also contain blood or purulent material. The amount, color, and contents of the sputum are important in the diagnosis of many illnesses, such as pneumonia and tuberculosis.

squad, 1. an emergency service agency or organization. **2.** a vehicle and two to four personnel equipped to provide a specific service, such as advanced life support, brush firefighting, first responder, light or medium rescue. Patient transport is not a normal function of this unit.

squamous cell /skwā´məs/, a flat, scaly cell.

squaw wood, the dead (dry) branches of an evergreen tree, generally located closer to the ground. This wood is useful for fire building.

squeeze, 1. gas within a space not equalizing fully with a higher pressure outside that space. Most often applied to divers, this phenomenon acts on the space within the facemask, middle ear, sinuses, teeth, and under a wetsuit. **2.** the edema, hemorrhage, pain, or rupture that accompanies a serious pressure differential between parts of the body and the outside environment. Also known as **barotrauma of descent.**

stabilization, the process of making firm or steady, such as with chocks under an overturned vehicle or medicating a patient to return physiological functioning toward normal.

stabilizer, any airfoil that increases the stability of an aircraft. Generally, this refers to the fixed, horizontal tail surfaces of an aircraft.

stack effect, the phenomenon seen in fires where the movement of smoke is more rapid and dangerous in tall buildings than in low ones. This is due to natural air movement within tall buildings, modified by temperature differences and external wind. This creates significant problems in the safe removal of those trapped within the fire structure.

staff of Aesculapius /es´kələ´pē·əs/, the symbol of medicine, consisting of a rod with one serpent encircling it. It also serves as the emblem of the American Medical Association, Royal Army Medical Corps (Britain), and the Royal Canadian Medical Corps. *See also caduceus.*

stages of dying, the five emotional and behavioral stages identified by Elizabeth Kubler-Ross as occurring after a patient first learns of approaching death: a period of denial, followed by anger, bargaining, depression and, finally, acceptance.

staging area. See **mobilization center.**

standard cubic foot, the amount of air in a cubic foot at sea level and at 70° F.

standardization. See **calibration.**

standard of care, the minimum accepted level of emergency care to be provided as set forth by law, administrative orders, guidelines, local protocols, and practice.

standing orders, emergency medical treatment protocols utilized without on-line medical control. These orders are created to avoid delay, which could harm the patient. Also known as **off-line medical control.** *See also on-line medical control.*

standing waves, water continuously piling upon itself in a narrowed portion of flowing water; usually found in a chute or downstream V. Also known as **haystack.**

stapes /stā´pēz/, one of the three small bones in the middle ear, resembling a tiny stirrup. It carries sound vibrations to the inner ear. *See also ear.*

staphylococcal infection /staf´ilōkok´əl/, an infection caused by any one of several disease-causing types of *Staphylococcus.* It commonly results in the formation of abscesses on the skin or other organs. Staphylococcal infections of the skin include carbuncles, folliculitis, and furuncles. Presence of the germ in the blood may result in endocarditis, meningitis, or osteomyelitis.

Staphylococcus /-kok´əs/, a type of bacteria. Some are normally found on the skin and in the throat; others cause infection or produce a toxin which may cause nausea, vomiting, and diarrhea. *See also staphylococcal infection.*

stare decisis /ster´ā dəsī´sis/, *(Latin)* "Let the decision stand"; the principle followed by the American justice system in which decisions in current cases adhere to decisions made in similar past cases.

Starling's law (Ernest Henry Starling, British physiologist, 1866-1927), the force of contraction in the heart is determined primarily by the stretched length of the muscle wall fibers during cardiac filling. The longer the fibers are stretched, the stronger the contraction.

startle reflex, a normal reflex in an infant caused by a sudden loud noise. It results in drawing up the legs, an embracing position of the arms, and usually a short cry.

START triage, **S**imple **T**riage **A**nd **R**apid **T**reatment, a field method for sorting large numbers of patients according to the severity of their conditions. This system assesses victims according to their ventilatory, circulatory, and neurological status. They are then rated dead-nonsalvageable, critical-immediate, or delayed. See Appendix 1-14.

starvation, **1.** a condition due to the lack of proper food over a long period of time and marked by numerous disorders of the body and metabolism. **2.** the act or state of starving or being starved. *See also malnutrition.*

stasis /stā´sis, stas´is/, **1.** a disorder in which the normal flow of a fluid through a vessel of the body is slowed or stopped. **2.** stillness.

statement of practical treatment, located on the front panel of a hazardous materials container, it is also referred to as the "first aid statement" or "note to physician." It may have precautionary information as well as emergency procedures for exposures. Antidote and treatment information may also be added.

static, without motion; at rest; in balance.

static electricity, sparking that occurs when an electrical charge accumulates on a surface exposed to a positive field and a negative field brought into close proximity.

static rope, type of kernmantle rope with minimal stretch (no more than 4% of its length) that is used in circumstances in which a large amount of stretch is undesirable. *See also rope.*

status, **1.** a specified state or condition. **2.** a continuing state or condition, as a long-lasting asthma attack (status asthmaticus).

status asthmaticus /azmat´ikəs/. See **asthma.**

status epilepticus /ep´ilep´tikəs/, repeated seizures occurring without intervals of consciousness. Causes include hypoglycemia, head injury, fever, or poisoning.

statutory law, the laws enacted by government bodies (federal and state legislatures) that derive their power from enabling constitutions. Also known as **legislative law.** *See also administrative law, common law, constitutional law.*

STCC number, the Standard Transportation Commodity Code number used in the rail industry; a seven-digit number assigned to a specific hazardous material or group of materials and used in determination of rates. For hazardous material, the STCC number will begin with the digits "49."

ST depression, downward deflection of the ST segment, thought to be due to myocardial ischemia. *See also ST elevation.*

steatorrhea /stē´ətorē´ə/, large amounts of fat in the feces; marked by frothy, foul-smelling fecal matter, as in celiac disease, some malabsorption syndromes, and any condition in which fats are poorly absorbed by the small intestine.

steering column, the metal shaft of a motor vehicle that connects the steering wheel with the steering assembly of the vehicle. These are generally divided into two types: solid and split.

ST elevation, upward deflection of the ST segment, believed to be due to myocardial infarction. *See also ST depression.*

stellate wound, a star-shaped wound.

stenosis, a narrowing or stricture of any canal. **Aortic** stenosis involves narrowing of the aortic valve, which restricts blood flow out of the left ventricle, decreasing cardiac output. **Cicatricial** /sik´ətrish´əl/ stenosis is a narrowing of a duct or tube due to scar tissue. Narrowing of any area of the larynx is known as **laryngeal** stenosis. **Mitral** stenosis occurs with narrowing of the mitral valve of the heart. Pulmonary artery narrowing as it leaves the right ventricle of the heart is **pulmonary** stenosis. Pulmonary hypertension and right ventricular hypertrophy can result. **Pyloric** stenosis is a narrowing of the pyloric sphincter, which can impede the flow of partly digested food into the small intestine.

stereotypy /ster´ē·ətī´pē, stir´-/, the continuous, improper repetition of actions, body postures, or speech patterns, usually occurring with a lack of variation in thought. It is often seen in patients with schizophrenia.

sterile /ster´il/, **1.** barren; unable to produce children because of a physical abnormality. Compare **impotence. 2.** aseptic.

sterilization, **1.** a process or act that makes a person unable to produce children. *See also hysterectomy, tubal ligation, vasectomy.* **2.** a technique for destroying microorganisms using heat, water, chemicals, or gases. **–sterilize,** *v.*

stern, the rear or back of a boat or ship.

sternal angle, the slight projection arising on the sternum at the junction of the manubrium and the body of the sternum. Also known as the **angle of Louis.**

sternoclavicular articulation /stur´nōkləvik´yə-lər/, the joint between the sternum and the clavicle.

sternocostal articulation /-kos´təl/, the flexible joint of the cartilage of each true rib and the sternum. Each sternocostal articulation also has five ligaments.

sternohyoideus /-hī·oi´dē·əs/, one of the four muscles of the anterior neck that extend from the clavicle to the larynx. It is used in swallowing and speaking.

sternothyroideus /-thīroi´dē·əs/, one of the four muscles of the anterior neck that extend from the clavicle to the larynx. It is used in swallowing and speaking.

sternum /stur´nəm/, the long, flat bone of the medial chest. Also known as **breastbone.**

sternutator, one of two classes of riot control agents, this one precipitates violent nausea and vomiting. The three primary agents in this class are DA (diphenylchloroarsine), DC (diphenylcyanarsine), and DM (diphenylaminochloroarsine). Although classed as vomiting agents, these gases also produce coughing, eye irritation, malaise, and sneezing. Effects are produced by direct action on the eyes or inhalation. These agents are dispersed as aerosols and cause a burning sensation in the eyes and throat, hypersalivation, and a violent frontal headache. *See also chemical agent, lacrimator.*

sterognosis /ster´ognō´-/, **1.** the sense of feeling and understanding the form and nature of objects by the sense of touch. **2.** perception by the senses of the solidity of objects.

steroid /stir´oid/. See **corticosteroid.**

stertorous /stur´tərəs/, breathing that is labored or struggling; having a snoring sound.

stethoscope (Rene Laennec, French physician, 1781-1826), an instrument, consisting of two earpieces connected to a diaphragm via flexible tubing, that is used to auscultate sounds. It is normally placed against the patient to listen to aneurysms, bowel sounds, breath sounds, bruits, heart sounds, and tracheal sounds. The most common instruments today use bell-shaped ends for low-pitched sounds, such as bowel sounds, and diaphragms for high-pitched sounds (breath sounds). Types include monaural (one earpiece), Sprague-Rapport (double earpiece/double hose), and compound, or training (two-person stethoscope terminating in one chestpiece). Variations include doppler and electronic amplification.

stigma, a moral or physical blemish that serves to label or socially isolate an individual or identifiable group, such as a contagious disease, religion.

stillbirth, the birth of a fetus that died before or during delivery.

stillborn, an infant that was born dead.

stimulant, any substance that increases the metabolism of a body system.

stimulus, *pl.* **stimuli,** anything that excites an organism or part to function, become active, or respond. **–stimulate,** *v.*

sting, an injury caused by a sharp, painful puncture of the skin, often accompanied by the toxin or venom of an insect or other animal. Stings that may be harmful to humans include bee, jellyfish, scorpion, sea urchin, and shellfish.

stingray, a flat, long-tailed fish that has barbed spines on its back that are connected to sacs of venom. The venom may precipitate dyspnea, severe local pain, seizures, and skeletal muscle spasm, if the skin is broken by the spines.

stink damp, hydrogen sulfide gas, as might be found in an underground mine. *See also damp.*

Stockholm syndrome, condition that can occur during hostage situations when kidnappers and/or their captives begin to identify or sympathize with the other's situation. A variation of this can occur in other involuntary captive situations, as between corrections officers and their prisoners and between soldiers and their prisoners-of-war. Extremes of this condition can result in providing money, weapons, or escape options.

Stokes-Adams syndrome (William Stokes, Irish physician, 1804-1878; Robert Adams, Irish physician, 1791-1875), syncope due to depressed cardiac output, precipitated by a transient third-degree atrioventricular (AV) block that reverts to a sinus rhythm or first-degree AV block. Also known as **Adams-Stokes disease, Adams-Stokes syncope, Morgagni's disease, Stokes-Adams attack.** *See also first-degree AV block, third-degree AV block.*

Stokes's litter, rescue stretcher for the movement of dead or injured from difficult-to-access locations. Originally constructed of welded tubular steel and wire mesh with a central leg divider, they are now also made of an aluminum frame and plastic body. Classed as a rigid transport vehicle, this litter is most commonly used in mountain, over-the-side, overwater, and rough terrain rescue. Also known as **Stokes, wire basket stretcher.** *See also rigid transport vehicle.*

stoma, **1.** a pore or opening on a surface. **2.** an artificial opening from an internal organ to the surface of the body, created surgically, as for a colostomy, ileostomy, or tracheostomy. **3.** a new opening created surgically, between two body structures, as for a gastroenterostomy.

stomach, the organ of digestion, which is divided into a body and a pylorus. It receives and partly digests food and drink funneled from the mouth through the esophagus and moves material into the intestine. The shape of the stomach is changed by the amount of contents, stage of digestion, development of the muscles, and condition of the intestine. It is lined with mucous membranes that have many blood vessels and nerves, and contains several important glands.

stomatitis /stō´mətī´-/, any inflammatory condition of the mouth, due to infection, exposure to certain chemicals or drugs, vitamin deficiency, or disease.

stool. See **feces.**

stope, the large room in underground mines where the mining occurs.

storm sewer, a pipeline that carries surface water.

strabismus, an inability of the eyes to converge on an object, seen in patients with impaired neurological function, as in head injury or substance abuse. An inward deviation of one eye in relation to the other is known as **convergent** strabismus or **esotropia.** The opposite condition is known as **divergent** strabismus or **exotropia.**

straight sinus, one of the six veins on the anterior portion of the brain, draining blood from the brain into the jugular vein. It has no valves.

strain, **1.** damage, usually muscular, that results from excessive physical effort. **2.** an emotional state reflecting mental pressure or fatigue.

strainer, flowing water obstruction that allows free movement of water but not larger objects. Animals, boats, and people tend to become trapped against the obstruction, due to the force of the current.

strait, a narrow channel or waterway connecting two large bodies of water.

strangulation, the tightening or closing of a tubular structure of the body, such as the throat, a section of bowel, or the blood vessels of a limb, that prevents function or slows circulation. *See also intestinal strangulation.*

strap, **1.** a band that is used to hold dressings in place or to attach one thing to another. **2.** to bind securely.

strapping, placing overlapping strips of adhesive tape on an arm, leg, or other body area to exert pressure and hold a structure in place.

stratum /strā´təm, strat´əm/, *pl.* **strata,** an even, thick sheet or layer, usually linked with other layers, such as the stratum basale.

stratum basale, the innermost layer of the epidermis.

stratum corneum, the outermost layer of the epidermis.

stratum granulosum, epidermal layer that lies beneath the stratum corneum, except in the hands and feet. *See also stratum lucidum.*

stratum lucidum, a layer of epidermis beneath the stratum corneum in the palms of the hand and the soles of the feet only. *See also stratum granulosum.*

stratum spinosum, the epidermal layer on top of the stratum basale and below the stratum granulosum.

strawberry mark. See **hemangioma.**

strawberry tongue, a symptom of scarlet fever, marked by a strawberry-like color of the tongue.

strep throat, *(informal)* an infection of the throat and tonsils caused by *Streptococcus.* Symptoms include sore throat, chills, fever, swollen lymph glands in the neck, and, sometimes, nausea and vomiting.

streptococcal infection /strep´təkok´əl/, an infection caused by bacteria of one of several types of *Streptococcus.* Almost any organ of the body may be involved. The infections occur in many forms, including endocarditis, erysipelas, impetigo, meningitis, pneumonia, scarlet fever, tonsillitis, and urinary tract infection. *See also strep throat.*

Streptococcus /-kok´əs/, a type of bacteria, causing many diseases in humans. **Beta-hemolytic streptococci** cause most of the acute streptococcal infection seen in humans, including rheumatic fever and many cases of pneumonia and septicemia.

streptokinase, a thrombolytic agent used in the presence of acute myocardial infarction. By combining with plasminogen, it produces plasmin, which degrades clotted blood. It is contraindicated in patients with trauma. Side effects include dysrhythmias, hypotension, and increased bleeding time. Use with caution in the presence of a recent cerebrovascular accident.

stress,   any emotional, physical, social, economic, or other factor that requires a response or change, such as severe loss of fluid, which can cause a rise in body temperature, or a separation from parents, which can cause a young child to cry. *See also general adaptation syndrome.*

stress fracture,   cracks or breaks in bone that is subjected to abnormal, prolonged, or repeated stresses. The feet (metatarsals) are most commonly affected.

stressor,   anything that causes wear and tear on the body's physical or mental resources, precipitating the general adaptation syndrome. *See also general adaptation syndrome.*

stress reaction,   a response to extreme anxiety, due to prolonged stress or a shocking or tragic event, such as a natural disaster or physical torture. Symptoms include an inability to concentrate, apathy, nightmares, restless sleep, and headaches. One form is **combat fatigue,** which results from the physical and mental stress of warfare. It is usually temporary but may lead to permanent neurosis. **Shell shock,** also caused by the stress of combat, may precipitate any number of disorders, ranging from extreme fear to dementia. Also known as **post-traumatic stress disorder, PTSD.** *See also general adaptation syndrome.*

stress test,   a test that measures a system of the body when subjected to carefully controlled stress. It is often used to test the heart, lungs, or health of the fetus in pregnant women.

stretcher,   1. a length of durable material stretched between two parallel poles and used for carrying victims of illness or injury; a litter. **2.** *(informal)* any moveable patient bed. *See also gurney, litter.*

stretch mark.   See **stria.**

stria /strī´ə/, *pl.* **striae,**   a streak or a narrow furrow in the skin that often results from a stretching of the skin, as seen on the stomach after pregnancy. Also known as **stretch mark.**

striated muscle /strī´ātid/.   See **muscle.**

stricture /strik´chər/,   narrowing of the lumen of a hollow organ, such as the throat or urethra, because of inflammation, pressure, or scarring. Compare **spasm.**

stridor /strī´dər/,   an abnormal, high-pitched respiratory breath sound, caused by partial blockage of the airway. It may indicate a tumor or inflammation. *See also breath sounds.*

strike team,   a group of five similar companies or units (resources) with common communications capability and leadership.

stroke.   See **cerebrovascular accident.**

stroke volume,   the volume of blood pumped from a ventricle during a single cardiac contraction. The volume pumped is dependent on cardiac contractility, preload, and afterload.

stroma /strō´mə/, *pl.* **stromata,**   the supporting tissue for an organ. An example is the vitreous stroma, which encloses the vitreous humor of the eye.

strongback.   See **upright.**

strongyloidiasis,   a disorder of the small intestine caused by the worm *Strongyloides stercoralis,* acquired when larvae from the soil penetrate intact skin, causing a pruritic rash. The larvae then penetrate the lungs via the circulation, move into the airway, and are swallowed, where they develop into adult worms in the small intestine. Diarrhea and intestinal disorders follow. Also known as **threadworm infection.**

structure,   a part of the body, such as heart, bone, or gland.

ST segment,   the portion of the cardiac complex between the S wave and the T wave. *See also ST depression, ST elevation.*

stump,   the part of a limb that is left after amputation. A **stump hallucination** is the feeling of the continued presence of an amputated limb. *See also phantom limb syndrome.*

stupor,   a condition in which a person seems unaware of his or her surroundings. The term is very subjective in nature.

sty,   infection on the edge of the eyelid formed in the root of an eyelash. Compare **chalazion.** Also known as **hordeolum.**

stylet,   any probe or rod that passes through a catheter, needle, or tube. These devices are used to stiffen an otherwise flexible tool to facilitate a puncture or insertion.

styloid process,   a bony protuberance located on the temporal bone, the distal radius, the distal ulna, and at the head of the fibula.

stylomandibular ligament/stī´lōmandib´yələr/, one of a pair of fibrous bands of tissue that forms part of the temporomandibular joint.

styptic /stip´tik/, **1.** a substance used to control bleeding. **2.** acting as an agent to control bleeding.

subacromial bursa /subəkrō´mē·əl/, the small fluid-filled sac in the shoulder joint.

subacute /-əkyo͞ot´/, relating to a disease or other abnormal condition present in a patient who appears to be well.

subarachnoid hemorrhage /-ərak´noid/, rapid bleeding into the space between the arachnoid and pia mater. The cause may be head trauma or an aneurysm. The first symptom is a painful headache that begins in one area and then spreads, becoming dull and throbbing. Other symptoms include dizziness, diaphoresis, and vomiting. It may result in prolonged unconsciousness and death. *See also sentinel headache, subdural hemorrhage.*

subclavian /-klā´vē·ən/, situated inferior to the clavicle, such as the subclavian artery.

subclavian artery, one of a pair of arteries that rise in the neck and supply blood to the vertebral column, spinal cord, ear, and brain.

subclavian steal syndrome, a disorder caused by a blockage in the subclavian artery near the beginning of the vertebral artery. This causes a change in blood pressure and blood flow. Symptoms include paralysis of the arm and occipital pain. Blood pressure in the arms may vary from one side to the other.

subclavian vein, the venous connection between the axillary vein of the arm and the internal jugular of the neck, where it forms the brachiocephalic vein. Located beneath the clavicle, it is a larger vessel, useful for central intravenous cannulation.

subclavius /-klā´vē·əs/, a short muscle of the chest wall. It moves the shoulder down and forward.

subclinical, relating to a disease or abnormal condition that is so mild it produces no symptoms.

subcutaneous, beneath the skin.

subcutaneous nodule, a small, solid bump beneath the skin that can be detected by palpation.

subcutaneous tissue, the layer of adipose tissue below the dermis. Also known as **hypodermis.**

subdural space, the potential space between the arachnoid and the dura mater meningeal layers.

subdural hemorrhage, bleeding between the dura mater and arachnoid, associated with injury to the underlying brain tissue. This type of bleeding (venous) may not be apparent for days or weeks after an injury, because of the slow buildup of pressure due to hemorrhage. Signs and symptoms include altered levels of consciousness, headache, and slurred speech. There is a high level of mortality associated with this injury. *See also sentinel headache, subarachnoid hemorrhage.*

subendocardial infarction. See **transmural infarction.**

subgaleal hematoma, a pooling of blood beneath the connective tissue joining the frontal and occipitofrontal muscles.

sublingual /-ling´gwəl/, beneath the tongue.

sublingual route, under the tongue. Medications placed here are absorbed into the venous circulation via the blood vessels of the tongue.

subluxation /-luksā´shən/, a partial dislocation, as a **shoulder subluxation** is an injury to the tissues around the shoulder joint.

submandibular duct /-mandib´yələr/, a tube through which a submandibular gland releases saliva. Also known as **submaxillary duct.**

submucous, beneath a mucous membrane.

subphrenic /-fren´ik/, referring to the area beneath or the inferior to the diaphragm.

substance abuse, the overuse of or addiction to a stimulant, depressant, or other chemical substance, leading to effects that are harmful to the patient's health, or the welfare of others.

substratum /-strā´təm/, any underlying layer; a foundation.

subthalamus /-thal´əməs/, a portion of the brain that serves as a center for signals from the eye. **–subthalamic,** *adj.*

subtle, not severe and having no serious results, as a mild infection.

subungual hematoma /-ung´gwəl/, a pool of blood beneath a nailbed, usually resulting from injury.

succinylcholine /suk´sənil kō´lēn/, a neuromuscular blocking agent used as an adjunct in endotracheal intubation. It causes muscle relaxation by blocking acetylcholine at the receptor site. Side effects include an increase in secretions, hypotension, and muscle fasciculation. A sedative should be used in conjunction with this medication because neuromuscular blockers do not alter level of consciousness.

succus /suk´əs/, *pl.* **succi** /suk´sī/, a juice or fluid, usually one released by an organ.

succussion splash /səkush´ən/, a sound heard in the body of a patient who has free fluid and air or gas in a hollow organ or body space. This sound may be heard over a normal stomach but may also be heard with hernias or blockage.

suckhole. See **hydraulic.**

suckle, 1. to provide nourishment, specifically to breastfeed. **2.** to take in as nourishment, especially by feeding from the breast.

sucrose /sōō´krōs/, sugar derived from sugar cane, sugar beets, and sorghum.

suction device, a device used to remove blood, secretions, or other fluids from a patient's mouth, throat, or stoma. Electrical, oxygen, and manually powered units are available.

sudden death, *(World Health Organization)* death occurring within 24 hours after the initial onset of illness or injury; *(American Heart Association)* death within one hour of the onset of signs or symptoms.

sudden infant death syndrome, the unexpected and sudden death of a seemingly normal and healthy infant that occurs during sleep and with no physical evidence of disease. It is the most common cause of death in children between 2 weeks and 1 year of age. The origin is unknown. Also known as **crib death, SIDS.**

sudoriferous gland /sōō´dôrif´ərəs/. See **sweat gland.**

sudorific /sōō´dôrif´ik/, referring to a drug, substance, or condition, such as heat or emotional tension, that causes sweating. Also known as **diaphoretic.**

suicide, the intentional taking of one's own life. Early signs of suicidal intent include depression, neglect of personal appearance, and direct or indirect threats to commit suicide.

sulcus /sul´kəs/, a depression or furrow on an organ or as in the chest cavity that holds up part of the lung.

sulfhemoglobin, a form of hemoglobin containing a bound sulfur molecule that stops normal oxygen binding. It is present in the blood in small amounts.

sulfiting agents, food preservatives used in processing of various foods and by restaurants to impart a fresh appearance to salad fruits and vegetables. The chemicals can cause a reaction in persons who are allergic to sulfites.

sulfur /sul´fər/, a tasteless, odorless chemical element that is used to make sulfuric acid and is used commercially in many industrial processes. The sulfonamides, or sulfa drugs, are used to treat various bacteria infections.

sulfuric acid /sulfyōōr´ik/, a clear, colorless, oily, highly dangerous liquid that creates great heat when mixed with water. A very poisonous substance, sulfuric acid causes severe skin burns, blindness on contact with the eyes, pulmonary injury, and death. It is used in various ways in industry, such as in the making of fertilizers.

summation, any cumulative action or effect, such as what might result from two stimuli.

sundowning, a condition in which elderly patients tend to become confused at the end of the day. Many of them have trouble seeing and have varying degrees of hearing loss. With less light, they lose visual cues that help them to make up for their sensory losses.

sun poisoning, systemic reaction to excessive ultraviolet radiation, which manifests as fever, headache, nausea, syncope, and vomiting. This syndrome generally occurs in the presence of first- and/or second-degree burns following prolonged exposure to sunlight.

sunstroke. See **heatstroke.**

superfecundation /sōō´pərfē´kəndā´shən/, the fertilization of two or more eggs released during one menstrual cycle by sperm from the same or different males during separate acts of sexual intercourse.

superfetation /-fētā´shən/, the fertilization of a second egg after the onset of pregnancy, resulting in the presence of two fetuses of different degrees of maturity developing within the uterus at the same time. Also known as **superimpregnation.**

superficial, 1. relating to the skin or another surface. **2.** not grave or dangerous.

superficial inguinal node, a lymph gland in one of two groups in the upper thigh that supply the skin of the penis, scrotum, perineum, buttocks, and abdominal wall inferior to the level of the umbilicus.

superficial reflex, any reflex begun by stimulation of the skin, such as the **abdominal reflex.** Compare **deep tendon reflex.**

superficial vein, one of the many veins between the layers of tissue just under the skin. Compare **deep vein.**

superinfection, an infection that occurs while treating another infection. It often results from change in the normal tissue favoring growth of some organisms by lowering the vitality and then the number of competing organisms, as yeast microbes thrive during penicillin therapy used to cure a bacterial infection.

superior, above or higher, as the head is superior to the torso. Compare **inferior.**

superior costotransverse ligament, one of five ligaments that help secure each rib to the spine.

superior mesenteric artery, a large artery in the abdomen that supplies blood to the small intestine and parts of the colon.

superior mesenteric vein, a branch of the vein that drains blood from the small intestine, cecum, and colon.

superior radioulnar joint, the pivot joint of the elbow. The joint allows the lower arm to move in circles. Also known as **proximal radioulnar articulation.**

superior sagittal sinus, one of six veins in the posterior portion of the dura mater that drains blood from the brain.

superior subscapular nerve /subskap´yələr/, one of two nerves on opposite sides of the body that supply the muscle of the anterior shoulder.

superior thyroid artery, one of a pair of arteries in the neck that supply the thyroid gland and several muscles in the head.

superior ulnar collateral artery, a division of the brachial artery that supplies the forearm.

superior vena cava, vein that receives deoxygenated blood from the upper body and routes it to the right atrium. *See also inferior vena cava.*

supervisor, **1.** an individual responsible for the activities of others. **2.** an incident command system title of an individual(s) responsible for command of a division or group.

supination /sōō´pinā´shən/, one of the movements allowed by certain joints, such as the elbow and the wrist joints, which allow the palm of the hand to turn up. *See also supine.* Compare **pronation. –supinate,** *v.*

supine /səpīn´, sōō´pīn/, lying flat on the back, face up. Compare **prone.**

supine hypotension syndrome, hypotension in pregnancy due to compression of the inferior vena cava by the gravid uterus when the woman is lying supine. The lowered blood pressure occurs as the result of diminished cardiac filling and subsequent output.

supplemental type certificate, a certification, provided by the FAA, that declares that certain equipment, installed on an aircraft after manufacture, meets required aviation standards. Also known as **STC.**

support branch, an incident command system level within the logistics section that is responsible for providing the equipment, personnel, and supplies needed to support incident operations.

suppository /səpoz´itôr´ē/, an easily melted cone or cylinder of material mixed with a drug for placing in the rectum, urethra, or vagina. Drugs given in this way are absorbed into the system.

suppurate /sup´yərāt/, producing purulent drainage.

supraclavicular /sōō´prəkləvik´yələr/, the area of the body above the clavicle.

supraclavicular nerve, one of a pair of nerves that run along the clavicle from the neck to the shoulder.

suprascapular nerve /-skap´yələr/, one of a pair of nerves that extends from the neck to the shoulder and scapula.

suprasternal notch, the landmark at the anterior base of the neck formed by the superior margin of the manubrium. Also known as **jugular notch.**

supraventricular tachycardia, **1.** rapid cardiac dysrhythmia with no visible P waves, narrow QRS complex, and a regular rhythm at rates generally greater than 150 beats per minute. Because the rate is fast enough to hide P waves within T waves, more accurate identification of the rhythm is not possible. Potential rhythm possibilities are atrial flutter with 1:1 response, atrial tachycardia, junctional tachycardia, and sinus tachycardia. Also known as **paroxysmal supraventricular tachycardia, PSVT, SVT.** *See also paroxysmal supraventricular tachycardia.* **2.** used to refer to all tachycardias originating above the ventricles.

surface-supplied diving equipment, diving equipment utilizing a mask with an air supply pumped from the surface. This equipment is useful in shallow water, where prolonged dive time or surface communication is necessary. Also known as **hookah rig, shallow water gear.**

surface tension, the tendency of a liquid to minimize its surface area by contracting.

surgery, a branch of medicine concerned with diseases and injuries requiring operations. **–surgical,** *adj.*

survey instrument, a portable instrument used for detecting and measuring radiation under varied physical conditions. The term covers a wide range of devices such as the CD V-700 Geiger counter, the CD V-715 ionization chamber, and many other similar instruments.

susceptibility /səsep´təbil´itē/, the condition of being more than normally likely to become ill from a disease or disorder. **–susceptible,** *adj.*

suspensory ligament, a band of peritoneum stretching from the ovary to the wall of the body.

Sutton's law, look for or suspect first those causes or diseases that are most likely where you are.

sutura /sŌŌtŌŌr´ə/, *pl.* **suturae,** an immoveable, fiberlike joint in which certain bones of the skull are connected by a thin layer of tissue. Suturae form as toothlike processes that interlock along the margins of connecting bones.

suture /sŌŌ´chər/, **1.** a border or a joint, as between the bones of the cranium. **2.** to stitch together cut or torn edges of tissue with suture material. **3.** material used for surgical stitches, such as absorbable or nonabsorbable silk, catgut, wire, or synthetic material.

swab, a stick or clamp for holding absorbent gauze or cotton, used for washing, cleansing, or drying a body surface, for collecting a specimen for laboratory tests, or for applying a topical medication.

swami belt, device used when climbing, consisting of several wraps of tubular webbing wrapped around the waist and securely tied. This device is very uncomfortable and cannot be used for prolonged periods of time. *See also seat harness.*

S wave, the first negative deflection in the EKG complex following the R wave.

sweat, **1.** the fluid, manufactured in the sweat glands, that is released through pores in the skin to assist in control of body temperature. It is composed of ammonia, phosphate, sodium, urea, and water. **2.** the release of sweat. Loss of fluid from the body by evaporation, as during respirations, is known as **insensible perspiration.** Also known as **diaphoresis, perspiration.** *See also diaphoresis.* **3.** the leaking of fluid, usually water, from containers under varying environmental conditions.

sweat duct, any one of the tiny tubes carrying sweat to the surface of the skin from the sweat glands throughout the body. The sweat ducts in the axilla and the groin are larger than in other parts of the body.

sweat gland, one of about 3 million tiny structures within the skin that produce sweat. The average quantity of sweat secreted in 24 hours varies from 700 to 900 g. The number of glands per square centimeter of skin varies in different parts of the body. They are found in great numbers on the palms of the hands and on the soles of the feet and fewest in the neck and the back. Also known as **sudoriferous gland.** Compare **sebaceous gland.**

sweating. See **diaphoresis.**

swimmer's ear, infection of the ear precipitated by the water of a swimming pool.

swimmer's harness, **1.** *(military)* device worn around the chest of helicopter aircrew personnel who enter the water during air-sea rescue. Constructed of double-stitched flat webbing, it provides attachment points for rescue equipment and helicopter hoisting. Also known as **rescue harness. 2.** any chest-waist harness worn by a water rescue swimmer, particularly in swift water, to provide a secure attachment point for safety lines used during a rescue.

swimmer's itch, a skin condition caused by sensitivity to tiny organisms (schistosome cercarias) that die under the skin, leading to reddening of the skin and the appearance of a rash lasting 1 or 2 days.

symmelia /simē´lyə/, a defect of the fetus marked by the growing together of the lower limbs with or without feet.

symmetrical, *(of the body or parts of the body)* equal in size or shape; very similar in placement about an axis. Compare **asymmetrical. –symmetry,** *n.*

sympathectomy, removal of the sheath that carries sympathetic nerves, from around an artery, relaxing the vessel and increasing blood flow. This procedure eases pain and improves circulation after skin grafts and in such vascular diseases as arteriosclerosis and Buerger's disease.

sympathetic amine /sim´pəthet´ik/, a drug that causes effects like those made by the sympathetic nervous system.

sympathetic nervous system, the division of the autonomic nervous system that functions during strenuous muscular work and other stresses. Sympathetic function dilates blood vessels in the skeletal muscle; increases adrenal secretion, heart rate, and pupillary size; and decreases digestive functions in preparation for fight-or-flight reactions. This system is balanced in function by the parasympathetic nervous system. *See also autonomic nervous system, central nervous system, parasympathetic nervous system, peripheral nervous system.*

sympathetic trunk, one of a pair of nerves that lie along the side of the spine from the base of the skull to the sacrum. Each trunk is part of the sympathetic nervous system.

sympatholytic /sim´pəthōlit´ik/. See **antiadrenergic.**

sympathomimetic /-mimet´ik/, a drug that causes effects like those of the sympathetic nervous system. *See also adrenergic.*

symphysis, a joint of cartilage in which bony surfaces lying next to one another are firmly united by fiberlike cartilage. Also known as **fibrocartilaginous joint.**

symphysis pubis, anterior joint of the pelvis, comprised of two ligaments forming the medial

ends of the pubis and ischium bones into a slightly moveable joint. Also known as **pubic symphysis.**

symptom, any subjective abnormality in body function indicative of disease, illness, or injury, such as headache, dizziness, nausea. A **delayed** symptom is one appearing sometime after its cause. **Local** symptoms indicate the specific location of a disease or injury process. **Prodromal** symptoms indicate an approaching illness or disease. **Withdrawal** symptoms occur when addicts are deprived of the focus of their addiction. *See also sign.*

synapse /sin´aps/, **1.** the point where one nerve signal jumps from one nerve cell to another. **2.** to form a synapse or connection between nerve cells. **–synaptic,** *adj.*

synaptic cleft, the space between the presynaptic and postsynaptic membranes.

synaptic vesicle, a sac in the presynaptic terminal that secretes neurotransmitter substances into the synaptic cleft when stimulated to propagate an impulse.

synchondrosis, any cartilaginous joint between two immovable bones, such as between the sternum and manubrium.

synchronized cardioversion, electrical discharge on the R wave of a rapid rhythm to convert it to a slower rhythm. This requires a timing device to calculate when the electrical discharge should occur (synchronizer).

syncope /sing´kəpē/, fainting. It may be caused by emotional stress, pooling of blood in the legs, heavy sweating, or sudden change in room temperature or body position. This condition may also result from any of a number of cardiopulmonary disorders.

syncytium, a group of cells in which the protoplasm of one cell is continuous with that of adjoining cells, as are cardiac muscle cells that act as one in response to an electrical impulse.

syndesmosis, an articulation between two bones connected by interosseous ligaments.

syndrome, a group of signs and symptoms that occur together and are typical of a particular disorder or disease.

synechia /sinek´ē·ə/, *pl.* **synechiae,** adhesion of the iris to the cornea or lens of the eye. It may develop from glaucoma, cataracts, or keratitis or as a complication of surgery or injury to the eye. Blindness may result.

synergism, 1. the combined action of two drugs, organs, or systems being greater than the sum of their individual actions. 2. working together.

synergist, 1. a muscle that assists other muscles to cause movement. 2. a remedy or treatment that stimulates the action of another.

synovia /sinō´vē·ə/, a clear, sticky fluid, resembling the white of an egg, released by synovial membranes and acting as a lubricant for joints, bursae, and tendons. It contains mucin, albumin, fat, and mineral salts. Also known as **synovial fluid. –synovial,** *adj.*

synovial joint. See **joint.**

synovial membrane /sinō´vē·əl/, the inner layer of the capsule surrounding a freely moveable joint. The synovial membrane secretes into the joint fluid that normally lubricates the joint, but can collect in painful amounts when the joint is injured.

synovitis /sin´əvī´-/, inflammation of the synovial membrane of a joint that results from a wound or an injury, such as a sprain. The joint is swollen, tender, and painful with limited motion.

synthetic, relating to a substance that is artificial instead of natural.

syphilis, a sexually transmitted disease caused by a type of bacteria (*Treponema pallidum*), marked by three clear stages over a period of years known as primary, secondary, and tertiary.

syringe /sir´inj/, a device for withdrawing, injecting, or instilling fluids.

syringomyelocele /siring´gōmī´əlōsēl´/, a condition in which a section of the spinal cord protrudes through a hole, present at birth, in the spinal column. It forms a fluid-filled sac. *See also spina bifida.*

system, a collection of parts that make a whole. Systems of the body, such as the cardiovascular or reproductive systems, are made up of structures specially adapted to perform functions necessary for life.

systemic /sistem´ik/, of or relating to the whole body rather than to a single area or part of the body.

systemic circulation, circulation of blood in the body from left ventricle to right atrium.

systemic lupus erythematosus. See **lupus erythematosus.**

systemic pressure, the pressure created by the left side of the heart, pumping against vascular resistance, which results in circulation of blood. Also known as **blood pressure.**

T

tabes dorsalis /tā´bēz dôrsā´lis/, a condition marked by deterioration of the body and the progressive loss of reflexes. This disease affects the spinal cord and destroys the large joints of affected extremities.

tablet, a small, solid dose form of a drug. It may be pressed or molded in its manufacture. Most tablets are meant to be swallowed whole. However, some may be dissolved in the mouth, chewed, or dissolved in liquid before swallowing.

tachycardia, heart rates exceeding 100 beats per minute; a rapid heart rate. *See also bradycardia.*

tachyphylaxis, a rapid decrease in the effectiveness of a drug after the administration of a few doses.

tachypnea /-pnē´ə/, rapid respirations.

tactical, **1.** thinking in a manner that advances a purpose or gains an advantage. **2.** pertaining to tactics.

tactics, **1.** carefully preplanned steps taken to achieve a purpose. **2.** the science and art of using force to its best advantage, considering the immediate situation.

tactile /tak´təl/, referring to the sense of touch.

tactile anesthesia, the absence or lack of the sense of touch in the fingers. It can result from injury or disease.

tactile corpuscle, any one of many small, oval end organs linked to the sense of touch. They are widely distributed throughout the body in peripheral areas, such as the hand, foot, forehead, lips, and tongue. Also known as **Meissner's corpuscle.**

tactile fremitus. See **vocal fremitus.**

tactile image, a mental concept of an object as perceived through the sense of touch. *See also image.*

tag line, lengths of small-diameter rope, used to move or steady an object being lifted or lowered.

tail rotor, the small, vertical rotor located to the aft of a helicopter. This device acts as a rudder for controlling the direction of forward flight of the helicopter. *See also main rotor.*

tail water, the slow-moving water downstream of the solid obstruction.

tail wind, wind blowing in the same general direction as the direction of travel of an airplane or boat.

tainos. See **tropical cyclone.**

talipes /tal´ipēz/, a deformity of the foot and ankle with the foot twisted and relatively fixed in an abnormal position.

talus, **1.** the ankle bone; *(historical)* astragalus. **2.** rock debris at the base of a cliff. **3.** a slope of rock fragments formed by and leading to a cliff face.

talus cave. See **speleogenesis.**

tampon, a pack of cotton, a sponge, or other material. Its purpose is to stem bleeding, absorb fluids in cavities or canals, or hold displaced organs in position.

tamponade /tam´pənād´/,   slowing or stopping blood flow to an organ or part of the body by pressure, as by a pressure dressing applied to stop hemorrhage.

tanker,   1. a railroad car, ship, or truck that carries liquids as its cargo, usually petroleum products. **2.** firefighting vehicle that carries water used to fight fires in areas without hydrants. It can be an aircraft or truck. *See also engine.*

tantrum,   a sudden outburst or violent display of rage, frustration, and temper. It usually occurs in a poorly adjusted child and certain emotionally disturbed persons. It is used primarily as an attempt to control others. Also known as **temper tantrum.**

tapeworm infection,   an intestinal infection by one of several species of parasitic worms called tapeworms or cestodes. The tapeworm species that most often infects human is *Taenia saginata*. It is in the tissues of cattle during its larval stage. It infects the intestine of humans in its adult form and may grow to a length of between 12 and 25 feet. **Pork tapeworm infection** is caused by the pork tapeworm (*Taenia solium*). Humans are usually infected with the adult worm after eating undercooked pork. **Fish tapeworm infection** is carried to humans when they eat raw or undercooked freshwater fish infected by *Diphyllobothrium latum*. It is common in warm areas throughout the world and is found in the Great Lakes area of the United States.

tardive dyskinesia,   involuntary, repetitious movements of muscles of the face, extremities, and trunk. This disorder most commonly affects older people who have been treated for extended periods with phenothiazine drugs to relieve the symptoms of parkinsonism. *See also antiparkinsonian.*

tardy peroneal nerve palsy,   a condition in which the peroneal nerve is compressed where it crosses the smaller leg bone. Such compression may occur when a person falls asleep with the legs crossed.

tardy ulnar nerve palsy,   atrophy of the hand muscles and difficulty in movement. It may be caused by injury of the ulnar nerve at the elbow. Symptoms include numbness of the small and ring finger.

target cell,   1. an abnormal red blood cell (leptocyte) that occurs after splenectomy and in blood diseases (anemias, hemoglobin C disease). **2.** any cell having a specific receptor that reacts with a specific hormone, antigen, antibody, antibiotic, sensitized tumor cell, or other substance.

target organ,   an organ most affected by a specific hormone, such as the thyroid gland, which is the target organ of thyroid-stimulating hormone released by the pituitary gland.

tarp,   a durable canvas or nylon cover, used to protect equipment from the elements.

tarsal /tär´səl/,   referring to the tarsus (ankle) or the eyelid.

tarsal bone,   any one of seven bones comprising the ankle, made up of the talus, calcaneus, cuboid, navicular, and the three cuneiforms.

tarsal gland,   one of numerous oil glands on the inner surfaces of the eyelids. Bacterial infection of a tarsal gland causes a sty. Compare **ciliary gland.**

tarsal tunnel syndrome,   pain and numbness in the sole of the foot. This may be caused by pressure on the posterior tibial nerve.

tarsus /tär´səs/, *pl.* **tarsi,   1.** the area between the foot and the leg (the ankle). **2.** a plate of cartilage (also known as **tarsal plate**) that forms each eyelid.

tartar /tär´tär/,   a hard, gritty deposit. It is made of organic matter, phosphates, and carbonates that collect on the teeth and gums. An excess of tartar may cause gum disease and other dental problems. *See also gingivitis, pyorrhea.*

task force,   a group of resources with common communications and a leader temporarily assembled for a specific mission.

taste,   the sense of perceiving different flavors in soluble substances that contact the tongue and send nerve impulses to special taste centers in the cortex and the thalamus of the brain. The sense of taste is linked with the sense of smell. The four basic taste sensations are sweet, sour, bitter, and salty. All other tastes are combinations of these four basic flavors. The front of the tongue is most sensitive to salty and sweet substances. The sides of the tongue are most sensitive to sour substances. The back of the tongue is most sensitive to bitter substances. The middle of the tongue produces virtually no taste sensation.

taste bud, any one of many outer taste organs distributed over the tongue and the roof of the mouth. Adults have about 9000 taste buds. Each taste bud rests in a spheric pocket. Taste (gustatory) cells and supporting cells form each bud. Also known as **gustatory organ.**

tattoo, 1. marking of the skin with pigments. **2.** imbedding of road surface material or other substances in the skin as a result of trauma.

taxonomy /takson´əmē/, a system for classifying organisms on the basis of natural relationships and giving them appropriate names.

Tay-Sachs disease /tā-saks´/, an inherited nerve disorder of fat processing. It is caused by the deficiency of an enzyme that results in the pooling of fats in the brain. It occurs foremost in families of Eastern European Jewish origin, specifically Ashkenazic Jews and causes progressive mental and physical retardation and early death. *See also lipidosis, Sandhoff's disease.*

T cell, a small circulating white blood cell (lymphocyte) made in the bone marrow. It matures in the thymus gland or as a result of exposure to a hormone (thymosin) released by the thymus. They have several functions but primarily involve immune responses, such as graft rejection and delayed allergy. One kind of T cell, the **helper cell,** affects the production of antibodies by B cells; a **suppressor T cell** supresses B cell activity. Compare **B cell.** *See also antibody, immune response.*

teaching hospital, a hospital with recognized programs in medical, nursing, or related health personnel education.

teardrop fracture, a tear-shaped break of one of the short bones, as a vertebra.

tear duct, any duct that carries tears, including the ducts in the eyelids and nose, and the ducts of the tear glands.

tearing, watering of the eye. It is usually caused by excess tear production from strong emotion, infection, or irritation by a foreign body. Tearing occurs when more tears are made than are drained by the ducts and sacs of the eyes.

technetium, a radioactive, metallic element. Isotopes of technetium are used in radioisotope scanning methods of internal organs, such as the liver and spleen.

technique, the method and details followed in performing a procedure, as in a physical examination.

telangiectasia /təlan´jē·ektā´zhə/, permanent widening of groups of capillaries and venules with occasional hemorrhage. Common causes include injury from excess sunlight, some skin diseases, as rosacea, and collagen blood vessel diseases.

telemetry, the science of measuring a quantity and then transmitting the results to be received, interpreted, and recorded. In emergency medical care, physiologic data is transmitted from the field via radio or telephone and received at the hospital to aid in patient evaluation and treatment. Also known as **biotelemetry.**

telephone coupler, communications device for transmitting electronic information via telephone lines to a computer or other decoding device. Electrocardiograms and other physiologic information can be transmitted in this fashion. Also known as **acoustic data coupler.**

telophase, completion of cell division, resulting in two identical cells; the last stage of mitosis. *See also anaphase, interphase, meiosis, mitosis, metaphase, prophase.*

temperature, 1. a measure of the tendency of heat to flow in a certain direction, using one of several scales, such as Celsius, Fahrenheit, Kelvin. **2.** the thermal condition or internal heat of a body. *See also body temperature, fever.*

template /tem´plit/, (in genetics) the strand of DNA that acts as a mold for the synthesis of messenger RNA. This messenger RNA has the same sequence of nucleic acids as the DNA strand. It carries the code to the ribosomes for the synthesis of proteins.

temporal arteritis /tem´pərəl/. See **arteritis.**

temporal artery, any one of three arteries on each side of the head: the superficial temporal artery, the middle temporal artery, and the deep temporal artery.

temporal bone, one of a pair of large bones forming part of the skull. It has many cavities and spaces linked to the ear, as the tympanic cavity and the auditory tube. Each temporal bone consists of four portions: the mastoid, the squama, the petrous, and the tympanic.

temporalis /tem´pôrā´lis/,   one of the four muscles of mastication. Upon contraction, it closes the mandible. Also known as **temporal muscle.**

temporal lobe.   See **brain.**

temporomandibular joint /-mandib´yələr/,   one of two joints connecting the mandible to the temporal bone of the skull. It is a combined hinge and gliding joint. Also known as **TMJ.**

temporomandibular joint syndrome,   facial pain and poor function of the mandible, caused by a defective or dislocated temporomandibular joint. Signs include clicking of the joint when the mandible moves, limitation of mandibular movement, and partial dislocation.

temporoparietalis /-pərī´ətā´lis/,   one of a pair of broad, thin muscles of the scalp that, upon contraction, wrinkle the forehead, widen the eyes, and raise the ears.

tenacious /tənā´shəs/,   referring to fluids that are sticky or adhesive or otherwise tend to hold together, such as mucus and sputum.

ten code,   radio transmission code utilizing 10 as the prefix for all coded transmissions. This code was originally developed when public service radio use became popular. Even though it provided a clearly stated method of describing emergency service situations, the code's meaning rapidly became clear to the general public and its value as a tool of confidentiality was diminished. Many services are today dropping their requirements for code usage. *See also clear text.*

tendon,   one of many white, fibrous bands of tissue that attach muscle to bone. Except at points of attachment, tendons are tubular shaped, fibroelastic connective tissue. Larger tendons have a thin inner septum, blood vessels, and specialized sterognostic nerves. Tendons are extremely strong, flexible, and inelastic and develop in various lengths and thicknesses. Compare **ligament.**

tendonitis /ten´dəni´-/,   inflammation of a tendon.

tenesmus /tənez´məs/,   persistent, ineffectual spasms of the rectum or bladder.

tenosynovitis /ten´ōsin´ōvī´-/,   inflammation of a tendon sheath usually caused by calcium deposits, repeated strain, or injury. In some instances, movement yields a crackling noise over the tendon.

tension,   1. the act of pulling or straining until strained. **2.** the condition of being tense, or under pressure. It is marked physically by a general increase in muscle tonus, heart rate, breathing, and alertness. *See also stress.*

tension crack,   cracks in the ground near a trench, indicating ground shift.

tension headache.   See **headache.**

tension pneumothorax,   positive-pressure air or gas accumulation within the pleural cavity, compressing the lungs and limiting the ability of the heart to function.

tensor,   any one of the muscles of the body that tenses a structure, the **tensor fasciae latae,** a muscle of the buttocks that acts to flex the thigh and rotate it slightly medial. Compare **abductor, adductor, depressor, sphincter.**

tentorial herniation /tentôr´e·əl/,   cerebral damage caused by increased pressure within the cranium. It results from edema, bleeding, or a tumor. Symptoms include altered levels of consciousness, diaphoresis, and hypotension.

tentorium /tentôr´ē·əm/, *pl.* **tentoria,**   any part of the body that looks like a tent.

tepid,   moderately warm to the touch.

teratism /ter´ətizm/,   any congenital or developmental anomaly that is produced by inherited or environmental factors, or by a combination of the two.

teratogen /ter´ətəjen/,   any substance, agent, or process that blocks normal growth of the fetus, causing one or more developmental abnormalities in the fetus. Teratogens act directly on the developing organism or indirectly, affecting such structures as the placenta. The type and extent of the defect are determined by the specific kind of teratogen, its mode of action, the embryonic process affected, and the stage of development at the time of exposure. Compare **mutagen. –teratogenic,** *adj.*

teratogenesis /ter´ətōjen´əsis/,   the development of physical defects in the embryo.

teres /tir´ēz/, *pl.* **teretes** /ter´ətēz/,   a long, cylindric muscle. The **teres major,** a shoulder muscle, acts to pull forward, extend, and rotate the arm to the midline. The **teres minor** acts to rotate the arm outwards, pull up the arm, and to strengthen the shoulder joint.

term, a pregnancy reaching 38 weeks of gestation.

terminal, *(of a structure or process)* near or approaching its end, as a terminal bronchiole or a terminal disease.

terminal bronchiole, the end of the conducting airway.

terminal control area, controlled airspace from the surface to specified altitudes, where all aircraft are subject to certain operating rules and pilot and equipment requirements. Also known as **TCA.**

terminal drop, a rapid decline in mental function and coping ability that occurs 1 to 5 years before death.

terminal sulcus of right atrium, a shallow channel on the outer surface of the right atrium between the upper and lower vena cava.

term infant, any newborn, regardless of birth weight, born after the end of the thirty-seventh and before the beginning of the forty-third week of gestation. Infants born at term usually measure from 48 to 53 cm from head to heel and weigh between 2700 and 4000 g.

termination of action, the end point of drug effectiveness.

tertian /tur´shən/, occurring every 48 hours or 3 days, including the first day of occurrence, such as tertian malaria, in which fever occurs every third day. Compare **quartan.** *See also malaria.*

tertiary /tur´shē·ər´ē/, /tursh´ərē/, third in frequency or in order of use; belonging to the third level of a system, as a tertiary health care facility.

tertiary health care, a specialized level of health care. It includes diagnosis and treatment of disease and disability in large hospitals with specialized intensive care units, advanced diagnostic support services, and highly specialized personnel. It offers highly centralized care to the population of a large region; in some cases, to the world.

tertiary injury, those injuries sustained from being thrown and impacting on other objects, including the surface, after an explosion. *See also blast injury, primary injury, secondary injury.*

tertiary segmental bronchus, an extension of the secondary bronchus, which conducts air to each lobe of the lung.

test, **1.** an examination or trial intended to establish a principle or determine a value. **2.** a chemical reaction or reagent that has clinical importance. **3.** to detect, identify, or conduct a trial.

testicle. See **testis.**

testicular /testik´yələr/, referring to the testicle.

testicular artery, one of a pair of long, slender branches of the abdominal aorta, arising posteria from the renal arteries and supplying the testicles.

testicular duct. See **vas deferens.**

testicular torsion, rotation of the spermatic cord, which occludes blood supply to testicular structures.

testicular vein, one of a pair of blood veins that arises from venous plexuses that drain blood from the testicles.

testis /tes´tis/, *pl.* **testes,** one of the pair of male gonads that produce semen. The adult testes are suspended in the scrotum by the spermatic cords. Each testis is an oval body about 4 cm long, 2.5 cm wide. It weighs about 12 g. The ducts in which the sperm is stored (epididymis) are located on the back of the testis.

testosterone /testos´tərōn/, a naturally occurring hormone that stimulates the growth of male characteristics (androgen).

tetanus, an acute infection of the central nervous system caused by an exotoxin produced by the anaerobic bacillus *Clostridium tetani.* More than 50,000 people worldwide die yearly from this infection. Commonly found in the top layers of soil, this bacillus is part of the normal flora of the intestinal tracts of cows and horses. It can be introduced into the human body from abrasions, burns, lacerations, or puncture wounds. Symptoms include fever, headache, irritability, and painful muscle spasms of such force that they are capable of fracturing bones. Also known as **lockjaw.**

tetany /tet´ənē/, a condition with cramps, seizures, and flexion of the wrist and ankle. These symptoms sometimes occur with respiratory stridor. Tetany is a sign of an abnormality in calcium processing.

tether, a cable, chain, or rope attached so as to limit one's movement.

tetrahydrocannabinol, the active substance of marijuana, it increases pulse rate, gives a feeling of excitement, and has variable effects on blood pressure, breathing, and pupil size. The drug affects memory, cognition, and the senses. It decreases motor coordination and increases appetite. Also known as **THC.** *See also cannabis.*

tetralogy of Fallot /tetral´-, falō´/, an inherited cardiac disorder made of four defects: pulmonic stenosis, ventricular septal defect, malposition of the aorta so that it arises from the septal defect or the right ventricle, and hypertrophy of the right ventricle. The primary symptoms in the infant are cyanosis and hypoxia, usually during crying and feeding. In older children a typical squatting position and clubbing of the fingers and toes are evident. Also known as **Fallot's syndrome.**

tetraploid /tet´rəploid/. See **euploid.**

Texas prusik /prus´ik/, a two-prusik method of self-rescue on a rope. One prusik runs from a rope to a waist harness, and the other runs from the same rope to both feet. This method is used when speed is essential, particularly when climbing on snow and ice.

thalamus /thal´əməs/, one of a pair of large, oval organs forming part of the brain. It is made up mainly of gray substance. It translates impulses from receptors for pain, temperature, and touch. It also joins in associating sensory impulses with pleasant and unpleasant feelings, in the arousal mechanisms of the body, and in the mechanisms that produce reflex movements. Compare **epithalamus, hypothalamus, subthalamus.**

thalassemia /thal´əsē´mē·ə/, a disease marked by abnormal and short-lived red blood cells. People of Mediterranean origin are more often affected than others. It is a genetically carried disease occurring in two forms. **Thalassemia major (Cooley's anemia)** causes anemia, fever, failure to thrive, and splenomegaly. **Thalassemia minor** causes a mild anemia and minimal red blood cell changes.

theca /thē´kə/, *pl.* **thecae** /thē´sē/, a sheath or capsule.

Theden's bandage /tā´dənz/, a roller bandage applied below the injury and continued upward over a compress. It is used to stop bleeding.

thelarche /thelär´kē/, the beginning of female pubertal breast growth that normally occurs before puberty at the beginning of phase of fast growth between 9 and 13 years of age. **Premature thelarche** is breast growth in a female without other evidence of sexual maturation. Compare **menarche.**

thenar /thē´när/, **1.** the ball of the thumb. **2.** referring to the thumb side of the palm.

therapeutic, 1. beneficial. **2.** referring to a treatment.

therapeutic abortion, legal termination of a pregnancy due to concerns about maternal health.

therapeutic action, the desired action of a drug.

therapeutic equivalent, a drug that has in essence the same effect in the treatment of a disease or condition as one or more other drugs. A drug that is a therapeutic equivalent may or may not be chemically or bioequivalent. *See also bioequivalent, chemical equivalent, generic equivalent.*

therapeutic index, a scale measuring a drug's safety.

therapeutic range, the range of a drug's concentration in the blood that is most likely to produce the desired effect, while minimizing toxicity.

therapy, the treatment of any disease or condition.

thermal /thur´məl/, referring to the production, application, or maintenance of heat.

thermal gradient, the temperature difference between the body and the environment.

thermal protective aid, an aluminum or Mylar™ cover designed to prevent and treat hypothermia by reflecting the wearer's body heat back to the body. Also known as a **space blanket.**

thermistor, a rescue device sensitive to variations in temperature below a surface. This device is most effectively utilized when searching for victims buried in snow.

thermocline, the division between warm and cold water. The warm water is generally in the upper level with cooler water below.

thermogenesis /thur´mōjen´əsis/, making of heat, especially by the cells of the body.

thermolabile /-lā´bil/, easily destroyed or changed by heat, as in stingray venom. Also known as **heat labile.**

thermolysis, body heat dissipated by conduction, convection, evaporation, or radiation.

thermometer, an instrument for measuring temperature. It is usually made of a sealed glass tube, marked in degrees of Celsius or Fahrenheit. It has a liquid, as mercury or alcohol. The liquid rises or falls as it expands or contracts according to changes in temperature. An **air thermometer** is one that uses air instead of mercury. An **electronic thermometer** gives temperature by electronic means. **Invasive thermometry** measures tissue temperature using probes directly in the tissue. A **surface thermometer** shows the temperature of the skin of any part of the body. A **thermistor** is a type of thermometer used for measuring very small changes in temperature. *See also thermistor.*

thermoneutral environment, 1. an environment that keeps body temperature at an optimum point at which the least amount of oxygen is consumed. **2.** an environment that enables a newborn to keep a body temperature of 36.5° C (97.7° F) with a minimal requirement of energy and oxygen.

thermopenetration, the use of heating techniques to create warmth within the body temperature for therapeutic purposes. Also known as **transthermia.**

thermoregulation, the control of heat production and heat loss; keeping the body temperature normal through physical mechanisms set off by the hypothalamus.

thermostat, a device for the automatic control of a heating or cooling system.

thermotaxis, 1. the normal adjustment and control of body temperature. **2.** the movement of an organism in response to heat, either toward the stimulus (positive thermotaxis) or away from the stimulus (negative thermotaxis). Also known as **thermotropism.**

thiamine, a vitamin essential for normal carbohydrate and fat metabolism. When used as a pharmacological agent, it is indicated in patients with altered levels of consciousness of unknown or alcoholic origin. After administration of dextrose, it prevents Wernicke-Korsakoff syndrome in the alcoholic or starving patient. There are no side effects or contraindications for field use. Also known as **vitamin B$_1$.**

thigh, the section of the lower limb between the hip and the knee.

thinking, the mental process for forming images or concepts, and problem-solving through the sorting, organizing, and classification of facts. **Concrete thinking** is a stage reached in a child between 7 and 11 years of age in which thought becomes more logical. Problem solving is based on what is seen. The literal meaning of words is still present. It is preceded by the ability to combine different beliefs (syncretic thinking). **Abstract thinking** is the last stage in the growth of the thought processes. This type of thinking appears from about 12 to 15 years of age.

third-degree heart block, dysrhythmia with the P wave having no relation to the QRS complex, due to a complete conduction block at the atrioventricular (AV) node. The atria and ventricles operate independently of each other via separate pacemaker sites. This AV dissociation diminishes the amount of blood pumped by the heart. The patient is usually symptomatic. Also known as **complete heart block, third-degree AV block.**

third stage of labor, from delivery of the infant to delivery of the placenta.

third ventricle, the fluid-filled space located between the halves of the thalamus in the center of the diencephalon.

thirst, a perceived desire for water or other fluid. The sensation of thirst is usually referred to the mouth and throat.

Thomas traction splint (Hugh Owen Thomas, British surgeon, 1834-1891). See **splint.**

Thompson carrier. See **rigid transport vehicle.**

thoracentesis, surgical puncture of the chest wall, usually with a large-bore needle, to allow removal of fluids. Also known as **thoracocentesis.**

thoracic /thôras´ik/, referring to the chest (thorax).

thoracic duct, a common trunk of many lymphatic vessels in the body. It begins superiorly in the abdomen, directed toward the second lumbar vertebra, enters the chest through the diaphragm, and extends into the neck. *See also lymphatic system.*

thoracic fistula, an opening in the chest wall that ends blindly or that communicates with the chest cavity.

thoracic medicine, the branch of medicine concerned with the diagnosis and treatment of disorders of the structures and organs of the chest, especially the lungs.

thoracic nerves, the 12 spinal nerves on each side of the thorax, including 11 intercostal nerves and one subcostal nerve. They are distributed mainly to the walls of the chest and abdomen. *See also autonomic nervous system.*

thoracic outlet syndrome, a type of nerve disorder, which causes an abnormal sensation of the fingers. It may be nerve root pressure from a vertebral disk or by pressure of the middle nerve in the carpal tunnel (carpal tunnel syndrome).

thoracic parietal node, one of the lymph glands in the chest. *See also lymphatic system, lymph node.*

thoracic vertebra. See **vertebra.**

thoracic visceral node, one of the lymph glands connected to the part of the lymphatic system that serves certain structures within the thorax, such as the pericardium, esophagus, lungs, and bronchi. *See also lymphatic system, lymph node.*

thoracocentesis. See **thoracentesis.**

thoracostomy /-kos´-/, surgical incision into the chest wall to provide an opening for drainage.

thoracotomy /-kot´-/, an incision into the chest cavity.

thorax, the chest area, with the bone and cartilage containing the principal organs of respiration and circulation and covering part of the abdominal organs. The thorax of women has less capacity and more movable upper ribs than that of men. Also known as **chest.**

thoroughfare channel, a route for blood through the capillary bed, which connects an arteriole with a venule.

threatened abortion, preterm uterine bleeding in an intrauterine pregnancy, when the cervical os is still closed. This may progress to an abortion or stabilize and allow a term delivery.

three-second rule, method of determining safe following distance when driving a vehicle larger than a car. Pick a spot that the vehicle in front just passed, and drive at a speed that will allow reaching that spot in no less than three seconds. *See also braking distance, following distance.*

threonine /thrē´ōnin/, an essential amino acid needed for proper growth in infants and for keeping the nitrogen balance in adults. *See also amino acid, protein.*

threshold, the point at which a stimulus is great enough to create an effect. For example, a pain threshold is the point at which a person first becomes aware of pain.

threshold limit value, the maximum concentration of a chemical to which workers can be exposed for a fixed period, such as 8 hours per day, without developing a health problem.

threshold limit value/ceiling, the maximum exposure to a toxin that should not be exceeded, even instantaneously.

threshold limit value/short term exposure limit (TLV/STEL), minute time-weighted average exposure that should not be exceeded at any time, nor repeatedly more than four times daily with a 60-minute rest period required between each STEL exposure. These short-term exposures can be tolerated without suffering from chronic or irreversible tissue damage, or narcosis of a sufficient degree to increase the likelihood of accidental injury, impair self-rescue, or reduce worker efficiency. TLV/STELs are expressed in ppm and mg/cu meter.

threshold limit value/time weighted average (TLV/TWA), the maximum airborne concentration of a material to which an average, healthy person may be exposed repeatedly for 8 hours each day, 40 hours per week without suffering adverse effects. Because TLVs involve an 8-hour exposure, they are difficult to adapt for emergency response operations. TLV/TWAs are expressed in ppm and mg/cu meter. (The lower the concentration, the more toxic the substance.)

threshold potential, the value reached as a result of cell depolarization, where an action potential is produced.

thrill, a vibration accompanying a cardiac or vascular murmur that can be palpated. *See also bruit, murmur.*

throat. See **pharnyx.**

throb, a deep, pulsating kind of discomfort or pain.

thrombectomy /thrombek´-/, the surgical removal of a thrombus from a blood vessel. Compare **embolectomy.**

thrombin /throm´bin/, an enzyme formed in blood during the clotting process from prothrombin, calcium, and thromboplastin. Thrombin causes fibrinogen to change to fibrin, essential in the formation of a clot. *See also blood clot, thrombus.*

thrombocytes, cell fragments.

thrombocytopenia /-sī´təpē´nē·ə/, a condition in which the number of platelets is reduced usually caused by breakdown of tissue in bone marrow. Thrombocytopenia is the most common cause of bleeding disorders.

thrombocytopenic purpura, a bleeding disorder marked by a decrease in the number of platelets. This results in petechiae and bleeding into the tissues. It may occur secondary to a number of causes, including infection, allergy, and poisoning. It is considered to be an immune response against one's own body tissues (autoimmunity).

thrombocytosis /-sītō´-/, an increase in the number of platelets in the blood. **Benign thrombocytosis,** or **secondary thrombocytosis,** has no specific symptoms. It usually occurs after splenectomy, hemolytic anemia, bleeding, or iron deficiency. Compare **thrombocytopenia.**

thromboembolism /-em´bōlizm/, a condition in which a blood vessel is blocked by an embolus. The area supplied by a blocked artery may tingle and become cyanotic. A thromboembolism in the vascular system of the lungs causes sharp chest pain, dyspnea, cough, fever, and hemoptysis.

thrombogenesis, formation of a clot.

thrombolytic agent, a drug that dissolves blood clots, usually via the breakdown of fibrin.

thrombolphelebitis /-fləbī´-/. See **phlebitis.**

thromboplastin, a complex substance that starts the clotting process by changing prothrombin to thrombin in the presence of calcium. It is found in most tissue cells and, in somewhat different form, in red and white blood cells. *See also blood clotting.*

thrombosis /thrombō´-/, *pl.* **thromboses,** condition in which a clot develops within a blood vessel. **Cerebral thrombosis** refers to a clot in any cerebral blood vessel. A **coronary thrombosis** blocks a coronary artery, causing myocardial infarction. *See also blood clotting, cavernous sinus syndrome.*

thrombus /throm´bəs/, *pl.* **thrombi,** a cluster of platelets, fibrin, clotting factors, and other cell elements of the blood attached to the interior wall of a vein or artery. Also known as **blood clot.** Compare **embolus.**

throw bag, a rope storage bag. When the bag is used as a rope carrier, the length of rope is coiled freely into the bag. When thrown, the free end of the line or rope is held in one hand, as the remaining rope feeds out due to momentum. Also known as **stuff bag.**

thrush, infection of the tissues of the mouth from a fungus.

thumb, the first digit of the hand. It is classified by some anatomists as one of the fingers. Other anatomists classify the thumb separately, regarding it as composed of one metacarpal bone and only two phalanges, while the fingers have three phalanges.

thymectomy, surgical removal of the thymus.

thymic /thī´mik/, referring to the thymus gland.

thymoma /thīmō´mə/, a usually benign tumor of the thymus gland, linked to myasthenia gravis or an immune deficiency disorder.

thymosin /thī´məsin/, **1.** a naturally occurring hormone released by the thymus gland. It is present in greatest amounts in young children and lessens in amount throughout life. **2.** an experimental drug derived from bovine thymus extracts. It is given as a drug that changes resistance to certain diseases.

thymus /thī´məs/,   a single, unpaired gland that is located in the superior thoracic cavity extending upwards into the neck to the lower edge of the thyroid gland. The thymus is the primary gland of the lymphatic system. The endocrine activity of the thymus is believed to depend on the hormone thymosin. This hormone is critical to the immune system. The size of the organ relative to the rest of the body is largest when the individual is about 2 years of age. The thymus usually attains its greatest absolute size at puberty. After puberty, the organ shrivels as fatty tissue replaces the receding thymic tissue. With aging, the gland may change in color from pinkish-gray to yellow. In the elderly individual it may appear as small islands of thymic tissue covered with fat. Compare **spleen.**

thyrocervical trunk /thī´rōsur´vikəl/,   one of a pair of short, thick arteries supplying muscles and bones in the head, neck, and back.

thyroid. See **thyroid gland, thyroid hormone.**

thyroid cartilage,   the largest cartilage of the larynx. It is made up of two thin flat plates fused together at an acute angle in the midline neck to form the larynx.

thyroidectomy /thī´roidek´-/,   the surgical removal of the thyroid gland.

thyroid gland,   an organ in the anterior neck. The thyroid gland is slightly heavier in women than in men. It becomes larger during pregnancy. The thyroid gland releases the hormone thyroxin directly into the blood. It is essential to normal body growth in infancy and childhood. Its removal may cause lowered bodily activity. The thyroid needs iodine to make thyroxine. Compare **parathyroid gland.**

thyroid hormone,   an iodine-containing compound released by the thyroid gland, mainly as thyroxine and in smaller amounts the four times more potent triiodothyronine. These hormones affect body temperature, regulate protein, fat, and carbohydrate catabolism in all cells. They keep up growth hormone release, skeletal maturation, and the heart rate, force, and output. They promote central nervous system growth, stimulate the making of many enzymes, and are necessary for muscle tone and vigor.

thyroiditis /thī´roidī´-/,   inflammation of the thyroid gland. **Fibrous thyroiditis** (Riedel's struma) is a disorder in which dense fiberlike tissue replaces normal thyroid tissue. It usually occurs in one lobe of the gland but sometimes in both lobes, the trachea, and surrounding muscles, nerves, and blood vessels. **Lymphocytic thyroiditis** (Hashimoto's disease) is a disorder of the immune system that attacks the thyroid gland. The disease seems to be inherited, but it is 20 times more common in women than in men. It occurs most often between 30 and 50 years of age but may arise in young children. The thyroid develops a goiter which can cause difficulty swallowing.

thyroid membrane,   the membrane joining the hyoid bone and the thyroid cartilages.

thyroid storm,   a crisis of uncontrolled hyperthyroidism caused by the release of large amounts of thyroid hormone. Symptoms include fever that may reach 106° F (41.1° C), tachycardia, dyspnea, restlessness, irritability, and exhaustion.

thyroid-stimulating hormone,   a substance released by the front lobe of the pituitary gland. It controls the release of thyroid hormone and is necessary for the growth and function of the thyroid gland. Also known as **rotropin.** *See also thyroid hormone.*

thyrotropin-releasing hormone,   a substance of the hypothalamus that stimulates the release of thyrotropin (thyroid-stimulating hormone) from the anterior pituitary gland.

tibia /tib´ē·ə/,   the second longest bone of the skeleton, located in the lower leg. It joins with the fibula and the femur, forming the knee joint. Also known as **shin bone.**

tibialis anterior /tib´ē·ā·lis/,   one of the lateral muscles of the lower leg.

tibial torsion,   a twisting style rotation of the tibia on its longitudinal axis.

tibial tuberosity,   the elevation at the proximal end of the tibia to which the ligament of the patella attaches.

tic,   unwilled movements of a small muscle group, as of the face. The movements are often caused by emotions rather than any physical disorder. A tic may be made worse by stress or anxiety.

tic douloureux /tēk dooloorœ´/. See **trigeminal neuralgia.**

tick, an arthropod of the class *Arachnida,* which is a major carrier of human disease in rural and wilderness areas. These blood-sucking parasites are divided into three families: the *Ixodidae* (hard-shell ticks), the *Argasidae* (soft-shell ticks), and the *Nuttalliellidae.* Ticks are vectors for such human afflictions as Lyme disease, Q fever, relapsing fever, the spotted fevers, and typhus.

tidal volume, the amount of air inhaled or exhaled in a single resting breath.

tide, an increase or decrease in the concentration of a particular component of body fluids, such as acid tide or fat tide.

tiered response, an emergency medical response system utilizing more than one vehicle and more than one level of training on each emergency response. An advanced life support unit located close to the call can be dispatched to assist a basic support unit or first responder.

Tietze's syndrome (Alexander Tietze, German surgeon, 1864-1927), inflammation of one or more rib cartilages (thorax). The chest pain caused may resemble that of myocardial infarction. Although the inflammation may be due to vigorous activity, its true etiology is unknown.

tight sheeting. See **solid sheeting.**

tilt test. See **orthostatic vital signs.**

timberline, the elevation or line on mountains and in arctic regions above which trees do not grow. Also known as **treeline.**

time of useful consciousness, the time that elapses from exposure to an oxygen-deficient environment until the point where loss of the ability to deliberately function occurs.

tinea /tin´ē·ə/, a group of fungal skin diseases, caused by several kinds of parasitical fungi. They cause itching, scaling, and painful sores. *See also athlete's foot, jock itch, ringworm.*

tinnitus /tinī´təs/, tinkling or ringing heard in one or both ears.

tissue, a collection of similar cells that act together in performing a particular function.

tissue binding, drug pooling in adipose tissue and bone.

tissue plasminogen activator, a clot-dissolving substance produced naturally by cells in the walls of blood vessels. It is used to remove clots blocking coronary arteries. Also known as **TPA.**

tissue response, any reaction or change in living cell tissue when it is acted on by disease, toxin, or other outer stimulus. Some kinds of tissue responses are **immune response, inflammation, necrosis.**

tissue typing, a series of tests to evaluate whether tissues of a donor and a recipient are compatible. It is done before a transplant by identifying and comparing a large series of human leukocyte antigens in the cells of the body. *See also human leukocyte antigen, immune system, transplant.*

titanium, a grayish, brittle, metallic element. Titanium dioxide is the active part in a number of skin ointments and lotions.

titer /tī´tər/, **1.** a measurement of the concentration of a substance in a solution. **2.** the quantity of a substance needed to obtain a reaction with another substance.

titubation /tich´əbā´shən/, unsteady posture with a staggering or stumbling style of walking. It may be caused by cerebral disease. Compare **ataxia.**

T lymphocyte, the lymphocyte produced in the thymus that is responsible for cell-mediated immunity.

toboggan, a long, narrow sled that curves upward at the front and is used for transport or travel on ice or snow.

Tobruk splint /tō´brook/, *(historical)* a Thomas full-ring traction splint that was applied to the affected leg and then immobilized with plaster of Paris casting material. First used during World War II, it was developed to immobilize the limb during hazardous movement, as movement from small to large boats. Named after the town in Libya where it was first used by the British.

tocodynamometer /tō´kōdī´nəmom´ətər/, an electronic device for monitoring and recording contractions of the uterus in labor.

tocolytic drug /tō´kōlit´ik/, any agent used to suppress premature labor.

tocopherol. See **vitamin E.**

toddler, a child between 12 and 36 months of age.

Todd's paralysis (Robert B. Todd, British physician, 1809-1860), a temporary paralysis involving one or more limbs, seen infrequently after seizures, particularly jacksonian seizures. Usually seen as a hemiplegia, it may mimic cerebral vascular accident or a transient ischemic attack, but it is preceded by seizure and is reversed with time.

toe, any one of the digits of the feet.

toenail, one of the heavy nail structures covering the end bones of the toes.

togaviruses /tō´gə-/, a family of viruses that includes organisms causing encephalitis, dengue, yellow fever, and rubella.

tolerance, the ability to live through hardship, pain, or ordinarily injurious substances, such as drugs, without apparent physical or mental injury.

tomography /təmog´rəfē/, an x-ray method that creates a film representing a detailed cross section of tissue structure at a predetermined depth. It is a valuable diagnostic tool for space-occupying tumors, as might be found in the brain, liver, pancreas, and gallbladder.

tone, an audio signal of controlled amplitude and frequency, used to alert or selectively activate a receiver, such as a pager.

tongue, the main organ for the sense of taste. It also assists in the chewing and swallowing of food. It is located in the floor of the mouth within the curve of the mandible. The anterior two thirds of the tongue are covered with small protrusions. The posterior third is smoother and has numerous mucous glands and lymph follicles. The use of the tongue as an organ of speech is a learned behavior. Also known as **lingua.**

tongues, waves formed by water flowing over obstacles that meet to form a V. These waves identify the beginning of most rapids, the largest of which can identify the safest point of entry into those rapids. *See also hydraulic, standing waves, rapids.*

tonicity /tōnis´itē/, the quality of possessing muscle tone or tonus.

tonic neck reflex /ton´ik/, a normal response in newborns to extend the arm and the leg on the side of the body to which the head is quickly turned while the infant is lying supine and to flex the limbs of the opposite side. The reflex prevents the infant from rolling over.

tonofibril /ton´əfī´bril/, a bundle of fine fibers found in the cytoplasm of epithelial cells.

tonometer /tōnom´ətər/, an instrument used in measuring tension or pressure, especially within the eye.

tonsil, a small, rounded mass of lymphoidal tissue. **Lingual tonsil** refers to a mass of small lymph nodes (nodules) that form part of the mucous membrane near the root of the tongue. The lingual tonsil is part of the body's defense system against infection. The **palatine tonsils** are a pair of almond-shaped masses of lymphoidal tissue on either side of the palatine arches. *See also adenoid.*

tonsillectomy /-ek´-/, the surgical removal of the palatine tonsils.

tonsillitis, an infection or inflammation of a tonsil, often caused by a streptococcal infection. Symptoms include sore throat, fever, headache, malaise, dysphagia, and large, tender lymph nodes in the neck. A **peritonsillar abscess,** also called **quinsy,** is an infection of tissue between the tonsil and throat, occurring most often after tonsillitis.

tonus /tō´nəs/, the normal state of balanced tension in the tissues of the body, especially the muscles. Tonus is essential from many normal body functions. For example, holding the spine erect, the eyes open, and the mandible closed. Also known as **tone.**

tooth, *pl.* **teeth,** one of numerous dental structures that develop in the jaws as part of the digestive system. They are used to cut, grind, and process food in the mouth for ingestion. Each tooth is made up of a crown above the gum; two to four roots in the sockets; and a neck, stretching between the crown and the root. Each tooth also has a cavity filled with pulp, richly supplied with blood vessels and nerves that enter the cavity through a small opening at the base of each root. The solid portion of the tooth consists of dentin, enamel, and a thin layer of bone on the surface of the root. The dentin comprises the bulk of the tooth. The enamel covers the exposed portion of the crown. A **deciduous tooth** is any of the 20 teeth that appear normally during infancy, often called baby teeth. A **permanent tooth** is any of the 32 teeth that appear during childhood and early adulthood. An **accessory tooth** is an extra one that does not look like a normal tooth in size, shape, or position. *See also dentition.*

tophus /tō´fəs/, *pl.* **tophi,** a stone (urate deposit) that forms in a joint, particularly in persons with gout.

topical /top´ikəl/, **1.** the surface of a part. **2.** a drug or treatment applied to the skin.

topographic map, a flat-surfaced, small-scale representation of part of the earth's surface that portrays landforms and terrain in a measurable form. The horizontal position of these features are shown as they are, and the vertical positions (relief) are represented by contour lines. The contours and elevation are usually measured from sea level. Also known as **relief map.**

tornado, a severe local storm, with winds up to 300 miles per hour, that concentrates its energy in a revolving vortex stretching from cloud to ground. This vortex is capable of destroying all that it touches, such as cars, houses, trees. The Fujita scale is used to measure the severity of a tornado by the amount of damage it causes (1 is minimal, 5 is catastrophic). *See also severe local storm.*

torque /tôrk/, a twisting force.

torr (Evangelista Torricelli, Italian physicist, 1608-1647), a unit of atmospheric pressure where 1 torr equals 1/760 millimeter of mercury.

torsades de pointes /tōrsäd´ də pwänt´/, bidirectional ventricular tachycardia. This dysrhythmia is often refractory to conventional treatments for ventricular tachycardia. Translated as "twisting of the points," it appears on EKG as ventricular tachycardia with bow-tie spiraling of complexes (QRS complexes varying between groups of positive and groups of negative deflections with a narrow waist between the series). These complexes have a varying R wave structure, which may frustrate the synchronizing capability of standard defibrillators. There is often an underlying electrolyte, metabolic, or pharmacological abnormality. *See also ventricular tachycardia.*

torsion /tôr´shən/, **1.** the process of twisting in a positive (clockwise) or negative (counterclockwise) direction. **2.** the state of being turned.

torticollis, unilateral neck pain and/or stiffness due to neck muscle spasm. Episodes of spasm (clonic) can occur due to infection, poor or uncomfortable sleeping positions, scars, or tumors. Often, no cause is apparent. Permanent (tonic) stiffness may occur in cases of spinal disease. Also known as **wryneck.**

torulopsosis /tôr´yəlop´səsis/, an infection with the yeast *Torulopsis glabrata.* This yeast is normally found in the throat, the intestinal and stomach tract, and the skin. However, it causes disease in severely weakened patients or in those who are immunosuppressed.

total body radiation, radiation that exposes the entire body so that, theoretically, all cells in the body receive the same radiation.

total body water, all the water within the body, including water in tissue cells as well as blood and lymph, plus the water in the stomach, intestines, and urinary tract.

total lung capacity, the volume of air in the lungs at the end of maximal inspiration.

total nitrogen, the nitrogen content of the feces. It is measured to detect various disorders, improper functioning of the pancreas, and blocked protein digestion.

total pressure, the combination of pressures exerted by all the gases in a mixture.

total renal blood flow, the total volume of blood that flows through the renal arteries. The average in a normal adults is 1200 ml per minute.

touch, **1.** the ability to feel objects; the tactile sense. **2.** the ability to note pressure when it is put on the skin or the mucosa of the body. **3.** to examine with the hand.

Tourette's syndrome. See **Gilles de la Tourette syndrome.**

tourniquet, **1.** a cloth or strap that, when tightened, stops circulation (therefore hemorrhage) in an extremity. This device should be used only when all other techniques for controlling hemorrhage fail. **2.** *(informal)* a constricting band, used to restrict venous or lymphatic flow for purposes of obtaining blood samples, starting an intravenous infusion, or restricting the flow of venom from an extremity into the central circulation.

toxemia, bodywide distribution of bacterial toxins from a specific site. This term is most often associated with toxemias of pregnancy. *See also eclampsia, preeclampsia, septicemia, shock.*

toxemias of pregnancy. See **preeclampsia, eclampsia.**

toxic, deadly; destructive; harmful; severe.

toxic atmosphere, any area, inside or outside a structure, where the air contains substances harmful to human life or health.

toxic dose, the amount of a substance that may be expected to produce a poisonous effect. A **median toxic dose** is the dose of a drug that causes side effects in one half of the patients to whom it is given.

toxic goiter. See **Graves' disease.**

toxicity /toksis´itē/, **1.** the degree to which something is poisonous. **2.** a condition that results from exposure to a poison or to poisonous amounts of a substance that does not cause side effects in smaller amounts.

toxicity signal words, indicates the relative degree of acute toxicity of a hazardous material. Located in the center of the front label panel of a container label, it is one of the most important label markings. The three toxic categories are high, moderate, and low toxicity.

toxic level, the concentration of a drug at which adverse side effects are likely to occur.

toxic nodular goiter. See **goiter.**

toxicokinetics /tok´sikōkinet´-/, the passage through the body of a poisonous substance or its products.

toxicologist /-kol´-/, a specialist in the scientific study of poisons and the diseases they bring about (toxicology).

toxicology /-kol´-/, the scientific study of poisons, their detection, their effects, and methods of treatment for conditions they produce. **–toxicologic, toxicological,** *adj.*

toxic products of combustion. See **products of combustion.**

toxic shock syndrome, hypotension due to vaginal growth of strains of *Staphylococcus aureus* bacteria. Associated with menstruation and tampon use, symptoms include elevated temperature, headache, joint pain, and urticaria. Also known as **TSS.**

toxin, a poisonous substance that, when produced naturally, occurs due to bacterial growth or as a by-product of metabolism. In animals, these substances are categorized as being crino-

toxins, as in jellyfish; oral toxins (botulism); and parenteral toxins (snakebite). Whether produced by plants or animals, all toxins are either poison or venoms.

toxoid, a toxin that has been treated with chemicals or with heat to lessen its poisonous effect but keeps its power to stimulate antibody formation. It is given to make immunity by stimulating the creation of antibodies. *See also toxin, vaccine.*

Toxoplasma /-plaz´mə/, a genus of protozoa with only one known species, *Toxoplasma gondii.* It is a parasite of cats and other hosts and causes toxoplasmosis in humans.

toxoplasmosis /-plazmō´-/, infection with the protozoan parasite *Toxoplasma gondii.* When transmitted to the fetus through the placenta, there are cerebral calcification, seizures, blindness, microcephaly, hydrocephaly, and retardation. Symptoms of an acquired form include rash, lymphadenopathy, fever, central nervous system disorders, and inflammation of the heart and lung. It may be acquired by eating inadequately cooked meat containing the parasite.

trabecula carnea /trəbek´yələ/, *pl.* **trabeculae carneae,** any one of the irregular bands and bundles of muscles that project from the inner surfaces of the cardiac ventricles. Some of these trabeculae are ridges of muscle along the ventricular walls. Compare **chordae tendineae.** *See also heart, ventricle.*

trace element, an element needed in tiny amounts for nutrition or mental processes.

tracer, a radioactive isotope that is used in diagnostic x-ray techniques to allow a biologic process to be seen.

trachea /trā´kē·ə/, a cylindrical tube extending from the larynx to the carina, through which air moves to the lungs. It is overlaid by the thyroid glands and various other structures.

tracheal stenosis, constriction of the trachea.

tracheitis /trā´kē·ī´-/, inflammation of the trachea.

tracheobronchitis /trā´kē·ōbrongkī´-/, inflammation of the trachea and bronchi.

tracheostomy /trā´kē·os´-/, a surgical opening into the trachea through which a tube may be inserted to allow unobstructed ventilations.

trachoma /trəkō´mə/, a chronic infectious disease of the eye, caused by the bacterium *Chlamydia trachomatis*. Trachoma is a significant cause of blindness.

tracking, the following of signs, such as clothing, damaged vegetation, and prints, to locate an animal or person. *See also sign cutting.*

tracking dog, a type of search dog that follows a scent on the ground, from a person's footsteps, in an effort to locate him or her. Prevailing wind has little effect on such dogs, and they closely follow the trail that the person has left. *See also scent dog, trailing dog.*

track trap, search areas that provide—due to their constricted or narrow nature (path along a canyon wall) or obvious ease of movement (trail through thick underbrush)—a location for hasty teams or other searches to look for clues (footprints) of lost subjects. *See also attraction.*

tract, a long group of tissues and structures that function together as a pathway, as the digestive tract.

tractor plow, any tracked vehicle with a plow.

trade name, any commercial or copyrighted name, as that of a drug. The commercial name is designated by the drug company that sells the drug. Also known as **brand name, proprietary name, trademark.** *See also generic name.*

tragsitz. See **soft transport vehicle.**

tragus, the projection at the opening of the external ear.

trailing dog, a type of search dog that follows a scent that has fallen onto the ground from the person being sought. This type of dog can follow the scent at a distance from the subject's actual path, but is more affected by the wind than is a tracking dog. *See also scent dog, tracking dog.*

trailing edge, the rear edge of an airfoil, such as a wing, propeller, tail surface. *See also leading edge.*

trait, **1.** a mode of behavior or any mannerism or physical feature that separates one individual or culture from another. **2.** any quality or condition that is inborn. *See also dominance, gene, Mendel's law, recessive.*

trance, **1.** a sleeplike state marked by the complete or partial loss of consciousness and the

loss or lack of muscle movement, as seen in hypnosis. **2.** a dazed or confused condition; stupor.

transcutaneous pacing, initiating a rhythmic electrical impulse through the chest wall when the natural pacemaker of the heart ceases to function properly. The artificial pacemaker is used in cases of asystole, heart block, symptomatic bradycardia, and torsade de pointes. Also known as **pacing, TCP.**

transdermal delivery system /-dur´məl/, applying a drug to unbroken skin. The drug is absorbed through the skin and enters the blood system. It is used to deliver nitroglycerin and scopolamine.

transect, to sever or cut across, as in doing a cross section of tissue.

transference /trans´fərəns, transfur´əns/, **1.** shifting symptoms from one part of the body to another, as occurs in conversion disorder. **2.** a way of shifting feelings that are linked to earlier events or people in one's life to others.

transferrin /transfer´in/, a protein in the blood that is needed to move iron from one place in the body to another.

transfusion. See **blood transfusion.**

transient dysphagia, temporary impairment of swallowing.

transient ischemic attack /tran´shənt/, a temporary cerebrovascular accident caused by a transient blockage of a cerebral blood vessel. The symptoms depend on where and how much of the brain is affected. The episode is most often brief, lasting a few minutes; rarely, symptoms continue for several hours. Also known as **TIA.** *See also cerebrovascular accident, ischemia.*

transillumination, shining a light through body tissue to look at its structure.

translational lift, the lift that develops in a helicopter as a result of forward to backward airflow over the main rotor blades. This lift is much more effective than that obtained in a vertical climb and occurs when the helicopter can first develop forward movement, while in ground effect. *See also ground effect.*

transmission, the transfer or carrying of a thing or condition, as a signal from the brain or an inherited trait, from one person or place to another.

transmural infarction, a myocardial infarction that has extended through the epicardium, endocardium, and myocardium. Also known as **subendocardial infarction.**

transom, the horizontal panel in the stern of a boat.

transplacental /-pləsen´təl/, across or through the placenta, especially referring to the exchange of nutrients, waste products, and other material between the growing fetus and the mother.

transplant, **1.** to transfer an organ or tissue from one person to another or from one body part to another in order to replace a diseased structure, to restore function, or to change appearance. **2.** a tissue or organ that is transplanted, or the patient who receives the donated tissue or organ. *See also corneal grafting, skin graft.*

transponder, signaling device, in an aircraft or satellite, that responds with identifiable information after receiving a designated signal.

transportation officer, an officer in the incident command system responsible for the operation of the transportation sector during a multiple casualty incident.

transportation sector, the section of the incident command system responsible for coordinating all patient transportation and destinations during a multiple (or mass) casualty incident.

transport index, the number placed on a radioactive materials package label that is indicative of the control required during transport. The transport index is the radiation level, in millirems per hour, at 3 feet from accessible external package surface or, for fissile class II packages, an assigned value based on criticality safety requirements for the package contents.

transposition, **1.** an abnormality occurring during growth in the womb in which a part of the body normally on the left is found on the right or vice versa. **2.** the shifting of genetic material from one chromosome to another at some point in the reproductive process, often resulting in a birth defect.

transposition of the great vessels, a birth defect in which the pulmonary artery arises from the left ventricle and the aorta from the right ventricle, the opposite of the normal positions. Signs of congestive heart failure develop rapidly, especially in infants with large ventricular defects. *See also tetralogy of Fallot.*

transthoracic resistance, the natural impediment of electrical flow through the chest, due to resistance of bone and skin. During defibrillation, this resistance can diminish the amount of current delivered to the heart.

transtracheal jet ventilation. See **jet insufflation.**

transudate /tran´sōōdāt/, fluid passed through a membrane or squeezed through a tissue or into the space between the cells of a tissue. It is thin and watery and contains few blood cells or other large proteins. *See also edema.*

transverse, at right angles to the long part of an object, as the planes that cut the long part of the body into upper and lower portions.

transverse colon, the portion of the large intestine that extends across the midabdomen and joins the ascending colon on the right and descending colon on the left.

transverse fissure, a crack dividing two surfaces of the brain.

transverse mesocolon, a broad fold of the bowel connecting the large intestine (transverse colon) to the wall of the abdomen. *See also colon.*

transverse plane, an anatomical view that divides the body into inferior and superior portions. This allows downward or upward views of body structures. Also known as **horizontal plane.**

transverse presentation. See **shoulder presentation.**

transverse process, the bony segment that extends laterally from each vertebra of the spine.

trapezius /trəpē´zē·əs/, a large flat triangular muscle of the shoulder and upper back. It raises the shoulder, and flexes the arm.

trapezoid bone /trap´əzoid/, the smallest wrist bone.

trauma /trou´mə, trô´mə/, **1.** physical injury caused by violent or disruptive action, or by a poisonous substance. **2.** mental or emotional injury. **–traumatic,** *adj.,* **traumatize,** *v.*

trauma center, a hospital equipped with the resources necessary to care for multitrauma victims from admission to discharge. All specialties of medicine must be accessible in a short period of time.

Trauma score, a scale for calculating injury severity in patients with blunt or penetrating trauma. This number is then used to determine transport destination and predict the patient's outcome. The score tabulates five categories for a number between 1 and 16. The lower the score, the higher the mortality. The five categories include systolic blood pressure, respiratory rate, respiratory expansion, capillary refill, and the Glasgow coma scale. *See also Glasgow coma scale, revised trauma score.*

traumatic anesthesia, absence of sensation in a part of the body, caused by injury.

traumatic iridoplegia, constriction or dilation of the pupil due to trauma.

travail /trəvāl´/, physical or mental effort, especially when it causes distress.

traveler's diarrhea, any of several diarrheal disorders commonly seen in people visiting regions of the world other than their own. Some strains of *Escherichia coli,* which produce a poison enzyme (exotoxin), are the common cause. Other organisms that cause the condition include *Giardia lamblia* and species of *Salmonella* and *Shigella.* Symptoms last for a few days and include abdominal and intestinal cramps, nausea, vomiting, fever, and watery stools.

Treacher Collins' syndrome, an inherited disorder marked by an incomplete head and facial defect (mandibulofacial dysostosis).

treatment, **1.** the care and assistance necessary to return a patient to health. **2.** a method of fighting, reducing, or preventing disease or injury. **Active** or **curative** treatment is designed to cure. **Causal** treatment focuses on the cause of a disorder. **Conservative** treatment avoids drastic measures and procedures. **Definitive** treatment refers to any that is generally accepted as the specific cure of a disease. **Empiric** treatment employs methods shown to work by experience. **Expectant** treatment relieves symptoms as they arise in the course of a disease, rather than treat-

ing the cause of the illness itself, as amputating a leg with gangrene in a patient with diabetes. **Palliative** treatment is directed to ease pain and distress, but not to cure. **Preventive** treatment is designed to keep a disease from occurring or mild disorder from getting more severe. **Prophylactic** treatment is for the prevention of a disease or disorder. **Rational** treatment is based on a knowledge of a disease process and the action of the measures used.

treatment officer, the person in the incident command system responsible for the operation of the treatment sector during a multiple casualty incident.

treatment protocols, guidelines for emergency medical practitioners, operating under the authority of a physician, which define their method of intervention and scope of care. *See also off-line medical control, on-line medical control.*

treatment sector, the section of the incident command system responsible, during a multiple casualty incident, for collecting and treating patients in a central treatment area(s).

Trechona /trikō´nə/, a genus of spiders, family Dipluridae, the bite of which is poisonous to humans.

tree belay /bilā´/, a simple belay utilizing several turns of rope around a large bush or tree. This belay provides enough friction to move equipment, rigid transport devices, or sleds up or down a slope.

trematode /trem´ətōd/. See **fluke.**

tremor /trem´ər, trē´mər/, rhythmic, quivering movements with no purpose caused by uncontrolled tightening and relaxing of groups of voluntary muscles attached to the skeleton. This disorder occurs in older patients, in certain families, and in patients with different nerve disorders.

tremulous /trem´yələs/, referring to tremors or uncontrolled muscular contractions.

trench, a temporary excavation in the ground, where the length of the bottom exceeds the width of the bottom. Generally, they are less than 20 feet deep and 15 feet wide at the bottom.

trench box, a structure placed in a trench to provide protection from trench collapse. This box, made of aluminum, fiberglass, or steel, is moved as work progresses.

trench fever,   an infection caused by *Rochalimaea quintana,* an organism in the Rickettsia group of microorganisms, carried by body lice. Symptoms include fever, leg pain, urticaria, and weakness.

trench foot.   See **immersion foot.**

trench lip,   the edge of a trench.

trench mouth.   See **gingivitis.**

Trendelenburg position (Friedrich Trendelenburg, German surgeon, 1844-1925),   elevation of the legs at a 45° angle while keeping the head lower than the hips and legs. This position is thought to improve circulation during hypovolemic states. Also known as **shock position.**

treponematosis /trep´ənē´mətō´-/,   any disease caused by spirochetes of the genus *Treponema,* such as syphilis, yaws.

trepopnea,   assuming a certain position to decrease shortness of breath.

triage,   the process of sorting sick or injured victims based on their urgency and condition, so that appropriate stabilization, transport, and treatment occur. See Appendix 1-15.

triage area,   the site(s) located near the incident to which injured victims are moved, prioritized, and stabilized prior to their movement to the treatment and/or transportation area(s).

triage officer,   the officer in the incident command system that is responsible, when handling casualties, for the operation of the triage sector.

triage sector,   the portion of the incident command system responsible for triage of all patients involved in a multiple casualty situation.

triage tag,   a preprinted form, attached to patients in multiple casualty situations, that allows triage categories and medical assessment and treatment information to be documented.

triage team,   a group of up to five members who have common communications, similar resources, and a designated person in charge.

triangular bandage,   muslin cloth material, cut or folded into a triangular shape. Used as a bandage, dressing, sling, splinting adjunct, restraint, and a multipurpose survival tool, it is one of the oldest and most versatile emergency medical devices.

triangular bone,   a wrist bone.

triaxial reference system,   the three intersecting lines of electrical reference used to define EKG configuration of the three standard limb leads, I, II, and III.

tributary,   a small river or stream that flows into a large body of water.

triceps brachii /trī´seps brak´ē·ī/,   a large muscle that extends along the length of the posterior upper arm. It extends the forearm and moves the arm toward the body.

triceps reflex.   See **deep tendon reflex.**

triceps surae limp,   abnormal walking, connected to a weakness in the triceps surae. The weakness keeps the triceps surae from raising the pelvis and carrying it forward while walking. As a result, the pelvis sags below its normal level and lags behind in the walking movement.

trichinosis /trik´inō´-/,   an infection caused by the parasitic roundworm *Trichinella spiralis,* acquired by eating raw or undercooked pork or bear meat. Early symptoms of infection include abdominal pain, nausea, fever, and fatigue.

trichologia /-lō´jē·ə/,   condition in which a person pulls out his or her own hair, usually seen only in a state of delirium.

trichomoniasis /-mənī´əsis/,   a vaginal infection caused by the microorganism *Trichomonas vaginalis,* marked by itching, burning, and vaginal discharge.

Trichophyton /trikof´iton/,   a genus of fungi that infects skin, hair, and nails. *See also dermatomycosis.*

trichostrongyliasis /-stron´jəlī´əsis/,   a condition of begin infested with *Trichostrongylus,* a genus of roundworm. Also known as **trichostrongylosis.**

trichuriasis /trik´yŏŏrī´əsis/   See **whipworm infection.**

tricuspid /trīkus´pid/,   referring to three points, as tricuspid valve of the heart.

tricuspid atresia,   a cardiac birth defect with the absence of the tricuspid valve between the right atrium and the right ventricle. Symptoms include cyanosis, dyspnea, and signs of right-sided heart failure.

tricuspid valve, the valve located between the right atrium and right ventricle of the heart. *See also mitral valve.*

tricyclic, a chemical substance used in the treatment of depression. It blocks the body's use of an adrenal gland hormone, norepinephrine. Overingestion of the drug causes tachycardias that may be life-threatening.

trigeminal nerve /trījem´inəl/, either of the largest pair of cranial nerves, necessary for chewing and general control of the face. The trigeminal nerves have sensory, motor, and intermediate roots and connect the three areas in the brain. Also known as **fifth nerve, trifacial nerve.**

trigeminal neuralgia, a nervous disorder of the trigeminal facial nerve. Symptoms include spasms and stabbing pain moving along the course of a branch of the nerve from the angle of the jaw. It is caused by breakdown of the nerve or by pressure on it. Any of the three branches of the nerve may be affected. Also known as **tic douloureux** /tick´dŌŌlŌŌroe´/.

trigeminy /trīgem´ənē/, grouping in threes, as that of two ventricular ectopics followed or preceded by a normal complex.

triglyceride /trīglis´ərīd/, a compound made up of a fatty acid (oleic, palmitic, or stearic) and glycerol. Triglycerides make up most animal and vegetable fats and appear in the blood bound to a protein, forming high- and low-density lipoproteins. *See also lipoprotein.*

trigone /trī´gōn/, the triangular area at the base of the bladder between the ureters and the urethra.

trigonitis /trī´gənī´-, trig´-/, inflammation of the trigone. This often occurs with urethritis.

triiodothyronine, a hormone that helps control growth and development, the body's chemical processes, and body temperature. It is used to treat hypothyroidism and goiter. *See also thyroid hormone.*

trimester /trīmes´tər/, one of the three periods of roughly 3 months into which pregnancy is divided. The first trimester includes the time from the first day of the last menstrual period to the end of 12 weeks. The second trimester, close to 4 months in length, extends from the twelfth to the twenty-eighth week of pregnancy. The third trimester begins at the twenty-eighth week and extends to the time of childbirth.

triple jaw thrust. See **jaw thrust.**

triplet, any one of three offspring born of the same gestation period during a single pregnancy.

triploid. See **euploid.**

trismus /trīz´məs/, spasm of the muscles of the jaw. Also known as *(informal)* **lockjaw.** *See also tetanus.*

trisomy /trī´səmē/, a birth defect resulting from the presence of three copies of a particular chromosome, rather than the normal pair. This defect occurs in Down's syndrome.

TRISS methodology, a retrospective trauma scoring system that determines the probability of survival for the patient. This system ties together the patient's age (≤54 and >54), the **TR**auma score, and the **I**njury **S**everity **S**core.

trocar /trō´kär/, a sharp, pointed rod that fits inside a tube. It is used to pierce the skin and the wall of a cavity or canal to guide the placement of a catheter. *See also cannula.*

trochanter /trōkan´tər/, one of the two bony structures of the proxima thigh. It provides for the attachment of various muscles.

troche /trō´kē/, a small oval, round, or oblong tablet that has a drug mixed in a flavored, sweetened base that dissolves in the mouth, releasing the drug. Also known as **lozenge.**

trochlea, the distal medial aspect of the humerus, which articulates with the ulna.

trochlear nerve /trok´lē·ər/, either of the smallest pair of cranial nerves, necessary for ocular movement. The trochlear nerves branch to supply the superior oblique muscle and link to the ophthalmic division of the trigeminal nerve, connecting with the brain. Also known as **fourth cranial nerve.**

trochoid joint /trō´koid/. See **pivot joint.**

trophic action /trof´ik/, the beginning of cell reproduction and enlargement by nurturing and causing growth.

trophoblast /trof´əblast/, the layer of tissue that forms the wall of the early embryo (blastocyst) of mammals with placentas in the early stages of the growth of the embryo. –**trophoblastic,** *adj.*

tropical cyclone, large, rotating storms that form over tropical oceans. Storm characteristics include winds faster than 75 miles per hour, a storm surge that causes flooding in coastal areas, heavy rain, and storm durations of 1 to 2 weeks. Cyclones that form in the Atlantic, Caribbean, and eastern Pacific Oceans are known as **hurricanes.** Cyclones of the western Pacific are known as **typhoons,** whereas in the Indian Ocean they are known as **cyclones.** Cultural names categorize cyclones even further: in Haiti they are known as **tainos,** in Mexico as **cordonazos,** and as **baguios** in the Philippines. Tropical cyclones are one of the most destructive natural phenomena known. *See also Saffir-Simpson hurricane scale.*

tropical medicine, the branch of medicine that deals with the diagnosis and treatment of diseases commonly occurring in tropic and subtropic regions of the world.

tropical sprue. See **sprue.**

truck, a fire department vehicle equipped with a variety of ladders, lighting, and ventilation equipment. Although some vehicles may have a limited water-pumping capability, most do not. They are often equipped with large amounts of rescue equipment, such as hydraulic rescue tools, litters, ropes. Also known as **ladder truck.** *See also engine, truck company.*

truck company, a truck and two to four assigned firefighting personnel. This unit's primary responsibilities include overhaul, rescue, and salvage. Also known as **ladder company.** *See also engine company, truck.*

true emergency, any situation where there is a high probability of death or significant injury to an individual(s) or a significant loss of property, which can be reduced by the actions of an emergency service.

truncal obesity, obesity of the trunk of the body.

trunking system, a radio connecting system with base stations on different channels connected together to allow simultaneous conversations.

Trypanosoma /trip´ənōsō´mə/, a genus of one-celled parasites that live in the body. Several species can cause serious diseases in humans. Most *Trypanosoma* organisms live part of their life-cycle in insects and enter humans by insect bites.

trypanosomiasis /-sōmī´əsis/, a parasitic disease caused by protozoal organisms carried to humans by the bite of bloodsucking insects.

tryptophan /trip´təfan/, an amino acid necessary for normal growth in infants and for nitrogen balance in adults. Tryptophan is the basis of several substances, including serotonin and niacin. Most of the body's need for trytophan is acquired from protein in foods, especially legumes, grains, and seeds. *See also amino acid, protein.*

tsunami /tso͞onä´mē/, a large sea wave generated by earthquake, volcano, or submarine landslide. Such a wave may travel at up to 600 miles per hour. As they reach shallow water, these waves grow from their open-ocean height of 2-4 feet to a height of up to 80 feet. The shore may be hit by a single wave or up to a dozen waves, 20-30 minutes apart. Destruction on the shore is massive, with loss of life much more significant than injuries. Also known as **tidal wave.**

tubal ligation, one of several sterilization methods in which both fallopian tubes are blocked to prevent conception from occurring.

tubal pregnancy, a pregnancy in which the embryo is implanted in the fallopian tube. The tube, which cannot hold the growing fetus for very long, breaks, causing bleeding in the peritoneal cavity. This hemorrhage can be severe enough to cause maternal death. *See also pregnancy.*

tube, a hollow, cylinder-shaped piece of equipment or structure of the body, such as a **chest tube.**

tubercle /to͞o´bərkəl/, **1.** a small group of cells or a bump (nodule), as that on a bone. **2.** a nodule, especially an elevation of the skin that is larger than a pimple. **3.** a small rounded nodule caused by infection with *Mycobacterium tuberculosis,* made up of a gray mass of small round cells.

tubercles of Montgomery, papillae on the surface of nipples and areolae that release a fatty lubricating substance.

tuberculoma /to͞obur´kyəlō´mə/, a tumorlike growth of tuberculous tissue in the central nervous system, marked by symptoms of an expanding cerebral or spinal mass.

tuberculosis, an airborne disease caused by the bacterial species *Mycobacterium tuberculosis,* after it enters the body (primarily by inhalation). Although the lung is the most common primary site of infection, the kidneys, liver, spine, or spleen can also be infected. Infected patients are contagious until treated and must be hospitalized with isolation procedures. Early signs and symptoms include decreased energy, night sweats, and weight loss. Advanced pulmonary symptoms include dyspnea, hemoptysis, and purulent sputum. Also known as **TB.**

tuberosity /tōō´bəros´itē/, a raised place, especially of a bone, such as **tuberosity of the tibia,** a large oblong elevation at the proximal end of the tibia that attaches to the ligament of the patella.

tube thoracostomy, insertion of a chest tube into the thoracic cavity to relieve hemothorax, pneumothorax, or tension pneumothorax. This is done by creating an incision in the fourth or fifth intercostal space of the affected side of the chest, inserting a chest tube, and attaching it to a water-seal drainage system to allow reexpansion of the collapsed lung. *See also needle thoracostomy.*

tubule /tōō´byōōl/, a small tube, such as one of the collecting tubules in the kidneys or the semen-producing tubules of the testicles.

tularemia /tōō´lərē´mē·ə/, an infectious disease of animals caused by the bacillus *Francisella (Pasteurella) tularensis,* which may be passed to humans by insect carriers or direct contact. Symptoms include fever, headache, and lymphadenopathy. Also known as **deerfly fever, rabbit fever.**

tumor, a new growth of tissue with continuing, uncontrolled spreading of cells. Also known as **neoplasm.**

tumorigenesis /tōō´mərijen´əsis/, the process of beginning the growth of a tumor. *See also carcinogen.* –**tumorigenic,** *adj.*

tunica, a covering membrane, such as the **tunica vaginalis testis,** the tissue surrounding the testicle and epididymis.

tunica adventitia, outer layer of a blood vessel or any other tubular structure. When applied to an artery, also known as **tunica externa.**

tunica intima, inner layer of a blood vessel. Also known as **tunica interna.**

tunica media, middle layer of a blood vessel.

tunnel vision, a defect in sight in which there is a great loss of peripheral vision, as if looking through a hollow tube or tunnel.

turbinate, cone-shaped; usually applied to the three conchae of the nasal cavity.

turbojet, a jet engine with a turbine-driven compressor supplying air to the engine. The turbine is activated by exhaust gas.

turboprop, a jet engine with a turbine-driven propeller.

turboshaft, a turbine engine utilizing a transmission to provide power to helicopter rotors.

turbulence, agitated air or water; rough flow due to pressure, speed, or temperature variables.

turgid /tur´jid/, swollen, hard; usually as a result of fluid.

turgor /tur´gər/, the strength and tension of the skin caused by the outward pressure of the cells and the fluid that surrounds them. Loss of body water causes decreased skin turgor, which appears as loose skin. Marked fluid gain causes increased turgor that appears as smooth, taut, shiny skin that cannot be grasped and raised.

turnout gear, *(informal)* firefighting and rescue protective clothing, usually including boots, gloves, helmet and visor, and protective coat and pants. This equipment should be worn by all personnel involved at an incident. Also known as **bunker gear.**

turret, a swivel-mounted firefighting nozzle, used for the application of foam or water from a fixed position.

T wave, deflection on an EKG that follows the QRS complex. It represents ventricular repolarization and refractory periods of the cardiac electrical cycle. The upward slope of the wave is the absolute refractory period. The downward slope is the relative refractory period.

twiddler's syndrome, condition in which a cardiac pacemaker wire is dislocated from its functional position. So named because of the occasions when a patient caused the movement of the wire due to "twiddling" with the pacemaker. Symptoms vary depending on the wire's new location and the patient's cardiac function.

twilight, **1.** faint light, usually that occurring after sunset. **2.** referring to faint or indistinct mental perception.

twilight narcosis, reduced awareness when driving in near-dark conditions, due to fatigue and poor lighting.

twin, either of two offspring born of the same pregnancy and developed from either a single egg or from two eggs that were released from the ovary and fertilized at the same time. Twin births occur approximately once in 80 pregnancies.

twinning, **1.** the development of two or more fetuses during the same pregnancy, either naturally or through outside control for experimental purposes on animals. **2.** the creation of two like structures or parts by division.

tympanic /timpan´ik/, referring to a structure that sounds when struck; drumlike, as a **tympanic abdomen** that sounds on percussion because the intestines are enlarged with gas.

tympanic membrane. See **ear.**

tympanic reflex, the reflection of a beam of light shining on the eardrum. In a normal ear a bright, wedge-shaped reflection is seen; its highpoint is at the end of the malleus, and its base is at the front of the eardrum. In disorders of the middle ear or eardrum, this shape may be distorted. Also known as **light reflex.**

Type A packaging, packaging designed to prevent the loss or dispersal of its radioactive contents under normal conditions of transport. This type of packaging carries radioactive materials that, because of their level of radioactivity or physical properties, constitute little hazard.

Type B packaging, packaging that meets the same criteria as Type A but in addition is designed to meet standards for performance under hypothetical accident conditions. This type of packaging is designed to carry greater quantities of radioactivity than Type A.

typhoid fever, a bacterial infection usually caused by *Salmonella typhi,* carries by contaminated milk, water, or food. Symptoms include headache, confusion and excitement, cough, watery diarrhea, rash, and fever. The incubation period may be as long as 60 days.

typhoon. See **tropical cyclone.**

typhus, any of a group of acute infectious diseases caused by various species of *Rickettsia* and usually carried from infected rodents to humans by the bites of lice, fleas, mites, or ticks. These diseases all involve headache, chills, fever, and red rash that covers much of the body. **Epidemic (classic) typhus** results from the bite of the body louse. The rickettsia is in the feces of the louse and enters the body when the bite is scratched. **Murine typhus** is carried by the bite of an infected flea. **Scrub typhus** occurs in Asia, India, northern Australia, and the western Pacific islands, and is carried from rats and mice to humans by mites.

typing, the process of determining the classification of a specimen of blood, tissue, or other substance. *See also blood typing, tissue typing.*

Tyrolean, **1.** any horizontal or lateral crossing by rope, as in traversing a canyon or rock face. **2.** the lateral belay and transfer systems that allow traversing in a horizontal direction. *See also Z rig.*

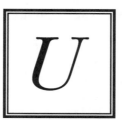

ulcer, a craterlike skin or mucous membrane lesion. The cause may be inflammation, infection, or malignant process. A **stress ulcer** is one that develops in the stomach or intestine of patients who are under heavy stress. **Serpent ulcer** refers to an open sore of the skin that heals in one place while growing in another. A **stasis ulcer** is a sore on the lower leg caused by chronic diminished blood flow, often from varicose veins. A **trophic ulcer** is a pressure sore caused by injury to an area of the body that is compromised by disease, diminished blood flow, or loss of innervation. *See also decubitus, peptic ulcer.*

ulceration, **1.** the formation of a pressure lesion on the mucous membranes or skin. **2.** wearing away of the surface due to friction or pressure.

ulcerative colitis /ul´sərā´tiv/, a chronic, inflammatory disease of the large intestine and rectum, marked by profuse watery diarrhea containing blood, mucus, and pus. Other symptoms include abdominal pain, fever, and weight loss. *See also colitis.*

ultra high frequency, radio frequency between 300 and 3000 megahertz.

ultrasound imaging, the use of high-frequency sound to map structures inside the body, such as fetuses, gallstones, cardiac defects, and tumors. Ultrasound imaging differs from x-ray imaging in that there is no radiation involved.

ultraviolet keratitis. See **snowblindness.**

ultraviolet light, light rays that are higher in frequency and shorter in wavelength than are visible to the human eye. They are lower in frequency and longer in wavelength than x-rays. Also known as **ultraviolet radiation, UV.**

umbilical cord, a flexible structure connecting the umbilicus with the placenta in the pregnant uterus, encapsulating the umbilical arteries and vein. In the newborn it is about 2 feet long and ½ inch in diameter. It is first formed during the fifth week of pregnancy.

umbilical fistula, an abnormal passage from the umbilicus to the intestine or another internal structure.

umbilical hernia. See **hernia.**

umbilicus, a depression in the middle of the abdomen, which is the scar from the former attachment of the umbilical cord to the fetus.

unconditioned response, a normal, instinctive, unlearned reaction to a stimulus. It is one occurring naturally, not acquired by association and training. Also known as **inborn reflex, instinctive reflex, unconditioned reflex.** Compare **conditioned response.**

unconscious, **1.** being unaware of the environment; insensible; unable to respond to sensory stimuli. **2.** *(psychiatry)* the part of mental function in which thoughts, ideas, emotions, or memories are beyond awareness and not subject to ready recall.

undercut rock, rock that has been worn such that water flow is directed both under and around it.

undertow, a retreating current from the beach toward open water, caused by water retreating rapidly down a slope under incoming waves. This current flow is usually of short duration and terminates with the next breaking wave.

undertruck nozzle, firefighting device located underneath an apparatus. Generally used on aircraft firefighting vehicles, this nozzle is designed to protect the vehicle's occupants from flame or fuel floating under the vehicle during operations.

undulant fever /unˊdyələnt/. See **brucellosis.**

unified command, a method for all agencies or individuals who have jurisdictional responsibility, and in some cases those who have functional responsibility at the incident, to contribute to determining overall objectives for the incident and selection of a strategy to achieve the objectives.

unifocal, occurring from one site or focus.

unilateral paralysis /yo͞oˊnēlatˊərəl/. See **hemiplegia.**

uniovular /-ovˊyələr/, developing from a single ovum, as in identical twins.

unipolar depressive response, a mental disorder marked by symptoms of depression only.

unipolar lead, an electrocardiogram lead composed of one positive electrode and a reference point.

unit, that organization element having functional responsibility for a specific incident planning, logistic, or finance activity.

United States Pharmacopeia, a drug encyclopedia with descriptions, uses, strengths, and standards of purity for certain drugs and their dosage. Also known as **USP.**

universal antidote, *(historical)* a mixture of 50% activated charcoal, 25% magnesium oxide, and 25% tannic acid, formerly thought useful as an antidote for most types of acid, heavy metal, alkaloid, and glycoside poisons. It is now known that there is no true universal antidote.

universal donor, a person with type O, Rh-negative blood.

universal precautions, procedures established by the Centers for Disease Control and Prevention to assist caregivers in protecting themselves from infectious disease. See Appendix 2-1.

universal recipient, a person with type AB blood, which allows transfusion using any other type of blood.

unmyelinated axon, nerve fiber without a myelin sheath.

untoward effect, a harmful side effect of a drug or treatment.

upcurrent, the direction opposite the water's flow; against the current.

upper esophageal sphincter, the muscle ring located at the superior opening of the esophagus. This muscle controls the passage of material into the esophagus.

uprights, planking that is held in place against sheeting sections with shores. These planks add strength by distributing pressure more evenly over the entire trench structure.

upstream, upcurrent from the present location; the direction from which the flow originated.

upstream V, water turbulence caused by a solid obstruction diverting water. The peak of the V is upstream.

upwelling, water rising from the bottom toward the surface.

upwind, away from the direction in which the wind is blowing; the direction from which the wind originates.

urate /yo͞orˊāt/, any salt of uric acid. Urates are found in the urine, blood, and in tissues. They may also be deposited as crystals in joints. *See also gout, uric acid.*

urea /yo͞orˊē·ə/, **1.** the nitrogen portion of urine made from protein breakdown. **2.** a sterile form of the chemical used as a diuretic.

uremia /yo͞orēˊmē·ə/, the presence of excessive amounts of urea and other waste products in the blood, as occurs in kidney failure.

uremic frost /yo͞orēˊmik/, a pale, frostlike deposit of white crystals on the skin caused by kidney failure and uremia. Urea compounds and other waste products that cannot be excreted by the kidneys are carried through capillaries to the skin, where they collect on the surface.

ureter /yo͞orēˊtər/, one of a pair of tubular structures that carry urine from the kidneys into the bladder.

ureteritis /yo͞orēˊtərīˊ-/, an inflammatory condition of a ureter caused by infection or kidney stone.

urethra /yo͞orēˊthrə/, a small tubular structure that drains urine from the bladder. In men, the urethra also serves as a passage for semen. *See also ureter.*

urethral /yŏŏrē´thrəl/, pertaining to the urethra.

urethritis /yŏŏr´ēthrī´-/, an inflammation of the urethra, often caused by infection in the bladder or kidneys.

uric acid /yŏŏr´ik/, a product of metabolism of protein present in the blood and excreted in the urine. *See also gout, urine.*

uricaciduria /yŏŏr´ikas´idŏŏr´ē·ə/, an increased amount of uric acid in the urine, often linked to kidney stones or gout.

urinalysis /yŏŏr´inal´isis/, a physical, microscopic, or chemical examination of urine.

urinary /yŏŏr´iner´ē/, pertaining to urine.

urinary bladder, the muscular membranous sac in the pelvis that stores urine for discharge through the urethra.

urinary calculus, a mineral deposit (stone) formed in the urinary tract, including the bladder. It may be large enough to block the flow of urine or small enough to be passed with the urine. *See also calculus, kidney stone.*

urinary frequency, an increase in the urge to void without an increase in the total daily volume of urine. It is a sign of inflammation in the bladder or urethra or of diminished bladder capacity or other structural abnormalities. *See also cystitis, cystocele.*

urinary hesitancy, a decrease in the force of the stream of urine, often with difficulty in starting the flow. Hesitancy is usually the result of a blockage or stricture between the bladder and the urethral opening; in men it may indicate a swelling of the prostate gland, in women, a tightening of the urethral opening.

urinary incontinence, involuntary passage of urine, with the failure of voluntary control over bladder and sphincters. Causes include bladder dysfunction stemming from lesions of the brain and spinal cord, or injury.

urinary output, the total volume of urine excreted daily. Various metabolic and renal diseases may change the normal urinary output. *See also anuria, oliguria, polyuria.*

urinary retention, an involuntary retention of urine in the bladder. This occurs due to a blockage in the urethra, narcotics, nerve or muscle injury, or other trauma.

urinary tract, all organs and ducts involved in the release and elimination of urine.

urinary tract infection, an infection of the urinary tract. Most of these infections are caused by bacteria. Symptoms include urinary frequency, burning, pain with voiding, and, if the infection is severe, visible blood and pus in the urine. It is more common in women than in men. Kinds of urinary tract infections include **cystitis, pyelonephritis, urethritis.** Also known as **UTI.**

urination, the act of passing urine. Also known as **micturition.**

urine, the fluid secreted by the kidneys, transported by the ureters, stored in the bladder, and voided through the urethra. Normal urine is clear, straw-colored, slightly acid, and odorless. It contains water, urea, sodium and potassium chloride, phosphates, uric acid, organic salts, and pigment. Abnormal substances in urine indicating disease include ketone bodies, protein, bacteria, blood, glucose, pus, and certain crystals. *See also bacteriuria, glycosuria, hematuria, ketoaciduria, proteinuria.*

urogenital system /yŏŏr´ōjen´ətəl/, the urinary and genital organs including the kidneys, ureters, bladder, urethra, and the genital structures of the male and female. In women these are the ovaries, uterine tubes, uterus, clitoris, and vagina. In men these are the testes, seminal vesicles, seminal ducts, prostate, and penis.

urogenital triangle, the anterior perianal region. The anatomical location of the base of the penis and the openings of the urethra and vagina.

urology /-ol´-/, the branch of medicine concerned with the anatomy and physiology, disorders, and care of the urinary tract in men and women. A licensed physician who specializes in urology is called a **urologist.**

uropathy /yŏŏrop´əthē/, any disease or abnormal state of the urinary tract. –**uropathic,** *adj.*

urticaria, a skin reaction, characterized by wheals, accompanied by itching. Allergy, drugs, heat, irritation, sunlight, and even water can be causative agents. Also known as **hives, nettle rash.** *See also pruritus.*

urushiol /ərŏŏ´shē·ôl/, a toxic resin in the sap of certain plants of the genus *Rhus,* such as poison ivy, poison oak, and poison sumac, that produces allergic contact dermatitis in many people.

useful load, the difference between empty weight and gross (maximum takeoff) weight in an aircraft. This is the amount of weight that an aircraft can safely carry and includes crew, fuel, and passengers.

uterine inversion, the uterus inverting and prolapsing outside the vaginal opening.

uterine rupture, rupture of the wall of the uterus.

uterine souffle /soo´fəl/, a quiet blowing sound that may be auscultated in the pregnant abdomen. It is created by blood passing through greatly enlarged uterine vessels. *See also fetal souffle.*

uterine tube, one of two ducts connecting the uterus and the peritoneal cavity. Also known as **fallopian tube.**

uteroovarian varicocele /yoo´tərōōver´e·ən/, a swelling of the veins of the female pelvis. Compare **ovarian varicocele, varicocele.**

uterosacral ligament, ligament retaining the uterus in position.

uterus /yoo´tərəs/, the hollow, pear-shaped inner female organ of reproduction in which the fertilized ovum is implanted and the fetus develops, and from which the menses flows. It is composed of three layers: the endometrium, the myometrium, and the parametrium. The endometrium lines the uterus and becomes thicker in pregnancy and during the second half of the menstrual cycle under the influence of the hormone progesterone. The myometrium is the middle muscular layer of the organ. After childbirth the fibers contract, creating natural ligatures that stop the flow of blood from the large blood vessels supplying the placenta. The parametrium is the outermost layer of the uterus. During pregnancy it becomes many times its usual size. The uterus is composed of the fundus, body, and cervix. The cervix has a vaginal portion bulging into the vagina.

uvea /yoo´ve·ə/, a layer of the eye that includes the iris, the ciliary body, and the choroid of the eye. Also known as **uveal tract. –uveal,** *adj.*

uveitis /yoo´ve·i´-/, inflammation of the uvea of the eye. Symptoms include an irregularly shaped pupil, irritation of the cornea, pain, and tearing. Causes include allergy, infection, injury, diabetes, and skin diseases. A major complication may be glaucoma.

uvula /yoo´vyələ/, *pl.* **uvulae,** the small, cone-shaped tissue suspended in the mouth posteriorly from the soft palate. –uvular, *adj.*

uvulitis /yoo´vyəli´-/, inflammation of the uvula. Common causes are allergy and infection.

U wave, a deflection following the T wave in the cardiac cycle. Although it may be associated with electrolyte abnormalities, it is not typically present and its origin is unclear.

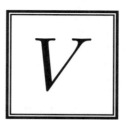

vaccination, the administration of deactivated, live-weakened, or nonliving bacteria or virus to stimulate the body to produce antibodies against a particular disease or infection, such as typhoid or whooping cough. This serves to decrease the severity of or eliminate the possibility of infection.

vaccine, the bacteria or viruses, administered orally or parenterally, to stimulate the production of antibodies, so as to protect against disease or infection.

vacuole /vak´yoo·ōl/, **1.** a clear or fluid-filled space within a cell, as when a drop of water is taken into the cell. **2.** a small space in the body enclosed by a membrane, usually containing fat or other matter.

vagal /vā´gəl/, of or concerning the vagus nerve.

vagina, the part of the female genitals that forms a canal from the external opening to the cervix. It is behind the bladder and in front of the rectum. The vagina is lined with mucous membranes covering a layer of tissue and muscle.

vaginal bleeding /vaj´inəl/, blood flow from the vagina at times other than menstruation. It may be caused by an abnormal pregnancy, glandular problems, or abnormalities of the ovaries or fallopian tubes. The following terms are commonly used in approximating the amount of vaginal bleeding: **heavy,** which is greater than heaviest normal menstrual flow; **moderate,** which is equal to heaviest normal menstrual flow; **light,** which is less than heaviest normal menstrual flow; **staining,** which is a very light flow of blood barely requiring the use of a sanitary napkin or tampon; and **spotting,** which is the passage of a few drops of blood. **Bloody show** refers to an episode of light vaginal bleeding as often occurs in early labor, during labor, and, particularly, at the end of the first stage of labor. **Breakthrough bleeding** is the escape of blood from the uterus between menstrual periods. This is an occasional side effect of birth control pills.

vaginismus /vaj´iniz´məs/, strong tightening of the muscles in the pelvic area and the vagina. *See also dyspareunia.*

vaginitis /vaj´inī´-/, an inflammation of the vaginal tissues, as in trichomoniasis.

vagolysis /vagol´əsis/, surgical removal of the esophageal branches of the vagus nerve to prevent cardiospasm.

vagotomy, surgical interruption of certain branches of the vagus nerve.

vagotonus /vā´gətō´nəs/, an increase in the activity of the vagus nerve, bradycardia, and syncope.

vagus nerve, the tenth cranial nerve. This mixed nerve has both motor and sensory functions that include gag reflex, parasympathetic control of the heart, speech, and swallowing. Also known as the **pneumogastric nerve.**

valgus /val´gəs/, position in which a limb is bent or twisted laterally. Compare **varus.**

valine /val´in/, an essential amino acid needed for growth in infants and nitrogen balance in adults. *See also amino acid.*

vallecula, a depression or crevice on the surface of an organ or structure. The **vallecula epiglottica** is the pharyngeal depression into which the tip of the curved laryngoscope blade is inserted during endotracheal intubation.

Valsalva's maneuver (Antonio Maria Valsalva, Italian anatomist, 1666-1723), **1.** attempted forced exhalation against a closed glottis. This causes increased intrathoracic pressure, which stimulates the vagus nerve, causing a slowing of heart rate. Side effects may include lightheadedness or syncope. **2.** blowing with an open glottis against closed lips and nares in order to inflate the middle ear through the eustachian tubes. This change in pressure in the nasopharynx equalizes internal and external air pressure when changing altitude or depth. *See also Frenzel maneuver.*

Valsalva's test, a method of determining whether the eustachian tubes are open. With mouth and nose kept tightly closed, the person breathes out very forcefully; if the eustachian tubes are open, air will enter into the middle ear cavities and the patient will hear a popping sound.

valve, a structure, either natural or artificial, that opens to allow fluid to flow in one direction, but closes to prevent it from flowing back in the other direction. Valves in veins are folds of membrane that prevent the backflow of blood. *See also heart valve.* **–valvular,** *adj.*

valvulitis /val´vyəlī´-/, inflammation of a valve.

vanadium, a grayish metallic element. Absorption of vanadium results in a condition called **vanadiumism.** Symptoms include anemia, conjunctivitis, pneumonitis, and irritation of the lungs.

vapor density, the weight of a given volume of gas or vapor compared to the weight of an equal volume of dry air, both measured at the same temperature and pressure. When the weight is less than 1, the material is lighter than air and will rise. If the weight is more than 1, the substance is heavier than air and will remain low to the ground.

vaporizing agents, liquid organic compounds, used to extinguish hydrocarbon fires. These agents, though applied as liquids, vaporize when exposed to heat and smother a fire as a gas (BCF, Halon, Tribromo). They are usually utilized in self-contained extinguishing systems onboard aircraft, ships, and isolated areas of buildings with high potential for fire.

vapor pressure, the pressure exerted by a gas. When dissolved in a liquid, it is also a measure of the tendency of the liquid to vaporize into a gas. Since this pressure is temperature dependent, when the temperature increases, so does the pressure. The lower the boiling point of a liquid, the greater the pressure at a given temperature. *See also partial pressure.*

varicella /ver´isel´ə/. See **chickenpox.**

varicella-zoster virus, a member of the herpesvirus family, which causes chickenpox (varicella) and shingles (herpes zoster). The virus is contagious and may be spread by direct contact or respiratory droplets. *See also chickenpox, herpes zoster.*

varicelliform /ver´isel´ifôrm/, resembling the rash of chickenpox.

varicocele /ver´ikōsēl´/, a disorder of the spermatic cord, which causes a soft, painful swelling in the scrotum. It is most common in men between 15 and 25 years of age. Compare **ovarian varicocele, uteroovarian varicocele.**

varicose /ver´ikōs/, abnormally and permanently distended.

varicose vein, a tortuous, distended vein. Causes include congenital defects of the valves or walls of the veins or increased pressure in the vessels resulting form prolonged standing, poor posture, pregnancy, and obesity.

variola /vərī´ōlə/. See **smallpox.**

varioloid /ver´ē·əloid´/, **1.** resembling smallpox. **2.** a mild form of smallpox in a vaccinated person or one who has previously had the disease.

varix, /ver´iks/, *pl.* **varices** /ver´isēz/, a twisted, widened vein, artery, or lymph vessel.

varus /ver´əs/, position in which a limb is turned medially. Compare **valgus.**

vas /vas/, *pl.* **vasa** /vā´sə/, any one of the many vessels of the body, especially those that carry blood, lymph, or sperm.

vascular /vas´kyələr/, relating to a blood vessel.

vascular insufficiency, poor blood circulation. Symptoms include variable skin color, tingling, muscle pain, and diminished or absent pulses. Causes are aneurysms, atherosclerosis, emboli, and fistulas. **Arterial insufficiency** is diminished blood flow in arteries.

vascularization, the process by which body tissue develops small blood vessels, especially capillaries.

vascular tunic, the choroid, ciliary body, and iris of the eye.

vasculitis /vas´kyəlī´-/, inflammation of blood vessels.

vas deferens /def´ərənz/, a tube passing from the testicles through the scrotum and joining the seminal vesicle. Also known as **deferent duct, spermatic duct, testicular duct.** *See also testis.*

vasectomy /vasek´-/, an operation that makes a man sterile by removing a section of the vas deferens.

vasoactive /vā´zō·ak´tiv, vas´-/, *(pharmacology)* tending to cause the widening or narrowing of a vessel.

vasoconstriction, constriction or narrowing of a blood vessel. Compare **vasodilatation.**

vasoconstrictor, relating to a process, condition, or substance that causes constriction of blood vessels. The hormones epinephrine and norepinephrine produced by the body cause blood vessels to contract. Also known as **vasopressor.**

vasodilatation /-dil´ətā´shən/, dilation or enlargement of blood vessels, usually caused by nerve impulses or drugs that relax smooth muscle in the walls of the blood vessels. Also known as **vasodilation.** Compare **vasoconstriction.**

vasodilator /-dī´lātər/, a nerve or agent that causes dilation or relaxation of blood vessel walls.

vasomotor, relating to the nerves and muscles that control constriction or dilation of blood vessels.

vasomotor system, the component of the nervous system that controls narrowing and widening of blood vessels. *See also vasoconstriction, vasodilation.*

vasopressin mechanism, increased secretion of antidiuretic hormone when blood pressure drops or plasma osmolarity increases. This has the effect of reducing urine output and increasing vasoconstriction.

vasopressor, a substance that stimulates contraction of the muscular walls of arteries and capillaries, increasing blood pressure.

vasospastic /-spas´-/, **1.** relating to spasms of blood vessels. **2.** any agent that produces spasms of blood vessels.

vasovagal reflex, fainting or lightheadedness resulting from reflex stimulation of the vagus nerve. Classically, this occurs in one who is exposed to a strong emotional stimulus. Also known as **vasodepressor syncope.**

vastus intermedius, one of the four muscles of the quadriceps femoris, situated in the center of the thigh. It functions with the other three muscles of the quadriceps to extend the leg.

vastus lateralis, the largest of the four muscles of the quadriceps femoris, situated on the lateral aspect thigh. It functions to help extend the leg.

vastus medialis, one of the four muscles of the quadriceps femoris, situated on the medial thigh. It functions together with other parts of the quadriceps femoris to extend the leg.

vector, **1.** any force whose quantity is specified by direction and magnitude. This quantity is usually represented by a line of appropriate direction and length, as in a cardiac vector. **2.** an animal that transmits disease organisms from reservoirs of infection to the noninfected.

vehicle warning placard, a sign, displayed on the outside of a carrier of hazardous material, indicating the nature of the cargo. The design and use of placards are specified by DOT regulations.

vehicular repeater. See **mobile repeater.**

vein, one of the many vessels that transports blood back to the heart from all parts of the body. Veins have thinner walls and are less elastic than arteries. Compare **artery.**

vein ligation and stripping, an operation that removes the saphenous vein in the leg. It is done to treat phlebitis or to graft in another site, as in a coronary bypass operation. *See also ligation, stripping.*

velocity never exceed, the highest speed at which an aircraft is rated as safe to fly; the outside limit of an aircraft's flight characteristics (envelope). Any speed in excess of this is unsafe and could cause destruction of the aircraft. Also known as **VNE.**

vena cava /vē´nə kā´və/, *pl.* **venae cavae,** one of two large veins returning blood from the body to the right chamber of the heart. The **inferior vena cava** is the vein that returns blood to the heart from below the diaphragm. The **superior vena cava** returns blood from the upper half of the body to the heart.

venereal /vənir´ē·əl/, relating to or caused by sexual intercourse or genital contact.

venereal disease. See **sexually transmitted disease.**

venereal sore. See **chancre.**

venereal wart, a soft, wartlike growth on the genitals. It is caused by a virus and is carried by sexual contact. Also known as **condyloma acuminatum.**

venipuncture, the puncture of a vein for any purpose.

venom /ven´əm/, a poisonous fluid secreted by some snakes, insects, spiders, and other animals and transmitted by their stings or bites.

venom extract therapy, the giving of antivenin as protection against the poisonous effects of the bite of a specific poisonous snake or spider, or other poisonous animal.

venostasis, diminished or retarded venous flow to an area.

venous /vē´nəs/, relating to a vein.

venous capillary, capillaries closest to venules.

venous insufficiency, circulatory condition with decreased return of blood from the legs to the trunk of the body.

venous pressure, the pressure of circulating blood on the walls of veins. Symptoms of increased pressure are continued distention of hand veins when raised above the rib cage and enlarging of neck veins when the individual is sitting with the head raised 30 to 45 degrees.

venous sinus, one of several sinuses that route blood to the internal jugular vein after collecting it from the dura mater.

ventilate, 1. moving gases in and out of the lungs. **2.** removing or releasing hot gases from a building that is in flames by the creation of air circulation within the structure (usually a hole in the roof).

ventilation, 1. the process of moving gases in and out of the lungs; breathing. **Mechanical** ventilation actively moves air (oxygen) into the lungs and allows passive exhalation. This usually involves the application of devices that simulate the work of the muscles of respiration. *See also artificial respiration, ventilator.* **2.** the amount of air inhaled each day (usually around 10,000 liters). **3.** the circulation of air within a structure; the amount of fresh air moved in and stale air moved out.

ventilator, 1. person(s) responsible for ventilation of the patient. **2.** any mechanical device that provides for artificial ventilation of the lungs, especially those devices used for the prolonged ventilation of patients in-hospital. *See also resuscitator.*

ventral /ven´trəl/, frontward; anterior. Compare **dorsal.**

ventral root, the nerve that carries efferent nerve impulses away from the spinal cord.

ventricle /ven´trikəl/, a small cavity, such as one of the cavities filled with cerebrospinal fluid in the brain, or the right and the left ventricles of the heart. In the heart, the **left ventricle** is a thick-walled lower chamber that pumps blood through the aorta to the body's tissues. It has walls about three times thicker than those of the right ventricle. The **right ventricle** pumps blood received from the right atrium into the pulmonary arteries to the lungs. The right ventricle is shorter and rounder than the long, conic left ventricle.

ventricular /ventrik´yələr/, relating to a ventricle.

ventricular bigeminy, cardiac electrical activity characterized by a ventricular ectopic occurring every other complex. The other complex is generally normal. This dysrhythmia indicates ventricular irritability.

ventricular fibrillation, lethal dysrhythmia producing chaotic ventricular activity, which causes ineffective cardiac muscle contraction. No measurable complexes appear on electrocardiogram; only a rapidly undulating, irregular baseline. This rhythm produces cardiac arrest. Also known as **V fib.**

ventricular flutter, ventricular tachycardia at rates exceeding 250 per minute. *See also ventricular tachycardia.*

ventricular quadrigeminy, cardiac electrical activity with a ventricular ectopic occurring every fourth complex. The other complexes remain normal. This dysrhythmia is indicative of ventricular irritability.

ventricular standstill, lethal dysrhythmia characterized by P waves without QRS complexes. The ventricles are not stimulated by electrical activity, do not depolarize, and have no mechanical contraction. The P waves are not conducted through the AV node. This rhythm produces cardiac arrest. Also known as **dying heart.**

ventricular tachycardia, a potentially lethal dysrhythmia, characterized by a cardiac rhythm exhibiting only wide ventricular complexes, depolarizing at a rate of 150-250 times a minute. Although typically regular, this rhythm may occur at rates below 150 and above 250. The heart may have mechanical contraction adequate to perfuse the brain with blood, allowing the patient to remain conscious, but symptomatic. There is no blood flow with the patient in cardiac arrest. Also known as **VT, V tach.** *See also slow ventricular tachycardia, torsade de pointes, ventricular flutter.*

ventricular trigeminy, cardiac electrical activity characterized by a ventricular ectopic occurring every third complex or two ventricular ectopics occurring with one normal complex. Even though the other complexes remain normal, this dysrhythmia is indicative of ventricular irritability.

ventrogluteal muscle, muscle overlying the anterior superior iliac spine and the iliac crest.

venule /ven´yo͞ol/, any one of the small blood vessels that gather blood from the capillary plexuses and join together to form the veins. **–venular,** *adj.*

verapamil, a calcium channel blocker effective in the treatment of supraventricular tachycardias with a narrow QRS complex. Side effects include asystole, bradycardia, heart blocks, and transient hypotension. Do not administer to patients in congestive heart failure. Also known as **Calan, Isoptin.**

vermiform appendix /vur´mifôrm/. See **appendix.**

vermifuge /vur´mifyo͞oj´/, an agent that causes parasitic worms to be flushed from the body.

vermis, /vur´mis/, *pl.* **vermes, 1.** a worm. **2.** a structure resembling a worm. **–vermiform,** *adj.*

vernix caseosa /vur´niks kas´ē·ō´sə/, a grayish-white substance that covers the skin of the fetus and newborn. It acts as a protection for the fetus while it is in the uterus and is thought to help keep it warm.

vertebra /vur´təbrə/, *pl.* **vertebrae,** any one of the 33 bones of the spinal column. The **cervical vertebrae** are the first seven segments of the spine. They are smaller than the thoracic and the lumbar vertebrae. The first cervical vertebra (**atlas**) supports the head. The second is the **axis.** The atlas rotates on the axis, allowing the head to turn, extend, and flex. The seventh cervical vertebra is above the clavicles. It has a very long, bony extension that is nearly horizontal and can be felt with the fingers. The 12 bony segments of the upper back are the **thoracic vertebrae.** They are named T1 to T12. T1 is just below the seventh cervical vertebra (C7). The vertebrae become thicker and heavier in descending order from T1 to T12 and are separated by intervertebral disks. The five largest segments of the movable part of the spinal column are the **lumbar vertebrae.** They are larger and heavier than vertebrae higher in the spinal column because they must support more weight. The body of each lumbar vertebra is flattened or slightly concave. **Sacral vertebrae** are five parts of the vertebral column that join together in the adult to form the **sacrum,** the large, triangle-shaped bone at the top of the pelvis. The sacrum is shorter and wider in women than in men. **Coccygeal vertebrae** are four vertebrae that join to form the adult **coccyx** at the very end of the spine. The coccyx fuses with the sacrum by adulthood.

vertebral arch, the dorsal arch of a vertebra, composed of laminae and pedicles.

vertebral artery, each of two arteries that carry blood to the neck, the spine, and parts of the brain.

vertebral body, the solid central portion of a vertebra that supports the weight of the body.

vertex /vur´teks/, **1.** the top of the head; crown. **2.** the highest point of any structure.

vertex presentation, *(obstetrics)* a birth in which the fetus is lying in the womb with its head downward. The head will be born first. *See also breech birth.*

vertigo /vur´tigō, vərtī´gō/, a feeling of faintness, dizziness or an inability to keep normal balance in a standing or seated position. Symptoms may include confusion, nausea, and weakness. **Postural vertigo** is dizziness brought on by moving the head to certain positions. There are many causes, among them ear infection or injury to the inner ear.

very high frequency, radio frequencies between 30 and 300 megahertz, divided into high and low bands. Also known as **VHF.**

very high frequency omnidirectional range, an aircraft ground navigational aid that generates directional information and transmits it to aircraft. This information consists of 360 courses (radials) oriented to the magnetic compass. There may also be plain voice transmissions from a ground facility. They operated at a range of around 40 nautical miles at normal minimum instrument flight rule altitudes. These facilities have a three-digit identifier that is transmitted in Morse code and printed on aviation maps. Also known as **VHF Omni-Range, VOR.**

very-low-density lipoprotein. See **lipoprotein.**

vesicants, war gas that produces large, painful blisters that are incapacitating; blister agent. Although classed as nonlethal, high doses can cause death. Common agents include lewisite, mustard, and nitrogen mustard.

vesicle /ves´ikəl/, a small sac or blister containing clear fluid. –**vesicular,** *adj.*

vesicle reflex, the sensation of a need to urinate when the bladder is partly full. *See also micturition reflex.*

vesicular follicle, the growth chamber for an oocyte.

vesicular sounds, breath sounds auscultated in the normal lung, particularly in the distal portions of the respiratory tree.

vesiculation, the formation of vesicles.

vesiculitis /vəsik´yəlī´-/, inflammation of any vesicle, particularly the seminal vesicles. It is usually linked with prostatitis.

vessel, any one of the many tubes throughout the body that convey fluids, as blood and lymph. The primary kinds of vessels are arteries, veins, and the lymphatic vessels.

vestibular /vestib´yələr/, relating to a vestibule, as the vestibular portion of the mouth, which lies between the cheeks and the teeth.

vestibular fold, one of two folds of mucous membrane in the laryngeal cavity that assists in glottic closure. Also known as **false vocal cord.**

vestibular gland, any one of four small glands, two on each side of the vaginal opening. The vestibular glands secrete a lubricating substance.

vestibule /ves´tibyo͞ol/, a space that serves as the entrance to a passageway, such as the vestibule of the ear.

vestibule of the ear, middle portion of the middle ear.

vestibule of the vagina, a cleftlike space containing the opening of the vagina, urethra, and the vestibular glands, behind the labia minora.

vestibulocochlear nerve, the combination of the cochlear and vestibular nerves; the eighth cranial nerve.

vestige /ves´tij/, a mainly useless organ or other structure of the body that was important at an earlier stage or in a simpler form of life, such as the appendix (vermiform). –**vestigial,** *adj.*

viable /vī´əbəl/, a capable of developing, growing, and otherwise sustaining life, as a normal human fetus at 28 weeks of pregnancy.

viaduct, a bridge constructed of short spans, supported on piers or towers.

vibration syndrome, finger blanching, numbness, and tingling after use of handheld vibration tools. This may persist without further exposure to vibration.

vibrio /vib´rē·ō/, any bacterium that is curved and able to move, as those belonging to the genus *Vibrio*. **Vibrio cholerae** is the species of comma-shaped, motile bacillus that is the cause of cholera.

vicarious liability. See **respondeat superior.**

victim, one who is the subject of a negative situation, with a resultant injury. *See also patient.*

villus, *pl.* **villi,** one of many tiny projections, barely visible to the naked eye, that cover the lining of the small intestine. The villi absorb and carry fluids and nutrients.

vindictive, inclined to cause harm or seek revenge against another.

viral hepatitis /vī´rəl/. See **hepatitis.**

viral pneumonia. See **pneumonia.**

viremia /vīrē´mē·ə/, viruses in the blood. Compare **bacteremia, fungemia, parasitemia.**

virgin soil, ground that has never been excavated.

virile /vir´əl/, **1.** of, relating to, an adult male; having masculine strength; capable of making a woman pregnant. Compare **virilism. –virility,** *n.*

virilism /vir´ilizm/, **1.** the growth of male secondary sexual characteristics in a female. This state is usually caused by an adrenal gland disorder, hormones, or tumors of the ovary. **2.** early development of masculine traits in the male.

virology /vīrol´-, virol´-/, the study of viruses and viral diseases.

virucide /vī´rəsīd/, any drug that destroys or renders a virus harmless. –**virucidal,** *adj.*

virulence /vir´yələns/, the power of a microbe to cause disease.

virus, an infectious microscopic complex of proteins and nucleic acids that can only grow in the cells of another animal. More than 200 viruses have been found to cause disease in humans. A **virion** is a simple virus particle. Types of viruses include **adenovirus, arenavirus, enterovirus, herpesvirus, rhinovirus.** *See also specific entry.* –**viral,** *adj.*

viscera /vis´ərə/, *sing.* **viscus** /vis´kəs/, the internal organs held within a space in the body, primarily the stomach and intestines.

visceral /vis´ərəl/, relating to the viscera, or internal organs in the body cavity.

visceral nervous system. See **central nervous system.**

visceral pain, dull pain arising from organs or smooth vasculature.

visceral pericardium, the serous tissue adhering to and covering the surface of the heart. Also known as **epicardium.**

visceral peritoneum, the tissue adhering to and covering the abdominal organs.

viscosity /viskos´itē/, the quality of a sticky or gummy fluid.

vision, 1. foresight; wisdom. **2.** an imagining. **3.** the ability to see with the eyes; sight. See **peripheral vision, photopic vision, purkinje shift, scotopic vision.**

visual field defect, one or more spots or defects in the vision that move with the eye, unlike a floater. This fixed defect may be caused by injuries to the eye, disease, or damage to the brain.

visual flight rules, the requirements governing air travel that occurs where flight is possible using visual references. These rules are more relaxed regarding types of equipment and training necessary to comply with federal regulations. This type of flight may occur day or night but only in weather conditions that do not obscure the ground or other aircraft. Also known as **VFR.** *See also instrument flight rules.*

visual pathway, a pathway over which a visual sensation is carried from the retina to the brain. A pathway consists of an optic nerve and other optic structures.

visual purple. See **rhodopsin.**

vital capacity, a measurement of the amount of air that can be breathed out slowly after the largest possible breath has been taken.

vital sign, a parameter of critical physiological body function. The classic vital signs are blood pressure, pulse, respirations, and temperature. Basic prehospital vital signs include level of consciousness. Advanced prehospital vital signs may also include EKG, lung sounds, and oxygen saturation. *See also specific entry.*

vital statistics, a numeric data on births, deaths, disease, injuries, and other factors affecting the general health and condition of human populations.

vitamin, a natural compound needed in small quantities for normal bodily functions. With few exceptions, vitamins must be obtained from the diet or dietary supplements. No one food contains all vitamins. *See also specific vitamins.*

vitamin A, vitamin needed for the growth of the skeleton. It is present in leafy green vegetables, yellow fruits and vegetables, the liver oils of the cod and other fish, liver, milk, cheese, butter, and egg yolk.

vitamin B$_1$. See **thiamine.**

vitamin B$_2$. See **riboflavin.**

vitamin B$_6$. See **pyridoxine.**

vitamin B$_{12}$. See **cyanocobalamin.**

vitamin B$_{17}$. See **amygdalin.**

vitamin B complex, a group of vitamins differing from each other in structure and their effect on the human body. All of the B vitamins are found in large quantities in liver and yeast, and they are present in many foods. *See also folic acid, and see specific B vitamins.*

vitamin C, a water-soluble, white crystalline vitamin, found in citrus fruits, tomatoes, berries, and potatoes. Fresh, green, leafy vegetables, such as broccoli, brussels sprouts, collards, turnip greens, parsley, sweet peppers, and cabbage also contain vitamin C. It is used by the body to form collagen and fiber for teeth, bone, cartilage, connective tissue, skin, and to fight bacterial infections. Also known as **ascorbic acid.**

vitamin D, a vitamin related to the steroids and needed for the normal growth of bones and teeth and for absorbing calcium and phosphorus from the intestines. The vitamin is present in saltwater fish, especially salmon, sardines, and herring, organ meats, fish-liver oils, and egg yolk. A lack of the vitamin results in rickets in children, and other bone diseases in adults. *See also calciferol, vitamin D_3.*

vitamin D_2. See **calciferol.**

vitamin D_3, a vitamin that is needed for calcium and phosphorus metabolism. It is found in most fish-liver oils, butter, brain, and egg yolk and is formed in the skin, fur, and feathers of animals and birds exposed to sunlight or ultraviolet rays. Also known as **activated 7-dehydrocholesterol, cholecalciferol.**

vitamin E, a vitamin needed for muscle development and various other bodily functions. Deficiency causes anemia and liver, muscle, and kidney damage. The richest dietary sources are wheat germ, soybean, cottonseed, peanut, and corn oils, margarine, whole raw seeds and nuts, soybeans, eggs, butter, liver, sweet potatoes, and the leaves of many vegetables, such as turnip greens. Also known as **tocopherol.**

vitamin H. See **biotin.**

vitamin K, a group of vitamins that are needed for proper liver function and to help blood clot. The vitamin is widely distributed in foods, especially leafy green vegetables, pork liver, yogurt, egg yolk, kelp, alfalfa, fish-liver oils, and is made by bacteria in the intestine. A deficiency of this vitamin is marked by blood disorders.

vitamin P. See **bioflavonoid.**

vitellin /vītel´in/, a protein containing lecithin, found in the yolk of eggs. Also known as **ovovitellin.**

vitelline circulation, the flow of blood and nutrients between the developing embryo and the yolk sac by way of the vitelline arteries and veins. *See also fetal circulation.*

vitellus /vītel´əs/, the yolk of an egg (ovum).

vitiligo /vit´ilī´gō, -lē´gō/, a skin disease of unknown cause, having uneven patches of various sizes totally lacking in color and often having very colorful borders. Exposed areas of skin are most often affected. Compare **albinism, piebald.**

vitreous cavity /vit´rē·əs/, the space behind the lens of the eyes that contains the vitreous humor and membrane that lines it.

vitreous hemorrhage, bleeding into the vitreous humor of the eye.

vitreous humor, a clear, jellylike substance contained in a thin membrane filling the space behind the lens of the eye. Also known as **vitreous body.**

vocal cord, either of two bands of yellow tissue in the larynx held by membranes called vocal folds. **False vocal cord** refers to either of two thick folds of mucous membrane in the larynx.

vocal fremitus, vibrations emitted by the vocal cords that are transmitted to the chest wall through bronchial air. In the presence of hemothorax or pneumothorax, these vibrations will be diminished on the affected side. To palpate, apply the anterior surface of the hand to each side of the chest and ascertain equality while the patient repeats "1, 2, 3". Also known as **tactical fremitus.**

voice box. See **larynx.**

void, to empty, as urine from the bladder.

volar /vō´lər/, relating to the palm of the hand or the sole of the foot.

volcano, a vent to the earth's surface from the earth's crust and the cone formed by it. This vent extends to a layer of molten material called *magma.* The cone is called a **volcanic edifice** and is formed by the material thrown from the vent. The four basic types are cinder cones, composite volcanoes, lava domes, and shield volcanoes. *See also coulee, magma.*

Volkmann's contracture (Richard von Volkmann, German surgeon, 1830-1899), a contraction of the fingers and wrist that develops soon after serious injury in the area of the elbow or after use of a tourniquet near the joint.

volt (Count Alessandro Volta, Italian physicist, 1745-1827), the electrical force required to produce one ampere of current through a resistance of one ohm.

voltage, the force that causes the flow of electricity. Low voltage is under 600 volts. High voltage is 600 volts and over.

volume, the amount of space occupied by an object, given in cubic units.

voluntary, actions or muscles subject to conscious impulse control.

volvulus /vol´vyələs/, a twisting of the bowel causing intestinal obstruction. Severe pain, nausea, and vomiting are symptoms. Compare **intussusception.**

vomer bone, the plow-shaped bone forming the inferior and posterior portion of the nasal septum.

vomit, 1. the act of forcing out the contents of the stomach through the esophagus and out of the mouth. **2.** *(informal)* the material forced out of the stomach. Also known as **emesis.**

von Willebrand's disease, an inherited disorder with slow blood clotting. *See also hemophilia.*

voting, a communications technique utilizing equipment to select the repeater station receiving the strongest signal and allow that station to rebroadcast the signal at greater strength.

voyeurism /voi´yərizm/, gaining sexual excitement and satisfaction from looking at naked bodies or seeing the sexual acts of others.

vulva /vul´və/, the outer genitals of a female, including the labia, the opening of the vagina, and the various glands.

vulvectomy /vəlvek´-/, removal by surgery of part or all of the tissues of the vulva.

vulvocrural /vul´vōkrŏŏr´əl/, relating to the vulva and the thigh.

vulvovaginitis /-vaj´inī´-/, an inflammation of the vulva and vagina, or their glands.

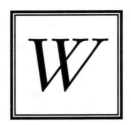

Waddell's triad, head, chest-abdominal, and lower leg injuries seen in pedestrian victims struck by a vehicle. Head injuries occur during contact with windshield or ground. Chest-abdominal injuries occur from contact with the hood. Lower leg injuries are sustained when struck by the bumper.

wake, the track left on the water's surface by a moving vessel.

wales, horizontal braces placed against panels and planks that support trench walls. Also known as **stringers, walers.**

walker, a very light, movable apparatus, made of metal tubing, used to assist a patient in walking. It has four widely placed legs. Compare **crutch**.

wall, 1. the vertical side of a mountain. Also known as **face. 2.** the side of a trench from the floor to the lip. Also known as **face. 3.** a divider within a structure, such as a cell wall or building wall.

wander, to move about without purpose or to cause to move back and forth in a searching manner.

wandering atrial pacemaker, a dysrhythmia in which the pacemaker site changes from the sinoatrial node to pacemaker sites in the atrium (AV junction) and back again. These changes do not generally follow a pattern, other than the alteration or presence of P waves. Also known as **WAP.**

wane, 1. to lose energy; dissipate; slow down. **2.** a defect on the edge of lumber, characterized by a lack of wood.

warfarin poisoning /wôr´fərin/, a toxic condition caused by swallowing warfarin. The poison results in internal bleeding.

warm-blooded, having a constant body temperature, despite changes in outside temperatures. Heat is made in the warm-blooded human body by the breakdown of foods. About 80% of the body heat that is lost in humans is lost through the skin. The rest is lost through the mucous membranes of the respiratory, digestive, and urinary systems. The average temperature of the healthy human is 98.6° F (37° C).

warm zone, forward control area for hazardous materials operation outside the hot zone. Personnel protection is not required. Restricted to operations and support personnel essential to hands-on work performed in the hot zone.

wart, a harmless growth (verruca) on the skin caused by a virus.

wash down, the removal of flammable or hazardous liquids from an area of operations by hosing away with water. This practice is now generally discouraged during extrication and rescue operations because it generally widens the area of hazard and increases danger to rescuers and victims.

wasp, a slender, narrow-waisted insect, belonging to the order, Hymenoptera, with two pairs of wings that are folded lengthwise when at rest. Many species are capable of painful stings, whose venom may cause allergic reaction or anaphylaxis.

wasting, a process of physiological breakdown marked by weight loss and decreased physical vigor, appetite, and mental activity.

water, a chemical compound, with a molecule of water having one atom of oxygen and two atoms of hydrogen. Almost three quarters of the earth's surface is covered by water. Water is essential to life as it exists on this planet. It comprises more than 70% of living organisms. Pure water freezes at sea level at 0° C (32° F) and boils at 100° C (212° F).

waterborne, carried or transmitted by water.

water ice, ice formed on surfaces by fog, groundwater, or rain, when the temperature drops to freezing. Also known as **live ice.**

water intoxication, an increase in the volume of free water in the body. This results in decreased sodium.

water-reactive materials, materials that will react and release energy after coming in contact with water.

water tender, any ground vehicle capable of transporting specified quantities of water.

watt (James Watt, Scottish engineer, 1736-1819), the power produced by 1 ampere of current flowing with a force or pressure of 1 volt; the work of 1 joule per second.

wavy flexibility, a condition often found in catatonic schizophrenia. The arms and legs stay for an indefinite period of time in the positions in which they are placed.

wean, to take from a patient something on which he or she is dependent.

weaver's bottom. See **bursitis.**

web, a network of fibers forming a tissue or a membrane.

webbing, nylon or polyester strap that, when tied together, form slings used for attaching to anchors and rope. Two major types of webbing are flat and tubular. Used extensively in mountaineering and caving, this material attaches climbers and equipment to rope and anchors.

wedge resection, the surgical removal of part of an organ. The segment removed is wedge-shaped.

weeping, 1. crying. **2.** slow-flowing fluid, as with a sore or rash.

weight belt, device used when scuba diving to provide an adequate amount of weight to offset the buoyancy of the diver and equipment. Premeasured weights may be added or removed when changing divers, equipment, or water. The goal is to achieve neutral buoyancy. All belts must be equipped with a quick-release device for rapid removal in the event of emergency.

Weil's disease /wīls/. See **leptospirosis.**

weir, a small dam. Also known as a **low-head dam.**

Wenckebach (Karel F. Wenckebach, Dutch physician, 1864-1940). See **Mobitz type I.**

Wernicke's encephalopathy (Karl Wernicke, German physician, 1848-1905), altered levels of consciousness, ataxia, hypothermia, and nystagmus due, in part, to a thiamine deficiency in alcoholic and malnourished patients. Research indicates that a congenital deficiency of the enzyme, transketolase, may contribute to this condition. Because the pathology is similar for Korsakoff's psychosis, these two conditions are often treated as one, known as **Wernicke-Korsakoff's syndrome** (or **encephalopathy**). See also Korsakoff's psychosis.

wet glacier, a glacier covered with snow.

wet lung, a respiratory condition with a persistent cough. It occurs in workers exposed to lung irritants, such as ammonia, chlorine, sulfur dioxide, organic acids, dusts, and vapors of corrosive chemicals. Compare **pulmonary edema.** See also pleural effusion, pleurisy.

wet suit, a thermal protective suit used by divers that allows a thin layer of water between the skin and suit. This water layer is rapidly warmed by the body, providing increased warmth in cooler water. Generally of two-piece construction, these suits also provide some protection against stinging animals and abrasion.

whale's tail, a descending device made of a solid piece of machined metal with several slots cut into it. The rope is run back and forth through the slots to increase friction. Primarily developed for caving, this device is used as a brake bar.

Wharton's jelly, a soft, jellylike substance of the umbilical cord.

wheal, a transient elevated lesion caused by injection or local edema.

wheeze, a whistling sound with a musical quality, resulting from narrowing of large or small airways. Although this is normally heard via auscultation of the chest, significant wheezing may be externally audible. Precipitating factors include bronchospasm, chronic obstructive pulmonary disease, pulmonary edema, foreign body obstruction, and tumors. When pulmonary edema is due to cardiac dysfunction, any wheezes that result are termed **cardiac asthma.**

whiplash, *(informal)* an injury to the cervical vertebrae or their supporting ligaments and muscles, causing pain and stiffness. It usually results from a violent movement of the head and neck. Also known as **cervical sprain.**

Whipple's disease, a rare intestinal disease with severe inability to absorb nutrients, anemia, weight loss, and joint pain. *See also malabsorption syndrome.*

whipworm infection, a condition of being infested with the roundworm *Trichuris trichiura.* Heavy infestation may cause nausea, abdominal pain, diarrhea, and anemia. It is common in tropic areas with poor sanitation. Prevention includes proper disposal of feces and good personal hygiene. Also known as **trichuriasis.**

white blood cell. See **leukocyte.**

white damp, carbon monoxide gas when found underground, as in a mine or sewer. *See also damp.*

whitehead. See **milia.**

white matter, the tissue surrounding the gray matter of the spinal cord. It consists of sheathed nerve fibers and is subdivided in each half of the spinal cord into three sections (funiculi): the anterior, posterior, and lateral white column. Compare **gray matter.** *See also spinal cord.*

whiteout, the loss of visual perception due to blowing snow. This condition is frequently encountered during helicopter operations in the snow, causing loss of visibility for the flight crew. Heavy wind or thick snowfall may also cause this condition.

whiteout syndrome, psychosis that can occur in those exposed to the stimulus deprivation of a snowy environment.

whitewater, a rapidly flowing body of water, which creates turbulence as it flows over and around natural obstacles and those made by humans.

whitlow, an inflammation of the end of a finger or toe. *See also felon.*

whole blood, blood that is unchanged except for the presence of an anti-clotting agent. It is generally used for transfusion.

whole-body exposure, an exposure of the body to radiation, where the entire body rather than an isolated part is irradiated.

whorl, a spiral turn, as in one of the ridges that form fingerprints.

will, **1.** the mental faculty that enables one consciously to choose or decide on a course of action. **2.** determination or purpose; willfulness. **3.** an expression or declaration in a legal document of a person's wishes as to the use of property, taking effect after death.

windchill, the loss of heat from the body when exposed to wind of a given speed at a given temperature and humidity. The **windchill index** is given in kilocalories per hour per square meter of skin surface. The **windchill factor** is the rate of cooling in kilogram-calories per square meter per hour of an unclad, inactive body when exposed to specific wind velocities and temperatures. See Appendices 3-18 and 3-19.

window, an opening in the surface of a structure.

wind sock, cone-shaped tube with both ends open, which is used for indicating wind direction and general windspeed. These devices are located at airports and helipads for use by pilots during landing and takeoff.

winter itch, pruritis occurring in cold weather in people who have dry skin, particularly with inflammation.

wipe sample, a sample taken for the purpose of determining the presence of removable radioactive contamination on a surface. It is taken by wiping a piece of soft filter paper over a representative surface area. Also known as **smear sample.**

wire ladder splint. See **ladder splint, splint.**

wire rope sling, a lifting device of wire rope with an eye at each end.

wire span, the distance between utility poles.

withdrawal, **1.** termination of drug administration to an individual that is addicted to the drug. **2.** syndrome that occurs when an addictive drug is suddenly discontinued after prolonged use.

Symptoms include altered level of consciousness, anxiety, chest pain, combativeness, fever, irritability, pain, and tremors.

Wolff-Parkinson-White syndrome (Louis Wolff, American physician, 1898-1972; Sir John Parkinson, British physician, twentieth century; Paul D. White, American physician, 1886-1973), a paroxysmal tachycardia that occurs because of the presence of an extra (accessory) conduction pathway, which bypasses the AV node. Characteristics of the syndrome are a rate of 150-300 beats per minute, a PR interval of less than 0.12 second, a QRS complex duration longer than 0.10 second, and the presence of a delta wave (slurred upstroke to the QRS complex). Also known as **WPW.** *See also delta wave, Lown-Ganong-Levine syndrome, preexcitation.*

wolf pack, clustered traffic with long stretches of open road between groups. Driving in these clusters is dangerous, because drivers tend not to leave enough maneuvering room for emergencies.

womb. See **uterus.**

word salad, a jumble of words and phrases that lacks meaning. It is often seen in seriously confused persons and schizophrenics.

working capacity over an edge, a rope's ability to absorb energy while hanging over an edge. The capacity for energy absorption while bent over an edge is less that the rope's static breaking strength and should not be forgotten when figuring safe load limits for a particular rope. Also known as **WCOE.**

work-up, the process of completing an initial evaluation of a patient, to include history, physical examination, laboratory tests, or other diagnostic techniques. The purpose is to establish a diagnosis and treatment plan.

World Health Organization, an agency of the United Nations, concerned with worldwide or regional health problems. Its tasks include offering technical assistance, advancing an investigation of diseases, recommending health regulations, and promoting cooperation among professional health groups. Also known as **WHO.**

wormian bone (Olaus Worm, Danish anatomist, 1588-1654), any of several smooth, segmented bones, usually found as the sawlike borders of the joints between the skull bones.

wound, **1.** any physical injury involving a break in the skin. **2.** to cause an injury, especially one that breaks the skin.

wound ballistics, the factors that determine the potential of a bullet (missile) to cause damage to the body. These factors include the amount of energy transmitted to the body, behavior on penetration, direction of transmitted energy, and velocity of the bullet.

wound irrigation, the cleansing of a wound or the cavity formed by a wound using a solution to remove fluid and dried blood.

wound repair, restoration of the normal structure after an injury, especially of the skin. *See also healing, intention.*

wrist, the joint between the forearm and the hand, of eight bones arranged in two rows. Also known as **carpus.**

writer's cramp, a painful involuntary tightening of the muscles of the hand after long periods of fine detail work.

wrongful death statute, *(in law)* a statute existing in all states that says that the death of a person allows for legal action against the person whose willful or negligent acts caused the death. Before the existence of these statutes, a civil suit could be brought only if the injured person survived the jury.

wryneck. See **torticollis.**

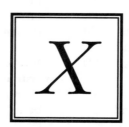

xanthine /zan´thēn/, a nitrogen compound normally found in the muscles, liver, spleen, pancreas, and urine.

xanthine derivative, any one of the closely linked alkaloids caffeine, theobromine, or theophylline. The xanthine derivatives stimulate the central nervous system.

xanthinuria /-oŏr´ē·ə/, **1.** the presence of excess quantities of xanthine in the urine. **2.** a rare disorder that results in the release of large amounts of xanthine in the urine.

xanthopsia /zanthop´sē·ə/, a visual condition in which everything appears with a yellow hue. It is often connected to liver disease or digitalis poisoning.

xanthosis /zanthō´-/, a yellowish discoloration of the skin. Sometimes seen in cancerous diseases, it is commonly caused by eating large amounts of yellow vegetables with carotene. The antimalarial drug quinacrine, if taken over a long period, may produce a similar skin color. Xanthosis can be differentiated from jaundice because the sclerae are yellow in jaundice but are not in xanthosis. *See also carotenemia.*

X chromosome, a sex chromosome that in humans is present in both sexes. It appears singly in the cells of males and in duplicate in the cells of females. Compare **Y chromosome.**

xenobiotic /zē´nōbī·ot´ik/, organic substances that are foreign to the body, as drugs or organic poisons.

xenogeneic /-jənē´ik/, individuals or cell types from different species and different genotypes.

xenophobia, an anxiety disorder with a fear of strangers.

xerophthalmia /zir´ofthal´mē·ə/, dry corneas, usually due to a lack of vitamin A and linked to night blindness.

xerostomia /-stō´mē·ə/, dryness of the mouth, a common side effect of drugs.

xiphoid process /zī´foid, zif´-/, the smallest of three sections of the sternum, near the seventh rib.

X-linked, referring to genes or to the traits or conditions they transmit that are carried on the X chromosome. Most X-linked traits and conditions, such as hemophilia, are recessive and therefore occur mostly in males, because they have only one X chromosome. Compare **Y-linked.**

x-ray, high-energy electromagnetic radiation in which wavelengths are shorter than ultraviolet radiation (0.1-100 angstroms). They are used for diagnostic and therapeutic purposes to destroy diseased tissues, ascertain the integrity of structures, and to create photographic images.

x-ray fluoroscopy, an examination that uses an x-ray source that projects through the patient onto a fluorescent screen or image intensifier.

XX, the designation for the normal sex chromosome complement in the human female. *See also X chromosome.*

XY, the normal sex chromosome complement in the human male.

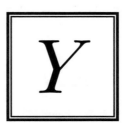

yaw, the vertical (sideways) axis of three-dimensional movement, usually relating to aircraft or ship motion. *See also pitch, roll.*

yaws /yôs/, a nonvenereal infection caused by a spirochete (*Treponema pertenue*). It is transmitted by direct contact. Symptoms include ulcer-like sores on the body with eventual tissue and bone destruction. It is a disease of unsanitary tropic living conditions.

Y chromosome, a sex chromosome that in humans is present singly in the male. It is carried as a sex determinant by one half of the male gametes and none of the female gametes. It has genes linked to triggering the development of male characteristics. Compare **X chromosome.**

yeast /yēst/, a fungus that reproduces by budding. *Candida albicans* is a kind of disease producing yeast.

yellow fever, an infection transmitted by mosquitoes. Symptoms include headache, fever, jaundice, vomiting, and hemorrhage.

yellow marrow, specialized adipose tissue found in the outer layer of the head of adult long bones. This tissue was red bone marrow, producing red blood cells, before age transformed it into inactive marrow.

Yersinia arthritis /yursin´ē·ə/, a joint inflammation occurring a few days to 1 month after an infection by either of two bacteria (*Yersinia enterocolitica* or *Y. pseudotuberculosis*). Knees, ankles, toes, fingers, and wrists are most often affected.

Y fracture, a **Y**-shaped fracture between the condyles at the end of a bone.

Y-linked, referring to genes or to traits or conditions they transmit that are carried on the Y chromosome. Compare **X-linked.**

yolk sac, a structure that develops in the inner cell mass of the embryo and expands into a sac. After supplying the nourishment for the embryo, the yolk sac usually disappears during the seventh week of pregnancy.

Z

Zahorsky's disease. See **roseola infantum.**

zero force current, *(electricity)* direct current (DC).

zero visibility, visibility restricted to 50 feet vertically or 165 feet horizontally; no visibility.

zinc, a bluish-white crystal-like metal. It is an essential nutrient in the body and is used in numerous drugs, such as zinc acetate, zinc oxide, zinc permanganate, and zinc stearate.

zinc salt poisoning, a toxic condition caused by eating or breathing a zinc salt. Symptoms include a burning sensation of the mouth and throat, vomiting, diarrhea and abdominal and chest pain. Hypotension and coma may follow.

Z line, the membrane-type structure found at both ends of a sarcomere.

zoanthropy /zō·an´thrəpē/, the false belief that one has the form and characteristics of an animal. *adj.*

Zollinger-Ellison syndrome, a condition marked by severe ulceration of the esophagus, stomach, or duodenum, excessive release of gastric fluid, and tumor of the pancreas or duodenum. The disorder is seen more often in patients between 20 and 50 years of age. *See also ulcer.*

zona pellucida /pəloō´sidə/, the thick, transparent membrane that encloses the egg (ovum). It is released by the ovum during its development in the ovary. It is kept until near the time of implantation. Also known as **oolemma.**

zone, an area with specific boundaries and traits, such as the epigastric zone of the stomach, the hot zone of a hazardous material spill.

zone of coagulation, the central area of a burn wound that has had the most intense thermal contact. The cells within this zone sustain coagulation necrosis and become nonviable. *See also zone of hyperemia, zone of stasis.*

zone of hyperemia, an area of increased blood flow due to inflammatory response to injury. This area is the outermost region affected by a burn injury. *See also zone of coagulation, zone of stasis.*

zone of stasis, an area of burn injury that surrounds the zone of coagulation. The tissue in this area is potentially viable. *See also zone of coagulation, zone of hyperemia.*

zonula ciliaris /zōn´yələ sil´ē·er´is/, a series of fibers connecting the ciliary body of the eye with the lens. It holds the lens in place. It relaxes by the contraction of the ciliary muscle. This allows the lens to become more rounded. *See also ciliary body, eye.*

zoology, the study of animal life.

zoonosis /zō´ənō´-, zō·on´əsis/, a disease of animals that can be carried to humans. Types of zoonoses include **equine encephalitis, leptospirosis, rabies, yellow fever.**

zooparasite /zō´əper´əsīt/, any parasitic animal organism. Kinds of zooparasites are **arthropods, protozoa, worms.**

zoophilia /zō´əfil´y·ə/, **1.** an abnormal fondness for animals. **2.** *(in psychiatry)* a sexual disorder in which sexual excitement occurs from the fantasy or act of sexual activity with animals.

zoophobia /zō´ə-/, an anxiety disorder. It is marked by a persistent, irrational fear of animals, particularly dogs, snakes, insects, and mice.

zoopsia /zō·op´sē·ə/, hallucination of seeing insects or other animals. This often occurs in delirium tremens.

zootoxicology /zō´ōtok´sikol´əjē/, the study of animal venoms, such as that from cone shells or snakes.

zootoxin /zō´ətok´sin/, a poisonous substance from an animal, such as the venom of snakes, spiders, and scorpions.

zoster. See **herpes zoster.**

Z rig, rope-lifting system utilizing pulleys that change rope direction up to 180°. This system utilizes the mechanical advantage obtained from the pulleys in configurations of 3:1 to 9:1 or greater. Larger loads can be safely lifted by fewer rescuers.

zygoma /zīgō´mə, zig-/, **1.** a long, slender projection from the temporal bone of the skull. **2.** the cheekbone (zygomatic bone).

zygomatic bone, one of the pair of bones that underlie the area of the cheek.

zygomatic process, one of two bones that form the lower orbit of the eye and the prominence of the cheek. Also known as **zygomatic bone.**

zygomaticus major /-mat´ikəs/, one of the 12 muscles of the mouth, used to smile or laugh.

zygomaticus minor, one of the 12 muscles of the mouth, used in making a frown.

zygomycosis /-mīkō´-/, a fungal infection caused by certain water molds. It is seen primarily in patients with long-term wasting diseases, especially uncontrolled diabetes mellitus. It often begins with fever and pain and may invade the eye and respiratory system. Also known as **mucormycosis.** Compare **phycomycosis.**

zygote /zī´gōt/, *(embryology)* the developing egg (ovum) from the time it is fertilized until, as a blastocyst, it is implanted in the uterus.

-zyme, a combining form meaning a ferment or enzyme.

APPENDICES

ASSESSMENT

1-1   Types of Lesions

Primary (earliest changes to appear and most important to recognize):

bulla circumscribed, elevated lesion greater than 5 mm in diameter, such as in friction injuries, second-degree burns. Also known as **blister.**

macule flat, discolored spot 10 mm or less in diameter, of varied shape, such as a freckle.

nodule palpable, solid lesion that may or may not be elevated, 5 to 10 mm in diameter, such as cysts, fibromas.

papule solid, elevated lesion 10 mm or smaller, such as a wart.

patch flat, discolored spot greater than 10 mm in diameter, of varied shape, such as a port-wine mark.

plaque solid, elevated skin lesion greater than 10 mm in diameter or a group of confluent papules, as in psoriasis, some acne.

pustule superficial lesion containing pus, such as carbuncles, impetigo.

telangiectasia dilated superficial blood vessels, as in rosacea, scleroderma.

tumor a solid and palpable lesion greater than 20 mm in diameter, either benign or malignant, such as lipoma, neoplasm.

vesicle circumscribed, elevated lesion 5 mm or less in diameter, containing serous fluid, as in herpes, insect bites.

wheal transient, elevated lesion caused by local edema, as in allergic reaction, insect sting.

Secondary (resulting from natural evolution of primary lesions or patient manipulation of primary lesions):

atrophy thinned, wrinkled skin.

crust dried blood, pus, or serum. Also known as **scab.**

erosion loss of all or part of the epidermis.

excoriation linear or hollowed-out crusted area due to picking, rubbing, or scratching.

lichenification thickened skin with accentuated skin markings.

scales heaped-up particles of horny epithelium.

scar result of healing after destruction of some dermis.

ulcer loss of epidermis and at least part of the dermis.

1-2   Cranial Nerves

Cranial Nerve	Dysfunction Caused by Damage
1st, Olfactory	Loss of ability to smell
2nd, Optic	Loss of sight
3rd, Oculomotor	Dilated, unreactive pupil; poor downward, medial, and upward gaze
4th, Trochlear	Difficulty with downward gaze when eye is located medially
5th, Trigeminal	Loss of corneal reflex and facial sensation
6th, Abducens	Loss of lateral eye movement
7th, Facial	Loss of taste on anterior portion of tongue; painful increase in sensation of sound; weakened facial muscles
8th, Auditory	Loss of hearing; nystagmus; vertigo
9th, Glossopharyngeal	Decreased oropharyngeal sensation
10th, Vagus	Impaired gag reflex and speech
11th, Accessory	Weakened sternocleidomastoid muscle and shoulder movement
12th, Hypoglossal	Difficulty with tongue movement

1-3 General Spinal Dermatomes

Sensory deficits follow these general patterns after nerve/spinal cord damage.

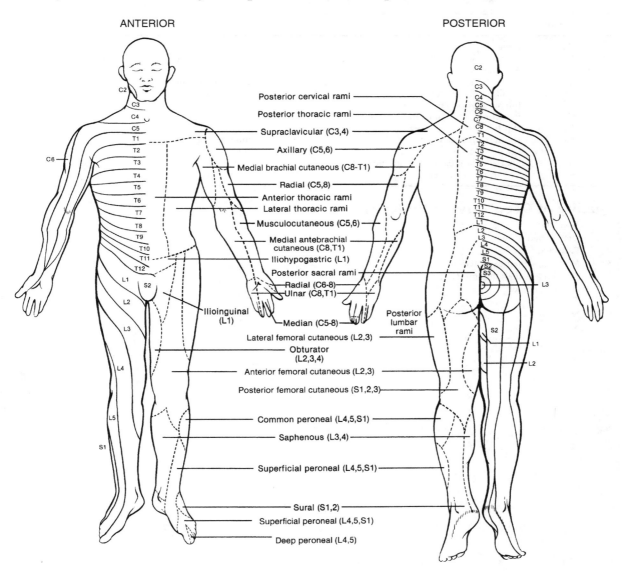

ANTERIOR

POSTERIOR

Posterior cervical rami
Posterior thoracic rami
Supraclavicular (C3,4)
Axillary (C5,6)
Medial brachial cutaneous (C8-T1)
Radial (C5,8)
Anterior thoracic rami
Lateral thoracic rami
Musculocutaneous (C5,6)
Medial antebrachial cutaneous (C8,T1)
Iliohypogastric (L1)
Posterior sacral rami
Radial (C6-8)
Ulnar (C8,T1)
Ilioinguinal (L1)
Median (C5-8)
Lateral femoral cutaneous (L2,3)
Obturator (L2,3,4)
Anterior femoral cutaneous (L2,3)
Posterior femoral cutaneous (S1,2,3)
Posterior lumbar rami
Common peroneal (L4,5,S1)
Saphenous (L3,4)
Superficial peroneal (L4,5,S1)
Sural (S1,2)
Superficial peroneal (L4,5,S1)
Deep peroneal (L4,5)

(From Mosby-Year Book, Inc. *Wilderness Medicine: Management of Wilderness and Environmental Emergencies,* Auerbach; "Wilderness Trauma Emergencies," Morris, Jr., et al., 3rd ed. pg. 316, St. Louis, MO, 1995)

1-4   Spinal Cord Injury Levels

		Function Lost		
Level of Lesion	*Motor*		*Sensory*	*Reflex*
C2	Breathing		occiput	none
C4	Spontaneous breathing, trapezius movement		suprasternal notch	none
C6	Arm flexion		thumb	biceps
C7	Arm extension		index/middle finger	triceps
C8	Small hand muscles		small finger	none
T4	Intercostal/abdominal muscles		nipple line	none
T10	Intercostal/abdominal muscles		umbilicus	none
L1	Hip flexion		groin	cremaster
L2	Hip flexion/adduction		anterior thigh	cremaster
L4	Knee extension		knee	patellar
S1	Foot and/or great toe plantar flexion		lateral foot	Achilles
S2	Rectal sphincter tone		perianal region	anal wink

Quality of Deep Tendon Reflexes

0	No response
1+	Diminished, sluggish
2+	Expected response
3+	More brisk than expected
4+	Hyperactive with intermittent or transient clonus

1-5 Signs

Aaron's (acute appendicitis) referred pain or feeling of distress in the epigastric or precordial regions with continuous firm pressure over McBurney's point.

accessory a finding frequently, though not consistently, present in a disease.

Allis's (fracture of the neck of the femur) riding up of the trochanter so that the fascia lata relaxes, allowing the finger to be inserted deeply between the great trochanter and iliac crest.

Auenbrugger's (marked pericardial effusion) an epigastric prominence.

Babinski's (pyramidal tract disease or injury) extension of the great toe with abduction of the other toes on stimulation of the plantar surface of the foot (positive Babinski), instead of the normal flexion reflex. (Although other signs use the same name, this is the one most commonly referred to in emergency medicine.) Also known as **Babinski's reflex, Babinski's phenomenon, paradoxical extensor reflex.**

Ballance's (ruptured spleen) dull percussion in both flanks, constant on the left, but shifting with change of position on the right (thought to be due to the presence of blood that is coagulated on the left, but fluid on the right).

Bamberger's (pericarditis with effusion) dullness to percussion at the angle of the scapula that clears when the patient leans forward.

Battle's (basilar skull and/or temporal bone fracture) ecchymosis over the mastoid process behind one or both ears.

Bechterew's (nervous system disease or injury) automatic facial movement paralysis, while capability for voluntary facial movement remains.

Beevor's (paralysis of the lower recti abdominis muscles) superior change in position of the umbilicus.

Biot's breathing (increased intracranial pressure) irregular periods of apnea that alternate with several deep breaths.

blue dot (torsion of a testicular appendage) a black or blue spot visible under the skin on the superior portion of epididymis or testis.

Blumberg's (peritonitis) pain occurring over a suspected area of abdomen on sudden release of steadily applied pressure.

Braxton Hicks's (pregnancy) irregular uterine contractions occurring after the third month of pregnancy.

Brudzinski's (meningitis) **1.** when the neck is passively flexed, leg flexion will also occur. Also known as **neck sign. 2.** when one leg is passively flexed, similar movement will occur in the other. Also known as **contralateral reflex, contralateral sign.**

burning drops (perforated gastric ulcer) a sensation similar to hot liquid falling into the abdominal cavity.

Byrant's (dislocation of the shoulder) an abnormal position of skin folds in the axilla develops.

Cantelli's (normal functioning brainstem) upward movement of the eyes as the head is lowered in the unconscious patient. See also **doll's eye sign.**

Carnett's (intraabdominal pain) the disappearance of abdominal tenderness on the contraction of the anterior abdominal muscles.

Castellani-Low (sleeping sickness) fine tremor of the tongue.

Chaddock's (corticospinal reflex disease) extension of the great toe when the skin in the area of the lateral malleolus is irritated.

chandelier (abdominal pain) *(informal)* pain of a severity that causes patients being examined to reach upward for relief, particularly in cases of pelvic inflammatory disease.

Chaussier's (preeclampsia) severe epigastric pain, indicating a deterioration toward eclampsia (may be due to liver capsule distention as a result of hemorrhage).

Chvostek's (tetany) facial irritability causing a unilateral spasm of the orbicularis oculi (oris) muscle when the facial nerve anterior to the external auditory meatus is tapped. Also known as **Weiss's sign.**

Claybrook's (rupture of abdominal viscus) transmission of breath and heart sounds into the abdominal cavity (may be auscultated over the abdomen).

Cleemann's (femur fracture) when the bone fragments override, wrinkling of the skin over the patella occurs.

clenched fist (angina and/or myocardial infarction) pressing with a fist against the chest in response to severe chest discomfort.

Comby's (measles) thin whitish patches on the mucous membranes of the cheek and gum.

commemorative pointing to the previous existence of a disease other than the one present.

Comolli's (fracture of the scapula) a triangular swelling, corresponding with the outline of the scapula.

Coopernail's (pelvic fracture) ecchymosis of the perineum and labia or scrotum.

Cullen's (intraabdominal hemorrhage, as in ectopic pregnancy, pancreatitis, trauma) an ecchymotic halo in the area around the umbilicus.

Danforth's (ruptured ectopic pregnancy) shoulder pain on inspiration, due to hemoperitoneum irritating the diaphragm.

doll's eye (normal functioning brainstem) eye movement in the opposite direction of head movement in the unconscious patient. Also known as **ocular vestibular reflex.** See also **Cantelli's sign.**

Drummond's (aortic aneurysm) a puffing sound from the nostrils that can be heard when the mouth is closed.

Duchenne's (paralysis of the diaphragm) collapse of the epigastrium during inspiration.

edema of lower lid (congestive heart failure, myxedema, nephrosis) swelling of the lower eyelid.

Ewing's (pericardial effusion) dullness to percussion of the inside angle of the medial left scapula.

eyelash (normal reflex function) movement of the eyelids when eyelashes are touched or stroked. Useful in determining the actual level of consciousness in patients who appear unconscious, this reflex will not occur in cases of serious cerebral compromise, such as CVA, seizures, subdural hematoma.

Faget's (yellow fever) elevated temperature with a slow pulse.

flag (kwashiorkor, protein depletion) hair discoloration occurring in bands or striations.

Forcheimer's (German measles) a reddish eruption of papules on the soft palate.

Graefe's (Graves's disease) sluggishness of upper eyelid movement in response to downward gaze.

Grasset's (hemiplegia) normal contraction on the paralyzed side of the sternocleidomastoid muscle.

Grey Turner's (retroperitoneal hemorrhage) ecchymosis of the area around the flanks and umbilicus.

Grocco's (hepatomegaly) extension of the percussive dullness of the liver to the left of the midline.

groove (lymphogranuloma venereum) hard, tender inguinal lymph nodes above and below the inguinal ligament, creating a groove along the ligament.

Hamman's (mediastinal emphysema) a crunching sound, auscultated over the chest, that is synchronous with the heartbeat. Also known as **Hamman's crunch, xiphisternal crunching.**

Hill's (aortic insufficiency) elevated systolic blood pressure in the legs. Normal systolic pressures are up to 20 millimeters higher in the legs than the arms. In the presence of this sign, those pressures may be elevated up to 90 millimeters higher in the legs. Also known as **Hill's phenomenon.**

Hoagland's (mononucleosis) edema of the eyelids.

Homan's (deep vein thrombosis of the lower extremities) pain in the calf or posterior knee on slow dorsiflexion of the ankle with the knee bent.

Hoover's (leg paralysis) while lying supine, a patient who attempts to lift a paralyzed leg will exert a counterpressure with the heel of the opposite foot. This does not occur if there is no paralysis present.

Hueter's (fractures) sound transmission that can be auscultated or palpated when tapping normal bone will not occur if fractured ends are separated by deformity or tissue. Also known as **Hillson's sign.**

Joffroy's (organ brain disease) an inability to do simple addition or multiplication when that faculty previously existed.

Kehr's (splenic rupture) severe left shoulder pain.

Landolfi's (aortic insufficiency) systolic contraction and diastolic dilation of the pupil.

Lasègue's (lumbar root or sciatic nerve irritation) while lying supine with the hip flexed, dorsiflexing the ankle will cause muscle spasm and/or pain in the posterior thigh.

Laugier's (fracture of the distal radius) the styloid processes of the radius and ulna will be located at the same level.

Legendre's (facial hemiplegia) when the eyelids of actively closed eyes are raised, there is decreased resistance on the affected side.

Leichtenstern's (spinal meningitis) gentle tapping of an extremity bone causes violent movement.

Magnan's (cocaine addiction) paresthesias that are imagined to feel like a grain of sand that changes position under the skin.

Mannkopf's (pain) acceleration of pulse rate when a painful location is palpated.

Marcus Gunn's (optic nerve defect) the pupil of one eye constricts poorly or dilates when exposed to light. Also known as **Gunn's sign.**

Masini's (mentally unstable children) significant dorsal extension of the fingers and toes.

McBurney's (appendicitis) tenderness two-thirds of the distance between the umbilicus and the superior iliac crest.

Murphy's (cholecystitis) pain when palpating the right costal margin during inspiration.

Musset's (aortic valve dysfunction) rhythmic nodding of the head, synchronized with the heartbeat.

Néri's (hemiplegia) the knee spontaneously bends when the leg is passively extended.

Osler's (bacterial endocarditis) painful, rounded areas of erythema on the hands and feet, ranging in size from a pinhead to a pea.

Payr's (thrombophlebitis) pain when pressure is applied to the sole of the foot.

Perez's (aortic arch aneurysm) crackles auscultated over the superior chest when the arms are raised and lowered.

physical those signs that are observed during auscultation, palpation, or percussion.

raccoon eyes (basilar skull or facial bone fracture) ecchymosis and edema around one or both eyes.

Ransohoff's (rupture of the common bile duct) yellowing of the umbilical region.

Revilliod's (hemiplegia) an inability to close the eye on the side of the paralysis unless the other eye is also closed. Also known as **sign of the orbicularis.**

Romberg's (intoxication, neurological illness or disease) increased unsteadiness when closing the eyes (after placing the feet together while standing with eyes open). Also known as **Romberg test, station test.**

Rotch's (pericardial effusion) dullness to percussion in the right fifth intercostal space.

Russell's (bulimia) abrasion or scars on the back of the hands due to attempts at self-induced vomiting.

spine (meningitis) resistance to flexion of the spine.

Sternburg's (pleurisy) tenderness of the shoulder muscles on palpation of the side with pleurisy.

Sumner's (early appendicitis, ovarian cyst, or renal calculi) slight increase in firmness or tone of the abdominal muscles when palpated over the left or right iliac fossa.

Thomson's (scarlet fever) pink or red lines in the antecubital space (bend of the elbow). Also known as **Pastia's sign.**

Westphal (central nervous system disease) loss of the patellar tendon reflex. Also known as **Erb's sign, Erb–Westphal sign, Westphal's phenomenon.**

wrist (Marfan's syndrome) when gripping the wrist with the opposite hand, the thumb and fifth finger will overlap significantly.

1-6 Odor Origins

acetone (breath, sweat): acetone or isopropyl alcohol ingestion, anorexia nervosa, diabetic ketoacidosis, diphtheria, lacquer ingestion, salicylate use

alcohol (breath, clothes, emesis): chloral hydrate, ethyl (drinking) alcohol, phenol ingestions

almond (breath): cyanide (in addition to the commercial type, it may also be ingested from the pits/seeds of apples (*Malus*), apricots, cherries (especially black/wild), peaches, and plums.

ammonia (breath, sweat, urine): bladder infection, kidney failure

bad breath: amphetamine abuse, dental disease and/or poor hygiene

baked bread (breath, sweat): typhoid

breath mint: odor to disguise alcohol

burned rope (breath, clothes): marijuana

disinfectants (breath, clothes, emesis): creosote, phenol

fecal/foul smell (breath, sputum): intestinal obstruction, lung abscess

fruit-like (breath, emesis): alcohol, amyl nitrate, diabetic ketoacidosis

garlic (breath, emesis, sweat): arsenic, garlic ingestion, organophosphates, phosphorus, selenium, tellurium, thallium

isopropyl alcohol (body smell): used as a remedy by some and rubbed on chest, neck

maple syrup (sweat, urine): Maple syrup disease (infant disease that causes deterioration of the central nervous system and death due to metabolic failure)

mothballs (breath, emesis): camphor products

necrosis (body smell): dead tissue

offensive, strong body odor: acromegaly, infected sweat glands,
poor hygiene

peanuts (breath, emesis): Vacor (rodenticide)

rotten apples (body smell): gas gangrene

rotten eggs (breath, sweat, stool): acetylcystine (Mucomyst), disulfiram (Antabuse), hydrogen sulfide, liver failure

shoe polish (breath, emesis): nitrobenzene

sweet, musty (breath, sweat): adult liver failure

urine (sweat, urine): incontinence, uremia

vinyl-like, pungent (breath, emesis): Placidyl

violets (breath, emesis, sweat, urine): turpentine poisoning

wintergreen (breath, body smell, emesis): breath mint, methyl salicylate

1-7 Urine Color Origins

blue, green: amitriptyline, indigo blue, methylene blue, Pseudomonas, triamterene (Dyazide)

brown, black: cascara, hemoglobin, melanin, methocarbamol (Robaxin), methyldopa (Aldomet), rhubarb

orange: dehydration, phenazopyridine (Pyridium), rifampin, sulfasalazine (Azulfdine)

red: beets, blackberries, hematuria, hemoglobinuria, iron, lead, mercury, myoglobinuria, phenothiazines, phenytonin (Dilantin), pyrvinium (Povan)

reddish-brown: furazolidone, metronidazole (Flagyl), nitrofurantoin (Macrodantin), porphyria, seaweed, urobilinogen

1-8   Dysrhythmias

Rhythm	Rate (per minute)	
	Atrial	Ventricular
normal sinus rhythm	60–100	60–100
sinus arrhythmia	60–100	60–100
sinus bradycardia	>60	>60
sinus tachycardia	100–160	100–160
atrial fibrillation	<350	varies
atrial flutter	250–350	varies
atrial tachycardia	150–250	150–250
supraventricular tachycardia	150–250	150–250
junctional rhythm	40–60	40–60
accelerated junctional rhythm	60–100	60–100
junctional tachycardia	100–180	100–180
first-degree block	60–100*	60–100*
Wenckebach	60–100*	45–75 (3:1)*
classical second-degree	60–100*	30–50 (2:1)*
third-degree	40–80*	varies
idioventricular rhythm	0	20–40
accelerated idioventricular rhythm	0	40–60
ventricular tachycardia	0	150–250
ventricular fibrillation	not discernible	
asystole	0	0

*depends on underlying rhythm and/or degree of block

1-9 Sounds

auscultatory bruits, crackles, murmurs, wheezes, or other sounds heard on auscultation.

bowel generally high-pitched abdominal sounds that occur when intestinal contents are moved through the intestine.

coconut sounds (resembling those made when tapping a cracked coconut) that occur when tapping the skull of an osteitis deformans patient.

eddy sounds that interrupt the continuous murmur caused by patent ductus arteriosus.

ejection clicking-type sounds that occur during blood flow through a hypertensive aorta or pulmonary artery. Aortic or pulmonic valve stenosis may cause similar sounds.

first heart sound caused by the closing of the atrioventricular valves, which occurs during ventricular systole. It is a normal heart sound. Also known as S_1.

fourth heart a low-frequency sound occurring in the left and/or right ventricles during late diastole while ventricular filling occurs. Although it may be a normal finding in older patients, it is usually abnormal in younger ages, particularly when palpable. It is seen in acute myocardial infarction

and may be found in ventricular hypertrophy with hypertension. Also known as **atrial sound, S_4.**

friction the creaking or rasping sound caused by two inflamed serous membranes rubbing against one another. Also known as **friction murmur, friction rub.** *See also pericardial friction, pleural friction,* in this list.

gallop a triple cadence rhythm caused by the addition of abnormal third or fourth heart sounds to the first and second.

heart noises created by the closing of heart valves and cardiac muscle contraction.

Korotkoff's arterial sounds that occur when pressure applied to the artery is reduced to below the artery's systolic pressure; sounds heard when a blood pressure is taken by auscultation.

percussion those sounds caused when sharply tapping any underlying structure or cavity of the body.

pericardial friction the grating or rasping sound caused when inflamed pericardial surfaces rub against one another during cardiac contraction or relaxation. Also known as **pericardial friction rub.**

pistol-shot a noise created when a large artery (brachial, femoral, radial) is lightly compressed during aortic insufficiency.

pleural friction a creaking or grating sound occurring when inflamed parietal and visceral pleura rub each other during respirations. Also known as **pleural friction rub.**

respiratory any of the sounds heard during auscultation of the upper or lower airways, such as crackles, bruits, fremitus, rhonchi, rubs, wheezes.

second heart the normal sound caused by the closing of the semilunar valves at the beginning of diastole. Also known as S_2.

succussion noises created by air and/or fluid mixtures when shaken, as in the stomach.

third heart the sound occurring at the end of ventricular filling during early diastole. It is normal in children and abnormal in adults. Also known as S_3.

waterwheel splashing noises occurring in the pericardial sac when air and fluid are present and agitated by cardiac motion.

water-whistle a bubbling whistle heard over a bronchial or pulmonary fistula.

Grading Intensity of Heart Murmurs

Grade I	Barely audible in a quiet room
Grade II	Quiet, but clearly audible
Grade III	Moderately loud
Grade IV	Loud, associated with a thrill
Grade V	Very loud, thrill easily palpable
Grade VI	Very loud, audible with ear to chest, thrill palpable and visible

(Modified from Mosby-Year Book, Inc., *Mosby's Guide to Physical Examination,* Seidel, Henry M. et al., 3rd ed., p. 403, St. Louis, 1995)

1-10 APGAR Score*

Sign	0	1	2
Appearance (Skin color)	Blue, pale	Body pink, blue extremities	Completely pink
Pulse Rate (Heart rate)	Absent	<100/minute	>100/minute
Grimace (Irritability)	No response	Grimace	Cough, sneeze, cry
Activity (Muscle tone)	Limp	Some flexion	Active motion
Respirations (Respiratory effort)	Absent	Slow, irregular	Good, crying

(From Mosby-Year Book, Inc., *Pediatric Advanced Life Support*, Aehlert, B., p. 192, St. Louis, 1994)

*The first letter of each category in the APGAR scoring system corresponds to the last name of the system's inventor, Virginia Apgar, MD (1909-1974).

1-11 Major Diabetic Events*

Findings	Hypoglycemia	Hyperglycemia	HHNK Coma*
History			
Food intake	Insufficient	Excessive	Excessive
Insulin dosage	Excessive	Insufficient	Insufficient
Onset	Rapid	Gradual	Gradual
Infection	Uncommon	Common	Common
Gastrointestinal tract			
Thirst	Absent	Intense	Intense
Hunger	Intense	Absent	Intense
Vomiting	Uncommon	Common	Uncommon
Respiratory system			
Breathing	Normal or rapid	Deep or rapid	Shallow/rapid
Breath odor	Normal	Acetone smell	Normal
Cardiovascular system			
Blood pressure	Normal	Low	Low
Pulse	Normal, rapid, or full	Rapid or weak	Rapid or weak
Skin	Pale or moist	Warm or dry	Warm or dry
Nervous system			
Headache	Present	Absent	Absent
Consciousness	Irritability	Restless	Irritable
	Seizure or coma	Coma (rare)	Seizure or coma
Urine			
Sugar level	Absent	Present	Present
Acetone level	Usually absent	Usually present	Absent
Serum glucose levels	Less than 60 mg/dl	Greater than 300 mg/dl	More than 600 mg/dl
Treatment response	Immediate (after glucose) (*note:* If the hypoglycemic episode is prolonged or severe, the response may be delayed and may require more than one dose.	Gradual (within 6-12 hours after medication and fluid replacement)	Gradual (within 6-12 hours after medication and fluid replacement)

(From Clarke: *Pharmacological Basis of Nursing*, ed. 4, 1993, St. Louis, Mosby-Year Book, Inc. Seen in Mosby-Year Book, Inc., *Mosby's Paramedic Textbook*, Sanders, Mick J. et al., p. 678, St. Louis, 1994)

*HHNK = Hyperosmolar (hyperglycemic) nonketotic.

1-12 Classes of Hypovolemia

	Class I	Class II	Class III	Class IV
Blood loss (ml)	Up to 750	750-1500	1500-2000	2000 or more
Blood loss (%BV)	Up to 15%	15%-30%	30%-40%	40% or more
Pulse rate	<100	>100	>120	140 or higher
Blood pressure	Normal	Normal	Decreased	Decreased
Pulse pressure (mm Hg)	Normal or increased	Decreased	Decreased	Decreased
Capillary blanch test	Normal	Positive	Positive	Positive
Respiratory rate	14-20	20-30	30-40	>35
Urine output (ml/hr)	30 or more	20-30	5-15	Negligible
CNS—Mental status	Slightly anxious	Mildly anxious	Anxious, confused	Confused, lethargic
Fluid replacement (3:1 rule)	Cyrstalloid	Crystalloid	Crystalloid plus blood	Crystalloid plus blood

(Values in table based on a 70-kg male)

Note: Applied blindly, these guidelines can result in excessive or inadequate fluid administration. For example, a patient with a crush injury to the extremity will have hypotension out of proportion to his or her blood loss and will require fluids in excess of the 3:1 guidelines. In contrast, a patient whose ongoing blood loss is being replaced will require less than 3:1. The use of bolus therapy with careful monitoring of the patient's response can moderate these extremes.

(From American College of Surgeons Committee on Trauma, *Advanced Trauma Life Support® Student Manual,* 1993 edition)

1-13 Systems of Triage

TWO-TIER SYSTEM

Immediate life-threatening conditions that are readily correctable at the scene and those conditions that are urgent

Delayed no injury, noncritical conditions, ambulatory victims; those who will die—even with care, and the dead

THREE-TIER SYSTEM

Life-threatening readily correctable conditions

Urgent treatment required within one to two hours

Delayed no injury, noncritical conditions or ambulatory

FOUR-TIER SYSTEM

Immediate serious condition with a reasonable chance of survival

Delayed can wait for care after simple aid

Expectant extremely critical; probably will die

Minimal no impairment of function; either self-treatment or first aid will suffice

FIVE-TIER SYSTEM (PRIMARILY MILITARY)

Life-threatening conditions that are readily correctable

Urgent must be treated within one to two hours

Delayed noncritical or ambulatory

No injury or no treatment necessary

Dead or will die

(Modified from Mosby-Year Book, Inc., *Wilderness Medicine: Management of Wilderness and Environmental Emergencies,* Auerbach; "Natural Disaster Management," Noji, Eric K., 3rd ed., p. 656, St. Louis, 1995)

1-14   **START Triage Protocol**

Step 1

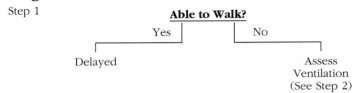

Able to Walk?

Yes → Delayed

No → Assess Ventilation (See Step 2)

Step 2

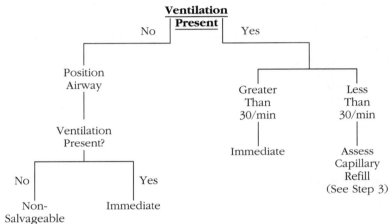

Ventilation Present

No → Position Airway → Ventilation Present?
- No → Non-Salvageable
- Yes → Immediate

Yes →
- Greater Than 30/min → Immediate
- Less Than 30/min → Assess Capillary Refill (See Step 3)

Step 3

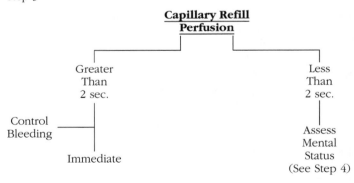

Capillary Refill Perfusion

Greater Than 2 sec. — Control Bleeding → Immediate

Less Than 2 sec. → Assess Mental Status (See Step 4)

Step 4

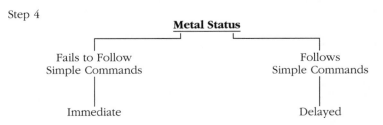

Metal Status

Fails to Follow Simple Commands → Immediate

Follows Simple Commands → Delayed

(From The C.V. Mosby Company, *Disaster Response,* Auf der Heide, Erik, p. 184-185, St. Louis, 1989, Adapted from Super, G.:
START Instructors Manual, Newport Beach, Presbyterian Hoag Memorial Hospital)

1-15   Triage Injury Classification by Categories

SIMPLE TRIAGE

Immediate (Priority I)
1. Asphyxia
2. Respiratory obstruction from mechanical causes
3. Sucking chest wounds
4. Tension pneumothorax
5. Maxillofacial wounds in which asphyxia exists or is likely to develop
6. Shock caused by major external hemorrhage
7. Major internal hemorrhage
8. Visceral injuries or evisceration
9. Cardio/pericardial injuries
10. Massive muscle damage
11. Severe burns *over* 25% BSA
12. Dislocations
13. Major fractures
14. Major medical problems readily correctable
15. Closed cerebral injuries with progressive loss of consciousness

Delayed (Priority II)
1. Vascular injuries requiring repair
2. Wounds of the genitourinary tract
3. Thoracic wounds without asphyxia
4. Severe burns *under* 25% BSA
5. Spinal cord injuries requiring decompression
6. Suspected spinal cord injuries without neurological signs
7. Lesser fractures
8. Injuries of the eye
9. Maxillofacial injuries without asphyxia
10. Minor medical problems
11. Victims with little hope of survival under the best circumstances of medical care

MASS CASUALTY TRIAGE WITH AN OVERWHELMING NUMBER OF INJURIES

Immediate (Priority I)
1. Asphyxia
2. Respiratory obstruction from mechanical causes
3. Sucking chest wounds
4. Tension pneumothorax
5. Maxillofacial wounds in which asphyxia exists or is likely to develop
6. Shock caused by major external hemorrhage
7. Dislocations
8. Severe burns *under* 25% BSA
9. Lesser fractures
10. Major medical problems that can be handled readily

Delayed (Priority II)
1. Major fractures (if able to stabilize)
2. Visceral injuries or evisceration
3. Cardio/pericardial injuries
4. Massive muscle damage
5. Severe burns *over* 25% BSA
6. Vascular injuries requiring repair
7. Wounds of the genitourinary tract
8. Thoracic wounds without asphyxia
9. Closed cerebral injuries with progressive loss of consciousness
10. Spinal cord injuries requiring decompression
11. Suspected spinal cord injuries without neurological signs
12. Injuries of the eye
13. Maxillofacial injuries without asphyxia
14. Complicated major medical problems
15. Minor medical problems
16. Victims with little hope of survival under the best circumstances of medical care

For use during re-triage by advanced life support personnel (Courtesy of Emergency Medical Services Authority, State of California)

1-16 Classification by Severity of High-Altitude Pulmonary Edema

Grade	Symptoms	Signs
1, Mild	Dyspnea on exertion Dry cough Fatigue while moving uphill	HR (rest) < 90-100 RR (rest) < 20 Dusky nailbeds Localized crackles, if any
2, Moderate	Dyspnea, weakness, fatigue on level walking Raspy cough, headache, anorexia	HR 90-100 RR 16-30 Cyanotic nailbeds Rhonchi present Ataxia may be present
3, Severe	Dyspnea at rest Productive cough Orthopnea Extreme weakness	HR > 110 RR > 30 Facial/nailbed cyanosis Bilateral rhonchi Ataxia and altered level of consciousness Blood-tinged sputum

(From Mosby-Year Book, Inc., *Wilderness Medicine: Management of Wilderness and Environmental Emergencies,* Auerbach; "High-Altitude Medicine," Hackett/Roach, 3rd ed., p. 20, St. Louis, 1995; modified from Dekker, *Lung Water and Solute Exchange: High-Altitude Pulmonary Edema,* Hultgren, H. N., New York, 1978)

1-17 Stages of Hypothermia

Stage	Core Temperature °C	°F	Characteristics
Mild	37.6	99.6	Normal rectal temperature
	37	98.6	Normal oral temperature
	35	95	Maximum heat production from shivering
	34	93.2	Amnesia, dysarthria, and poor judgment develop; normal BP; maximum respiratory stimulation
	33	91.4	Apathy/ataxia develop; J wave associated with QRS complex; cardiac output down 30%
Moderate	32	89.6	Altered level of consciousness; 25% decrease in oxygen consumption
	31	87.8	Heat production from shivering is extinguished
	30	86	Atrial fibrillation and other dysrhythmias develop; pulse and cardiac output $\frac{2}{3}$ of normal; poikilo-thermia
	29	85.2	Progressive decrease in level of consciousness, pulse, and respiration; pupils dilate
	28	82.4	Decreased ventricular fibrillation threshold; 50% decrease in oxygen consumption and pulse
	27	80.6	Loss of reflexes and voluntary motion
Severe	26	78.8	No reflexes or response to pain; major acid-base disturbances
	25	77	Pulmonary edema may develop; cardiac output 45% of normal; cerebral blood flow $\frac{1}{3}$ of normal
	24	75.2	Significant hypotension
	23	73.4	No corneal or oculocephalic reflexes
	22	71.6	Maximum risk of ventricular fibrillation; 75% decrease in oxygen consumption
	20	68	Pulse 20% of normal; lowest level of resumption of cardiac electromechanical activity
	19	66.2	Flat electroencephalogram
	18	64.4	Asystole

(Modified from Mosby-Year Book, Inc., *Emergency Medicine,* Rosen et al.; "Accidental Hypothermia," Danzl, D. F., 3rd ed., p. 917, St. Louis, 1992)

2-1   Body-Substance Isolation

The prevention of contact with blood and other potentially infectious materials is important for both current and future patients and caregivers. Limiting contact with infectious substances uses a technique previously known as universal precautions. But because contact with infectious substances in the field cannot easily be anticipated, it is safer to go beyond universal precautions and consider all body substances as potentially infectious. The presumption that wet is bad is the thought process behind body substance isolation. Though circumstances occur that make the wearing of current personal protective equipment (eye/face protection, gloves, pocket masks, etc.) impractical, the use of such equipment in the field should not be considered optional.

Gloves should be worn when contact is anticipated with blood/body fluids, mucous membranes, and skin that is not intact. In addition, contact with items or surfaces with fluid spills on them, routine interior vehicle cleaning, and any respiratory/vascular access procedures necessitate glove use. Remember that neither latex nor vinyl gloves are absolute barriers to infection and routine handwashing after glove removal is necessary. When facilities for immediate handwashing are not available, "waterless" antiseptic hand cleaner should be used until such facilities are reached.

When wearing gloves, health care providers should remember to avoid touching their faces with their hands until after adequate handwashing. The mere wearing of gloves does not protect from hazards being transmitted via gloves to the face. If a glove becomes torn during patient care, it should be replaced as promptly as patient safety permits.

When extrication, broken glass, sharp edges, or other hazardous situations are anticipated, structural firefighting gloves meeting OSHA firefighter glove standards should be worn. Patient care gloves are not a substitute for this increased protection. Patients may be cared for while wearing safety gloves with the provision that adequate glove cleaning be accomplished after the incident is over.

Faceshields or **mask/eyewear** should be worn when procedures generating droplets of blood/body fluids are performed, such as endotracheal intubation or intravenous punctures.

Disposable jumpsuits or gowns should be worn if blood/body fluid splashes can be anticipated. Primary work uniforms/flightsuits are not adequate for this purpose. Firefighting-type overwear can provide protection, but it must be adequately cleaned/decontaminated after a response.

Health care providers who have skin conditions that generate exudate should refrain from direct patient care until the condition is resolved.

Perform all procedures so as to minimize splashing or spattering of potentially infectious material.

All amputated/avulsed tissue, fluid samples, and other biological material should be transported in leak-proof containers. Glass tubes are best transported in sealable plastic bags.

Do not apply cosmetics, eat/chew, drink, or use tobacco products in areas in which patient care is performed, during patient care, or in areas where contaminated equipment is cleaned or stored.

Maintain up-to-date immunizations because they provide a great deal of protection from specific diseases.

Follow your organization's exposure reporting and follow-up procedures whenever you believe you have had a significant exposure.

2-2 Aircraft/Ambulance Sanitation

Daily sanitation reduces the possibility of cross infection. All patient contact areas should be cleaned with a solution described below once a day. (Windows and doors on aircraft need not be cleaned so often.) In addition, cleaning should occur after each patient transport. Properly dispose of all disposable patient care items, thoroughly remove all blood/body fluid secretions, and clean the floor.

Centers for Disease Control and Prevention recommend using a germicidal/virucidal solution effective against tuberculosis. Premixed or concentrated commercial solutions are available that meet these recommendations. A mixture of 1:10 bleach/water or Lysol/water, mixed daily, will also meet these parameters. If the solution is not packaged in a commercially available spray device, a plastic spray bottle will provide the necessary spray dispersal for proper decontamination. Remember to wear disposable gloves and use either disposable or washable wipes.

EQUIPMENT SANITATION

If it is not known how the germicide being used will act on a particular material, consult the manufacturer. **Always wear gloves to clean equipment.**

Anti-shock garment/trousers Remove any gauges and close all valves. Scrub with soap/hot water (or wash in an industrial washer), gas sterilize or cold sterilize, as for respiratory equipment, and allow to air dry.

Backboards/straps Scrub with soap/hot water, wash down with germicidal solution, and allow to air dry. Wooden backboards should be in good repair with no splintered or worn areas exposed that may absorb body fluids. Replace if not repairable.

Blood spills Wear eye protection. Apply germicidal solution, soak up with disposable material, and appropriately dispose as infectious waste.

Equipment bags Cordura nylon bags or covers should be removed once every two weeks, washed with a germicidal solution or a manufacturer's recommended detergent, and allowed to air dry. Any body fluids contacting the material necessitate immediate cleaning, as described above.

Extrication collars Scrub with soap/hot water. Rinse with water and air dry. Discard as contaminated material when excessively soiled.

Linen Disposable and durable linens should be appropriately bagged after use, while being handled as little as possible. Dispose of per standard operating policy.

Monitoring devices Wipe the cables and case with germicidal solution and allow to air dry. If nylon is used to cover the device, clean as for equipment bags.

Needles/other sharps Do not bend or recap any needles or other sharp items. When recapping is necessary (multiple doses from same syringe), use a one-handed scoop technique to avoid injury. Broken glassware should be picked up mechanically (no use of hands or vacuum cleaners) and disposed of, as all sharps, in approved containers. Have suitable containers available in all patient care vehicles. Dispose of containers frequently according to local rules and regulations.

Respiratory equipment Use disposable devices when possible. Dispose of properly after single-patient use. If reuseable bag/valve mask devices or laryngoscopes must be used, disassemble after use, wash with a broad-spectrum soap/hot water solution, and cold sterilize in liquid sterilization solution for twenty minutes or gas sterilize and air dry.

Splints Scrub with soap/hot water, wipe down with germicidal solution, and allow to air dry.

Stretchers Remove all body secretions as detailed under blood spills, as possible. Wipe down the device with a germicidal solution, and allow to air dry. These devices have a large number of irregular surfaces and require meticulous attention to detail to be adequately cleaned. Any mattresses or straps may be cleaned as above, but contaminated straps should first be cleaned, soaked in germicidal solution for six hours, and then air dried.

Suction devices Remove disposable canisters and dispose as contaminated waste. If not disposable, pour out liquid in sink in dirty holding room of hospital, wash with soap/hot water, wash with germicidal solution, and air dry. Wipe down all surfaces with germicidal solution and also allow to air dry.

Uniforms/protective equipment Contaminated clothes or uniforms should be laundered per agency's specifications. Boots and other leather goods should be scrubbed with a brush, using a high-level disinfectant soap/hot water and allowed to air dry.

Waste materials All contaminated waste material should be placed in leakproof red containers that are labeled as biological hazards. Disposal should be accomplished as set forth by standard operating policies in compliance with appropriate laws.

2-3   **Communicable and Infectious Diseases**

Name	Synopsis of symptoms	Incubation period	Mode of transmission	Period of communicability
Acanthamebiasis of eye, skin, and vagina	Lesions of conjunctiva, cornea, and inner structures of eye. Granulomatous lesions of the skin have been recorded. Also secondary invasion of central nervous system and occasionally of vagina. (See also Meningoencephalitis caused by Acanthamoeba.)			
Acquired Immune Deficiency Syndrome (AIDS)	A secondary immunodeficiency syndrome caused by the human immunodeficiency virus (HIV). Formerly referred to as human T-lymphotropic virus type III (HTLV III). It is characterized by severe compromise of the immune system. This results in opportunistic infections (pneumocystis carinii pneumonia, tuberculosis, cytomegalovirus), neurologic abnormalities (acute and chronic aseptic meningitis, encephalopathy with seizures, progressive dementia), and malignancies (Kaposi's sarcoma, non-Hodgkin's lymphoma) in individuals not known to be previously immunologically compromised. Clinical manifestations are variable, but may include weight loss, malaise, intermittent fever, anemia, generalized lymphadenopathy, oral candidiasis (thrush). The AIDS patient with a fully involved syndrome displays any of the above symptoms and the presence of any of the opportunistic infections, neurologic disorders, or secondary cancers mentioned.	Within 2 to 4 weeks after infection, some patients may develop a viral syndrome with fever, malaise, arthralgias; usually followed in 1 to 3 months by seroconversion. However, most patients are asymptomatic during this time, and may remain so while antibody positive for years. Among homosexual men, about 25% developed AIDS-related conditions, and around 15% developed full-blown AIDS, within 6 years of seroconversion. Among patients with transfusion-associated AIDS, the average time from infection to diagnosis is around 20 to 30 months.	Invasive or intimate contact with the blood or body fluids of an infected individual primarily through sexual contact, blood transfusions, or sharing contaminated needles for IV drug administration.	From time of infection with the human immunodeficiency virus (HIV) until postmortem.
Actinomycosis	Chronic disease most frequently localized in jaw, thorax, or abdomen; septicemic spread with generalized disease may occur. Lesions are firmly indurated areas of purulence and fibrosis.	Irregular; probably years after colonization in oral tissues, plus days or months after precipitating trauma and actual penetration of tissues.	Contact from person to person as part of normal oral flora.	Time and manner in which A. israelii becomes part of normal flora is unknown.

Disease	Description	Incubation period	Mode of transmission	Period of communicability
Amebiasis	Infection with a protozoan parasite that exists in two forms: the hardy, infective cyst and the more fragile, potentially invasive trophozoite. Parasite may act as a commensal or invade tissues, giving rise to intestinal or extraintestinal disease.	Variation—from a few days to several months or years. Commonly 2 to 4 weeks.	Contaminated water or food containing cysts from feces of infected persons, often as complication of another infection such as shigellosis.	During period of cyst passing, which may continue for years.
Ancylostomiasis (hookworm disease, uncinariasis, necatoriasis)	Chronic, debilitating disease with vague symptoms varying greatly, usually in proportion to degree of anemia and hypoproteinemia.	Symptoms may develop after a few weeks to many months.	Eggs in feces are deposited on ground, and under favorable environmental conditions, hatch; larvae develop to third stage, becoming infective in 7 to 10 days. Human infection occurs when infected larvae penetrate skin, usually foot.	Not transmitted from person to person, but infected persons can contaminate soil for several years in absence of treatment.
Arenaviral hemorrhagic fever	Acute febrile illnesses, duration 7 to 15 days. Onset is gradual with malaise, headache, retroorbital pain, conjunctival injection, sustained fever, and diaphoresis. An exanthem appears on thorax and flanks 3 to 5 days after onset.	Commonly 7 to 16 days.	Saliva and excreta of infected rodents contain virus. May be airborne transmission by dust contaminated by infected rodent excreta.	Probably not often directly transmitted from person to person (although this has occurred in the Bolivia disease).
Arthropod-borne viral diseases (arboviral diseases)				
1. Arthropod-borne viral arthritis and rash	Acute self-limited disease characterized by arthritis, primarily in small joints of extremities that lasts from 2 days to 8 months.	10 to 11 days.	Culicine mosquitoes.	No evidence of transmission from person to person.
2. Arthropod-borne viral encephalitides a. Mosquito-borne	Group of acute inflammatory diseases of short duration. Mild cases often occur as aseptic meningitis. Severe infections are usually marked by acute onset, headache, high fever, meningeal signs, stupor, disorientation, coma, seizures, and spastic paralysis.	Usually 5 to 15 days.	Infective mosquitoes.	Not directly transmitted from person to person. Virus is not usually demonstrable in blood of humans after onset of disease. Mosquitoes remain infective for life.
b. Tick-borne	Group of diseases resembling mosquito-borne encephalitides, except Russian spring-summer type often is associated with flaccid paralysis, particularly of the shoulder girdle.	Usually 7 to 14 days.	By infective ticks or by consuming milk from infected animals.	Not directly transmitted from person to person. Tick infected at any stage remains infective for life.

Communicable and Infectious Diseases—cont'd

Name	Synopsis of symptoms	Incubation period	Mode of transmission	Period of communicability
Angiostrongyliasis (eosinophilic meningoencephalitis, eosinophilic meningitis)	Disease of central nervous system caused by a nematode. Invasion may be asymptomatic or mildly symptomatic; more commonly characterized by severe headache, stiffness of neck and back, and various paresthesias. Temporary facial paralysis and low-grade fever may be present.	Usually 1 to 3 weeks.	Ingestion of raw or insufficiently cooked snails, slugs, or land planarians, which are intermediate or transport hosts harboring infective larvae.	Not transmitted from person to person.
Anisakiasis	Disease of human gastrointestinal tract manifested by intestinal colic, fever, and eosinophilic abscesses resulting from ingesting uncooked fish containing larval nematodes of the family Anisakidae.	Stomach involvement may develop within a few hours of ingestion.	Infective larvae live in organs of fish until its death when they invade somatic muscles. When ingested by humans and liberated by digestion in stomach they penetrate gastric or intestinal mucosa.	No direct transmission from person to person.
Anthrax	Acute bacterial disease usually affecting skin but may rarely involve mediastinum or intestinal tract.	Within 7 days, usually 2 to 5 days.	Infection of skin is by contact with tissues of animals dying of the disease or with contaminated animal by-products (e.g., wool or hides).	No evidence of transmission from person to person. Articles and soil contaminated with spores may remain infective for years.
Arthropod-borne viral fevers 1. Mosquito-borne a. Yellow fever	Acute infectious disease of short duration and varying severity. Mildest cases are clinically indeterminate; typical attacks are characterized by denguelike illness, i.e., sudden onset, fever, headache, backache, prostration, nausea, and vomiting.	3 to 6 days.	In urban and certain rural areas transmitted by infective *Aedes aegypti* mosquitoes.	Blood is infective for mosquitoes shortly before onset of fever and for first 3 to 5 days of illness. Highly communicable where many susceptible persons and abundant vector mosquitoes coexist.
b. Dengue (breakbone fever)	Characterized by sudden onset, fever for about 5 days, and intense headache, retroorbital pains, joint and muscle pains, and rash.	3 to 15 days; commonly 5 to 6 days.	Infective mosquitoes.	Not directly transmitted from person to person.
c. Venezuelan equine fever	Clinical manifestations of infection are influenza-like, with abrupt onset of severe headache, chills, fever, myalgia, retroorbital pain, nausea, and vomiting.	Usually 2 to 6 days; can be as short as 1 day.	Infected mosquitoes.	Person-to-person transmission may occur but has not been demonstrated.

Disease	Clinical features	Incubation period	Mode of transmission	Period of communicability
2. Tick-borne a. Colorado tick fever and other tick-borne fevers	Acute febrile, diphasic, denguelike disease with infrequent rash. Brief remission is usual, followed by second bout of fever lasting 2 or 3 days; neutropenia almost always occurs on fourth or fifth day of fever.	Usually 4 to 5 days.	Infective vector ticks.	Not directly transmitted from person to person except by transfusion. Virus is present during course of fever and, in Colorado tick fever, from 2 to 16 weeks or more after onset.
Ascariasis (roundworm infection)	Helminthic infection of small intestine. Symptoms are variable, often vague or absent, and ordinarily mild; live worms, passed in stools or regurgitated, are frequently first recognized sign of infection.	Worms reach maturity about 2 months after ingestion of embryonated eggs.	By ingestion of infective eggs from soil contaminated with human feces containing eggs, but not directly from person to person.	As long as mature female worms live in intestine. Maximum lifespan of adult worms is under 18 months; however, female produces up to 200,000 eggs a day that can remain viable in soil for months or years.
Aspergillosis	Variety of clinical syndromes can be produced by several *Aspergillus* species.	2 to 5 days.	Inhalation of air-borne spores.	Not directly transmitted from person to person.
Babesiosis	Fever, fatigue, and hemolytic anemia lasting several days to a few months.	1 to 12 months.	During the summer months by bite of nymphal *Ixodes* ticks carried by voles or deer mice. Adult tick is normally found on deer.	Transmission from person to person is unlikely except by blood transfusion.
Balantidiasis	Disease of colon characteristically producing diarrhea or dysentery accompanied by abdominal colic, tenesmus, nausea, and vomiting.	Unknown; may be only a few days.	By ingestion of cysts from feces of infected hosts; in epidemics, mainly by fecally contaminated water.	As long as infection persists.
Blastomycosis	Chronic granulomatous mycosis primarily of lungs or skin. *Acute pulmonary blastomycosis* begins with fever and symptoms of respiratory infection and can progress gradually with fever, weight loss, cachexia, cough, and purulent sputum.	Indefinite; probably a few weeks or less to months.	Conidia, typical of the mold or saprophytic growth form, probably are inhaled in spore-laden dust.	Not transmitted directly from humans or from animals to humans.
Botulism, infant	Illness typically begins with constipation followed by lethargy, listlessness, poor feeding, ptosis, dysphagia, loss of head control, hypotonia, generalized weakness, and in some cases, respiratory arrest. Wide spectrum of clinical severity ranging from mild illness to sudden infant death.	Usually unknown, because it cannot be determined precisely when the infant ingested the botulinal spores.	By ingestion of botulinal spores. Sources of spores for infants probably are multiple.	Excretion of *C. botulinum* toxin and organisms. Continues at high levels in patient's feces for weeks to months. No instances of secondary person-to-person transmission have been documented.
Brucellosis (undulant fever)	Systemic disease with acute or insidious onset characterized by continued, intermittent, or irregular fever of variable duration, headache, weakness, diaphoresis, chills, arthralgia, depression, and generalized aching.	Highly variable—usually 5 to 30 days; sometimes several months.	By contact with tissues, blood, urine, vaginal discharges, aborted fetuses, and especially placentas, and by ingestion of raw milk or dairy products from infected animals. Air-borne infection occurs in humans in laboratories and slaughterhouses.	No evidence of communicability from person to person.

Communicable and Infectious Diseases—cont'd

Name	Synopsis of symptoms	Incubation period	Mode of transmission	Period of communicability
Candidiasis (moniliasis, thrush, candidosis)	Mycosis usually confined to superficial layers of skin or mucous membranes with oral thrush, intertrigo, vulvovaginitis, paronychia, or onychomycosis.	Variable; 2 to 5 days in thrush of infants.	Through contact with excretions of mouth, skin, vagina, and especially feces from patients or carriers, from mother to infant during childbirth, and by endogenous spread.	Presumably for duration of lesions.
Capillariasis A. Intestinal capillariasis	Enteropathy with massive protein loss and a malabsorption syndrome that lead to progressive weight loss and extreme emaciation.	Unknown in humans.	Uncertain. Often obtain history of ingesting raw or inadequately cooked fish.	Not transmitted directly from person to person.
B. Hepatic capillariasis (also a pulmonary capillariasis—but only 10 documented cases of human infection recorded).	Uncommon and occasionally fatal disease in humans caused by presence of adult *Capillaria hepatica* in liver. Acute or subacute hepatitis with marked eosinophilia resembling visceral larva migrans.	3 to 4 weeks.	Ingesting liver of infected animal.	Not transmitted directly from person to person.
Carditis, Coxsackie (viral carditis, enteroviral carditis)	Acute or subacute myocarditis or pericarditis, which occurs as the only manifestation, or may occasionally be associated with other manifestations.	Usually 3 to 5 days.	Fecal-oral or respiratory droplet contact with infected person.	Apparently during acute stage of disease.
Cat-scratch disease	Subacute, self-limited infectious disease characterized by malaise, granulomatous lymphadenitis, and variable patterns of fever.	Variable; usually 3 to 14 days from inoculation to primary lesions.	90% of patients report history of scratch, bite, lick, or other exposure to healthy cat or kitten.	Unknown. Not directly transmitted from person to person.
Chancroid (ulcus molle, soft chancre)	Acute, localized, genital infection characterized by single or multiple painful necrotizing ulcers at site of inoculation, frequently accompanied by painful inflammatory swelling and suppuration of regional lymph nodes. Extragenital lesions have been reported.	From 3 to 5 days; up to 14 days.	By direct sexual contact with discharges from open lesions and pus from buboes; suggestive evidence of asymptomatic infections in women. Multiple sexual partners and uncleanliness favor transmission.	As long as infectious agent persists in original lesion or discharging regional lymph nodes; usually until healed—a matter of weeks.
Chickenpox, herpes zoster (varicella shingles)	Acute generalized viral disease with sudden onset of slight fever, mild constitutional symptoms, and a skin eruption that is maculopapular for a few hours, vesicular for 3 to 4 days, and leaves a granular scab.	From 2 to 3 weeks; commonly 13 to 17 days.	From person to person by direct contact, droplet, or air-borne spread of secretion of respiratory tract of chickenpox cases or of vesicle fluid of patients with herpes zoster.	As long as 5 days but usually 1 to 2 days before onset of rash and not more than 6 days after appearance of first crop of vesicles.

Disease	Description	Incubation period	Mode of transmission	Period of communicability
Cholera	Acute intestinal disease with sudden onset, profuse watery stools, occasional vomiting, rapid dehydration, acidosis, and circulatory collapse. Death may occur within a few hours.	From a few hours to 5 days; usually 2 to 3 days.	Through ingestion of food or water contaminated with feces or vomitus of infected persons or with feces of carriers.	Thought to be for duration of stool-positive stage, usually only a few days after recovery. Carrier stage may last for several months.
Chromoblastomycosis (chromomycosis, dermatitis verrucosa)	Chronic spreading mycosis of skin and subcutaneous tissues, usually of a lower extremity. Hematogenous spread to brain has been reported.	Unknown; probably months.	Contact with contaminated wood or other materials.	Not directly transmitted from person to person.
Clonorchiasis (Chinese or oriental liver-fluke disease)	Symptoms result from local irritation of bile ducts by flukes, from toxemia, and possibly from secondary bacterial invaders. Loss of appetite, diarrhea, and sensation of abdominal pressure are early common symptoms.	Unpredictable, varies with the number of worms present; flukes reach maturity within 1 month after encysted larvae are ingested.	Humans infected by ingesting freshwater fish containing encysted larvae (*Clonorchis sinensis*).	Not directly transmitted from person to person, but infected individual may pass viable eggs for as long as 30 years.
Coccidioidomycosis (valley fever, desert fever, desert rheumatism, coccidiodal granuloma)	Internal mycosis that begins as respiratory infection. *Primary infection* may be entirely asymptomatic or resemble acute influenza illness with fever, chills, cough, and pleural pain.	1 to 4 weeks in primary infection.	Inhalation of spores from soil and in laboratory accidents from cultures.	Not directly transmitted from humans or animals to humans.
Conjunctivitis, acute bacterial	Clinical syndrome beginning with lacrimation, irritation, and hyperemia of the palpebral and bulbar conjunctivae of one or both eyes, followed by edema of lids, photophobia, and mucopurulent discharge.	Usually 24 to 72 hours.	Contact with discharges from conjunctivae or upper respiratory tract of infected persons through contaminated fingers, clothing, or other articles.	During course of active infection.
Conjunctivitis, epidemic hemorrhagic (Apollo 11 disease)	Virus infection with sudden onset of pain or sensation of a foreign body in eye. Disease rapidly progresses (1 to 2 days) to full case of swollen eyelids, hyperemia of the conjunctivae, often with a cirumcorneal distribution, seromucous discharge, and frequent subconjunctival hemorrhages.	1 to 2 days or even shorter.	Through direct or indirect contact with discharge from infected eyes and possibly by droplet infection from those with virus in throat.	Unknown, but assumed to be for period of active disease, usually 1 to 2 weeks.
Conjunctivitis, inclusion (swimming-pool conjunctivitis, paratrachoma)	In the newborn, acute papillary conjunctivitis with abundant mucopurulent discharge. In children and adults, acute follicular conjunctivitis with preauricular lymphadenopathy, often with superficial corneal involvement.	5 to 12 days.	During sexual intercourse; genital discharges of infected persons are infectious. Also from mother to infant during childbirth.	While genital infection persists; can be longer than 1 year in female.

Communicable and Infectious Diseases—cont'd

Name	Synopsis of symptoms	Incubation period	Mode of transmission	Period of communicability
Contagious pustular dermatitis	Primarily a proliferative cutaneous disease of sheep and goats transmissible to humans and usually a solitary lesion located on hands, arms, or face that is maculopapular or pustular.	Generally 3 to 6 days.	By direct contact with mucous membranes of infected animals.	Unknown. Human lesions show a decrease in number of virus particles as disease progresses.
Crimean-Congo hemorrhagic fever (viral hemorrhagic fever)	Chest pain, cough, fever, sore throat, and vomiting that can lead to encephalopathy, hemorrhage, shock, and death.	3 to 12 days.	Bites from infected ticks or exposure to infected blood/secretions of infected people or butchered animals.	Unknown, though infected ticks probably infective for life.
Cryptococcosis (torulosis, European blastomycosis)	Mycosis, usually subacute or chronic meningoencephalitis. Infection of lung, kidney, prostate, bone, or liver.	Unknown. Pulmonary disease may precede brain infection by months or years.	Presumably by inhalation.	Not directly transmitted from humans or animals to humans.
Cutaneous larva migrans caused by *Ancylostoma braziliense*	Infective larvae of dog and cat hookworm that causes dermatitis in humans.	Each larva causes serpiginous track, advancing several mm to a few cm a day.	Larva, which enter skin from contact with contaminated soil, migrate intracutaneously for long periods, but eventually penetrate to deeper tissues.	Disease is self-limited, with spontaneous cure after several weeks or months.
Cytomegalovirus infections: Congenital cytomegalovirus infection Cytomegalic inclusion disease	Most severe form of disease occurs in perinatal period, following congenital infection, with signs and symptoms of severe generalized infection especially involving central nervous system and liver.	Information inexact. 3 to 8 weeks following transfusion with infected blood. 3 to 12 weeks after birth.	Intimate exposure to infectious secretions or excretions. Virus is excreted in urine, saliva, cervical secretions, breast milk, and semen.	Virus is excreted in urine or saliva for months and may persist for several years following primary infection.
Dermatophytosis				
A. Ringworm of scalp and beard (tinea capitis, tinea kerion, favus)	Begins as small papule and spreads peripherally, leaving scaly patches of temporary baldness. Infected hairs become brittle and break off easily. Kerions sometimes develop.	10 to 14 days.	Direct or indirect contact with articles infected with hair from humans or infected animals.	As long as lesions are present and viable fungus persists on contaminated materials.
B. Ringworm of nails (tinea unguium, onychomycosis)	Chronic infectious disease involving one or more nails of hands or feet. Nail thickens becoming discolored and brittle with an accumulation of caseous-appearing material beneath nail.	Unknown.	Presumably by direct extension from skin or nail lesions of infected persons. Low rate of transmission.	Possibly as long as infected lesion is present.
C. Ringworm of groin and perianal region (dhobie itch, tinea cruris)	Characteristically appears as flat, spreading, ring-shaped lesions. Periphery is usually reddish, vesicular, or pustular and may be dry and scaly or moist and crusted.	4 to 10 days.	Direct or indirect contact with skin and scalp lesions of infected persons or animals.	As long as lesions are present and viable fungus persists on contaminated materials.

	Description	Incubation period	Mode of transmission	Period of communicability
D. Ringworm of the body (tinea corporis)	Ring-shaped lesion with a raised border that first improves centrally.	8 to 12 days.	Direct or indirect contact with lesions of infected persons.	Possibly as long as infected lesions are present.
E. Ringworm of the foot (tinea pedis, athlete's foot)	Scaling or cracking of skin, especially between toes, or blisters containing watery fluid are characteristic. In severe cases vesicular lesions appear on various parts of body.	Unknown.	Direct or indirect contact with skin lesions of infected persons or contaminated floors or shower stalls.	As long as lesions are present and viable spores persist on contaminated materials.
Diarrhea, acute				
A. Diarrhea caused by *Escherichia coli*	May be invasive, enterotoxigenic, and enteropathogenic. *Invasive*—fever and mucoid and occasionally bloody diarrhea occur. *Enterotoxigenic*—profuse watery diarrhea without blood or mucus. *Enteropathogenic*—associated with outbreaks of acute diarrhea disease in newborn nurseries.	12 to 72 hours.	Fecal contamination of food, water, or fomites. Persons with diarrhea excrete large numbers of organisms and constitute greatest hazard.	Not known; presumably for duration of fecal excretion, which may be several weeks or longer.
B. Diarrhea caused by *Campylobacter* (vibriosis, vibrionic enteritis)	Acute enteric disease characterized by diarrhea, abdominal pain, malaise, fever, nausea, vomiting, and constitutional complaints.	Range is 1 to 10 days with a usual period of 3 to 5 days.	By ingestion of organisms in food or contaminated water; contact with contaminated animals; drinking unpasteurized milk.	Throughout course of infection from several days to several weeks.
Diphtheria	Characteristic lesion marked by patch or patches of grayish membrane with surrounding dull-red inflammatory zone. Throat is moderately sore in faucial diphtheria, with cervical lymph nodes enlarged and tender; occasionally swelling and edema of neck.	2 to 5 days, sometimes longer.	Contact with patient or carrier; more rarely with articles soiled with discharges from lesions of infected persons. Raw milk has been a vehicle.	Variable, until virulent bacilli have disappeared from discharge and lesions. Usual period is 2 to 4 weeks but chronic carriers may shed organisms for 6 months or more.
Diphyllobothriasis	Symptoms commonly are trivial or absent; depending on severity, vitamin B_{12} deficiency anemia, diarrhea, and toxic symptoms may be present.	From 3 to 6 weeks from ingestion to passage of eggs in stool.	From eating raw or inadequately cooked fish.	Not directly transmitted from person to person.
Dracontiasis	Infection of subcutaneous and deeper tissues by large nematode. Blister appears, usually on a lower extremity, as gravid, meter-long adult female prepares to discharge her larvae.	About 12 months.	Humans swallow infected copepods by drinking water from contaminated stepwells and ponds.	Not directly transmitted from person to person.
Ebola fever (viral hemorrhagic fever)	Chest pain, cough, fever, sore throat, and vomiting that can lead to encephalopathy, hemorrhage, shock, and death.	2 to 21 days.	Direct contact with infected blood, organs, and secretions. Parenteral contact via contaminated needles/syringes is uniformly fatal.	As long as virus can be found in blood or secretions.

Communicable and Infectious Diseases—cont'd

Name	Synopsis of symptoms	Incubation period	Mode of transmission	Period of communicability
Echinococcosis multilocularis infection (alveolar hydatid disease)	Disease primarily of liver caused by poorly circumscribed microvesicular larval masses of *Echinococcus multilocularis*; may be found also in lungs and other organs.	Variable from months to years, depending on number and location of cysts and how rapidly they grow.	By ingestion of infective eggs or by fecally soiled dog fur, harnesses, and environmental fomites.	Not directly transmitted from person to person or from one intermediate host to another.
Enterobiasis (pinworm disease, oxyuriasis)	Intestinal infection with mild or nonspecific symptoms, if any. May be anal itching, disturbed sleep, irritability, and local irritation with secondary infection of scratched skin.	Life cycle of *Enterobius vermicularis* is 4 to 6 weeks.	Direct transfer of infective eggs by hand from anus to mouth of the same or new host, or indirectly through materials contaminated with eggs of parasite. Dust-borne infection by inhalation is possible.	As long as gravid females are discharging eggs on perianal skin. Continuous reinfection occurs by ano-oral transfer of eggs from self or infected others.
Food poisoning				
A. Staphylococcal food poisoning	Intoxication (not infection) of abrupt and sometimes violent onset, with severe nausea, cramps, vomiting, diarrhea, and prostration; sometimes with subnormal temperature and lowered blood pressure.	Interval between eating food and onset of symptoms is 1 to 6 hours, but usually 2 to 4 hours.	By ingesting food contacted by food-handler's hands without subsequent cooking or inadequately heated, such as pastries, custards, salads, and meat products.	Not applicable.
B. Botulism	Severe intoxication (not infection as in infant botulism) characterized by clinical manifestations relating primarily to the nervous system. Ptosis, visual difficulty, dry mouth, and sore throat are often first complaints.	Symptoms usually appear within 12 to 36 hours, sometimes several days, after eating contaminated food.	By ingestion of food in which toxin had been formed, primarily from jars or cans inadequately heated during canning, and eaten without subsequent adequate cooking.	Not applicable.
C. Clostridial food poisoning (*C. welchii*)	Intestinal disorder characterized by sudden onset of abdominal colic followed by diarrhea. Nausea is common but vomiting and fever are usually absent.	From 6 to 24 hours, usually 10 to 12 hours.	Ingestion of food contaminated by soil or feces in which conditions have permitted multiplication of organism.	Not applicable.
D. *Vibrio parahaemolyticus* food poisoning	Intestinal disorder characterized by watery diarrhea and abdominal cramps; nausea, vomiting, fever, and headache are variably present.	Usually 12 to 24 hours, but can range from 4 to 96 hours.	Ingestion of raw or inadequately cooked seafood.	Not communicable from person to person.
E. *Bacillus cereus* food poisoning	Gastrointestinal disorder characterized in some cases by sudden onset of nausea and vomiting and in others by intense abdominal colic and diarrhea.	From 1 to 5 hours in cases when vomiting is predominant symptom; from 6 to 16 hours when diarrhea is predominant.	Ingestion of food that has been kept at ambient temperatures after cooking, permitting multiplication of organisms.	Not communicable from person to person.

Disease	Clinical characteristics	Incubation period	Mode of transmission	Period of communicability
Gastroenteritis, viral A. Epidemic viral gastroenteritis	Usually self-limited mild disease that often occurs in outbreaks with clinical symptoms of nausea, vomiting, diarrhea, abdominal pain, myalgia, headache, malaise, low-grade fever, or a combination thereof.	24 to 48 hours; in volunteer studies with Norwalk agent, range was 10 to 51 hours.	Unknown; probably by fecal-oral route. Several outbreaks strongly suggest food-borne and water-borne transmission.	During acute stage of disease and shortly thereafter.
B. Rotavirus gastroenteritis (sporadic viral gastroenteritis of infants and children)	Sporadic severe gastroenteritis of infants and young children characterized by diarrhea and vomiting, often with severe dehydration and occasional deaths.	Approximately 48 hours.	Probably fecal-oral and possibly respiratory routes.	During acute stage of disease and later while virus shedding continues. Virus is not usually detectable after eighth day of illness.
Giardiasis (*Giardia* enteritis, lambliasis)	Protozoan infection principally of upper small bowel; often asymptomatic, it may also be associated with a variety of intestinal symptoms such as chronic diarrhea, steatorrhea, abdominal cramps, bloating, frequent loose and pale, greasy, malodorous stools, fatigue, and weight loss.	In a water-borne epidemic in United States, clinical illnesses occurred 1 to 4 weeks after exposure; average 2 weeks.	Localized outbreaks occur from contaminated water supplies, by ingestion of cysts in fecally contaminated water, and occasionally by fecally contaminated food.	Entire period of infection.
Gonococcal infections A. Gonococcal infection of genitourinary tract (gonorrhea, gonococcal urethritis)	*Males*—purulent discharge from anterior urethra with dysuria appears 2 to 7 days after infecting exposure. *Females*—few days after exposure initial urethritis or cervicitis occurs, frequently so mild as to pass unnoticed. About 20% of patients have uterine invasion at the first, second, or later menstrual period with symptoms of endometritis, salpingitis, or pelvic peritonitis.	Usually 2 to 7 days, sometimes longer.	By contact with exudates from mucous membranes of infected persons, almost always results after sexual activity.	May extend for months if untreated, especially in females, who frequently are asymptomatic. Specific therapy usually ends communicability within hours except with penicillin-resistant strains.
B. Gonococcal conjunctivitis neonatorum (gonorrheal ophthalmia neonatorum)	Acute redness and swelling of conjunctiva of one or both eyes, with mucopurulent or purulent discharge in which gonococci are identifiable by microscopic and cultural methods.	Usually 1 to 5 days.	Contact with infected birth canal during childbirth.	While discharge persists if untreated; for 24 hours following initiation of specific treatment.
Granuloma inguinale (donovanosis)	Mildly communicable, nonfatal, chronic and progressive, autoinoculable bacterial disease of skin and mucous membranes of external genitalia, inguinal, and anal region. Small nodule, vesicle, or papule is present.	Unknown; probably 8 to 80 days.	Presumably by direct contact with lesions during sexual activity.	Unknown and probably for duration of open lesions on skin or mucous membranes.
Hemorrhagic nephroso-nephritis	Acute infectious disease characterized by abrupt onset of fever of 3- to 8-day duration, conjunctival injection, prostration, anorexia, and vomiting.	Usually 12 to 16 days, but varying from 9 to 35 days.	Unknown; transmission from rodent excreta is presumed.	Apparently not directly transmitted from person to person.

Communicable and Infectious Diseases—cont'd

Name	Synopsis of symptoms	Incubation period	Mode of transmission	Period of communicability
Hepatitis, viral				
A. Viral hepatitis A (infectious hepatitis, epidemic hepatitis, epidemic jaundice, catarrhal jaundice, Type A hepatitis)	Onset is usually abrupt with fever, malaise, anorexia, nausea, and abdominal discomfort, followed within a few days by jaundice.	From 15 to 50 days, with average 28 to 30 days.	Person to person by fecal-oral route. Common-vehicle outbreaks have been related to contaminated water and food.	Studies indicate maximum infectivity during latter half of incubation period, continuing for a few days, after onset of jaundice.
B. Viral hepatitis B (Type B hepatitis, serum hepatitis)	Onset is usually insidious with anorexia, vague abdominal discomfort, nausea, and vomiting, sometimes arthralgias and rash, often progressing to jaundice. Fever may be absent or mild.	Usually 45 to 160 days, average 60 to 90 days. Variation is related in part to amount of virus in inoculum, mode of transmission, and host factors.	Parenteral or sexual via blood/blood products, body fluids, or maternal-fetal contact.	Before onset of symptoms through clinical course of disease; carrier state can last for lifetime.
C. Viral hepatitis C (post-transfusion non-A, non-B hepatitis, Type C hepatitis)	Chronic infection may be symptomatic or asymptomatic. Differential diagnosis depends on exclusion of hepatitis types A and B.	2 weeks to 6 months, model 6 to 8 weeks.	Parenteral via blood/blood products and unknown exposures.	Before onset of symptoms through clinical course of disease; carrier state can last for lifetime.
D. Viral hepatitis D (delta virus, HDV)	Can only exist in the presence of hepatitis B. Symptoms similar to hepatitis B.	15 to 64 days.	Similar to hepatitis B. Most commonly seen in Africa, the Middle East, and South America.	Unknown.
E. Viral hepatitis E (enteric non-A, non-B hepatitis, HEV)	Symptoms similar to hepatitis A. Doesn't progress to chronic hepatitis.	15 to 50 days.	Fecal-oral route via fecal-contaminated water. Endemic in developing countries. Rare in United States.	Unknown.
Herpangina; hand-foot-and-mouth disease, acute lymphonodular pharyngitis	*Herpangina*—grayish papulovesicular pharyngeal lesions on an erythematous base. *Hand-foot-and-mouth disease*—more diffuse oral lesions on buccal surfaces of cheeks, gums, and tongue. *Acute lymphonodular pharyngitis*—lesions are firm, raised, discrete, whitish to yellowish nodules.	3 to 5 days for herpangina and hand-foot-and-mouth disease. 5 days for acute lymphonodular pharyngitis.	Direct contact with nose and throat discharges and feces of infected (possibly asymptomatic) persons and by droplet spread.	During acute stage of illness and longer because virus persists in stools for as long as several weeks.
Herpes simplex	Viral infection characterized by localized primary lesion, latency, and a tendency to localized recurrence. In perhaps 10% of primary infections overt disease may appear as illness of varying severity marked by fever and malaise lasting 1 week or more.	2 to 12 days.	HSV Type 1: Direct contact with virus in saliva of carriers. HSV Type 2: Sexual contact.	Secretion of virus in saliva has been reported for as long as 7 weeks after recovery from stomatitis. Patients with primary lesions are infective for about 7 to 12 days, with recurrent disease for 4 days to 1 week.

Disease	Description	Incubation period	Mode of transmission	Period of communicability
Histoplasmosis, histoplasma capsulatum (Darling's disease, American histoplasmosis)	Systemic mycosis of varying severity with primary lesion, usually in lung. Whereas infection is common, overt clinical disease is not. Five clinical forms are recognized.	Symptoms appear within 5 to 18 days after exposure, commonly 10 days.	Inhalation of airborne spores.	Not transmitted from person to person.
Influenza	Acute viral disease of respiratory tract characterized by fever, chilliness, headache, myalgia, prostration, coryza, and mild sore throat. Cough is often severe and protracted.	Usually 24 to 72 hours.	By direct contact through droplet infection; possibly airborne among crowded populations in enclosed spaces.	Probably limited to 3 days from clinical onset.
Keratoconjunctivitis, epidemic	Acute viral disease of eye. Onset is sudden with pain, photophobia, blurred vision, occasionally low-grade fever, headache, malaise, and tender preauricular lymphadenopathy.	Probably 5 to 12 days.	Direct contact with eye secretions of infected person or indirectly through contaminated instruments or solutions.	From late in incubation period to 14 days after onset.
Lassa fever (viral hemorrhagic fever)	Acute viral illness with duration of 7 to 31 days. Onset is gradual with malaise, fever, headache, sore throat, cough, nausea, vomiting, diarrhea, myalgia, and chest or abdominal pain; fever is persistent or intermittent-spiking.	Commonly 7 to 21 days.	Primarily through direct or indirect contact with urine of infected rodents in dust or on food.	Person-to-person infections occur during acute febrile phase when virus is present in throat. Virus may be excreted in urine of patients for 3 weeks or as long as 70 days.
Legionellosis (Legionnaire's disease, Legionnaire's pneumonia, Pontiac fever)	Characterized initially by anorexia, malaise, myalgia, and headache. Within 1 day is usually rapidly rising fever associated with chills. Nonproductive cough, abdominal pain, and diarrhea often occur.	Legionnaire's disease: 2 to 10 days; most often 5 to 6 days. Pontiac fever: 5 to 66 hours; most often 24 to 48 hours.	Evidence supports airborne transmission.	Person-to-person transmission has not been documented.
Leishmaniasis, cutaneous	Polymorphic disease of skin and mucous membranes characterized by ulcerating lesions that may be single or multiple and self-limited or indolent or multiple nodular lesions.	From a few days to many months.	Bite of infective sandfly.	As long as parasites remain in lesions; in untreated cases, 1 year or more.
Leishmaniasis, visceral	Chronic systemic infectious disease characterized by fever, hepatosplenomegaly, lymphadenopathy, anemia with leukopenia, and progressive emaciation and weakness.	Generally 2 to 4 months; range is 10 days to 2 years.	Bite of infective sandfly.	As long as parasites persist in circulating blood or skin. Transmission from person to person, and by blood transfusion, sexual contact, and bites of infected laboratory animals have been reported.
Leprosy (Hansen's disease)	Chronic bacterial disease characterized by lesions of skin and mucous membranes, by involvement and often palpable enlargement of peripheral nerves with consequent anesthesia, muscle weakness, paralysis, and trophic changes in skin, muscle, and bone.	Shortest known is 7 months. Average is probably 3 to 6 years.	Not clearly established, but household and prolonged intimate contact are important. Organisms may gain entrance through broken skin and respiratory tract.	As long as morphologically normal bacilli are demonstrable, infectiousness should be considered possible.

Communicable and Infectious Diseases—cont'd

Name	Synopsis of symptoms	Incubation period	Mode of transmission	Period of communicability
Listeriosis	Bacterial disease usually manifested as acute meningoencephalitis with or without associated septicemia, less frequently septicemia only; very often neonatal. Onset of meningoencephalitis is usually sudden with fever, intense headache, nausea, vomiting, and signs of meningeal irritation.	Unknown; probably 4 days to 3 weeks. Fetus is usually infected within several days after maternal disease.	Largely neonatal; infection is transmitted from mother to unborn infant in utero or during its passage through infected birth canal.	Mothers of infected newborn infants may shed infectious agent in vaginal discharges or urine for 7 to 10 days after delivery. Period of person-to-person communicability is unknown.
Lyme disease	Characterized by distinctive skin lesion (ECM), systemic symptoms, polyarthritis, and neurological and cardiac involvement in varying combination.	From 3 to 21 days after tick exposure.	Presumably tick-borne.	No evidence of transmission from person to person.
Lymphocytic choriomeningitis (LCM, benign or serous lymphocytic meningitis)	Viral disease of animals, especially mice, transmissible to man with marked diversity of clinical manifestations. At times it begins with influenza-like attack followed by complete recovery; or after 1 to 2 weeks of remission, meningeal symptoms suddenly appear.	Probably 8 to 13 days; 15 to 20 days for meningeal symptoms.	Virus is excreted in urine, saliva, and feces of infected animals, usually mice transmission to humans, usually through contaminated food or dust.	Not known to be directly transmitted from person to person.
Lymphogranuloma venereum (lymphogranuloma inguinale, esthiomene, climatic bubo, tropical bubo)	Venereally acquired infection, beginning with painless evanescent erosion, papule, nodule, or herpetiform lesion on penis or vulva, frequently unnoticed. Regional lymph nodes undergo suppuration followed by extension of inflammatory process to adjacent tissues.	Usually 7 to 12 days, with a range of 4 to 21 days for primary lesion. If bubo is first manifestation, 10 to 30 days, sometimes several months.	Direct contact with open lesions of infected persons usually during sexual intercourse.	Variable, from weeks to years, during presence of active lesions.
Malaria	Fever, chills, diaphoresis, and headache that may progress to icterus, coagulation defects, shock, renal and liver failure, acute encephalitis, and coma are symptoms of most serious form (falciparum malaria). Symptoms difficult to differentiate in the four human malarias, so laboratory confirmation is needed by demonstration of malaria parasites in blood films.	Average 12 days for *P. falciparum*, 12 days for *P. vivax* and *P. ovale*, and 30 days for *P. malariae*.	By infective female anopheline mosquito.	For infection of mosquitoes, as long as infective gametocytes are present in blood of patients; varies with species and strain of parasite and with response to therapy.

Disease	Characteristics	Incubation period	Mode of transmission	Period of communicability
Measles (rubeola, hard measles, red measles, morbilli)	Acute, highly communicable viral disease with prodromal fever, conjunctivitis, coryza, bronchitis, and Koplik's spots on the buccal mucosa. A characteristic red blotchy rash appears on third to seventh day, beginning on face, becoming generalized, lasting 4 to 7 days, and sometimes ending in branny desquamation. Leukopenia is common.	About 10 days, varying from 8 to 13 days from exposure to onset of fever; about 14 days until rash appears; uncommonly longer or shorter. Human normal immune globulin (IG), given later than third day of incubation period for passive protection, may extend the incubation period to 21 days instead of preventing disease.	By droplet spread or direct contact with nasal or throat secretions of infected persons. Measles is one of most readily transmitted communicable diseases.	From slightly before beginning of prodromal period to 4 days after appearance of rash; communicability is minimal after second day of rash.
Melioidosis	Range of clinical manifestations from apparent infection or asymptomatic pulmonary consolidation to rapidly fatal septicemia. May simulate typhoid fever or even tuberculosis.	As short as 2 days; however, several months or years may elapse between presumed exposure and appearance of clinical disease.	Usually by contact with contaminated soil or water through overt or inapparent skin wounds, by aspiration or ingestion of contaminated water, or by inhalation of dust from soil.	Person-to-person transmission and laboratory-acquired infections are uncommon.
Meningitis, aseptic (viral meningitis, serous meningitis, nonbacterial or abacterial meningitis)	Common, rarely fatal, clinical syndrome with multiple causes, most commonly viral, characterized by sudden onset of febrile illness with signs and symptoms of meningeal involvement. Spinal fluid findings of pleocytosis (usually mononuclear but may be polymorphonuclear in early stages), increased protein, normal sugar, and absence of bacteria. Active illness seldom exceeds 10 days.	Varies with specific infectious agent (refer to specific diseases).	Varies with specific infectious agent (refer to specific diseases).	Varies with specific infectious agent (refer to specific diseases).
Meningitis, bacterial	Clinical signs and symptoms may be indistinguishable from those caused by meningococci including rash. Differentiation is based on smears and bacteriological studies.	24 to 72 hours.	By droplet infection and close contact.	Varies with specific infectious agent (refer to specific diseases).
Meningitis, meningococcal (cerebrospinal fever, meningococcemia)	Characterized by sudden onset of fever, intense headache, nausea and often vomiting, nuchal rigidity, and frequently a petechial rash with pink macules or, very rarely, vesicles. Delirium and coma often appear; occasional fulminating cases exhibit sudden ecchymoses and shock at onset.	Varies from 2 to 10 days, commonly 3 to 4 days.	By direct contact, including droplets and discharges from nose and throat of infected persons.	Until meningococci are no longer present in discharges from nose and throat. If organisms are sensitive to sulfonamides, meningococci usually disappear from nasopharynx within 24 hours after institution of treatment. They are not fully eradicated from oronasopharynx by penicillin.

Communicable and Infectious Diseases—cont'd

Name	Synopsis of symptoms	Incubation period	Mode of transmission	Period of communicability
Meningitis, hemophilus (meningitis caused by *Heamophilus influenzae*)	Most common bacterial meningitis in children 2 months to 3 years old in U.S. Otitis media or sinusitis may be precursor. Almost always associated with bacteremia. Onset is sudden with symptoms of fever, vomiting, lethargy, and meningeal irritation.	Probably short—within 2 to 4 days.	By droplet infection and discharges from nose and throat during infectious period. May be purulent rhinitis. Portal of entry is most commonly nasopharyngeal.	As long as organisms are present, which may be for prolonged period even without nasal discharge.
Meningitis, pneumococcal	High fatality rate is associated with this disease. Usually fulminant and occurs with bacteremia but not necessarily with another focus, although there may be otitis media or mastoiditis. Symptoms such as fever, lethargy, or coma and signs of meningeal irritation usually signal onset.	Within 48 hours.	By droplet infection and close contact.	As long as organisms are present.
Meningitis, neonatal	Patients exhibit symptoms of lethargy, seizures, apneic episodes, poor feeding, hypothermia or hyperthermia, and sometimes respiratory distress in first week of life.	Hours to days.	Acquired from birth canal. For prevention of early onset form, ampicillin treatment at onset of labor has been recommended for mothers known to be infected with Group B *Streptococcus.*	Directly transmitted only during childbirth.
Meningoencephalitis caused by *Naegleria* and *Acanthamoeba*	*Naegleria*—Disease organisms cause a typical syndrome of fulminating pyogenic meningoencephalitis with severe frontal headache, occasional olfactory hallucinations, nausea, vomiting, high fever, nuchal rigidity, and somnolence.	3 to 7 days in documented cases.	*Naegleria*—Infection acquired by forcing infected water into nasal passages. *Naegleria* trophozoites colonize nasal tissues, then invade brain and meninges by extension along olfactory nerves.	No person-to-person transmission has been observed.
	Acanthamoeba—Disease organisms invade the brain and meninges, usually without involvement of nasal and olfactory tissues, causing disease characterized by insidious onset and prolonged course. (*See also* Acanthamebiasis of eye, skin, and vagina.)	Weeks to months.	*Acanthamoebae* trophozoites reach central nervous system by metastasis from skin lesion or other site of primary colonization.	No person-to-person transmission has been observed.

Disease	Characteristics	Incubation period	Mode of transmission	Period of communicability
Molluscum contagiosum	Viral disease of skin that results in pearly pink to white papules with prominent central core. Papules vary in size from less than 1 mm to 10 mm. Usually multiple lesions, most frequently in the genital area in adults; may occur anywhere in children. Eruption usually clears spontaneously in 6 to 9 months.	2 to 7 weeks.	Usually by direct contact, but transmission by fomites is possible. Sexual transmission occurs.	Unknown, but probably as long as lesions persist.
Mononucleosis, infectious (glandular fever, EBV mononucleosis)	Characterized by fever, sore throat (often with exudative pharyngotonsillitis), and lymphadenopathy (especially posterior cervical). Jaundice occurs in about 4% of infected young adults and splenomegaly in 50%. Duration is from 1 to several weeks.	From 4 to 6 weeks.	Person-to-person spread by oropharyngeal route via saliva. Spread may also occur via blood transfusion to susceptible recipients.	Prolonged; pharyngeal excretion may persist for 1 year after infection; 15% to 20% of healthy adults are oropharyngeal carriers.
Mumps (infectious parotitus)	Acute viral disease characterized by fever, swelling, and tenderness of one or more salivary glands, usually parotid and sometimes sublingual or submaxillary glands.	About 2 to 3 weeks, commonly 18 days.	By droplet spread and by direct contact with saliva of an infected person.	Virus has been isolated from saliva from 6 days before salivary gland involvement to as long as 9 days thereafter; but height of infectiousness occurs about 48 hours before swelling begins. Urine may be positive for as long as 14 days after onset of illness.
Mycetoma, actinomycotic (mycetomia, mycotic)	Characterized by swelling and suppuration of subcutaneous tissues, and formation of sinus tracts with visible granules in pus draining from sinus tracts. Lesions usually are on foot or lower leg.	Usually months.	Subcutaneous implantation of spores or hyphal elements from a saprophytic source by penetrating wounds (thorns, splinters).	Not transmitted from person to person.
Nocardiosis	Chronic disease often originating in lungs, with hematogenous spread to produce abscesses of brain, subcutaneous tissue, and other organs; high fatality rate.	Unknown; probably weeks.	Nocardia are presumed to enter body principally by inhalation of contaminated dust into lung.	Not directly transmitted from humans or animals to humans.
Onchocerciasis	Chronic, nonfatal filarial disease with fibrous nodules in subcutaneous tissues, particularly head and shoulders.	Microfilariae are found in skin usually about 1 year or more after infection.	By infected female blackflies.	Not directly transmitted from person to person; however, humans infect flies as long as living microfilariae occur in skin; i.e., for 10 to 15 years if untreated.

Communicable and Infectious Diseases—cont'd

Name	Synopsis of symptoms	Incubation period	Mode of transmission	Period of communicability
Ornithosis (psittacosis, parrot fever)	Acute generalized infectious disease with variable clinical presentations; fever, headache, myalgia, chills, and upper or lower respiratory tract disease are commonly present.	From 4 to 15 days, commonly 10 days.	Infection is usually acquired by inhaling agent from desiccated droppings of infected birds. Turkeys are usually involved but ducks and pigeons are occasionally responsible for human disease. Household birds are frequent source.	Person-to-person transmission is rare but can occur, especially with paroxysmal coughing.
Paracoccidioidomycosis	Chronic mycosis characterized by patchy pulmonary infiltrates or ulcerative lesions of mucosa (oral, nasal, gastrointestinal) and of skin. Lymphadenopathy is frequent. In disseminated cases all viscera may be affected; adrenal gland is especially susceptible.	Highly variable, from 1 month to many years.	Presumably acquired through inhalation of contaminated soil and dust.	Not known to be transmitted directly from person to person.
Paragonimiasis (pulmonary distomiasis, lung fluke disease)	Clinical signs depend on path of migration and organs parasitized. Lungs are most frequently involved; symptoms are cough and hemoptysis.	Flukes mature and begin to lay eggs approximately 6 weeks after humans ingest infective larvae. Interval until symptoms appear is long and variable depending on organ invaded and number of worms involved.	Infection occurs when raw or partially cooked flesh of freshwater crabs or crayfish containing infective larvae (metacercariae) are eaten.	Not directly transmitted from person to person, but eggs may be discharged by the human host for 20 years or more.
Paratyphoid fever	Frequently generalized bacterial enteric infection, often with abrupt onset, continued fever, enlargement of spleen, sometimes rose spots on trunk, usually diarrhea, and involvement of lymphoid tissues of mesentery and intestines.	1 to 3 weeks for enteric fever; 1 to 10 days for gastroenteritis.	Direct or indirect contact with feces or urine of patient or carrier. Spread is by food, especially milk, milk products, and shellfish. Flies may be vectors.	As long as infectious agent persists in excreta, which is from appearance of prodromal symptoms, throughout illness, and for periods up to several weeks or months. Commonly 1 to 2 weeks after recovery.
Pediculosis (lousiness)	Infestation of head, hairy parts of body, or clothing with adult lice, larvae, or nits (eggs), which results in severe itching and excoriation of scalp or scratch marks of body.	Under optimum conditions, eggs of lice hatch in 1 week, reach sexual maturity in approximately 2 weeks.	Direct contact with infected person and indirectly by contact with personal belongings, especially clothing and headgear. Crab lice are usually transmitted through sexual contact.	Communicable as long as lice remain alive on infested person or in clothing, and until eggs in hair and clothing have been destroyed.

Disease	Clinical description	Incubation period	Mode of transmission	Period of communicability
Pinta (carate)	Scaling papule with satellite lymphadenopathy appears within 1 to 8 weeks after infection, usually on hands, legs, or dorsum of feet. In 3 to 12 months, a maculopapular, erythematous secondary rash appears and may evolve into tertiary dyschromic macules of variable size. Organ systems are not involved.	3 to 60 days.	Presumably person-to-person transmission by direct and prolonged contact with initial and early dyschromic skin lesions; location of primary lesions suggests that trauma provides portal of entry.	Unknown; potentially communicable while dyschromic skin lesions are active, sometimes for many years.
Plague (pest)	Specific zoonosis involving rodents and their fleas that transfer infection to various animals including humans. Initial response is commonly lymphadenitis in node receiving drainage from site of flea-bite. Nodes become swollen and tender and fever is often present. Secondary involvement of lungs may result in severe pneumonia with mediastinitis and pleural effusion.	From 2 to 6 days; may be longer in vaccinated individuals.	Plague in humans occurs as result of intrusion into zoonotic transmission cycle or by entry of sylvatic infected animals and their infected fleas into human habitat.	Fleas may remain infected for days, weeks, or months under suitable conditions of temperature and humidity.
Pleurodynia, epidemic	Acute viral disease characterized by acute onset of severe pain localized in chest or abdomen that may be intensified by movement, usually accompanied by fever and frequently by headache.	Usually 3 to 5 days.	Probably fecal-oral or respiratory droplet contact with infected person or with articles freshly soiled with feces or throat discharges of infected person who may or may not have symptoms.	Apparently during acute stage of disease.
The pneumonias A. Pneumococcal pneumonia	Acute bacterial infection characterized by sudden onset with single shaking chill, fever, pleural pain, dyspnea, cough productive of "rusty" sputum, and leukocytosis.	Not well determined; believed to be 1 to 3 days.	By droplet spread; by direct oral contact, or indirectly, through articles freshly soiled with respiratory organisms.	Presumably until discharges of mouth and nose no longer contain virulent pneumococci in significant numbers. Penicillin will render patient noninfectious within 24 to 48 hours.
B. Mycoplasmal pneumonia (primary atypical pneumonia)	Predominantly afebrile lower respiratory infection. Onset is gradual with headache, malaise, cough—often paroxysmal, and usually substernal pain (not pleuritic). Sputum, scant at first, may increase later.	14 to 21 days.	Probably by droplet inhalation, direct contact with infected person, or with articles freshly soiled with discharges of nose and throat from acutely ill and coughing patient.	Probably less than 10 days; occasionally longer with persisting febrile illness or persistence of the organisms in convalescence (as long as 13 weeks is known).

Communicable and Infectious Diseases—cont'd

Name	Synopsis of symptoms	Incubation period	Mode of transmission	Period of communicability
C. Pneumocystis pneumonia (interstitial plasmacell pneumonia)	Acute pulmonary disease occurring early in life, especially in malnourished, chronically ill, or premature infants. Characterized by progressive dyspnea, tachypnea, and cyanosis; fever may not be present.	Analysis of data from institutional outbreaks among infants indicates 1 to 2 months.	Unknown.	Unknown.
D. Chlamydial pneumonia (pertussoid eosinophilic pneumonia)	Subacute pulmonary disease occurring in early infancy, primarily in infants of mothers with infection of uterine cervix with causative organism. Characterized by insidious onset, cough, lack of fever, patchy infiltrates on chest x-ray with hyperinflation; eosinophilia, elevated IgM and IgG.	Not known, but pneumonia may occur in infants from 1 to 18 weeks of age (more commonly between 4 and 12 weeks). Nasopharyngeal infection is usually not present before 2 weeks of age.	Presumed to be transmitted from infected cervix to infant during birth, with resultant nasopharyngeal infection (and occasionally conjunctival infection as inclusion conjunctivitis). Direct contact or respiratory transmission has not been established.	Unknown, but length of nasopharyngeal excretion can be at least 2 months.
Poliomyelitis (infantile paralysis)	Acute viral infection with symptoms that include fever, malaise, headache, nausea, vomiting, and nuchal rigidity with or without paralysis.	Commonly 7 to 14 days for paralytic cases, with a range from 3 to possibly 35 days.	Direct contact through close association. In rare instances milk, foodstuffs, and fecally-contaminated materials have been incriminated as vehicles. Fecal-oral is major route when sanitation is poor, but during epidemics and when sanitation is good, pharyngeal spread becomes relatively more important.	Not accurately known. Cases are probably most infectious during first few days after onset of symptoms.
Q fever (query fever)	Acute febrile rickettsial disease; onset may be sudden with chills, retrobulbar headache, weakness, malaise, and diaphoresis. Pneumonitis occurs in many cases with cough, scanty expectoration, chest pain, and minimal physical findings. Chronic endocarditis, pericarditis, hepatitis, and generalized infections have been reported.	Usually 2 to 3 weeks.	Commonly by airborne dissemination of rickettsiae in dust from premises contaminated by placental tissues, birth fluids, and excreta of infected animals.	Direct transmission from person to person is very rare, but may occur in cases of pneumonia.

Disease	Clinical features	Incubation period	Mode of transmission	Period of communicability
Rabies (hydrophobia, lyssa)	Almost invariably fatal acute encephalomyelitis; onset is with sense of apprehension, headache, fever, malaise, and sensory changes often referred to site of animal bite. Disease progresses to paresis or paralysis; spasm of deglutition muscles with attempts to swallow, fear of water, and seizures.	Usually 2 to 8 weeks, occasionally as short as 10 days or as long as 1 year or more depending on severity and site of wound.	Virus-laden saliva of a rabid animal is introduced by bite or, very rarely, through intact mucous membranes.	In dogs and most other biting animals, for 3 to 5 days before onset of clinical signs and during course of disease.
Rat-bite fever A. Streptobacillary fever	Abrupt onset with chills and fever, headache, and muscle pain is shortly followed by maculopapular or sometimes petechial rash. One or more joints may be swollen, red, and painful. Bacterial endocarditis and focal abscesses may occur late in untreated cases.	3 to 10 days, rarely longer.	Infection is transmitted by secretions of mouth, nose, or conjunctival sac of infected animal, most frequently introduced by biting.	Not directly transmitted from person to person.
B. Spirillum fever	Symptoms rarely include arthritic symptoms, but distinctive rash of reddish or purplish plaques is evident.	1 to 3 weeks.	Rat or mouse secretions introduced by biting.	Not directly transmitted from person to person.
Relapsing fever	Systemic spirochetal disease in which periods of fever lasting 2 to 9 days alternate with afebrile periods of 2 to 4 days; number of relapses varies from 1 to 10 or more.	5 to 15 days; usually 8 days.	Not directly transmitted from person to person.	Louse becomes infective 4 to 5 days after ingestion of blood from infected person and remains so for life (20 to 40 days) of the louse.
Respiratory disease (excluding influenza) A. Acute febrile respiratory disease	Viral diseases of respiratory tract are characterized by fever and one or more constitutional reactions such as chills or chilliness, headache, general aching, malaise, and anorexia; in infants by occasional gastrointestinal disturbances.	From a few days to 1 week or more.	Directly by oral contact or by droplet spread, indirectly by hands or other materials soiled by respiratory discharges of infected person.	For duration of active disease; little is known about subclinical or latent infections.
B. Common cold (acute coryza)	Acute catarrhal infections of upper respiratory tract characterized by sneezing, lacrimation, irritated nasopharynx, and malaise lasting 2 to 7 days. Fever is uncommon in children and rare in adults.	1 to 3 days.	Presumably by direct oral contact or by droplet spread; indirectly by hands and articles freshly soiled by discharges of nose and throat of infected person.	Generally 3 to 8 days, but varies with specific infectious agent.

Communicable and Infectious Diseases—cont'd

Name	Synopsis of symptoms	Incubation period	Mode of transmission	Period of communicability
Rickettsioses, tick-borne (spotted fever group)				
A. Rocky Mountain spotted fever	Characterized by sudden onset with moderate to high fever that ordinarily persists for 2 to 3 weeks, significant malaise, deep muscle pain, severe headache, chills, and conjunctival injection. A maculopapular rash appears about the third day. Petechiae and hemorrhages are common.	From 3 to about 14 days.	Ordinarily by infected tick.	Not directly transmitted from person to person. Tick remains infective for life; commonly as long as 18 months.
B. Boutonneuse fever (African tick typhus, Queensland tick typhus, North Asian tick fever, rickettsial pox)	Mild to moderately severe febrile illness of a few days to 2 weeks; characterized by primary lesion at site of tick bite. Lesion (tache noire), usually present at onset of fever, is small ulcer 2 mm to 5 mm in diameter with black center and red areola; regional lymph nodes are enlarged.	Usually 5 to 7 days.	By infected ticks.	Same as in Rocky Mountain spotted fever.
Rubella (German measles, three-day measles)				
A. Congenital rubella	Mild febrile infectious disease with diffuse punctate and macular rash. Sometimes resembling that of measles, scarlet fever, or both. May be few or no constitutional symptoms in children but adults may experience 1- to 5-day prodrome characterized by low-grade fever, headache, malaise, mild coryza, and conjunctivitis. As many as 20% to 50% of infections may occur without evident rash; overall 50% are not recognized.	From 16 to 18 days with a range of 14 to 21 days.	Contact with nasopharyngeal secretions of infected person. Infection is by droplet spread or direct contact with patients and indirect contact.	For about 1 week before and at least 4 days after onset of rash. Highly communicable. Infants with congenital rubella syndrome may shed virus for months after birth.
B. Erythema infectiosum (fifth disease)	Mild nonfebrile erythematous eruption occurring as epidemics among children. Characterized by striking erythema of cheeks, reddening of skin, and lacelike serpiginous rash of body.	4 to 12 days.	By airborne droplets or close direct/indirect contact.	Unknown.
C. Exanthema subitum (roseola infantum, pseudorubella)	Acute illness of probable viral cause characterized by high fever that suddenly appears and lasts 3 to 5 days. A maculopapular rash on trunk and later on rest of body ordinarily follows lysis of fever.	5 to 15 days.	Not known.	Unknown.

Disease	Description	Incubation period	Mode of transmission	Period of communicability
Salmonellosis	Commonly manifested by acute gastroenteritis. Acute infectious disease with sudden onset of abdominal pain, diarrhea, nausea, and, sometimes, vomiting. Dehydration may be severe. Fever is nearly always present.	6 to 72 hours, usually about 12 to 36 hours.	By ingestion of organisms in food contaminated by feces of infected person or animal.	Throughout course of infection—extremely variable.
Scabies (sarcoptic acariasis)	Infectious disease of skin caused by mite whose penetration is visible as papules or vesicles, or as tiny linear burrows containing mites and their eggs.	2 to 6 weeks before onset of itching in persons without previous exposure. Person who have been previously infested develop symptoms 1 to 4 days after reexposure.	Transfer of parasites is by direct skin-to-skin contact and to limited extent from undergarments or soiled bedclothes freshly contaminated by infected persons; frequently acquired during sexual contact.	Until mites and eggs are destroyed by treatment, ordinarily after one or occasionally two courses of treatment 1 week apart.
Shigellosis (bacillary dysentery)	Acute bacterial disease primarily involving large intestine, characterized by diarrhea, accompanied by fever, nausea, sometimes vomiting, abdominal pain, and tenesmus. In severe cases stools contain blood, mucus, and pus.	1 to 7 days, usually 1 to 3 days.	By direct or indirect fecal-oral transmission from patient or carrier. Infection may occur after ingestion of very few organisms.	During acute infection and until infectious agent is no longer present in feces, usually within 4 weeks of illness.
Slow virus infections of central nervous system A. Kuru	Signs include cerebellar ataxia, tremors, rigidity, progressive wasting, and variable cranial nerve signs in patients 4 years of age or older.	8 to 9 years in childhood cases; range is 4 to more than 30 years.	Exact route of transmission not firmly established. Principally by traditional mortuary practices with intimate contact with infected tissues.	CNS tissues are infectious throughout symptomatic illness.
B. Jakob-Creutzfeldt disease	Insidious onset of confusion, progressive dementia, and variable ataxia in patients 25 years of age or older.	Unknown in most cases.	Unknown.	While illness is symptomatic.
Smallpox	Systemic disease with usually characteristic exanthem. Onset is sudden, with fever, malaise, headache, severe backache, prostration, and occasionally abdominal pain. Rash appears after 2 to 4 days and goes through stages of macules, papules, vesicles, pustules, and finally scabs.	From 7 to 17 days; commonly 10 to 12 days to onset of illness and 2 to 4 days more to onset of rash.	Transmission normally through close contact with respiratory discharges and skin lesions of patients and with material they had recently contaminated. Airborne spread occurs infrequently.	From a few days before development of earliest lesions to disappearance of all scabs; about 3 weeks. Most communicable during first week.
Sporotrichosis	Fungal disease, usually of skin, which begins as nodule. As nodule grows, lymphatics draining area becomes firm and cordlike and forms a series of nodules, which in turn may soften and ulcerate.	Lymphatic form may develop 1 week to 3 months after injury.	Introduction of fungus through skin following pricks by thorns or barbs, handling of sphagnum moss, or by slivers from wood or lumber.	Not transmitted from person to person. Environment presumably may be contaminated for duration of active lesion.

Communicable and Infectious Diseases—cont'd

Name	Synopsis of symptoms	Incubation period	Mode of transmission	Period of communicability
Staphylococcal disease				
A. Staphylococcal disease in community (boils, carbuncles, furuncles, impetigo)	Staphylococci produce variety of syndromes with clinical manifestations that range from single pustule to impetigo to septicemia to death.	Variable and indefinite. Commonly 4 to 10 days.	Major site of colonization is anterior nares. Autoinfection is responsible for at least one third of infections.	As long as purulent lesions continue to drain or carrier state persists.
(cellulitis, abscesses, Staphylococcal septicemia, Staphylococcal pneumonia, osteomyelitis, endocarditis)	Lesion or lesions containing pus is primary clinical finding; abscess formation is typical.	Variable.	Person with draining lesion or any purulent lesion or who is asymptomatic (usually nasal) carrier of pathogenic strain. Airborne spread is rare.	As long as purulent lesions continue to drain or carrier state persists.
B. Staphylococcal disease in hospital nurseries (impetigo, abscess of breast)	Characteristic lesions develop secondary to colonization of nose or umbilicus, conjunction, circumcision site, or rectum of infants with pathogenic strain.	Commonly 4 to 10 days but may occur several months after colonization.	Spread by hands of hospital personnel is primary mode of transmission within hospitals; to a lesser extent, airborne.	As long as purulent lesions drain.
C. Staphylococcal disease in medical and surgical wards of hospitals	Lesions vary from simple furuncles or stitch abscesses to extensively infected bedsores or surgical wounds, septic phlebitis, chronic osteomyelitis, fulminating pneumonia, endocarditis, or septicemia.	Variable and indefinite. Commonly 4 to 10 days.	Major site of colonization is anterior nares. Autoinfection is responsible for at least one third of infections. Person with a draining lesion or any purulent lesion or who is an asymptomatic (usually nasal) carrier of a pathogenic strain. Airborne spread is rare.	As long as purulent lesions continue to drain or carrier state persists.
D. Toxic shock syndrome	Characterized by sudden onset of fever, vomiting, profuse watery diarrhea, and myalgia, followed by hypotension, and in severe cases, shock. An erythematous "sunburnlike" rash is present during acute phase.	Often within 48 hours.	Related to use of tampons; other modes of transmission are under investigation.	Not directly transmitted from person to person.
Streptococcal diseases caused by group A (beta hemolytic) streptococci				
A. Streptococcal sore throat	Fever, sore throat, exudative tonsillitis or pharyngitis, and tender anterior cervical lymph nodes.	Short, usually 1 to 3 days, rarely longer.	Transmission results from direct or intimate contact with patient or carrier, rarely by indirect contact through objects or hands. Nasal carriers are particularly likely to transmit diseases.	In untreated uncomplicated cases 10 to 21 days; in untreated conditions with purulent discharges, weeks or months.

Disease	Description	Incubation	Transmission	Period of communicability
B. Streptococcal skin infections	Usually superficial, may proceed through vesicular, pustular, and encrusted stages.	3 to 5 days.	Usually via direct contact with patient or carrier.	As long as purulent lesions drain.
C. Scarlet fever (scarlatina)	Skin rash and symptoms similar to streptococcal sore throat, enanthem, strawberry tongue, and exanthem. Rash is usually fine erythema.	2 to 4 days.	Usually via direct contact with patient or carrier.	24 hours before symptom onset, continuing until 3 or more weeks after symptoms resolve.
D. Erysipelas	Acute cellulitis characterized by fever, constitutional symptoms, leukocytosis, and red, tender, edematous, spreading lesion of skin with definite raised border.	Indefinite.	Direct contact with patient or carrier.	As long as purulent lesions drain or a carrier state exists.
E. Streptococcal puerperal fever	Acute disease, usually febrile, accompanied by local and general symptoms and signs of bacterial invasion of genital tract and sometimes bloodstream in postpartum or postabortion patient.	24 to 72 hours.	Results from contamination of genital tract after childbirth.	Not directly transmitted from person to person.
Streptococcal (group B) disease of the newborn	Produces diseases of newborn infants including cases of septicemia, evidence of pulmonary involvement and meningeal involvement.	Within seven days when vaginally acquired.	Acquired during passage through birth canal. Some cases are acquired through environment.	Directly transmitted only during childbirth; otherwise acquired only from environment.
Strongyloidiasis	Helminthic infection of duodenum and upper jejunum, asymptomatic in majority of cases. Clinical manifestations include dermatitis, cough, and abdominal symptoms.	From penetration of skin by filariform larvae until rhabitiform larvae appear in feces is about 2 to 3 weeks; period until symptoms appear is variable.	Infective larvae that develop in moist soil contaminated with feces penetrate skin, enter venous circulation, and are carried to lungs.	As long as living worms remain in intestine; up to 35 years.
Syphilis, venereal (lues)	Acute and chronic treponematosis characterized clinically by primary lesion, secondary eruption involving skin and mucous membranes, long periods of latency, and late lesions of skin, bone, viscerae, and central nervous and cardiovascular systems. Papule appears 3 weeks after exposure at site of initial invasion; after erosion, most common form is indurated chancre.	10 days to 10 weeks, usually 3 weeks.	By direct contact with infectious exudates from obvious or concealed lesions of skin and mucous membrane, body fluids, and secretions of infected persons during sexual contact.	Variable and indefinite during primary and secondary stages and also in mucocutaneous recurrences; some cases may be intermittently communicable for 2 to 4 years.
Syphilis, nonvenereal endemic	Acute disease of limited geographical distribution, characterized clinically by eruption of skin and mucous membrane, usually without evident primary sore.	2 weeks to 3 months.	Direct or indirect contact with infectious early lesions of skin and mucous membranes. Congenital transmission does not occur.	Until moist eruptions of skin and mucous patches disappear—sometimes several weeks or months.

Communicable and Infectious Diseases—cont'd

Name	Synopsis of symptoms	Incubation period	Mode of transmission	Period of communicability
Taeniasis and cysticercosis *Taenia solium* infection, intestinal form (pork tapeworm) Cysticercosis (cysticerciasis, infection by *Cysticercus cellulosae*) *Taenia saginata* infection (beef tapeworm)	Taeniasis is intestinal infection with adult stage of large tapeworms. Cysticercosis is somatic infection with larvae stage of one species, *Taenia solium*. Clinical manifestations of infection with adult worm are variable and may include nervousness, insomnia, anorexia, weight loss, abdominal pain, and digestive disturbance. Cysticercosis is serious somatic disease that may involve many different organs. Eggs of tapeworm, when swallowed, hatch in small intestines and larvae migrate throughout the body.	For adult tapeworm, from 8 to 14 weeks.	Ova of *Taenia saginata* passed in stool of infected person are infectious only to cattle. Infection of man follows ingestion of raw or inadequately cooked beef containing cysticerci. Ova of *Taenia solium* are infectious to both man and pigs. Human infection occurs by direct transfer of eggs in feces of person harboring adult worm to own or another's mouth, or indirectly through ingestion of food or water contaminated with eggs, resulting in somatic cysticercosis. Intestinal infection of humans (taeniasis) follows ingestion of raw or inadequately cooked infected pork.	*Taenia saginata* is not directly transmitted from person to person but *Taenia solium* may be; eggs of both species are disseminated into environment as long as worm remains in intestines, sometimes more than 30 years; eggs may remain viable for months.
Tetanus (tetanus neonatorum, lockjaw)	Acute disease induced by tetanus bacillus that grows anaerobically at site of injury and produces neurotoxin. Characterized by painful muscular contractions, abdominal rigidity, and generalized spasms. Symptoms usually appear between fifth and twelfth day, most frequently about seventh day.	4 to 21 days, dependent on character, extent, and location of wound; average 10 days. Most cases occur within 14 days.	Tetanus spores introduced into body during injury, usually puncture wound contaminated with soil, street dust, or animal or human feces, but also through lacerations, burns, and trivial or unnoticed wounds.	Not directly transmitted from person to person.
Toxocariasis (larva migrans visceralis, *Toxocara* [Canis] [Cati] infection, visceral larva migrans syndrome)	Chronic and usually mild disease of young children caused by migration of certain nematode larvae in organs and tissues. Characterized by eosinophilia of variable duration, hepatomegaly, hyperglobulinemia, pulmonary symptoms, and fever.	Probably weeks or months, depending on intensity of infection and sensitivity of patient.	By direct or indirect transmission of infectious *Toxocara* eggs from contaminated soil to mouth; directly related to eating of dirt by young children. Eggs reach soil in feces from infected cats and dogs.	Not directly transmitted from person to person.

Disease	Identification	Incubation period	Mode of transmission	Period of communicability
Toxoplasmosis (congenital toxoplasmosis)	Systemic protozoal disease. Primary infection is frequently asymptomatic; acute disease may occur with fever, lymphadenopathy, and lymphocytosis persisting for days or weeks. Rare severe manifestations include cerebral signs, pneumonitis, generalized muscle involvement, and death.	Unknown; 10 to 23 days in one outbreak in which larva vehicle was undercooked meat, and 5 to 20 days in an outbreak associated with infected cats.	Transplacental infection may occur in women with primary infection. Postnatal infections might be acquired by eating raw or undercooked infected meat or more often by ingesting infective oocysts. Drinking water contaminated with feces of *Felidae* has been incriminated.	Not directly transmitted from person to person except in utero.
Trachoma	Communicable keratoconjunctivitis characterized by conjunctival inflammation with papillary hyperplasia, associated with vascular invasion of cornea and in later stages by conjunctival scarring that may eventually lead to blindness.	5 to 12 days (based on volunteer studies).	By direct contact with ocular discharges and possibly mucoid or purulent discharges of nasal mucous membranes of infected persons or materials. Flies (*Musca sorbens*) may contribute to spread of disease.	As long as active lesions are present in the conjunctivae and adnexal mucous membranes.
Trench fever (Wollhynian fever, quintan fever)	Nonfatal, febrile disease of protean manifestations characterized by headache, malaise, pain, and tenderness, especially in shins; onset either sudden or slow with fever, which may be relapsing, typhoid-like, or limited to single short febrile episode lasting several days.	Generally 7 to 30 days.	Not directly transmitted from person to person. Humans infected by inoculation of organism in louse feces through a skin break from either bite of louse or other means.	Organisms may circulate in blood (by which lice can be infected) for weeks, months, or years and may recur with or without symptoms. History of trench fever is permanent contraindication to blood donation.
Trichinosis (trichiniasis, trichinellosis)	Disease caused by larvae of *Trichinella spiralis* that migrate to and become encapsulated in muscles. Clinical manifestations usually include mild febrile disease, but can range from inapparent infection to fulminating, fatal disease.	Usually about 10 to 14 days after ingestion by humans of infective meat; varies between 1 and 45 days.	Eating raw or insufficiently cooked flesh of animals containing viable encysted trichinae, chiefly pork and pork products.	Not transmitted directly from person to person. Animal hosts remain infective for months as does meat from such animals for appreciable periods unless processed to kill larvae.
Trichomoniasis	Common disease of genitourinary tract, characterized in women by vaginitis, with small petechial or sometimes punctate hemorrhagic lesions and profuse, thin, foamy, yellowish discharge with foul odor; frequently asymptomatic. In men, the infectious agent invades and persists in prostate, urethra, or seminal vesicles, but rarely produces symptoms or demonstrable lesions.	Generally 2 to 15 days, but can be longer in some patients. In men, 4 to 20 days with an average of 7 days.	By contact with vaginal and urethral discharges of infected persons during sexual intercourse and possibly by contact with contaminated articles.	For duration of infection.

Communicable and Infectious Diseases—cont'd

Name	Synopsis of symptoms	Incubation period	Mode of transmission	Period of communicability
Trichuriasis (trichocephaliasis)	Nematode infection of large intestine, often asymptomatic. Heavy infections result in bloody stools and diarrhea. Rectal prolapse may occur in very heavily infected children.	1 to 2 weeks.	Poor sanitation, allowing ingestion of soil containing roundworm eggs.	Not directly transmitted from person to person. Environment may be continuously contaminated.
Trypanosomiasis (African sleeping sickness)	In early stages chancre usually appears at primary tsetse fly bite site with fever, intense headache, insomnia, lymph node enlargement, anemia, local edema, and rash. In late stage is body wasting, somnolence, and signs referable to central nervous system.	In *T. rhodesiense* infection, usually 2 to 3 weeks; in *T. gambiense* infection, usually longer and extremely variable—months or even years.	By bite of infective *Glossina*, the tsetse fly. Congenital transmission can occur in humans, as well as direct mechanical transmission by blood on proboscis of *Glossina* and other human-biting flies, or in laboratory accidents.	As long as parasite is present in blood of infected person or animal. Parasitemia is extremely variable in untreated cases and occurs in late and early stages of disease.
Trypanosomiasis, American (Chagas' disease)	Acute disease usually occurs in children; chronic manifestations generally appear later in life. Acute disease is characterized by variable fever, malaise, lymphadenopathy, and hepatosplenomegaly. Inflammatory response at site of infection (chagoma) may last up to 8 weeks. Unilateral bipalpebral edema occurs in significant percentage of acute cases. Life-threatening or fatal manifestations include myocarditis and meningoencephalitis.	About 5 to 14 days after bite of insect vector; 30 to 40 days if infected by blood transfusion.	By fecal material passed when bitten by infected vectors. Infection is through contamination of conjunctiva, mucous membranes, abrasions, or skin wounds by fresh infected insect feces. Transmission also may occur by blood transfusion and organisms may pass through placenta to cause congenital infection.	Organisms are present regularly in blood during acute period and may persist in very small numbers throughout life in symptomatic and asymptomatic persons. Vector becomes infective 10 to 30 days after biting an infective host and remains so for life (as long as 2 years).
Tuberculosis	Mycobacterial disease. Initial infection usually goes unnoticed; tuberculin sensitivity appears within a few weeks; lesions commonly heal, leaving no residual changes except pulmonary or tracheobronchial lymph node calcification. May progress to pulmonary tuberculosis or, by lymphohematogenous dissemination of bacilli, to produce miliary, meningeal, or other extrapulmonary involvement.	From infection to demonstrable primary lesion, about 4 to 12 weeks. Whereas subsequent risk of progressive pulmonary or extrapulmonary tuberculosis is greatest within 1 or 2 years after infection, it may persist for a lifetime as a latent infection.	Exposure to bacilli in airborne droplet nuclei from sputum of persons with infectious tuberculosis. Bovine tuberculosis results from exposure to tubercular cattle and ingestion of unpasteurized dairy products.	As long as infectious tubercle bacilli are being discharged.

Disease	Clinical characteristics	Incubation period	Mode of transmission	Period of communicability
Tularemia (rabbit fever, deerfly fever, Ohara's disease)	Clinical manifestations related to route of introduction and virulence of strain. Most often ulcer, often on hand, accompanied by swelling of regional lymph nodes. May be no apparent primary ulcer but only enlarged and painful lymph nodes that may suppurate.	Related to virulence of infecting strain and to size of inoculum; 2 to 10 days, usually 3 days.	Inoculation of skin, conjunctival sac, or oropharyngeal mucosa with blood or tissue while handling infected animals; or by fluids from infected flies, ticks, or other animals; or through bite of arthropods.	Not directly transmitted from person to person. Unless treated, infectious agent may be found in blood during first 2 weeks of disease, and in lesions for 1 month from onset—sometimes longer.
Typhoid fever (enteric fever, typhus abdominalis)	Systemic infectious disease characterized by sustained fever, headache, malaise, anorexia, relative bradycardia, enlargement of spleen, rose spots on trunk, nonproductive cough, constipation more commonly than diarrhea, and involvement of lymphoid tissues.	Depends on size of infecting dose; usual range 1 to 3 weeks.	By food or water contaminated by feces or urine of patient or carrier.	As long as typhoid bacilli appear in excreta; usually first week throughout convalescence; variable thereafter. About 10% of untreated patients will discharge bacilli for 3 months after onset of symptoms; 2% to 5% become permanent carriers.
Typhus fever, epidemic louse-borne (exanthematic typhus, classical typhus fever)	Onset is variable, often sudden and marked by headache, chills, fever, and general pains. Macular eruptions appear on fifth or sixth day, initially on upper trunk followed by spread to entire body but usually not to face, palms, or soles. Toxemia is usually pronounced and disease terminates by rapid lysis after about 2 weeks of fever.	From 1 to 2 weeks, commonly 12 days.	The body louse, *Pediculus humanis corporis*, is infected by feeding on blood of patient with acute typhus fever. Humans are infected by rubbing feces or crushed lice into bites of louse or other superficial abrasions. Inhalation of infective louse feces as dust may account for some infections.	Disease is not directly transmitted from person to person. Patients are infective for lice during febrile illness and possibly for 2 or 3 days after temperature returns to normal.
Typhus fever, flea-borne (murine typhus, endemic typhus fever, shop typhus)	Course of flea-borne typhus fever resembles that of epidemic louse-borne typhus, but is milder. Fatality rate is about 2%, but increases with age.	From 1 to 2 weeks, commonly 12 days.	Infective rat fleas (usually *Xenopsylla cheopis*) defecate rickettsiae while sucking blood and contaminate bite site and other fresh skin wounds. Occasional case may follow inhalation of dried infective flea feces.	Not directly transmitted from person to person. Once infected, fleas remain so for life.
Typhus, scrub (tsutsugamushi disease, mite-borne typhus fever)	Often characterized by primary skin ulcer (eschar) corresponding to site of attachment of infected mite. Acute febrile onset follows within several days, along with headache, diaphoresis, conjunctival injection, and lymphadenopathy.	Usually 10 to 12 days; varies from 6 to 21 days.	By infected larval mites; nymphs and adults do not feed on vertebrate hosts.	Not directly transmitted from person to person.

Communicable and Infectious Diseases—cont'd

Name	Synopsis of symptoms	Incubation period	Mode of transmission	Period of communicability
Urethritis, chlamydial (urethritis, nongonorrheal and nonspecific)	Sexually transmitted urethritis of males caused by chlamydial agent. Clinical manifestations are usually indistinguishable from gonorrhea but are often milder and include opaque discharge of moderate or scanty quantity, urethral itching and burning on urination. Infection of women results in cervicitis and salpingitis; infections are often asymptomatic.	5 to 7 days or longer.	Sexual contact.	Unknown.
Verruca vulgaris (warts)	Viral disease manifested by variety of skin and mucous membrane lesions. Include the common wart, a circumscribed, hyperkeratotic, rough textured, painless papule varying in size from pinhead to large masses; also filiform warts, venereal warts, and plantar warts.	About 4 months; range is 1 to 20 months.	Usually by direct contact, but contaminated floors and fomites are frequently implicated. Warts may be autoinoculated. *Condyloma accuminatum* is usually sexually transmitted.	Unknown, but probably as long as visible lesions persist.
Whooping cough (pertussis)	Acute bacterial disease involving tracheobronchial tree. Initial catarrhal stage has insidious onset with irritating cough that gradually becomes paroxysmal, usually within 1 to 2 weeks, and lasts for 1 to 2 months.	Commonly 7 days; almost uniformly within 10 days, and not exceeding 21 days.	Primarily by direct contact with discharges from respiratory mucous membranes of infected persons by airborne route, probably by droplets. Frequently brought into home by older sibling.	Highly communicable in early catarrhal stage before paroxysmal cough stage. For control purposes, communicable stage extends from 7 days after exposure to 3 weeks after onset of typical paroxysms in patients not treated with antibiotics; in patients treated with erythromycin, period of infectiousness extends only 5 to 7 days after onset of therapy.
Yaws (frambesia, pian, bouba, parang)	Chronic relapsing nonvenereal treponematosis characterized by early cutaneous lesions and noncontagious late, destructive lesions. Typical initial lesion (mother yaw) is papilloma on face or extremities that persists for several weeks or months.	From 2 weeks to 3 months.	Principally by direct contact with exudates of early skin lesions of infected persons. Indirect transmission by contamination from scratching, skin piercing articles, and by flies on open wounds is probable but of undetermined importance.	Variable; may extend intermittently over several years while moist lesions are present. Infectious agent is not usually found in late ulcerative lesions.

Yersinia (pseudotuberculosis)	Acute enteric disease manifested by diarrhea, enterocolitis, acute mesenteric lymphadenitis mimicking appendicitis, fever, headache, pharyngitis, anorexia, vomiting, erythema nodosum, arthritis, cutaneous ulceration, abscesses, and septicemia.	Probably 3 to 7 days, generally less than 10 days.	Fecal-oral transmission takes place by contact with infected persons or animals (hand-to-mouth), or by eating and drinking contaminated food and water.	Fecal shedding as long as symptoms exist. Chronic carrier state probably exists.
Zygomycosis (mucormycosis, phycomycosis)	Group of mycoses usually caused by fungi of the family Mucoraceae of the class Zygomycetes. These fungi have affinity for blood vessels, causing thrombosis and infarction. In its craniofacial form, is usually nasal or paranasal sinus infections, most often during ketoacidotic episodes of diabetes mellitus.	Unknown. Fungus spreads rapidly in susceptible tissues.	By inhalation or ingestion of fungus by susceptible individuals. Direct inoculation by minor trauma, intravenous catheters, and cutaneous burns are occasionally implicated.	Not directly transmitted from human or animal to human.

REFERENCE

3-1 | Normal Lab Values

Values vary according to lab technique used.

Acetone 0.3-2 mg/dl
Alanine aminotransferase (ALT) 5-30 U/L (37° C)
Albumin 3.5-5.0 gm/dl
Alcohol 0%
   legal intoxication 0.08% or higher (usually 0.10%)
   marked intoxication 0.3-0.4%
   unconsciousness 0.4-0.5%
Alkaline phosphatase (serum) 20-90 U/L (30° C)
Ammonia 80-110 µg/dl
Amylase 25-125 U/L (serum)
   1-17 unit/h (urine)
Aspartate aminotransferase (AST) 10-30 U/L
   (37° C)
Base excess, blood 0 ± 2 mEq/L
Bicarbonate (HCO$_3$) 8-23 mEq/L
Bilirubin 0.1-1.2 mg/dl (total)
Bleeding coagulation time (IVY) 1-6 minutes
BUN (blood urea nitrogen) 11-23 mg/dl
Calcium (serum) 8.4-10.2 mg/dl
Carbon monoxide 0-2%; symptoms seen with saturation over 20%
Carbon dioxide (arterial) 35-45 mm/Hg (pCO$_2$)
   (venous) 24-32 mEq/L
Chloride 96-106 mEq/L
Cholesterol <200 mg/dl
Cholinesterase (serum) 0.5-1.3 pH units
Coagulation time (Lee-White) 5-15 minutes (glass)
   19-60 minutes (siliconized)
Copper (serum) (M) 70-140 µg/dl
   (F) 85-155 µg/dl
CPK (creatine phosphokinase) (M) 5-55 mU/ml
   (F) 5-35 mU/ml
Creatine (serum) 0.6-1.5 mg/dl
Creatinine (plasma or serum) (M) 0.7-1.3 mg/dl
   (F) 0.6-1.1 mg/dl
Fibrinogen 200-400 mg/dl (plasma)
Folic acid 6-15 ng/ml
Globulin 1.5-3 gm/dl
Glucose 65-110 mg/dl
Hematocrit (M) 42-52 ml/dl
   (F) 37-47 ml/dl
Hemoglobin (M) 14.0-18.0 gm/dl
   (F) 12.0-18.0 gm/dl
Immunoglobulins (serum) IgA—69-382 mg/dl
   IgD—0.5-3.0 mg/dl
   IgE—<500 mg/ml
   IgG—550-1900 mg/dl
   IgM—45-145 mg/dl

Iron (serum) (Male) 67-170 µg/dl
   (Female) 50-170 µg/dl
Lactic acid 3-7 mg/dl (arterial)
   9-16 mg/dl (venous)
Lactic dehydrogenase (LDH) 100-190 U/L
Lipase (serum) 10-40 U/L (37° C)
Lithium 0.5-1.0 mEq/L
Leukocyte count *see WBC*
Magnesium 1.8-3.0 mEq/L
MCH (Mean Corpuscular Hemoglobin) 27-32 pg/RBC
MCHC (Mean Corpuscular Hemoglobin Concentration) 33-38%
MCV (Mean Corpuscular Volume) 80-94 cubic microns (µm^3)
Osmolality (serum) 280-295 mOsm/kg serum water
Oxygen (arterial) 83-108 mm/Hg (pO$_2$)
   saturation—95-98%
   (venous) 35-45 mm/Hg
   saturation—60-85%
Partial thromboplastin time, activated (ADTT) 20-35 sec.
pH (arterial) 7.35-7.45
   (urine) 4.6-8.0 (diet dependent)
Phosphate, inorganic (serum) 2.7-4.5 mg/dl
Platelets 150,000-350,000/mm^3
pO$_2$ 80-100 mm/Hg
Potassium (serum) 3.5-5.1 mEq/L
Protein (serum)—total 6.4-8.3 gm/dl
   globulin 3.5-5.0 gm/dl
Prothrombin time (one stage) 12.0-14.0 sec
Pyruvate (whole blood) 0.3-0.9 mg/dl
RBC (erythrocyte) count (Male) 4,600,000-6,200,000/mm^3
   (Female) 4,200,000-5,400,000/mm^3
SGOT *see Aspartate aminotransferase*
SGPT *see Alanine aminotransferase*
Sodium 136-147 mEq/L
Triglycerides (serum, fasting) (Male) 40-160 mg/dl
   (Female) 35-135 mg/dl
Urea nitrogen *see BUN*
Uric acid (serum, enzymatic) (Male) 2.5-8.0 mg/dl
   (Female) 1.5-7.0 mg/dl
Urine—glucose < 250 mg/24 h
   potassium 40-65 mEq/24 h
   protein up to 150 mg/24 h
   sodium 130-260 mEq/24 h
specific gravity 1.002-1.030
WBC 5,000-10,000/mm^3

3-2 Table of the Elements

The left number in each box is the atomic number. (positive charge of the nucleus in multiples of the unit charge e).

The right number in each box is atomic mass (atomic mass units), averages by isotopic abundance in the earth's surface. Atomic masses for radioactive elements shown in parentheses are the whole number nearest the most stable isotope of that element.

Key:
- atomic number: 14
- atomic weight: 28.09
- symbol: Si
- name: Silicon

IA	IIA	IIIB	IVB	VB	VIB	VIIB	VIII	VIII	VIII	IB	IIB	IIIA	IVA	VA	VIA	VIIA	0
1 1.0080 **H** Hydrogen																	2 4.003 **He** Helium
3 6.940 **Li** Lithium	4 9.013 **Be** Beryllium											5 10.82 **B** Boron	6 12.011 **C** Carbon	7 14.008 **N** Nitrogen	8 16.000 **O** Oxygen	9 19.00 **F** Fluorine	10 20.183 **Ne** Neon
11 22.991 **Na** Sodium	12 24.32 **Mg** Magnesium											13 26.98 **Al** Aluminum	14 28.09 **Si** Silicon	15 30.975 **P** Phosphorus	16 32.066 **S** Sulfur	17 35.457 **Cl** Chlorine	18 39.944 **Ar** Argon
19 39.100 **K** Potassium	20 40.08 **Ca** Calcium	21 44.96 **Sc** Scandium	22 47.90 **Ti** Titanium	23 50.95 **V** Vanadium	24 52.01 **Cr** Chromium	25 54.94 **Mn** Manganese	26 55.85 **Fe** Iron	27 58.94 **Co** Cobalt	28 58.71 **Ni** Nickel	29 63.54 **Cu** Copper	30 65.38 **Zn** Zinc	31 69.72 **Ga** Gallium	32 72.60 **Ge** Germanium	33 74.91 **As** Arsenic	34 78.96 **Se** Selenium	35 79.916 **Br** Bromine	36 83.80 **Kr** Krypton
37 85.47 **Rb** Rubidium	38 87.63 **Sr** Strontium	39 88.92 **Y** Yttrium	40 91.22 **Zr** Zirconium	41 92.91 **Nb** Niobium	42 95.95 **Mo** Molybdenum	43 (99) **Tc** Technetium	44 101.1 **Ru** Ruthenium	45 102.91 **Rh** Rhodium	46 106.4 **Pd** Palladium	47 107.880 **Ag** Silver	48 112.41 **Cd** Cadmium	49 114.82 **In** Indium	50 118.70 **Sn** Tin	51 121.76 **Sb** Antimony	52 127.61 **Te** Tellurium	53 126.91 **I** Iodine	54 131.30 **Xe** Xenon
55 132.91 **Cs** Cesium	56 137.36 **Ba** Barium	57 138.92 **La** Lanthanum ▲	72 178.50 **Hf** Hafnium	73 180.95 **Ta** Tantalum	74 183.86 **W** Wolfram	75 186.22 **Re** Rhenium	76 190.2 **Os** Osmium	77 192.2 **Ir** Iridium	78 195.09 **Pt** Platinum	79 197.0 **Au** Gold	80 200.61 **Hg** Mercury	81 204.39 **Tl** Thallium	82 207.21 **Pb** Lead	83 209.00 **Bi** Bismuth	84 (210) **Po** Polonium	85 (210) **At** Astatine	86 (222) **Rn** Radon
87 (223) **Fr** Francium	88 (226) **Ra** Radium	89 (227) **Ac** Actinium ▲▲	104 (261) **Rf** Rutherfordium	105 (262) **Ha** Hahnium	106 (266) **Sg** Seaborgium	107 (262) **Ns** Nielsbohrium	108 (262) **Hs** Hassium	109 (266) **Mt** Meitnerium									

Lanthanide series ▲

58 140.12 **Ce** Cerium	59 140.91 **Pr** Praseodymium	60 144.24 **Nd** Neodymium	61 (145) **Pm** Promethium	62 150.40 **Sm** Samarium	63 151.96 **Eu** Europium	64 157.25 **Gd** Gadolinium	65 158.93 **Tb** Praseodymium	66 162.50 **Dy** Dysporsium	67 164.93 **Ho** Holmium	68 167.26 **Er** Erbium	69 168.93 **Tm** Thilium	70 173.04 **Yb** Ytterbium	71 174.97 **Lu** Lutetium

Actinide series ▲▲

90 232.04 **Th** Thorium	91 231.04 **Pa** Protactinium	92 238.03 **U** Uranium	93 237.05 **Np** Neptunium	94 (244) **Pu** Plutonium	95 (243) **Am** Americium	96 (247) **Cm** Curium	97 (247) **Bk** Berkelium	98 (249) **Cf** Californium	99 (252) **Es** Einsteinium	100 (257) **Fm** Fermium	101 (260) **Md** Mendelevium	102 (254) **No** Nobelium	103 (262) **Lr** Lawrencium

3-3 | Conversion Equivalents

LENGTH

1 inch = 25.4 millimeters
1 inch = 2.54 centimeters
1 foot = 0.3048 meter
1 yard = 0.9144 meter
1 mile = 1.609 kilometers
1 nautical mile = 1.1507 miles
1 nautical mile = 1.852 kilometers
1 foot = 12 inches
1 mile = 1,760 yards

1 millimeter = 0.0394 inch
1 centimeter = 0.3937 inch
1 meter = 3.2808 feet
1 meter = 1.0936 yards
1 kilometer = 0.6215 mile
1 mile = 0.8689 nautical mile
1 kilometer = 0.5399 nautical mile
1 yard = 3 feet

AVOIRDUPOIS WEIGHTS

1 grain = 64.8 milligrams
1 ounce = 28.35 grams
1 pound = 0.4536 kilogram
1 pound = 16 ounces

1 milligram = 0.0154 grain
1 gram = 0.0353 ounce
1 kilogram = 2.2046 pounds

APOTHECARY WEIGHTS/MEASURES

1 pound = 0.3732 kilogram
1 fluid ounce = 29.5737 milliliters
1 pint = 0.4732 liter
1 quart = 0.9464 liter
1 gallon = 3.7854 liters

1 kilogram = 2.6792 pounds
1 milliliter = 0.0338 fluid ounce
1 liter = 2.1134 pints
1 liter = 1.0567 quarts
1 liter = 0.2642 gallon

Continued

Conversion Equivalents—cont'd

TEMPERATURE CONVERSION TABLE

Fahrenheit to Celsius				Celsius to Fahrenheit	
°F	°C	°F	°C	°C	°F
−40	−40.0	95	35.0	−40	−40.0
−35	−37.2	96	35.5	−35	−31.0
−30	−34.4	97	36.1	−30	−22.0
−25	−31.7	98	36.6	−25	−13.0
−20	−28.9	98.6	37.0	−20	−4.0
−15	−26.6	99	37.2	−15	5.0
−10	−23.3	100	37.7	−10	14.0
−5	−20.6	101	38.3	−5	23.0
0	−17.7	102	38.8	0	32.0
1	−17.2	103	39.4	1	33.8
5	−15.0	104	40.0	5	41.0
10	−12.2	105	40.5	10	50.0
15	−9.4	106	41.1	15	59.0
20	−6.6	107	41.6	20	68.0
25	−3.8	108	42.2	25	77.0
30	−1.1	109	42.7	30	86.0
31	−0.5	110	43.3	31	87.8
32	0	115	46.1	32	89.6
33	0.5	120	48.8	33	91.4
34	1.1	125	51.6	34	93.2
35	1.6	130	54.4	35	95.0
40	4.4	135	57.2	36	96.8
45	7.2	140	60.0	37	98.6
50	10.0	145	62.7	38	100.4
55	12.7	150	65.5	39	102.2
60	15.5	155	68.3	40	104.0
65	18.3	160	71.1	41	105.8
70	21.1	165	73.8	42	107.6
75	23.8	170	76.6	43	109.4
80	26.6	175	79.4	44	111.2
85	29.4	180	82.2	45	113.0
86	30.0	185	85.0	50	122.0
87	30.5	190	87.7	55	131.0
88	31.0	195	90.5	60	140.0
89	31.6	200	93.3	65	149.0
90	32.2	205	96.1	70	158.0
91	32.7	210	98.8	75	167.0
92	33.3	211	99.4	80	176.0
93	33.8	212	100	85	185.0
94	34.4			90	194.0
				95	203.0
				100	212.0

To convert Fahrenheit to Celsius: (temperature − 32) × 5/9

To convert Celsius to Fahrenheit: (temperature × 9/5) + 32

3-4 | Med-Math Simplified

Courtesy Steve McGraw, REMT-P, MHSA, assistant professor, The George Washington University, EMS Program

For the most part, med-math can be summarized as three categories of calculations: (1) weights and measures, (2) concentrations, and (3) IV drips. Although a number of different methods exist for solving each of these categories of problems, one method (and in some cases a refinement of the methods) will be presented here. If you have a different process than what is shown here and, most importantly, if it works, stick with your method. How you get to the correct answer is not as important as consistently getting the correct answer.

WEIGHTS AND MEASURES

All med-math problems involve weights and measures. Some may require volume (the space occupied by a substance), such as one cup or 5 milliliters (ml). Other calculations may require weight (the heaviness or mass of an object), such as ten pounds or 3 kilograms (kg). Another measurement is distance, but this has limited application to med-math calculations.

Several different systems are used to measure medications: (1) the household system, (2) the apothecary system, and (3) the metric system.

Household System

The household system, the least exact of the three systems, is used primarily for home medication administration. Also, most people are not familiar with the other systems and do not have the appropriate measuring devices. Most medication that is administered orally does not require exact measurement, so "close" is sufficient.

Volume measurement under the household system utilizes the drop (gtt), ounce (oz), teaspoon (tsp), tablespoon (tbsp), and cup (c). (The pint, quart, and gallon are historically apothecary measurements and have limited applicability to med-math calculations.) Weight measurement under the household system includes ounces (oz), pounds (lbs), and tons. Distance is measured in inches (in), feet (ft), yards (yd), and miles.

It is important for the health care provider to be able to convert household measurements to metric calculations. For example, a child should receive 15 ml of ipecac, which is equivalent to one tablespoon.

The most common conversions in the household system are listed below:

16 oz = 1 lb	4 quarts = 1 gallon
1kg = 2.2 lb	1 inch = 2.54 centimeters
1 lb = 0.45 kg	60 gtts = 1 fluid oz
1 tsp = 5 ml	1 tbsp = 15 ml
3 tsp = 1 tbsp	2 tbsp = 30 ml
16 tbsp = 1 cup (liquid)	1 cup = approximately 240 ml
16 fluid oz = 1 pint	1 pint = approximately 500 ml
2 pints = 1 quart	1 quart = approximately 1,000 ml, or 1 liter

One method of performing the conversion from household to metric (or any other conversion for that matter) is in the form of a ratio of known-to-unknown. For example, your patient is taking 3 tablespoons of a particular drug and you want to know how many milliliters that is. First set up your known (the conversion factor).

$$\text{KNOWN}$$
$$\frac{15 \text{ ml}}{1 \text{ tbsp}}$$

Then on the other side of the equal sign, set up your unknown (what you want to know), inserting your given factor. x will equal the amount you wish to solve for. Be sure to remember to keep like units together, i.e., ml with ml, tbsp with tbsp, etc.

$$\frac{\overset{\text{KNOWN}}{15 \text{ ml}}}{1 \text{ tbsp}} = \frac{\overset{\text{UNKNOWN}}{x \text{ ml}}}{3 \text{ tbsp}}$$

Now solve for x by cross-multiplying, that is, by multiplying diagonally across the equal sign of the known-to-unknown equation.

$$3 \times 15 = 1 \times x \text{ ml}$$
$$45 \text{ ml} = x$$

To convert from pounds to kilograms, divide the number of pounds by 2.2; e.g., 150 lb is equal to 68 kg (150/2.2 = 68). Another method is to divide the number of pounds by 2; e.g., one half of 150 is 75. Then subtract 10% of that number; e.g., 10% of 75 is about 7, 7 from 75 is 68.

Apothecary System

The apothecary system was once the only system used for drugs in this country. Occasionally, you will come across a drug (e.g., aspirin or nitroglycerin) that is still measured in apothecaries or you may run into an older physician who gives orders in apothecary measurements (e.g., orders for morphine sulfate).

Volume measurement in the apothecary system is the minim (M). Rarely does anyone other than a pharmacist use minims, and they will not be discussed here. The grain (gr) is the basic unit of weight in the apothecary system. Conversions form grains to metric is performed as follows:

$$1 \text{ gr} = 65 \text{ mg}$$
$$1 \text{ mg} = 0.015 \text{ gr}$$

An easy way to remember this is to keep in mind that a 5-gr aspirin contains 325 mg of the drug.

Metric System

Generally all medications have the dosage presented in metric units. Therefore, it is imperative to become thoroughly familiar with the metric system.

The basic unit of metric measurement for volume is the liter (L or l), the basic unit of weight is the gram (g or gm), and the basic unit of distance is the meter (m). The metric system is based on units of 10, with prefixes to indicate the fraction or multiple of ten that we are dealing with:

kilo	= 1000	centi	= 0.01
hecto	= 100	milli	= 0.001
deca	= 10	micro	= 0.000001
deci	= 0.1		

Note that a cubic centimeter (cc) is similar to a milliliter (ml), and they are used interchangeably.

To convert liters (or grams or meters) to ml (or mg or mm) multiply the liters by 1000; e.g., 2 l is 2000 ml (2 × 1000 = 2000). To convert ml (or mg or mm) to liters (or g or m), divide the ml by 1000; e.g., 500 ml = 0.5 l (500/1000 = 0.5).

To convert grams to micrograms (μg), multiply the grams by 1,000,000 (move the decimal point six places to the right); e.g., 0.25 gm is 250,000 mcg (0.25 × 1,000,000 = 250,000). To convert mcg to gm, divide the mcg by 1,000,000 (move the decimal point six places to the left).

To convert mg to μg, multiply the mg by 1000 (move the decimal point three places to the right). To convert μg to mg, divide μg by 1000 (move the decimal point three places to the left).

It is very important to ensure that your decimal point is in the proper position. A decimal point misplaced by one position results in a drug dosage either over or short by a factor of 10 (enough to make the drug lethal or ineffective).

Making Weight-Dependent Calculations

Many drug dosages are dependent on the weight of the patient. This type of problem is usually expressed as follows: "You are to administer x amount (mg, ml, etc.) of a drug per kilogram of body weight." The notation of x mg/kg is usually used. If the equation does not numerically state how much of a given unit should be used, as 2 mg/1 kg, then assume one unit of measure; thus 2 mg/1 kg could be 2 mg/kg. To perform this type of calculation, two steps are required. First convert the patient's weight from pounds to kilograms (divide by 2.2). Second, multiply the weight in kilograms by the amount that you are to administer.

For example, you have a patient who weighs 160 lb and medical control orders you to administer 0.5 mg/kg of lidocaine. How much of the drug are you to administer?

First, convert the pounds to kilograms.

$$\frac{160 \text{ lbs}}{2.2 \text{ lbs/kg}} = 72 \text{ kg.}$$

Next, multiply the weight by the dosage.

$$72 \text{ kg} \times 0.5 \text{ mg/kg} = 36 \text{ mg of lidocaine.}$$

CONCENTRATIONS

A concentration is how much of one substance is present in another. For example, 12 students per classroom, 4 wheels per car, or 200 mg of a drug in 500 cc of solution.

Each drug is packaged as a particular concentration: 5 mg per tablet, 2 mg/cc, etc. The health care provider must be able to compute how much of a drug with a certain concentration is to be administered.

In pharmacology, a concentration is generally expressed as x amount of mg (or milliequivalents (mEq), μg, or gm) per ml of solution. To compute the concentration, one simply divides the total number of mg of drug in the package by the total number of ml of solution in the package.

Drug packages are labeled according to the concentration of the drug; e.g., epinephrine 1:10,000 is labeled as containing 1 mg in 10 ml of solution; epinephrine 1:1000 contains 1 mg in 1 ml of solution. It is important for the provider to carefully read the package to ensure that the concentration is correct before administering the drug.

You may be ordered to administer 0.3 mg of epinephrine to a patient. Use the following formula:

Packaged mg/packaged ml = concentration (mg per 1 ml)
Dose to be given/concentration = ml to administer

In this case, using the epinephrine 1:1000,

$$1 \text{ mg/1 ml} = 1 \text{ mg/ml}$$

$$\frac{0.3 \text{ mg}}{1 \text{ mg/ml}} = 0.3 \text{ ml to be administered}$$

Using the epinephrine 1:10,000,

$$1 \text{ mg/10 ml} = 0.1 \text{ mg/ml}$$

$$\frac{0.3 \text{ mg}}{0.1 \text{ mg/ml}} = 3 \text{ ml to be administered}$$

The computations involved are relatively easy, but notice how important it is to keep a close watch on the decimal place and to be sure of the concentration of the drug.

A shortcut for computation of a bolus administration is to use the "block" method. Lay out your problem using four blocks:

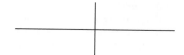

Each of the blocks then has a number inserted in it:

Ordered/ Desired Drug Dose	Volume (ml) in syringe of drug available	
Amount (mg, μg, etc.) in syringe of drug available	1	= ml to be administered

The only restriction is that all measurements must be in the same units; i.e., desired dose and amount must be in the same units (mg, grams, mEq, etc.).

So to compute our problem with the 0.3 mg 1:10,000 epinephrine,

$$\frac{0.3 \text{ mg} \quad | \quad 10 \text{ ml}}{1 \text{ mg} \quad | \quad 1} = \text{ml}$$

Multiply across the top two blocks and across the bottom two blocks, and then divide:

$$\frac{0.3 \times 10}{1 \times 1} = \frac{3}{1} = 3 \text{ ml}$$

IV DRIPS

An IV is a method of administering either a volume of fluid over a period of time (such as in fluid resuscitation due to hypovolemia) or administering a particular amount of a drug over a period of time. The health care provider must be able to do this with a high degree of accuracy since an error could mean life or death to your patient.

Each type of IV administration set is calibrated to deliver x amount of drops per cc of fluid. For example, most "mini-drip" sets are calibrated to deliver 60 drops (gtts) per cc of fluid. Most standard (or "macrodrip") administration sets are calibrated to administer 15 or 20 drops per cc. It is important for the provider to ascertain the calibration of the administration set.

Volume Administration

To compute an IV drip rate for volume administration, you need the following pieces of information: calibration of the administration set (gtts/cc), the volume of solution to be administered (in cc), and the time (in minutes) over which the fluid is to be administered. The computation is performed using the formula:

$$\text{gtts/min} = \frac{\substack{\text{Amount to be administered} \\ \text{(in ml or cc)}} \times \substack{\text{Calibration of} \\ \text{administration set}}}{\text{Time in minutes}}$$

Remember when performing your calculations to keep the units similar: The amount to be administered should be in cc because most administration sets are calibrated in gtts/cc. Also remember that there are 60 minutes to an hour.

Using the box method,

Ordered/ desired dose (cc)	Administration set (gtts/cc)	
Time, in minutes	1	= gtts/min

For example, you want to administer 1 L of lactated Ringer's solution over a 3-hour period using a standard (20 gtts/cc) administration set.

The first step is to get everything into common units:

$$1 \text{ L} = 1000 \text{ cc (or ml)}$$
$$3 \text{ h} = 180 \text{ min}$$

Now, plug in the numbers:

$$\frac{1000 \text{ cc} \quad | \quad 20 \text{ gtts/cc}}{180 \text{ min} \quad | \quad 1} = \text{gtts/min}$$

Cancel the zeros in the 20 and the 180 leaving:

$$\frac{1000 \quad | \quad 2}{18 \quad | \quad 1} = \frac{1000 \times 2}{18 \times 1} = \frac{2000}{18} = 111 \text{ gtts/min}$$

Drip Infusion

Drugs are often administered over time utilizing an IV drip. This allows for a constant dosage to be administered and therapeutic blood levels to be maintained.

To compute the drip rate for a drip infusion, one needs the following items of information: calibration of the drip chamber (gtts/cc), the concentration of the drug after the drug is placed into the solution (mg/cc), and the amount of the drug to be administered per minute (mg/min).

$$\text{gtts/min} = \frac{\text{Desired dose} \times \substack{\text{Calibration of} \\ \text{administration set}}}{\text{Concentration on hand}}$$

Using the box method,

Ordered/ desired drug dose (mg/min)	Administration set (gtts/cc)	
Concentration on hand (mg/cc)	1	= gtts/min

For example, you are ordered to place 2 grams of lidocaine into 500 cc of D_5W and administer 2 mg/min using a mini-drip (60 gtts/cc) administration set.

First of all, ensure that all numbers are in similar units:

$$2 \text{ grams} = 2000 \text{ mg}$$

Next, plug in the numbers:

$$\frac{2 \text{ mg/min} \quad | \quad 60 \text{ gtts/cc}}{2000 \text{ mg/}500 \text{ cc} \quad | \quad 1} = \text{gtts/min}$$

Note that it is always a good idea to label your units to avoid confusion and to ensure that all numbers in the formula are in similar units. This also will simplify rechecking of your calculations when necessary.

Now simplify the concentration: 2000 mg/500 cc = 4 mg/cc.

Multiply the top numbers together and the bottom numbers together. Then divide to get your final answer:

$$\frac{2 \times 60}{4 \times 1} = \frac{120}{4} = 30 \text{ gtts/min (or 1 gtt every 2 seconds)}$$

THE BOX METHOD SUMMARIZED

The box method of computing med-math is a simple way to remember the formula. Note that the upper left-hand box is always the desired dose and that the bottom right-hand box is always 1. The upper right-hand box is either the volume in the syringe (ampule, vial, etc.) or the calibration of the administration set. The bottom left-hand box is either the concentration in the syringe, bag, etc. or the time over which the fluid is to be administered.

Bolus administration:

$$\frac{\text{Ordered/desired drug dose}}{\text{Amount (mg) in syringe of drug available}} \times \frac{\text{Volume (ml) in syringe of drug available}}{1} = \text{ml to be administered}$$

Volume Administration:

$$\frac{\text{Ordered/desired drug dose (cc)}}{\text{Time in minutes}} \times \frac{\text{Administration set (gtts/cc)}}{1} = \text{gtts/min}$$

Drip infusion:

$$\frac{\text{Ordered/desired drug dose (mg/min)}}{\text{Concentration on hand (mg/cc)}} \times \frac{\text{Administration set (gtts/cc)}}{1} = \text{gtts/min}$$

MISCELLANEOUS

Drug Concentrations Expressed as a Percentage

Some drug concentrations are expressed as a percentage, e.g., 10% calcium chloride, 4% lidocaine. The percentage indicates the number of parts in 100. In the case of a drug concentration, the percentage is the number of grams present in 100 ml of solution. Another way to express this concentration is

$$\frac{\text{grams}}{100 \text{ ml}}$$

For example, to determine the concentration of 10% calcium chloride,

$$10\% = \frac{10 \text{ grams}}{100 \text{ ml}} = \frac{10,000 \text{ mg}}{100 \text{ cc}} = 100 \text{ mg/cc}$$

Drug Concentrations Expressed as a Ratio

A ratio is the relative magnitude of two quantities. The concentration of some drugs is expressed as a ratio, most notably, epinephrine 1:1000 and epinephrine 1:10,000. Like the percentage, the ratio is an expression of the number of parts present in a given amount of solution, in this case, the number of grams present in a number of ml of solution.

For example, to determine the concentration of 1:10,000 epinephrine,

$$1\!:\!10,\!000 = \frac{1 \text{ gram}}{10,\!000 \text{ cc}} = \frac{1000 \text{ mg}}{10,\!000 \text{ cc}} = 1 \text{ mg/10 cc}$$

Conversion of Fahrenheit Degrees to Centigrade Degrees

The Fahrenheit temperature measurement system uses 32 degrees as the freezing point of water and 212 degrees as the boiling point of water. Normal body temperature under the Fahrenheit system is 98.6 degrees F.

The Centigrade (or Celsius) system, the metric temperature measurement system, uses 0 degrees as the freezing point of water and 100 degrees as the boiling point of water. Normal body temperature is 37 degrees C.

To convert Fahrenheit degrees to Centigrade degrees, subtract 32 from the number of Fahrenheit degrees, and multiply the difference by 5/9. For example, $150°$ F $= (150 - 32) \times 5/9 = 118 \times 5/9 = 65.5°$ C .

To convert Centigrade degrees to Fahrenheit degrees, multiply the Centigrade degrees by 9/5, and add 32 to the result. For example, $65°$ C $= (65 \times 9/5) + 32 = 117 + 32 = 149°$ F.

3-5 Prescription and Nonprescription Drugs and General Classification

Listed alphabetically; **boldface type** = trade name.

ACCUPRIL/quinapril: antihypertensive

ACCURBRON/theophylline: xanthine bronchodilator

ACCUTANE/isotretinoin: antibacterial (acne)

ACETA with CODEINE/acetaminophen, codeine: narcotic analgesic

acetaminophen/**TEMPRA, TYLENOL**: analgesic, antiinflammatory

acetaminophen, codeine/**TYLENOL with CODEINE**: narcotic analgesic

acetazolamide/**DIAMOX**: anticonvulsant, diuretic

acetohexamide/**DYMELOR**: oral hypoglycemic

acetophenazine/**TINDAL**: phenothiazine tranquilizer

acetylcysteine/**MUCOMYST**: mucolytic

ACHROMYCIN/tetracycline: antibiotic

ACHROMYCIN V/tetracycline: antibiotic

ACLOVATE/alclometasone: steroidal antiinflammatory

ACTIBINE/yohimbine: alpha blocker

ACTIDIL/ triprolidine: antihistamine

ACTIFED/ triprolidine, pseudoephedrine: antihistamine, decongestant

ACTIGALL/ursodiol: bile acid (dissolves gall stones)

acyclovir/**ZOVIRAX**: antiviral

ADALAT/nifedipine: antianginal, antihypertensive

ADAPIN/doxepin: tricyclic antidepressant

ADIPEX-P/phentermine: appetite suppressant

ADRENALIN/epinephrine: bronchodilator

ADRUCIL/fluorouracil: anticancer

ADVIL/ibuprofen: analgesic, antiinflammatory

AEROBID/flunisolide: steroidal antiinflammatory

AEROLATE/theophylline: xanthine bronchodilator

AEROLONE/isoproteronol: bronchodilator

AEROSPORIN/polymycin: antibiotic

AFTATE/tolnaftate: antifungal

A-HYDROCORT/hydrocortisone: steroidal antiinflammatory

AKINETON/biperiden: antiparkinsonian, antiextrapyramidal symptoms

albuterol/**PROVENTIL, VOLMAX**: bronchodilator

ALDACTAZIDE/HCTZ/spironolactone: antihypertensive, diuretic

ALDACTONE/ spironolactone: diuretic (potassium sparing)

ALDOCHLOR/methyldopa, clorothiazide: antihypertensive, diuretic

ALDOMET/ methyldopa: antihypertensive

ALDORIL/ methyldopa/HCTZ: antihypertensive/diuretic

ALLEREST/APAP, chlorpheniramine, phenylpropanolamine: antihistamine, decongestant

ALLERNADE/chlorpheniramine, phenylpropanolamine: antihistamine, decongestant

ALLERTOC/pyrilamine: antihistamine

allopurinol/**LOPURIN, ZYLOPRIM**: uricosuric

alphaprodine/**NISENTIL**: narcotic analgesic

alprazolam/**XANAX**: benzodiazepine tranquilizer

ALTACE/ramipril: antihypertensive

aluminum hydroxide/**AMPHOJEL**: antacid

ALUPENT/metaproterenol: bronchodilator

amantadine/**SYMMETREL**: antiparkinsonian, antiviral

AMBIEN/zolpidem: tranquilizer

AMCILL/ampicillin: antibiotic

AMICAR/aminocaproic acid: vasoconstrictor

amikacin/**AMIKIN**: antibiotic

AMIKIN/amikacin: antibiotic

amiloride/**MIDAMOR**: diuretic (potassium sparing)

amiloride, HCTZ/**MODURETIC**: antihypertensive, diuretic

aminocaproic acid/**AMICAR**: vasoconstrictor

AMINODUR/aminophylline: xanthine bronchodilator

aminophylline/**AMINODUR, MUDRANE**: xanthine bronchodilator

amiodarone/**CORDARONE**: antidysrhythmic

AMITRIL/amitriptyline: tricyclic antidepressant

amitriptyline, chlordiazepoxide/**LIMBITROL**: antidepressant, tranquilizer

amitriptyline/**ELAVIL, NORPRAMIN**: tricyclic antidepressant

amitriptyline, perphenazine/**ETRAFON, TRIAVIL**: tricyclic antidepressant

amlodipine/**NORVASC**: antianginal, antihypertensive

AMNESTROGEN/esterified estrogens: hormone

amobarbital/**AMYTAL**: barbiturate

AMOBELL/belladonna, amobarbital: antispasmodic

amodiaquine/**CAMOQUIN**: antimalarial

amoxicillin/**AMOXIL, WYAMOX**: antibiotic

AMOXIL/amoxicillin: antibiotic

amphetamine/**BENZEDRINE**: stimulant

AMPHICOL/chloramphenicol: antibiotic

AMPHOJEL/aluminum hydroxide: antacid

amphotericin B/**FUNGIZONE**: antibiotic

ampicillin/**OMNIPEN, POLYCILLIN**: antibiotic

AMYTAL/amobarbital: barbiturate

ANAFRANIL/clomipramine: tricyclic antidepressant

ANAPROX/naproxen: analgesic, antiinflammatory

ANASPAZ PB/belladonna, phenobarbital: antispasmodic

ANCEF/cefazolin: antibiotic

ANCOBON/flucytosine: antifungal

ANEXSIA/hydrocodone, APAP: narcotic analgesic

ANHYDRON/cyclothiazide: antihypertensive, diuretic

anisindione/**MIRADON**: anticoagulant

ANSAID/flurbiprofen: analgesic, antiinflammatory

ANSPOR/cephradine: antibiotic

ANTABUSE/disulfiram: alcohol antagonist

ANTI-TUSS/guaifenesin: expectorant

ANTI-TUSS DM/guaifenesin, dextromethorphan: antitussive, expectorant

ANTIVERT/meclizine: antiemetic

ANTURANE/sulfinpyrazone: uricosuric

ANUSOL-HC/hydrocortisone, bismuth, benzyl benzoate: antiinflammatory

APAP/acetaminophen: analgesic, antiinflammatory

APAP, aspirin/**GEMNISYN**: analgesic, antiinflammatory

APAP, codeine/**CAPITAL with CODEINE**: narcotic analgesic

APAP, codeine, salicylamide/**CODALAN**: narcotic analgesic

APC (aspirin, phenacetin, caffeine) codeine/**EMPIRIN with CODEINE, SALATIN with CODEINE:** narcotic analgesic

APC, dihydrocodeine, promethazine/**SYNALGOS-DC:** narcotic analgesic

APOGEN/gentamicin: antibiotic

A-POXIDE/chlordiazepoxide: benzodiazepine tranquilizer

APRESAZIDE/HCTZ, hydralazine: antihypertensive, diuretic

APRESOLINE/hydralazine: antihypertensive, diuretic

aprobarbital/**ALURATE:** barbiturate

AQUACHLORAL/chloral hydrate: tranquilizer

AQUASTAT/benzthiazide: antihypertensive, diuretic

AQUATAG/benzthiazide: antihypertensive, diuretic

AQUATENSEN/methychlothiazide: antihypertensive, diuretic

ARALEN/chloroquine: antimalarial

ARISTOCORT/ triamcinolone: steroidal antiinflammatory

ARISTOSPAN/ triamcinolone: steroidal antiinflammatory

ARLIDIN/nylidrin: peripheral vasodilator

ARTANE/trihexyphenidyl: antiparkinsonian, antiextrapyramidal symptoms

ASA/acetylsalicylic acid: analgesic, antiinflammatory

ASA AND CODEINE/APC, codeine: narcotic analgesic

ASA COMPOUND/aspirin, phenacetin, caffeine: analgesic, antiinflammatory

ASBRON G/ theophylline, guaifenesin: bronchodilator, expectorant

ASENDIN/amoxapine: tricyclic antidepressant

ASMA/ theophylline, guaifenesin: bronchodilator, expectorant

ASMA-LIEF/theophylline, ephedrine, phenobarbital: bronchodilator, expectorant

ASMINOREL/theophylline, ephedrine, hydroxyzine: bronchodilator, expectorant

ASMINYL/theophylline, ephedrine, phenobarbital: bronchodilator, expectorant

aspirin (coated)/**ECOTRIN:** analgesic, antiinflammatory

astemizole/**HISMANAL:** antihistamine

ASTHMAHALER/epinephrine: bronchodilator

ASTHMANEFRIN/racepinephrine: bronchodilator

ASTRAMORPH PF/morphine: narcotic analgesic

ATARAX/hydroxyzine: antihistamine, tranquilizer

ATIVAN/lorazepam: benzodiazepine tranquilizer

atovaquone/**MEPRON:** antiprotozoal

ATROBARB/belladonna, phenobarbital: antispasmodic

ATROMID-S/clofibrate: antilipid

ATROVENT/ipratropium: bronchodilator

AUGMENTIN/amoxicillin, clavulanate potassium: antibiotic

auranofin/**RIDAURA:** antiarthritic

AVENTYL/nortriptyline: tricyclic antidepressant

AVLOSULFON/dapsone: antileprosy

AXID/nizatidine: histamine antagonist

AXOTAL/butalbital, ASA: analgesic

azatadine/**OPTIMINE:** antihistamine

azathioprine/**IMURAN:** immunosuppressant

AZMACORT/triamcinolone acetonide: steroidal antiinflammatory

AZODINE/phenazopyridine: urinary tract analgesic

AZO GANTANOL/sulfamethoxazole, phenazopyridine: antibacterial, analgesic

AZO GANTRISIN/sulfamethoxazole, phenazopyridine: antibacterial, analgesic

AZOLID/phenylbutazone: analgesic, antiinflammatory

AZOLID-A/buffered phenylbutazone: analgesic, antiinflammatory

AZO-100/phenazopyridine: urinary tract analgesic

AZO SOXAZOLE/ sulfamethoxazole, phenazopyridine: antibacterial, analgesic

AZO-STANDARD/ phenazopyridine: urinary tract analgesic

AZOSUL/sulfamethoxazole, phenazopyridine: antibacterial

AZO-SULFIZIN/ sulfamethoxazole, phenazopyridine: antibacterial, analgesic

AZT/azidothymidine: antiviral

AZULFIDINE/ sulfsalazine: antibacterial

bacampicillin/**SPECTROBID:** antibiotic

BACTOCILL/oxacillin: antibiotic

BACTRIM/trimethoprim: antibiotic

BACTROBAN/mupirocin: antibiotic

BANCAP-HC/hydrocodone, APAP: narcotic analgesic

BARBIDONNA/belladonna, phenobarbital: antispasmodic

beclomethasone /**BECLOVENT, VANCERIL:** steroidal antiinflammatory

BECLOVENT/ beclomethasone: steroidal antiinflammatory

BECONASE/ beclomethasone: steroidal antiinflammatory

BEEPEN-VK/penicillin: antibiotic

BELLADENAL/belladonna, phenobarbital: antispasmodic

belladonna/**BELLADENAL:** antispasmodic

belladonna, amobarbital/**AMOBELL:** antispasmodic

belladonna, butabarbital/**MINABEL, BUTIBEL:** antispasmodic

belladonna, phenobarbital/**DONNATAL, SPALIX:** antispasmodic

BELLERGAL/belladonna, ergotamine, phenobarbital: analgesic, antispasmodic

BELLO-PHEN/belladonna, phenobarbital: antispasmodic

benactyzine, meprobamate/**DEPROL:** antidepressant, tranquilizer

BENADRYL/diphenhydramine: antihistamine, tranquilizer

benazepril/**LOTENSIN:** antihypertensive

BENDOPA/levodopa, carbidopa: antiparkinsonian

bendroflumethiazide/**NATURETIN:** antihypertensive, diuretic

bendroflumethiazide, nadolol/**CORZIDE:** antihypertensive, diuretic

BENDYLATE/diphenhydramine: antihistamine

BENEMID/probenecid: prolongs action of penicillin, uricosuric

BENTYL/dicyclomine: antispasmodic

BENYLIN/diphenhydramine: antihistamine

BENZEDRINE/amphetamine: stimulant

benzphetamine/**DIDREX:** appetite suppressant

benzthiazide/**AQUASTAT, HYDREX:** antihypertensive, diuretic

benztropine/**COGENTIN:** antiparkinsonian, antiextrapyramidal symptoms

bepridil/**VASCOR:** antianginal

betamethasone/**CELESTONE, VALISONE:** steroidal antiinflammatory

BETAPACE/sotalol: antidysrhythmic

BETAPAR/mepredisone: steroidal antiinflammatory

BETAPEN-VK/penicillin: antibiotic

betaxolol/**KERLONE:** antihypertensive

bethanechol/**DUVOID, URECHOLINE:** vagomimetic (urinary retention)

BETOPTIC/betaxolol: antiglaucoma
BICILLIN/penicillin: antibiotic
biperiden/**AKINETON:** antiparkinsonian, antiextrapyramidal symptoms
BIPHETAMINE/dextroamphetamine, amphetamine: stimulant
bisacodyl/**CODYLAX, DULCOLAX:** laxative
bishydroxycoumarin/**DICUMAROL:** anticoagulant
BLOCADREN/timolol: antihypertensive, beta blocker
BONTRIL PDM/phendimetrazine: appetite suppressant
BREONESIN/guaifenesin: expectorant
BRETHAIRE/terbutaline: bronchodilator
BRETHINE/terbutaline: bronchodilator
BRICANYL/terbutaline: bronchodilator
BRISTACYCLINE/tetracycline: antibiotic
BRISTAGEN/gentamicin: antibiotic
BRISTAMYCIN/erythromycin: antibiotic
BROMATAPP/brompheniramine, phenylephrine: antihistamine, decongestant
bromocriptine/**PARLODEL:** antiparkinsonian
BROMPHEN / brompheniramine: antihistamine
brompheniramine / **BROMPHEN, DIMETANE:** antihistamine
BROMPHENIRAMINE COMPOUND/ brompheniramine, phenylephrine: antihistamine, decongestant
brompheniramine, phenylephrine /**DIMETANE, DIMETAPP:** antihistamine, decongestant
brompheniramine, phenylephrine, codeine/**DIMETANE DC, MIDATANE DC:** antihistamine, narcotic antitussive
BRONCHOLATE/theophylline, guaifenesin, phenobarbital: bronchodilator, expectorant
BRONDECON/oxtriphylline, guaifenesin: bronchodilator, expectorant
BRONDELATE/oxtriphylline, guaifenesin: bronchodilator, expectorant
BRONITIN/epinephrine: bronchodilator
BRONKAID/epinephrine: bronchodilator
BRONKEPHRINE/ethylnorepinephrine: bronchodilator
BRONKODYL/theophylline: xanthine bronchodilator
BRONKOLIXIR/ theophylline, guaifenesin, phenobarbital: bronchodilator, expectorant
BRONKOMETER/isoetharine: bronchodilator
BRONKOSOL/isoetharine: bronchodilator
BRONKOTABS/theophylline, guaifenesin, phenobarbital: bronchodilator, expectorant
BRONTEX/codeine, guaifenesin: narcotic antitussive, expectorant
BUCLADIN-S/buclizine: antiemetic
buclizine/**BUCLADIN-S:** antiemetic
buffered phenylbutazone/**AZOLID-A, BUTAZOLIDIN ALKA:** analgesic, antiinflammatory
bumetanide/**BUMEX:** diuretic
BUMEX/bumetanide: diuretic
BUSPAR/buspirone: tranquilizer
buspirone/**BUSPAR:** tranquilizer
butabarbital/**BUTICAPS, BUTISOL:** barbiturate
butalbital, APAP/**SEDAPAP:** analgesic
butalbital, APC/**FIORINAL:** analgesic
butalbital, ASA/**AXOTAL:** analgesic
butaperizine/**REPOISE:** phenothiazine tranquilizer
BUTAZOLIDIN/phenylbutazone: analgesic, antiinflammatory

BUTAZOLIDIN ALKA/buffered phenylbutazone: analgesic, antiinflammatory
BUTIBEL/belladonna, butabarbital: urinary antispasmodic
BUTICAPS/butabarbital: barbiturate
BUTISOL/butabarbital: barbiturate
butorphanol/**STADOL:** narcotic analgesic
CAFERGOT/ergotamine, caffeine: cerebral vasoconstrictor
CAFERGOT-PB/ergotamine, belladonna, caffeine, phenobarbital: cerebral vasoconstrictor
CAFERMINE/ergotamine, caffeine: cerebral vasoconstrictor
CAFETRATE/ergotamine, caffeine: cerebral vasoconstrictor
CALAN/verapamil: antihypertensive, antidysrhythmic
CALCIDRINE/codeine, calcium iodide: narcotic antitussive, expectorant
CALCIFEROL/vitamin D: vitamin (hypoparathyroidism)
CAMOQUIN/amodiaquine: antimalarial
CAPADE/chlorpheniramine, phenylpropanolamine: antihistamine, decongestant
CAPASTAT/capreomycin: antibiotic
CAPITAL with CODEINE/APAP, codeine: narcotic analgesic
CAPOTEN/captopril: antihypertensive
CAPOZIDE/captopril, HCTZ: antihypertensive, diuretic
capreomycin/**CAPASTAT:** antibiotic
capsaicin/**ZOSTRIX:** analgesic
captopril/**CAPOTEN:** antihypertensive
captopril, HCTZ/**CAPOZIDE:** antihypertensive, diuretic
CARAFATE/sucralfate: antiulcer
carbamazepine/**TEGRETOL:** anticonvulsant
carbenicillin/**GEOCILLIN, GEOPEN:** antibiotic
CARBRITAL/pentobarbital, carbromal: tranquilizer
CARDENE/nicardipine: antianginal, antihypertensive
CARDILATE/erythrityl tetranitrate: antianginal, vasodilator
CARDIOQUIN/quinidine: antidysrhythmic
CARDIZEM/diltiazem: antianginal, antihypertensive
CARDURA/doxazosin: antihypertensive
carisoprodol/**RELA, SOMA:** muscle relaxant
carphenazine/**PROKETAZINE:** phenothiazine tranquilizer
carteolol/**CARTROL:** antihypertensive
CARTROL/carteolol: antihypertensive
CATAFLAM/diclofenac: antiinflammatory
CATAPRES/clonidine: antihypertensive
CECLOR/cefaclor: antibiotic
CEDILANID/lanatoside C: cardiac glycoside (CHF, SVT)
CEDILANID-D/deslanoside: cardiac glycoside (CHF, SVT)
cefaclor/**CECLOR:** antibiotic
cefadroxil/**DURICEF, ULTRACEF:** antibiotic
CEFADYL/cephapirin: antibiotic
cefamandole/**MANDOL:** antibiotic
cefazolin/**ANCEF, KEFZOL:** antibiotic
cefotaxime/**CLAFORAN:** antibiotic
cefoxitin/**MEFOXIN:** antibiotic
ceftazidime/**FORTAZ:** antibiotic
CEFTIN/cefuroxime: antibiotic
ceftriaxone/**ROCEPHIN:** antibiotic
cefuroxime/**CEFTIN, KEFUROX:** antibiotic
CELBENIN/nafcillin: antibiotic
CELESTONE/betamethasone: steroidal antiinflammatory
CELONTIN/methsuximide: anticonvulsant (petit mal)
CENTRAX/prazepam: benzodiazepine tranquilizer

cephalexin/**KEFLEX:** antibiotic

cephaloglycin/**KAFOCIN:** antibiotic

cephaloridine/**LORIDINE:** antibiotic

cephalothin/**KEFLIN NEUTRAL:** antibiotic

cephapirin/**CEFADYL:** antibiotic

cephradine/**ANSPOR, VELOSEF:** antibiotic

CEREBID/papaverine: cerebral/peripheral vasodilator

CERESPAN/papaverine: cerebral/peripheral vasodilator

CERYLIN/theophylline, guaifenesin: bronchodilator, expectorant

CHARDONNA-2/belladonna, phenobarbital: antispasmodic

CHERACOL/guaifenesin, codeine: antitussive, expectorant

CHERACOL D/guaifenesin, dextromethorphan: antitussive, expectorant

CHLORAMEAD/chlorpromazine: phenothiazine tranquilizer

chloramphenicol/**AMPHICOL, CHLOROMYCETIN:** antibiotic

chloral hydrate/**AQUACHLORAL, NOCTEC:** tranquilizer

chloralidone, reserpine/**DEMI-REGROTON:** antihypertensive, diuretic

chlordiazepoxide/**A-POXIDE, LIBRIUM:** benzodiazepine tranquilizer

chlordiazepoxide, clidinium/**LIBRAX:** antispasmodic, tranquilizer

chlordiazepoxide, estrogen/**MENRIUM:** benzodiazepine tranquilizer

CHLOROFON-F/chlorzoxazone, acetaminophen: muscle relaxant, analgesic

CHLOROMYCETIN/chloramphenicol: antibiotic

chloroquine/**ARALEN:** antimalarial

chlorothiazide/**DIURIL, SK-CHLOROTHIAZIDE:** antihypertensive, diuretic

chlorotrianisene/**TACE:** hormone

chlorpheniramine/**CHLOR-TRIMETON, TELDRIN:** antihistamine

chlorpheniramine, phenylephrine, methscopolamine/
DALLERGY, EXTENDRYL: antihistamine, decongestant

chlorpheniramine, phenylpropanolamine/**CAPADE, ORNADE:** antihistamine, decongestant

chlorpheniramine, pseudoephedrine/**CODIMAL LA:** antihistamine, decongestant

chlorpheniramine, pseudoephedrine, codeine/**NOVAHISTINE DH:** narcotic antitussive, decongestant

chlorphentermine/**PRE-STATE:** appetite suppressant

chlorpromazine/**PROMAPAR, THORAZINE:** phenothiazine tranquilizer

chlorpropamide/**DIABENESE:** oral hypoglycemic

chlorprothixene/**TARACTAN:** tranquilizer

chlorthalidone/**HYGROTON, URIDON:** antihypertensive, diuretic

CHLOR-TRIMETON/chlorpheniramine: antihistamine

CHLORZONE FORTE/chlorzoxazone, acetaminophen: muscle relaxant

chlorzoxazone/**PARAFLEX:** muscle relaxant

chlorzoxazone, acetaminophen/**LOBAC, PARAFON FORTE:** muscle relaxant

CHOLEDYL/oxtriphylline: xanthine bronchodilator

cholestyramine/**CHOLYBAR, QUESTRAN:** decreases serum cholesterol

CHOLOXIN/dextrothyroxine: decreases serum cholesterol

CHOLYBAR/cholestyramine: decreases serum cholesterol

CIBALITH-S/lithium carbonate: antidepressant

cimetidine/**TAGAMET:** antiulcer

CIN-QUIN/quinidine: antidysrhythmic

CIPRO/ciprofloxacin: antibiotic

ciprofloxacin/**CIPRO:** antibiotic

CITRATE OF MAGNESIA/magnesium citrate: laxative

CLAFORAN/cefotaxime: antibiotic

clemastine/**TAVIST:** antihistamine

CLEOCIN/clindamycin: antibiotic

clidinium/**QUARZAN:** antiulcer

clindamycin/**CLEOCIN:** antibiotic

CLINORIL/sulindac: antiinflammatory

clofibrate/**ATROMID-S:** antilipid

clomipramine/**ANAFRANIL:** tricyclic antidepressant

clonazepam/**KLONOPIN:** benzodiazepine tranquilizer

clonidine/**CATAPRES:** antihypertensive

clonidine, chlorthalidone/**COMBIPRES:** antihypertensive, diuretic

clorazepate/**TRANXENE-SD:** benzodiazepine tranquilizer

clortermine/**VORANIL:** appetite suppressant

clotrimazole/**LOTRIMIN, MYCELEX:** antifungal

cloxacillin/**CLOXAPEN, TEGOPEN:** antibiotic

CLOXAPEN/cloxacillin: antibiotic

clozapine/**CLOZARIL:** antischizophrenia

CLOZARIL/clozapine: antischizophrenia

COADVIL/ibuprofen, pseudoephedrine: analgesic, decongestant

COCO-QUININE/quinine: antimalarial

CODALAN/APAP, codeine, salicylamide: narcotic analgesic

codeine, butalbital, APAP/**SEDAPAP #3:** narcotic analgesic

codeine, calcium iodide/**CALCIDRINE:** narcotic antitussive, expectorant

codeine, guaifenesin/**BRONTEX:** narcotic antitussive, expectorant

CODIMAL LA/chlorpheniramine, pseudoephedrine: antihistamine, decongestant

CODONE/hydrocodone: narcotic analgesic, antitussive

CODYLAX/bisacodyl: laxative

COGENTIN/benztropine: antiparkinsonian, antiextrapyramidal symptoms

COGESIC/hydrocodone, acetaminophen: narcotic analgesic

COHIDRATE/chloral hydrate: tranquilizer

COLACE/docusate sodium: laxative

COLAX/docusate sodium: laxative

ColBENEMID/colchicine, probenecid: uricosuric

colchicine/**COLSALIDE IMPROVED:** uricosuric

colchicine, probenecid/**ColBENEMID:** uricosuric

COLESTID/colestipol: decreases serum cholesterol

colestipol/**COLESTID:** decreases serum cholesterol

COLONIL/diphenoxylate, atropine: narcotic antidiarrheal, antispasmodic

COLSALIDE IMPROVED/colchicine: uricosuric

COMBID/prochlorperazine, isopropamide: antiemetic, antispasmodic

COMBIPRES/clonidine, chlorthalidone: antihypertensive, diuretic

COMPAZINE/prochlorperazine: phenothiazine tranquilizer

conjugated estrogens/**PREMARIN:** hormone

CORDARONE/amiodarone: antidysrhythmic

CORGARD/nadolol: beta blocker

CORT-DOME/hydrocortisone: steroidal antiinflammatory

CORTEF/hydrocortisone: steroidal antiinflammatory

CORTENEMA/hydrocortisone: steroidal antiinflammatory

cortisone/**CORTONE:** steroidal antiinflammatory

CORTONE/cortisone: steroidal antiinflammatory

CORTUSSIS/terpin hydrate, codeine: narcotic antitussive, expectorant

CORZIDE/bendroflumethiazide, nadolol: antihypertensive, diuretic

COTRIM/sulfamethoxazole, trimethoprim: antibacterial

COUMADIN/warfarin: anticoagulant

cromolyn/**INTAL:** antiasthma

cryptenamine/**UNITENSEN:** antihypertensive

CRYSTICILLIN/penicillin G: antibiotic

CRYSTODIGIN/digitoxin: cardiac glycoside (CHF, SVT)

CUPRIMINE/penicillamine: chelating agent (for heavy metal poisoning)

CUTIVATE/fluticasone: steroidal antiinflammatory

CYANTIN/nitrofurantion: antibacterial

cyclacillin/**CYCLAPEN-W:** antibiotic

cyclandelate/**CYCLOSPASMOL:** vasodilator

CYCLAPEN-W/cyclacillin: antibiotic

cyclizine/**MAREZINE:** antimotion sickness

cyclobenzaprine/**FLEXERIL:** muscle relaxant

CYCLOSPAR/tetracycline: antibiotic

CYCLOSPASMOL/cyclandelate: vasodilator

cyclosporine/**SANDIMMUNE:** immunosuppressant

cyclothiazide/**ANHYDRON:** antihypertensive, diuretic

cycrimine/**PAGITANE:** antiparkinsonian, antiextrapyramidal symptoms

CYLERT/pemoline: antihyperactive, antinarcoleptic

CYPRODINE/cyproheptadine: antihistamine

cyproheptadine/**CYPRODINE, PERIACTIN:** antihistamine

CYSTOSPAZ/hyoscyamine: urinary antispasmodic

CYSTOSPAZ-M/hyoscyamine: urinary antispasmodic

CYSTOSPAZ-SR/belladonna, butabarbital: urinary antispasmodic

CYTOTEC/misoprostol: antiulcer

CYTOVENE/ganciclovir: antiviral

DALGAN/dezocine: narcotic analgesic

DALLERGY/chlorpheniramine, phenylephrine, methscopolamine: antihistamine, decongestant

DALMANE/flurazepam: benzodiazepine tranquilizer

DAMASON-P/hydrocodone, ASA, caffeine: narcotic analgesic

DANTRIUM/dantrolene: muscle relaxant

dantrolene/**DANTRIUM:** muscle relaxant

dapsone/**AVLOSULFON:** antileprosy

DARANIDE/dichlorphenamide: decreases intraocular pressure

DARBID/isopropamide: antiulcer

DARVOCET-N/propoxyphene, acetaminophen: narcotic analgesic

DARVON/propoxyphene: narcotic analgesic

DARVON COMPOUND/propoxyphene, ASA, caffeine: narcotic analgesic

DARVON with ASA/propoxyphene, ASA: narcotic analgesic

DATRIL/acetaminophen: analgesic, antiinflammatory

DAYPRO/oxaprozin: antiinflammatory

DDAVP/desmopressin: antidiuretic hormone

DECADRON/dexamethasone: steroidal antiinflammatory

DECAPRYN/doxylamine: antihistamine

DECLOMYCIN/demeclocycline: antibiotic

DELAXIN/methocarbamol: skeletal muscle relaxant

DELESTROGEN/ estradiol: hormone

DELSYM/dextromethorphan: antitussive

DELTA-CORTEF/prednisolone: steroidal antiinflammatory

DELTASONE/prednisone: steroidal antiinflammatory

demeclocycline/**DECLOMYCIN:** antibiotic

DEMEROL/meperidine: narcotic analgesic

DEMI-REGROTON/chloralidone, reserpine: antihypertensive, diuretic

DEMSER/metyrosine: antihypertensive

DEPAKENE/valproic acid: anticonvulsant

DEPAKOTE/divalproex: anticonvulsant

DEPEN/penicillamine: antiarthritic, chelating agent (for heavy metal poisoning)

DEPROL/benactyzine, meprobamate: antidepressant, tranquilizer

DES/diethylstilbestrol: hormone

deserpidine/**HARMONYL:** antihypertensive

DESIPRAMINE/amitriptyline: tricyclic antidepressant

deslanoside/**CEDILANID-D:** cardiac glycoside (CHF, SVT)

desmopressin/**DDAVP:** antidiuretic hormone

DESOXYN/methamphetamine: stimulant

DESYREL/trazodone: tricyclic antidepressant

dexamethasone/**DECADRON, HEXADROL:** steroidal antiinflammatory

DEXAPEX/dextroamphetamine: stimulant

DEXASONE/dexamethasone: steroidal antiinflammatory

dexbrompheniramine, pseudoephedrine/**DISOPHROL, DRIXORAL:** antihistamine

dexchlorpheniramine/**POLARAMINE:** antihistamine

DEXEDRINE/dextroamphetamine: stimulant

dextroamphetamine/**DEXEDRINE, SPANCAP:** stimulant

dextroamphetamine, amphetamine/**BIPHETAMINE:** stimulant

dextromethorphan/**DELSYM:** antitussive

dextromethorphan, guaifenesin /**DEXTRO-TUSS GG:** antitussive, expectorant

dextrothyroxine/**CHOLOXIN:** decreases serum cholesterol

DEXTOR-TUSS GG/dextromethorphan, guaifenesin: antitussive, expectorant

dezocine/**DALGAN:** narcotic analgesic

DIABENESE/chlorpropamide: oral hypoglycemic

DIABETA/glyburide: oral hypoglycemic

DIAFEN/diphenylpyraline: antihistamin

DIALIXIR/theophylline, guaifenesin: bronchodilator, expectorant

DIALOSE/docusate: laxative

DIAMOX/acetazolamide: anticonvulsant, diuretic

diazepam/**VALIUM, VALRELEASE:** benzodiazepine tranquilizer

DI-AZO/phenazopyridine: urinary tract analgesic

diazoxide/**PROGLYCEM:** oral hypoglycemic

DIBENZYLINE/phenoxybenzamine: antihypertensive

dichlorphenamide/**DARANIDE:** decreases intraocular pressure diclofenac/**CATAFLAM, VOLTAREN:** analgesic, antiinflammatory

dicloxacillin/**DYCILL, DYNAPEN:** antibiotic

DICODID/hydrocodone: antitussive, narcotic analgesic

DICUMAROL/bishydroxycoumarin: anticoagulant

dicyclomine/**BENTYL, DYSPAS:** antispasmodic

DIDREX/benzphetamine: appetite suppressant

diethylpropion/**TENUATE, TEPANIL:** appetite suppressant

diethylstilbestrol/**DES, STILPHOSTROL:** hormone

difenoxin, atropine/**MOTOFEN:** narcotic antidiarrheal

diflorasone/**FLORONE:** steroidal antiinflammatory

DIFLUCAN/fluconazole: antifungal

diflunisal/**DOLOBID:** analgesic

DIGIFORTIS/digitalis: cardiac glycoside (CHF, SVT)

digitalis/**DIGIFORTIS, PIL-DIGIS:** cardiac glycoside (CHF, SVT)

digitoxin/**CRYSTODIGIN, PURODIGIN:** cardiac glycoside (CHF, SVT)

digoxin/**LANOXIN:** cardiac glycoside (CHF, SVT)

DILACOR/diltiazem: antianginal, antihypertensive

DILANTIN/phenytoin: anticonvulsant

DILATRATE-SR/isosorbide dinitrate: antianginal

DILAUDID/hydromorphone: narcotic analgesic

DILOR/dyphylline: xanthine bronchodilator

diltiazem/**CARDIZEM, DILACOR:** antianginal, antihypertensive

dimenhydrinate/**DRAMAMINE, ELDODRAM:** antimotion sickness

DIMETANE/brompheniramine: antihistamine

DIMETANE DC/brompheniramine, phenylephrine, codeine: antihistamine, narcotic antitussive

DIMETANE EXPECTORANT/brompheniramine, phenylephrine: antihistamine, expectorant

DIMETAPP/brompheniramine, phenylephrine: antihistamine, decongestant

dimethindene/**FORHISTAL, TRITEN:** antihistamine

DIPAV/papaverine: cerebral/peripheral vasodilator

DI-PHEN/phenytoin: anticonvulsant

diphenidol/**VONTROL:** antiemetic

diphenhydramine/**BENEDRYL, VALDRENE:** antihistamine

diphenoxylate, atropine/**COLONIL, LOMOTIL:** narcotic antidiarrheal

DIPHENYLAN/phenytoin: anticonvulsant

DIPHENYLHYDANTOIN/phenytoin: anticonvulsant

diphenylpyraline/**DIAFEN, HISPRIL:** antihistamine

dipyridamole/**PERSANTINE:** vasodilator

DIRENIUM/triamterene: diuretic

DISALCID/salsalate: antiinflammatory

diserpidine, hydrochlorothiazide/**ORETICYL:** antihypertensive, diuretic

diserpidine, methyclothiazide/**ENDURONYL:** antihypertensive, diuretic

DISOPHROL/dexbrompheniramine, pseudoephedrine: antihistamine

disopyramide/**NORPACE:** ventricular antidysrhythmic

disulfiram/**ANTABUSE:** alcohol antagonist

DITROPAN/oxybutynin: antispasmodic

DIUCARDIN/hydroflumethiazide: antihypertensive, diuretic

DIULO/metolazone: antihypertensive, diuretic

DIUPRES/reserpine, chlorothiazide: antihypertensive, diuretic

DIURIL/chlorothiazide: antihypertensive, diuretic

DIUTENSEN-R/reserpine, methyclothiazide: antihypertensive, diuretic

divalproex/**DEPAKOTE:** anticonvulsant

docusate/**DIALOSE, DSS:** laxative

docusate calcium/**SURFAK:** laxative

docusate danthron/**DOXIDAN:** laxative

docusate sodium/**COLACE, COLAX:** laxative

DOLACET/propoxyphene, acetaminophen: narcotic analgesic

DOLENE/propoxyphene: narcotic analgesic

DOLENE AP-65/propoxyphene, acetaminophen: narcotic analgesic

DOLOBID/diflunisal: analgesic, antiinflammatory

DOLOPHINE/methadone: narcotic analgesic

DONNABARB/belladonna, phenobarbital: antispasmodic

DONNAGEL-PG/kaolin, belladonna, opium: antidiarrheal, antispasmodic

DONNATAL/belladonna, phenobarbital: antispasmodic

DONPHEN/belladonna, phenobarbital: antispasmodic

DOPAR/levodopa, carbidopa: antiparkinsonian

DOPRAM/doxapram: respiratory stimulant

DORAL/quazepam: benzodiazepine hypnotic

DORIDEN/glutethimide: tranquilizer

DORMTABS/glutethimide: tranquilizer

DORYX/doxycycline: antibiotic

doxapram/**DOPRAM:** respiratory stimulant

doxazosin/**CARDURA:** antihypertensive

doxepin/**ADAPIN, SINEQUAN:** tricyclic antidepressant

DOXIDAN/docusate, danthron: laxative

DOXYCHEL/doxycycline: antibiotic

doxycycline/**DORYX, VIBRAMYCIN:** antibiotic

doxylamine/**DECAPRYN:** antihistamine

DOXY-TABS/doxycycline: antibiotic

DRAMAMINE/dimenhydrinate: antiemetic

DRIXORAL/dexbrompheniramine, pseudoephedrine: antihistamine, decongestant

droperidol/**INAPSINE:** tranquilizer

DSS/docusate: laxative

DULCOLAX/bisacodyl: laxative

DUOCET/hydrocodone, APAP: narcotic analgesic

DUO-MEDIHALER/isoproterenol, phenylephrine: bronchodilator, decongestant

duotrate/**ISOBID, ISORDIL:** vasodilator (angina)

DUOVENT/theophylline, guaifenesin, phenobarbital: bronchodilator, expectorant

DURACILLIN/penicillin G: antibiotic

DURADYNE/hydrocodone APAP: narcotic analgesic

DURAGESIC/fentanyl: narcotic analgesic

DURALONE/methylprednisolone: steroidal antiinflammatory

DURAMORPH/morphine: narcotic analgesic

DURAQUIN/quinidine: antidysrhythmic

DURETIC/methyclothiazide: antihypertensive, diuretic

DURICEF/cefadroxil: antibiotic

DUVOID/bethanechol: vagomimetic (urinary retention)

DYAZIDE/triamterene, HCTZ: antihypertensive, diuretic

DYCILL/dicloxacillin: antibiotic

DYLATE/papaverine: cerebral/peripheral vasodilator

DYMELOR/acetohexamide: oral hypoglycemic

DYNACIRC/isradipine: antihypertensive

DYNAPEN/dicloxacillin: antibiotic

dyphylline/**DILOR, LUFYLLIN:** xanthine bronchodilator
DYREMIUM/triantamterene: diuretic
DYSPAS/dicyclomine: antispasmodic
ECOTRIN/aspirin (coated): analgesic, antiinflammatory
ECTASULE MINUS/ephedrine: bronchodilator
EDECRIN/ethacrynic acid: diuretic
EES/erythromycin: antibiotic
EFFEXOR/venlafatine: antidepressant
ELAVIL/amitriptyline: tricyclic antidepressant
ELDADRYL/diphenhydramine: antihistamine
ELDATAPP/brompheniramine, phenylephrine: antihistamine, decongestant
ELDEPRYL/selegiline: antiparkinsonian
ELDODRAM/dimenhydrinate: antiemetic
ELIMITE/permethrin: topical scabicide
ELIXICON/theophylline: xanthine bronchodilator
ELIXOPHYLLIN/theophylline: xanthine bronchodilator
EME-NIL/pyrilamine, pentobarbital: antiemetic
EMPIRIN with CODEINE #2, #3, #4/aspirin, codeine: narcotic analgesic
EMPIRIN COMPOUND with CODEINE/APC, codeine: narcotic analgesic
EMPRACET with CODEINE/acetaminophen, codeine: narcotic analgesic
E-MYCIN/erythromycin: antibiotic
E-MYCIN E/erythromycin: antibiotic
enalapril/**VASOTEC:** antihypertensive, diuretic
enalapril, HCTZ/**VASERETIC:** antihypertensive, diuretic
encainide/**ENKAID:** ventricular antidysrhythmic
ENDEP/amitriptyline: tricyclic antidepressant
ENDURON/methyclothiazide: antihypertensive, diuretic
ENDURONYL/diserpidine, methyclothiazide: antihypertensive, diuretic
ENKAID/encainide: ventricular antidysrhythmic
ENTEX LA/phenylpropanolamine, guaifenesin: decongestant, expectorant
ephedrine/**ECTASULE MINUS, EPHEDSOL:** bronchodilator
EPHEDSOL/ephedrine: bronchodilator
epoetin alfa/**PROCIT:** hormone (red blood cell production)
EPOGEN/erythropoietin: bone marrow RBC stimulator
EPSOM SALTS/magnesium sulfate: laxative
EQUAGESIC/meprobamate, ethoheptazine, ASA: analgesic, tranquilizer
EQUANIL/meprobamate: tranquilizer
ERGOCAF/ergotamine, caffeine: cerebral vasoconstrictor
ERGOCAFFEINE/ergotamine, caffeine: cerebral vasoconstrictor
ergoloid mesylates/**ERGOTRATE, HYDERGINE:** improved mental function
ERGOMAR/ergotamine tartrate: antimigraine, oxytocic
ergonovine maleate/**ERGOTRATE MALEATE:** oxytocic
ERGOSTAT/ergotamine tartrate: antimigraine, oxytocic
ergotamine, belladonna, phenobarbital/
    BELLERGAL: analgesic, antispasmodic
ergotamine, belladonna, phenobarbital, caffeine/**CAFERGOT-PB:** cerebral vasoconstrictor
ergotamine, caffeine/**CAFERGOT, WIGRAINE:** cerebral vasoconstrictor
ergotamine tartrate/**ERGOMAR, GYNERGEN:** antimigraine, oxytocic

ERGOTRATE/ergoloid mesylates: improved mental function
ERGOTRATE MALEATE/ergonovine maleate: oxytocic
ERYPAR/erythromycin: antibiotic
ERYC/erythromycin: antibiotic
ERYTAB/erythromycin: antibiotic
erythrityl tetranitrate/**CARDILATE:** antianginal, vasodilator
ERYTHROCIN/erythromycin: antibiotic
erythromycin/**E-MYCIN, PEDMYCIN:** antibiotic
ESGIC/APAP, caffeine, butalbital: analgesic, muscle relaxant
ESIDRIX/hydrochlorothiazide (HCTZ): antihypertensive, diuretic
ESIMIL/guanethidine, HCTZ: antihypertensive, diuretic
ESKALITH/lithium carbonate: antidepressant
esterifed estrogens/**AMNESTROGEN:** hormone
ESTINYL/ethinyl estradiol: hormone
ESTRACE/estradiol: hormone
estradiol/**ESTRACE, PROGYNON:** hormone
estrone/**THEELIN:** hormone
estropipate/**OGEN, PIPERZINE SULFATE:** hormone
ESTROVIS/quinestrol: hormone
ethacrynic acid/**EDECRIN:** diuretic
ethambutol/**MYAMBUTOL:** antibiotic
ETHATAB/ethaverine: smooth muscle relaxant, vasodilator
ethaverine/**ETHATAB:** smooth muscle relaxant, vasodilator
ethchlorvynol/**PLACIDYL:** tranquilizer
ETH COMPOUND/theophylline, ephedrine, hydroxyzine: bronchodilator
ethinamate/**VALMID:** tranquilizer
ethinyl estradiol/**ESTINYL, FEMINONE:** hormone
ethionamide/**TRECATOR-SC:** antibiotic
ETHMOZINE/moricizine: ventricular antidysrhythmic
ethopropazine/**PARSIDOL:** antiparkinsonian, antiextrapyramidal symptoms
ethosuximide/**ZARONTIN:** anticonvulsant (petit mal)
ethotoin/**PEGANONE:** anticonvulsant
ETHRIL/erythromycin: antibiotic
ethylnorepinephrine/**BRONKEPHRINE:** bronchodilator
etodolac/**LODINE:** analgesic, antiinflammatory
ETRAFON/amitriptyline, perphenazine: tricyclic antidepressant, tranquilizer
EUTHROID/liotrix: thyroid hormone
EUTONYL/pargyline: antihypertensive
EUTRON/methyclothiazide, pargyline: antihypertensive, diuretic
EXNA/benzthiazide: antihypertensive, diuretic
EXNA-R/reserpine, benzthiazide: antihypertensive, diuretic
EXTENDRYL/chlorpheniramine, methscopolamine: antihistamine, decongestant
famotidine/**PEPCID:** antiulcer
FASTIN/phentermine: appetite suppressant
FELDENE/piroxicam: analgesic, antiinflammatory
felodipine/**PLENDIL:** antihypertensive
FEMINONE/ethinyl estradiol: hormone
fenfluramine/**PONDIMIN:** appetite suppressant
fenoprofen/**NALFON:** analgesic, antiinflammatory
fentanyl/**DURAGESIC, SUBLIMAZE:** narcotic analgesic
FEOSOL/ferrous sulfate: iron supplement
FERNDEX/dextroamphetamine: stimulant
ferrous sulfate/**FEOSOL:** iron supplement

FIORINAL/butalbital, APC: analgesic
FLAGYL/metronidazole: antifungal
flavoxate/**URISPAS:** urinary antispasmodic
FLEXERIL/cyclobenzaprine: muscle relaxant
FLEXOJET/orphenadrine: analgesic, antiinflammatory
FLEXON/orphenadrine: analgesic, antiinflammatory
FLORONE/diflorasone: steroidal antiinflammatory
fluconazole/**DIFLUCAN:** antifungal
flucytosine/**ANCOBON:** antifungal
flunisolide/**NASALIDE:** steroidal antiinflammatory
fluocinolone/**LIDEX:** steroidal antiinflammatory
fluorouracil/**ADRUCIL:** anticancer
fluoxetine/**PROZAC:** antidepressant
fluphenazine/**PERMITIL, PROLIXIN:** phenothiazine tranquilizer
flurazepam/**DALMANE:** benzodiazepine tranquilizer
fluticasone/**CUTIVATE:** steroidal antiinflammatory
FORBAXIN/methocarbamol: muscle relaxant
FORHISTAL/dimethindene: antihistamine
FORTAZ/ceftazidime: antibiotic
fosinopril/**MONOPRIL:** antihypertensive
FULVICIN P/G/griseofulvin: antifungal
FULVICIN U/F/griseofulvin: antifungal
FUNGIZONE/amphotericin B: antibiotic
FURADANTIN/nitrofurantin: antibacterial
furosemide/**LASIX, NEO-RENAL:** diuretic
ganciclovir/**CYTOVENE:** antiviral
GANTANOL/sulfamethoxazole: antibacterial
GANTRISIN/sulfisoxazole: antibacterial
GARAMYCIN/gentamicin: antibiotic
gemfibrozil/**LOPID:** decreases serum lipids
GEMNISYN/APAP, aspirin: analgesic, antiinflammatory
GEMONIL/metharbital: barbiturate
GENETUSS/guaifenesin: expectorant
gentamycin/**APOGEN, GARAMYCIN:** antibiotic
GEOCILLIN/carbenicillin: antibiotic
GEOPEN/carbenicillin: antibiotic
GITALIGIN/gitalin: cardiac glycoside (CHF, SVT)
gitalin/**GITALIGIN:** cardiac glycoside (CHF, SVT)
glipizide/**GLUCOTROL:** oral hypoglycemic
GLUCOTROL/glipizide: oral hypoglycemic
glutethimide/**DORIDEN, DORMTABS:** tranquilizer
GLYBRON/theophylline, guaifenesin: bronchodilator, expectorant
glyburide/**DIABETA:** oral hypoglycemic
GLYCERYL TRINITRATE/nitroglycerin: antianginal, vasodilator
GLYTUSS/guaifenesin: expectorant
GRIFULVIN V/griseofulvin: antifungal
GRISACTIN/griseofulvin: antifungal
griseofulvin/**GRIFULVIN V, GRIS-PEG:** antifungal
GRISOWEN/griseofulvin: antifungal
GRIS-PEG/griseofulvin: antifungal
G-TUSS DM/guaifenesin, dextromethorphan: antitussive, expectorant
guaifenesin/**NORTUSSIN, ROBITUSSIN:** expectorant
guaifenesin, codeine/**CHERACOL, ROBITUSSIN A-C:** antitussive, expectorant
guanabenz/**WYTENSIN:** antihypertensive

guanadrel/**HYLOREL:** antihypertensive
guanethidine/**ISMELIN:** antihypertensive
guanethidine, HCTZ/**ESIMIL:** antihypertensive, diuretic
GYNE-LOTRIMIN/clotrimazole: antifungal
GYNERGEN/ergotamine tartrate: antimigraine, oxytocic
halazepam/**PAXIPAM:** benzodiazepine tranquilizer
HALCION/triazolam: benzodiazepine tranquilizer
HALDOL/haloperidol: tranquilizer
haloperidol/**HALDOL:** tranquilizer
HARMONYL/deserpidine: antihypertensive
HASP/belladona, phenobarbital: antispasmodic
HCTZ/hydrochlorothiazide: antihypertensive, diuretic
heparin/**HEPRINAR, PANHEPRIN:** anticoagulant
HEPRINAR/heparin: anticoagulant
HEPTOGESIC/meprobamate, ethoheptazine, ASA: analgesic, tranquilizer
HERPLEX/idoxuridine: antiviral
hetacillin/**PATHOCIL, VERSAPEN:** antibiotic
HEXADROL/dexamethasone: steroidal antiinflammatory
hexobarbital/**SOMBULEX:** barbiturate
HIPREX/methenamine hippurate: antibacterial
HISMANAL/astemizole: antihistamine
HISPRIL/diphenylpyraline: antihistamine
HISTASPAN/chlorpheniramine: antihistamine
HYBAR/belladonna, phenobarbital: antispasmodic
HYCODAN/hydrocodone, homatropine: narcotic antitussive
HYDERGINE/ergoloid mesylates: improved mental function
hydralazine/**APRESOLINE:** antihypertensive
HYDREX/benzthiazide: antihypertensive, diuretic
HYDRO-AQUIL/hydrochlorothiazide: antihypertensive, diuretic
HYDROCET/hydrocodone, APAP: narcotic analgesic
hydrochlorothiazide/**ESIDRIX, HCTZ:** antihypertensive, diuretic
hydrocodone/**CODONE, DICODID:** antitussive, narcotic analgesic
hydrocodone, acetaminophen/**COGESIC, VICODIN:** narcotic analgesic
hydrocodone, ASA, caffeine/**DAMASON-P:** narcotic analgesic
hydrocodone, chlorpheniramine/**TUSSIONEX:** narcotic antitussive
hydrocodone, homatropine/**HYCODAN:** narcotic antitussive
hydrocodone, pseudoephedrine, guaifenesin/**TUSSEND EXPECTORANT:** expectorant, narcotic antitussive
hydrocortisone/**PROCTOCORT, SOLU-CORTEF:** steroidal antiinflammatory
hydrocortisone, belladonna, ephedrine/**WYANOIDS HC:** steroidal antiinflammatory
hydrocortisone, bismuth, benzyl benzoate/**ANUSOL-HC:** steroidal antiinflammatory
HYDROCORTONE/hydrocortisone: steroidal antiinflammatory
HYDRODIURIL/hydrochlorothiazide: antihypertensive, diuretic
hydroflumethiazide/**DIUCARDIN, SALUTENSIN:** antihypertensive diuretic
hydromorphone/**DILAUDID:** narcotic analgesic
HYDROMOX/quinethazone: antihypertensive, diuretic

HYDROMOX-R/reserpine, quinethazone: antihypertensive, diuretic

HYDROPHED/theophylline, ephedrine, hydroxyzine: bronchodilator

HYDROPRES/reserpine, hydrochlorothiazide: antihypertensive, diuretic

hydroxychloroquine/**PLAQUENIL:** antimalarial

hydroxyzine/**ATARAX, VISTARIL:** antihistamine, tranquilizer

HYGROTON/chlorthalidone: antihypertensive, diuretic

HYLATE/theophylline, guaifenesin: bronchodilator, expectorant

HYLOREL/guanadrel: antihypertensive

HYOBID/papaverine: cerebral/peripheral vasodilator

hyoscyamine/**CYSTOSPAZ, LEVSIN:** antispasmodic

HYOSOPHEN/belladonna, phenobarbital: antispasmodic

HYTRIN/terazosin: antihypertensive

HYTUSS/guaifenesin: expectorant

ibuprofen/**ADVIL, NUPRIN:** analgesic, antiinflammatory

ibuprofen, pseudoephedrine/**COADVIL:** analgesic, decongestant

idoxuridine/**HERPLEX, STOXIL:** antiviral

ILOSONE/erythromycin: antibiotic

ILOTYCIN/erythromycin: antibiotic

IMAVATE/imipramine: tricyclic antidepressant

imipramine/**IMAVATE, TOFRANIL:** tricyclic antidepressant

IMODIUM/loperamide: antidiarrheal

IMURAN/azathioprine: immunosuppressant

INAPSINE/droperidol: tranquilizer

indapamide/**LOZOL:** antihypertensive, diuretic

INDERAL/propranolol: antidysrhythmic, antimigraine

INDERIDE/propranolol, HCTZ: antihypertensive, diuretic

INDOCIN/indomethacin: analgesic, antiinflammatory

indomethacin/**INDOCIN:** analgesic, antiinflammatory

INFUMORPH/morphine: narcotic analgesic

INH/isoniazid: antibiotic (tuberculosis)

INTAL/cromolyn: antiasthma

interferon/**ROFERON-A:** immune system stimulant

INVERSINE/mecamylamine: antihypertensive

iodoquinol/**MOEBIQUIN, YODOXIN:** amebicide

IONAMIN/phentermine: appetite suppressant

IPRENOL/isoproteronol: bronchodilator

iron/**SLOW FE:** iron supplement

ISMELIN/guanethidine: antihypertensive

ISOBID/isosorbide dinitrate: antianginal, vasodilator

isocarboxazid/**MARPLAN:** antidepressant

ISOCOM/isometheptene, dichloralphenazone, APAP: analgesic, cerebral vasoconstrictor

isoetharine/**BRONKOMETER, BRONKOSOL:** bronchodilator

isometheptene/**MIDRIN:** analgesic, tranquilizer

isometheptene, dichloralphenazone, APAP/**ISOCOM:** analgesic, cerebral vasoconstrictor

isoniazid/**INH, NYDRAZID:** antibiotic (tuberculosis)

isopropamide/**DARBID:** antiulcer

isoproterenol/**ISUPREL, NORISODRINE AEROTROL:** bronchodilator

isoproterenol, phenylephrine/**DUO-MEDIHALER:** bronchodilator, decongestant

ISOPTIN/verapamil: antianginal, antihypertensive, antidysrhythmic

ISORDIL/isosorbide dinitrate: antianginal, vasodilator

isosorbide dinitrate/**DILATRATE-SR, SORBATE:** antianginal, vasolidator

ISOTRATE/isosorbide dinitrate: antianginal, vasolidator

isoxsuprine/**VASODILAN:** vasodilator

isradipine/**DYNACIRC:** antihypertensive

ISUPREL/isoproterenol: bronchodilator

JANIMINE/imipramine: tricyclic antidepressant

KAFOCIN/cephaloglycin: antibiotic

kanamycin/**KANTREX, KLEBCIL:** antibiotic

KANTREX/kanamycin: antibiotic

KAOCHLOR-EFF/potassium chloride: potassium supplement

kaolin, belladonna, opium/**DONNAGEL-PG:** antidiarrheal, antispasmodic

kaolin, paregoric/**PAREPECTOLIN:** antidiarrheal, antispasmodic

KAON/potassium chloride: potassium supplement

KAON-CL/potassium chloride: potassium supplement

KATO/potassium chloride: potassium supplement

KAVRIN/papaverine: cerebral/peripheral vasodilator

KAY-CIEL/potassium chloride: potassium supplement

K-DUR/potassium chloride: potassium supplement

KEFF/potassium chloride: potassium supplement

KEFLEX/cephalexin: antibiotic

KEFLIN NEUTRAL/cephalothin: antibiotic

KEFUROX/cefuroxime: antibiotic

KEFZOL/cefazolin: antibiotic

KEMADRIN/procyclidine: antiparkinsonian, antiextrapyramidal symptoms

KENACORT/triamcinolone: steroidal antiinflammatory

KENALOG/triamcinolone: steroidal antiinflammatory

KERLONE/betaxolol: antihypertensive

ketoconazole/**NIZORAL:** antifungal

ketoprofen/**ORUDIS:** analgesic, antiinflammatory

KLEBCIL/kanamycin: antibiotic

KLONOPIN/clonazepam: benzodiazepine tranquilizer

K-LOR/potassium chloride: potassium supplement

KLOR-CON/potassium chloride: potassium supplement

KLORVESS/potassium chloride: potassium supplement

KLOTRIX/potassium chloride: potassium supplement

K-LYTE/potassium chloride: potassium supplement

KOLYUM/potassium chloride: potassium supplement

K-TAB/potassium chloride: potassium supplement

KWELL/lindane: parasiticide

labetalol/**NORMODYNE, TRANDATE:** antihypertensive

labetalol, HCTZ/**NORMOZIDE, TRANDATE HCT:** antihypertensive

lanatoside C/**CEDILANID:** cardiac glycoside (CHF, SVT)

LANATRATE/ergotamine, caffeine: cerebral vasoconstrictor

LANOPHYLLIN-GG/theophylline, guaifenesin: bronchodilator, expectorant

LANOXIN/digoxin: cardiac glycoside (CHF, SVT)

LARADOPA/levodopa, carbidopa: antiparkinsonian

LAROTID/amoxicillin: antibiotic

LASIX/furosemide: diuretic

LAUDANUM/opium, tincture of: narcotic analgesic

LEDERCILLIN/penicillin: antibiotic

levallorphan/**LORFAN:** narcotic analgesic

LEVATOL/penbutolol: antihypertensive

levorphanol/**LEVO-DROMORAN:** narcotic analgesic

levodopa, carbidopa/**DOPAR, SINEMET:** antiparkinsonian
LEVO-DROMORAN/levorphanol: narcotic analgesic
LEVOTHROID/levothyroxine: thyroid hormone
levothyroxine/**LEVOTHROID, SYNTHROID:** thyroid hormone
LEVSIN/hyoscyamine: antispasmodic
LIBRAX/chlordiazepoxide, clidinium: antispasmodic, benzodiazepine tranquilizer
LIBRIUM/chlordiazepoxide: benzodiazepine tranquilizer
LIDEX/fluocinolone: steroidal antiinflammatory
LIMBITROL/amitriptyline, chlordiazepoxide: antidepressant, benzodiazepine tranquilizer
LINCOCIN/lincomycin: antibiotic
lincomycin/**LINCOCIN:** antibiotic
lindane/**KWELL:** parasiticide
LIORSAL/baclofen: muscle relaxant
liotrix/**EUTHROID, THYROLAR:** thyroid hormone
LIPO GANTRISIN/sulfisoxazole: antibacterial
LIPO-HEPIN/heparin: anticoagulant
LIQUAEMIN/heparin: anticoagulant
LIQUIPRIN/acetaminophen: analgesic
lisinopril/**PRINIVIL, ZESTRIL:** antihypertensive
lisinopril, HCTZ/**PRINZIDE, ZESTORETIC:** antihypertensive, diuretic
LITHANE/lithium carbonate: antidepressant
lithium carbonate/**ESKALITH, LITHANE:** antidepressant
LITHONATE/lithium carbonate: antidepressant
LIXAMINOL/aminophylline: xanthine bronchodilator
LOBAC/chlorzoxazone, acetaminophen: muscle relaxant, analgesic
LODINE/etodolac: analgesic, antiinflammatory
LOMOTIL/diphenoxylate, atropine: narcotic antidiarrheal, antispasmodic
LONITEN/minoxidil: antihypertensive
loperamide/**IMODIUM:** antidiarrheal
LOPID/gemfibrozil: decreases serum lipids
LOPRESSOR/metoprolol: antihypertensive
LOPURIN/allopurinol: uricosuric
lorazepam/**ATIVAN:** benzodiazepine tranquilizer
LORCET PLUS/hydrocodone, APAP: narcotic analgesic
LORELCO/probucol: anticholesterol
LORFAN/levallorphan: narcotic analgesic
LORIDINE/cephaloridine: antibiotic
LORTAB/hydrocodone, APAP: narcotic analgesic
LORTAB ASA/hydrocodone, ASA: narcotic analgesic
LOTESIN/benazepril: antihypertensive
LOTRIMIN/clotrimazole: antifungal
LOTUSATE/talbutal: barbiturate
lovastatin/**MEVACOR:** anticholesterol
loxapine/**LOXITANE:** tranquilizer
LOXITANE/loxapine: tranquilizer
LOZOL/indapamide: antihypertensive, diuretic
LUFTODIL/theophylline, guaifenesin, phenobarbital: bronchodilator, expectorant
LUFYLLIN/dyphylline: xanthine bronchodilator
LUMINAL/phenobarbital: anticonvulsant
MACRODANTIN/nitrofurantion: antibacterial
MAGAN/magnesium salicylate: analgesic, antiinflammatory
magnesium citrate/**CITRATE OF MAGNESIA:** laxative

magnesium salicylate/**MAGAN:** analgesic, antiinflammatory
magnesium sulfate/**EPSOM SALTS:** laxative
MALOTUSS/guaifenesin: expectorant
MANDELAMINE/methnamine: antibacterial
MANDOL/cefamandole: antibiotic
MARAX/theophylline, ephedrine, hydroxyzine: bronchodilator
MAREZINE/cyclizine: antiemetic
MARFLEX/orphenadrine: analgesic
MARPLAN/isocarboxazid: antidepressant
MATULANE/procarbazine: anticancer
MAXAIR/pirbuterol: bronchodilator
mazindol/**SANOREX:** appetite suppressant
MEBARAL/mephobarbital: anticonvulsant
mebendazole/**VERMOX:** antihelminthic
mecamylamine/**INVERSINE:** antihypertensive
meclizine/**ANTIVERT, BONINE:** antiemetic
meclofenamate/**MECLOMEN:** analgesic, antiinflammatory
MECLOMEN/meclofenamate: analgesic, antiinflammatory
MEDIHALER-EPI/epinephrine: bronchodilator
MEDIHALER ERGOTAMINE/ergotamine tartrate: antimigraine, oxytocic
MEDIHALER-ISO/isoproteronol: bronchodilator
MEDRALONE/methylprednisolone: steroidal antiinflammatory
MEDROL/methylprednisolone: steroidal antiinflammatory
medroxyprogesterone/**PROVERA:** hormone
mefenamic acid/**PONTSEL:** antiinflammatory
MEFOXIN/cefoxitin: antibiotic
MEGACE/megestrol: hormone
megestrol/**MEGACE:** hormone
MELLARIL/thioridazine: phenothiazine tranquilizer
MENRIUM/chlordiazepoxide, estrogen: benzodiazepine tranquilizer
MEPERGAN/meperidine, promethazine: antiemetic, narcotic analgesic
meperidine/**DEMEROL, PETHADOL:** narcotic analgesic
meperidine, promethazine/**MEPERGAN:** antiemetic, narcotic analgesic
mephenytion/**MESANTOIN:** anticonvulsant
mephobarbital/**MEBARAL:** anticonvulsant
meprednisone/**BETAPAR:** steroidal antiinflammatory
meprobamate/**EQUANIL, MILTOWN:** tranquilizer
meprobamate, ethoheptazine, ASA/**EQUAGESIC, MEPROGESIC:** analgesic
MEPRO COMPOUND/meprobamate, ethoheptazine, ASA: analgesic, tranquilizer
MEPROGESIC/meprobamate, ethoheptazine, ASA: analgesic, tranquilizer
MEPRON/atovaquone: antiprotozoal
MEPROSPAN/meprobamate: tranquilizer
MESANTOIN/mephenytion: anticonvulsant
mesoridazine/**SERENTIL:** phenothiazine tranquilizer
METAHYDRIN/trichlormethiazide: antihypertensive, diuretic
METAMUCIL/psyllium: laxative
METAPREL/metaproterenol: bronchodilator
metaproterenol/**ALUPENT, METAPREL:** bronchodilator
METATENSIN/reserpine, trichlormethiazide: antihypertensive, diuretic
metaxalone/**SKELAXIN:** muscle relaxant
methacycline/**RONDOMYCIN:** antibiotic

methadone/**DOLOPHINE, WESTADONE:** narcotic analgesic
METHAMPEX/methamphetamine: stimulant
methamphetamine/**DESOXYN, METHAMPEX:** stimulant
metharbital/**GEMONIL:** barbiturate
methazolamide/**NEPTAZANE:** decreases intraocular pressure
methenamine hippurate/**HIPREX, UREX:** antibacterial
METHERGINE/methylergonovine: oxytocic
methicillin/**VERSAPEN-K:** antibiotic
methnamine/**MANDELAMINE, PROV-U-SEP:** antibacterial
methocarbamol/**ROBAMOL, ROBAXIN:** muscle relaxant
METHOXAL/sulfamethoxazole: antibacterial
methoxalen/**OXSORALEN:** improves melanin production (vitiligo)
METHOXANOL/sulfamethoxazole: antibacterial
methsuximide/**CELONTIN:** anticonvulsant (petit mal)
methyclothiazide/**AQUATENSEN, ENDURON:** antihypertensive, diuretic
methyclothiazide, pargyline/**EUTRON:** antihypertensive, diuretic
methyldopa/**ALDOMET:** antihypertensive
methyldopa, chlorothiazide/**ALDOCOR:** antihypertensive, diuretic
methyldopa, hydrochlorothiazide/**ALDORIL:** antihypertensive, diuretic
methylergonovine/**METHERGINE:** oxytocic
METHYLONE/methylprednisolone: steroidal antiinflammatory
methylpenidate/**RITALIN:** antihyperactive, antinarcoleptic
methylprednisolone/**DURALONE, MEDROL:** steroidal antiinflammatory
methyprylon/**NOLUDAR:** tranquilizer
methysergide/**SANSERT:** serotonin inhibitor (headaches)
METICORTEN/prednisone: steroidal antiinflammatory
metoclopramide/**OCTAMIDE, REGLAN:** antiulcer
metolazone/**DIULO, ZAROXOLYN:** antihypertensive, diuretic
metoprolol/**LOPRESSOR:** antihypertensive
metronidazole/**FLAGYL:** antifungal
metyrosine/**DEMSER:** antihypertensive
MEVACOR/lovastatin: anticholesterol
mexiletine/**MEXITIL:** antidysrhythmic
MEXITIL/mexiletine: antidysrhythmic
MICATIN/miconazole: antifungal
MICRO-K/potassium chloride: potassium supplement
MICRONASE/glyburide: oral hypoglycemic
miconazole/**MICATIN, MONISTAT:** antifungal
MICRONEFRIN/racepinephrine: bronchodilator
MICRONOR/norethindrone: hormone
MIDAMOR/amiloride: diuretic (potassium sparing)
MIDATANE DC/brompheniramine, phenylephrine, codeine: narcotic antitussive, antihistamine
MIDRIN/isometheptene: analgesic, tranquilizer
MIGRASTAT/ergotamine, caffeine: cerebral vasoconstrictor
MILFLEX/chlorzoxazone, acetaminophen: muscle relaxant, analgesic
MILONTIN/phensuximide: anticonvulsant (petit mal)
MILTOWN/meprobamate: tranquilizer
MINABEL/belladonna alkaloids, butabarbital: antispasmodic
MINI-LIX/aminophylline: xanthine bronchodilator
MINIPRESS/prazosin: antihypertensive
MINIZIDE/polythiazide, prazosin: antihypertensive
MINOCIN/minocycline: antibiotic

minocycline/**MINOCIN:** antibiotic
monoxidil/**LONITEN:** antihypertensive
MIRADON/anisindione: anticoagulant
misoprostol/**CYTOTEC:** antiulcer
MOBAN/molindone: tranquilizer
MODURETIC/amiloride, HCTZ: antihypertensive, diuretic
MOEBIQUIN/iodoquinol: amebicide
molindone/**MOBAN:** tranquilizer
MONISTAT/miconazole: antifungal
MONOPRIL/fosinopril: antihypertensive
moricizine/**ETHMOZINE:** ventricular antidysrhythmic
morphine/**ASTRAMORPH PF, DURAMORPH:** narcotic analgesic
MOTOFEN/difenoxin, atropine: narcotic antidiarrheal
MOTRIN/ibuprofen: analgesic, antiinflammatory
MS CONTIN/morphine: narcotic analgesic
MSIR/morphine: narcotic analgesic
MUCOMYST/acetylcysteine: mucolytic
MUDRANE/aminophylline: xanthine bronchodilator
MUDRANE GG/theophylline, guaifenesin, phenobarbital: bronchodilator, expectorant
MYAMBUTOL/ethambutol: antibiotic
MYCELEX/clotrimazole: antifungal
MYCIFRADIN/neomycin: antibiotic
MYCOBUTIN/rifabutin: antibiotic
MYCOSTATIN/nystatin: antifungal
MYKROX/metolazone: antihypertensive, diuretic
MYOBID/papaverine: cerebral/peripheral vasodilator
MYOLIN/orphenadrine: analgesic
MYOTONACHOL/bethanechol: vagomimetic (urinary retention)
MYSOLINE/primidone: anticonvulsant
nadolol/**CORGARD:** antianginal, antihypertensive
NAFCIL/nafcillin: antibiotic
nafcillin/**STAPHCILLIN, UNIPEN:** antibiotic
naftifine/**NAFTIN:** antifungal
NAFTIN/naftifine: antifungal
nalbuphine/**NUBAIN:** narcotic analgesic
NALDECON/phenylpropanolamine, phenylephrine, chlorpheniramine: antihistamine, decongestant
naldixic acid/**NEG GRAM:** antibiotic
NALFON/fenoprofen: analgesic, antiinflammatory
naltrexone/**TREXAN:** narcotic antagonist
NAPROSYN/naproxen: analgesic, antiinflammatory
naproxen/**ANAPROX, NAPROSYN:** analgesic, antiinflammatory
NAQUA/trichlormethiazide: antihypertensive, diuretic
NAQUIVAL/reserpine, trichlormethiazide: antihypertensive, diuretic
NARDIL/phenelzine: tranquilizer
NASALIDE/flunisolide: steroidal antiinflammatory
NATURETIN/bendroflumethiazide: antihypertensive, diuretic
NAVANE/thiothixene: tranquilizer
NEBCIN/tobramycin: antibiotic
NEG GRAM/naladixic acid: antibiotic
NEMBUTAL/pentobarbital: barbiturate
NEOBIOTIC/neomycin: antibiotic
NEOCYTEN/orphenadrine: analgesic
neomycin/**MYCIFRADIN, NEOBIOTIC:** antibiotic

NEO-RENAL/furosemide: diuretic
NEOTHYLLINE/dyphylline: xanthine bronchodilator
NEO-VADRIN/guaifenesin, dextromethorphan: antitussive, expectorant
NEPTAZANE/methazolamide: decreases intraocular pressure
NIA-BID/niacin: decreases serum cholesterol
niacin/NIA-BID, NICOLAR: decreases serum cholesterol
nicardipine/CARDENE: antianginal, antihypertensive
NICOLAR/niacin: decreases serum cholesterol
nifedipine/PROCARDIA: antianginal, antihypertensive
NILSTAT/nystatin: antifungal
nimodipine/NIMOTOP: decreases neurological deficits
NIMOTOP/nimodipine: decreases neurological deficits
NISENTIL/alphaprodine: narcotic analgesic
NITRO-BID/nitroglycerin: antianginal, vasodilator
NITROCINE/nitroglycerin: antianginal, vasodilator
nitrofurantion/FURADANTIN, MACRODANTIN: antibacterial
nitroglycerin/NITRO-BID, NITROSTAT: antianginal, vasodilator
NITROGLYN/nitroglycerin: antianginal, vasodilator
NITROL/nitroglycerin: antianginal, vasodilator
NITRONG/nitroglycerin: antianginal, vasodilator
NITROSPAN/nitroglycerin: antianginal, vasodilator
NITROSTAT/nitroglycerin: antianginal, vasodilator
NIZORAL/ketoconazole: antifungal
NOCTEC/chloral hydrate: tranquilizer
NOLUDAR/methyprylon: tranquilizer
norethindrone/MICRONOR, NORLUTIN: hormone
NORFLEX/orphenadrine: muscle relaxant
norfloxacin/NOROXIN: antibacterial
NORGESIC/orphenadrine and APC: analgesic
NORGESIC FORTE/orphenadrine and APC: analgesic
NORISODRINE AEROTROL/isoproterenol: bronchodilator
NORLUTIN/norethindrone: hormone
NORMATENE DC/brompheniramine, phenylephrine, codeine: narcotic antitussive, antihistamine
NORMATENE EXPECTORANT/brompheniramine, phenylephrine: antihistamine, decongestant
NORMODYNE/labetalol: antihypertensive
NORMOZIDE/labetalol, HCTZ: antihypertensive
NOROXIN/norfloxacin: antibacterial
NORPACE/disopyramide: antidysrhythmic (ventricular)
NORPRAMIN/amitriptyline: tricyclic antidepressant
nortriptyline/AVENTYL, PAMELOR: tricyclic antidepressant
NORTUSSIN/guaifenesin: expectorant
NORTUSSIN with CODEINE/guaifenesin, codeine: narcotic antitussive, expectorant
NORVASC/amlodipine: antianginal, antihypertensive
NOVAHISTINE DH/chlorpheniramine, pseudoephedrine, codeine: narcotic antitussive, decongestant
NUBAIN/nalbuphine: narcotic analgesic
NUMORPHAN/oxymorphone: narcotic analgesic
NUPRIN/ibuprofen: analgesic, antiinflammatory
NYDRAZID/isoniazid: antibiotic
nylidrin/ARLIDIN: vasodilator
nystatin/MYCOSTATIN, NILSTAT: antifungal
OBOTAN/dextroamphetamine: stimulant
OCTAMIDE/metoclopramide: antiulcer
OGEN/estropipate: hormone
omeprazole/PRILOSEC: decreases gastric acid

OMNIBEL/belladonna, butabarbital: antispasmodic
OMNIPEN/ampicillin: antibiotic
opium/PANTOPON: narcotic analgesic
opium, tincture of/LAUDANUM: narcotic analgesic
OPTIMINE/azatadine: antihistamine
ORADRATE/choral hydrate: tranquilizer
ORAMORPH SR/morphine: narcotic analgesic
ORAPAV/papaverine: cerebral/peripheral vasodilator
ORASONE/prednisone: steroidal antiinflammatory
ORETIC/hydrochlorothiazide: antihypertensive, diuretic
ORETICYL/diserpidine, hydrochlorothiazide: antihypertensive, diuretic
ORINASE/tolbutamide: oral hypoglycemic
ORNADE/chlorpheniramine, phenylpropanolamine: antihistamine, decongestant
orphenadrine/NORFLEX, TEGA-FLEX: muscle relaxant
orphenadrine and APC/NORGESIC, NORGESIC FORTE: muscle relaxant, analgesic
ORUDIS/ketoprofen: analgesic, antiinflammatory
ouabain/STROPHANTHIN-G: cardiac glycoside (CHF, SVT)
oxacillin/BACTOCIL, PROSTAPHLIN: antibiotic
OXALID/oxyphenbutazone: analgesic, antiinflammatory
oxaprozin/DAYPRO: antiinflammatory
oxazepam/SERAX: benzodiazepine tranquilizer
oxiconazole/OXISTAT: antifungal
OXISTAT/oxiconazole: antifungal
oxtriphylline/CHOLEDYL: xanthine bronchodilator
oxtriphylline, guaifenesin/BRONDECON, BRONDELATE: bronchodilator
oxybutynin/DITROPAN: antispasmodic
oxycodone/ROXICODONE: narcotic analgesic
oxycodone, acetaminophen/PERCOCET-5, TYLOX: narcotic analgesic
oxycodone, APAP/ROXIDCET: narcotic analgesic
oxycodone, aspirin/PERCODAN, PERCODAN-DEMI: narcotic analgesic
OXYDESS/dextroamphetamine: stimulant
oxymorphone/NUMORPHAN: narcotic analgesic
oxyphenbutazone/OXALID, TANDEARIL: analgesic, antiinflammatory
oxytetracycline/TERRAMYCIN, TETRAMINE: antibiotic
PABALATE/salicylate, aminobenzoate: analgesic
P-A-C COMPOUND/aspirin, phenacetin, caffeine: analgesic
P-A-C COMPOUND with CODEINE/APC, codeine: narcotic analgesic
PAGITANE/cycrimine: antiparkinsonian, antiextrapyramidal symptoms
PALBAR/belladonna alkaloids, butabarbital: antispasmodic
PAMELOR/nortriptyline: tricyclic antidepressant
PANHEPRIN/heparin: anticoagulant
PANMYCIN/tetracycline: antibiotic
PANTOPON/opium: narcotic analgesic
PANWARFIN/warfarin: anticoagulant
papaverine/PAVABID, VASOSPAN: cerebral/peripheral vasodilator
PARACHLOR/chlorzoxazone, acetaminophen: muscle relaxant, analgesic
PARADIONE/paramethadione: anticonvulsant (petit mal)
PARAFLEX/chlorzoxazone: muscle relaxant

PARAFON FORTE/chlorzoxazone, acetaminophen: muscle relaxant, analgesic
PARAL/paraldehyde: tranquilizer
paraldehyde/PARAL: tranquilizer
paramethadione/PARADIONE: anticonvulsant (petit mal)
PAREPECTOLIN/kaolin, paregoric: antidiarrheal, antispasmodic
PARGESIC 65/propoxyphene: narcotic analgesic
pargyline/EUTONYL: antihypertensive
PARLODEL/bromocriptine: antiparkinsonian
PARNATE/tranylcypromine: monoamine oxidase inhibitor
paroxetine/PAXIL: antidepressant
PARSIDOL/ethopropazine: antiparkinsonian, antiextrapyramidal symptoms
PATHOCIL/hetacillin: antibiotic
PAVABID/papaverine: cerebral/peripheral vasodilator
PAVACON/papaverine: cerebral/peripheral vasodilator
PAVADON/acetaminophen, codeine: narcotic analgesic
PAVADUR/papaverine: cerebral/peripheral vasodilator
PAVASED/papaverine: cerebral/peripheral vasodilator
PAVASULE/papaverine: cerebral/peripheral vasodilator
PAVATRAN/papaverine: cerebral/peripheral vasodilator
PAVEROLAN/papaverine: cerebral/peripheral vasodilator
PAXIL/paroxetine: antidepressant
PAXIPAM/halazepam: benzodiazepine tranquilizer
PBZ/tripelennamine: antihistamine
PCE/erythromycin: antibiotic
PEDIAMYCIN/erythromycin: antibiotic
PEGANONE/ethotoin: anticonvulsant
pemoline/CYLERT: antihyperactive, antinarcoleptic
PENAPAR VK/penicillin V: antibiotic
penbutolol/LEVATOL: antihypertensive
penicillamine/CUPRIMINE, DEPEN: antiarthritic, chelating agent (for heavy metal poisoning)
penicillin G/BICILLIN, WYCILLIN: antibiotic
penicillin V/PEN-VEE K, VEETIDS: antibiotic
PENSYN/ampicillin: antibiotic
pentaerythritol tetranitrate/PENTRITOL, PERITRATE: antianginal, vasodilator
pentazocine/TALWIN: narcotic analgesic
pentazocine, acetaminophen/TALACEN: narcotic analgesic
pentazocine, ASA/TALWIN COMPOUND: narcotic analgesic
pentazocine, naloxone/TALWIN NX: narcotic analgesic
PENTIDS/penicillin G: antibiotic
pentobarbital/NEMBUTAL: barbiturate
pentobarbital, carbromal/CARBRITAL: tranquilizer
pentoxifylline/TRENTAL: decreases blood viscosity
PENTRITOL/pentaerythritol tetranitrate: antianginal, vasodilator
PEN-VEE K/penicillin V: antibiotic
PEPCID/famotidine: antiulcer
PERCOCET/oxycodone, acetaminophen: narcotic analgesic
PERCODAN/oxycodone, aspirin: narcotic analgesic
PERCODAN-DEMI/ oxycodone, aspirin: narcotic analgesic
pergolide/PERMAX: antiparkinsonian
PERIACTIN/cyproheptadine: antihistamine
PERITRATE/pentaerythritol tetranitrate: antianginal, vasodilator
PERMAPEN/penicillin G: antibiotic
PERMAX/pergolide: antiparkinsonian

permethrin/ELIMITE: topical scabicide
PERMITIL/fluphenazine: phenothiazine tranquilizer
perphenazine/TRILAFON: phenothiazine tranquilizer
PERSANTINE/dipyridamole: vasodilator
PERTOFRANE/amitriptyline: tricyclic antidepressant
PETHADOL/meperidine: narcotic analgesic
PFIZER-E/erythromycin stearate: antibiotic
PHEDRAL/theophylline, ephedrine, barbiturate: bronchodilator, expectorant
phenacemide/PHENURONE: anticonvulsant
PHENAPHEN/acetaminophen: analgesic, antiinflammatory
PHENAPHEN with CODEINE/acetaminophen, codeine: narcotic analgesic, antiinflammatory
PHEN-AZO/phenazopyridine: urinary tract analgesic
PHENAZODINE/phenazopyridine: urinary tract analgesic
phenazopyridine/AZODINE, PYRIDIUM: urinary tract analgesic
PHENDIET/phendimetrazine: appetite suppressant
phendimetrazine/BONTRIL PDM, PHENDIET: appetite suppressant
phenelzine/NARDIL: antidepressant
PHENERGAN/promethazine: antiemetic, phenothiazine tranquilizer
PHENETRON/chlorpheniramine: antihistamine
phenmetrazine/PRELUDIN: appetite suppressant
phenobarbital/LUMINAL, SOLFOTON: barbiturate
PHENOBEL/belladonna alkaloids, phenobarbital: antispasmodic
phenoxybenzamine/DIBENZYLINE: antihypertensive
phensuximide/MILONTIN: anticonvulsant (petit mal)
phentermine/FASTIN, IONAMIN: appetite suppressant
PHENURONE/phenacemide: anticonvulsant
phenylbutazone/AZOLID, BUTAZOLIDIN: analgesic, antiinflammatory
phenylpropanolamine/PROPAGEST, RHINDECON: decongestant
phenylpropanolamine, caramiphen/TUSS-ORNADE: antitussive, decongestant
phenylpropanolamine, guaifenesin/ENTEX LA: decongestant, expectorant
phenylpropanolamine, phenylephrine, chlorpheniramine/NALDECON: antihistamine, decongestant
phenylpropanolamine, phenyltoloxamine, APAP/SINUBID: decongestant
PHENYLZONE-A/buffered phenylbutazone: analgesic, antiinflammatory
phenytoin/DILANTIN, DIPHENYLAN: anticonvulsant
PHYSPAN/theophylline: xanthine bronchodilator
PIL-DIGIS/digitalis: cardiac glycoside (CHF, SVT)
pindolol/VISKEN: antihypertensive
piperacetazine/QUIDE: phenothiazine tranquilizer
PIPERZINE ESTRONE/estropipate: hormone
PIPERZINE SULFATE/estropipate: hormone
pirbuterol/MAXAIR: bronchodilator
piroxicam/FELDENE: analgesic, antiinflammatory
PLACIDYL/ethchlorvynol: tranquilizer
PLAQUENIL/hydroxychloroquine: antimalarial
PLEGINE/phendimetrazine: appetite suppressant
PLENDIL/felodipine: antihypertensive

POLARAMINE/dexchlorpheniramine: antihistamine
POLYCILLIN/ampicillin: antibiotic
POLYMOX/amoxicillin: antibiotic
polythiazide/**RENESE**: antihypertensive, diuretic
polythiazide, prazosin/**MINIZIDE**: antihypertensive
PONDIMIN/fenfluramine: appetite suppressant
PONTSEL/mefenamic acid: antiinflammatory
potassium chloride/**KLORVESS, SLOW-K**: potassium supplement
prazepam/**CENTRAX, VERSTRAN**: benzodiazepine tranquilizer
prazosin/**MINIPRESS**: antihypertensive
prednisolone/**DELTA-CORTEF, STERONE**: steroidal antiinflammatory
prednisone/**METICORTEN, ORASONE**: steroidal antiinflammatory
PRELONE/prednisolone: steroidal antiinflammatory
PRELUDIN/phenmetrazine: appetite suppressant
PREMARIN/conjugated estrogens: hormone
PRE-STATE/chlorphentermine: appetite suppressant
PRILOSEC/omeprazole: decreases gastric acid
PRIMATENE MIST/epinephrine: bronchodilator
primidone/**MYSOLINE**: anticonvulsant
PRINCIPEN/ampicillin: antibiotic
PRINIVIL/lisinopril: antihypertensive
PRINZIDE/lisinopril, HCTZ: antihypertensive, diuretic
PROBALAN/probenecid: prolongs action of penicillin, uricosuric
PRO-BANTHINE/propantheline: antiulcer
probenecid/**BENEMID, PROBALAN**: prolongs action of penicillin, uricosuric
probucol/**LORELCO**: anticholesterol
procainamide/**PROCAN, PRONESTYL**: antidysrhythmic
PROCAMIDE/procainamide: antidysrhythmic
PROCAN/procainamide: antidysrhythmic
PROCAN SR/procainamide: antidysrhythmic
procarbazine/**MATULANE**: anticancer
PROCARDIA/nifedipine: antianginal, antihypertensive
prochlorperazine/**COMPAZINE, STEMETIL**: phenothiazine tranquilizer
prochlorperazine, isopropamide/**COMBID**: antiemetic, antispasmodic
PROCIT/epoetin alpha: hormone (red blood cell production)
PROCO/guaifenesin: expectorant
PROCOPAN/procainamide: antidysrhythmic
PROCRIT/erythropoietin: bone marrow RBC stimulator
PROCTOCORT/hydrocortisone: steroidal antiinflammatory
procyclidine/**KEMADRIN**: antiparkinsonian, antiextrapyramidal symptoms
progesterone/**PROLUTON**: hormone
PROGLYCEM/diazoxide: oral hypoglycemic
PROGYNON/estradiol: hormone
PROKETAZINE/carphenazine: phenothiazine tranquilizer
PROLIXIN/fluphenazine: phenothiazine tranquilizer
PROLUTON/progesterone: hormone
PROMAPAR/chlorpromazine: phenothiazine tranquilizer
promazine/**SPARINE**: phenothiazine tranquilizer
promethezine/**PHENERGAN, REMSED**: antiemetic, phenothiazine tranquilizer
PRONESTYL/procainamide: antidysrhythmic

PROPACET/propoxyphene, APAP: narcotic analgesic
propafenone/**RHYTHMOL**: ventricular antidysrhythmic
PROPAGEST/phenylpropanolamine: decongestant
propantheline/**PRO-BANTHINE**: antiulcer
propoxyphene/**DARVON, DOLENE**: narcotic analgesic
propoxyphene, acetaminophen/**DARVOCET-N, WYGESIC**: narcotic analgesic
propoxyphene, APAP/**PROPACET**: narcotic analgesic
propoxyphene, ASA /**DARVON with ASA, DARVON-N with ASA**: narcotic analgesic
propoxyphene, ASA, caffeine/**DARVON COMPOUND**: narcotic analgesic
propranolol/**INDERAL**: antidysrhythmic, antimigraine
propranolol, HCTZ/**INDERIDE**: antihypertensive, diuretic
PROSTAPHLIN/oxacillin: antibiotic
PROTERNOL/isoproteronol: bronchodilator
protriptyline/**VIVACTIL**: tricyclic antidepressant
PROTROPIN/somatrem: hormone
PROVAL/acetaminophen, codeine: narcotic analgesic
PROVENTIL/albuterol: bronchodilator
PROVERA/medroxyprogesterone: hormone
PROV-U-SEP/methnamine: antibacterial
PROXAGESIC/propoxyphene: narcotic analgesic
PROXENE/propoxyphene: narcotic analgesic
PROZAC/fluoxetine: antidepressant
psyllium/**METAMUCIL**: laxative
PURETANE/brompheniramine: antihistamine
PURETAPP/brompheniramine, phenylephrine: antihistamine, decongestant
PURODIGIN/digitoxin: cardiac glycoside (CHF, SVT)
PYRIBENZAMINE/tripelennamine: antihistamine
PYRIDIATE/phenazopyridine: urinary tract analgesic
PYRIDIUM/phenazopyridine: urinary tract analgesic
pyrilamine/**ALLERTOC, THYLOGEN**: antihistamine
pyrilamine, pentobarbital/**EME-NIL, WANS**: antiemetic
PYRODINE/phenazopyridine: urinary tract analgesic
quazepam/**DORAL**: benzodiazepine tranquilizer
QUARZAN/clidinium: antiulcer
QUELTUSS/guaifenesin, dextromethorphan: antitussive, expectorant
QUESTRAN/cholestyramine: decreases serum cholesterol
QUIBRON/theophylline, guaifenesin: bronchodilator, expectorant
QUIBRON PLUS/theophylline, guaifenesin, barbiturate: bronchodilator, expectorant
QUIDE/piperacetazine: phenothiazine tranquilizer
QUINAGLUTE DURA-TABS/quinidine: antidysrhythmic
QUINE/quinine: antimalarial
quinestrol/**ESTROVIS**: hormone
quinethazone/**HYDROMOX**: antihypertensive, diuretic
QUINIDEX EXTENTABS/quinidine: antidysrhythmic
quinidine/**QUINAGLUTE DURA-TABS, QUINIDEX EXTENTABS**: antidysrhythmic
quinine/**COCO-QUININE, QUINE**: antimalarial
QUINORA/quinidine: antidysrhythmic
racepinephrine/**MICRONEFRIN, VAPONEFRIN**: bronchodilator
ramipril/**ALTACE**: antihypertensive
ranitidine/**ZANTAC**: antiulcer
RAUDIXIN/rauwolfia serpentina: antihypertensive

RAULFIA/rauwolfia serpentina: antihypertensive

RAUPIOD/rauwolfia serpentina: antihypertensive

RAU-SED/reserpine: antihypertensive

RAUSERPA/rauwolfia serpentina: antihypertensive

rauwolfia serpentina/**RAULFIA, RAUSERPA:** antihypertensive

rauwolfia serpentina, bendroflumethiazide/**RAUZIDE:** antihypertensive

RAUZIDE/rauwolfia serpentina, bendroflumethiazide: antihypertensive

REGLAN/metoclopramide: antiulcer

REGROTON/reserpine, chlorthalidone: antihypertensive, diuretic

RELA/carisoprodol: muscle relaxant

REMSED/promethazine: antiemetic, tranquilizer

RENESE/polythiazide: antihypertensive, diuretic

RENESE-R/reserpine, methyclothiazide: antihypertensive, diuretic

RENOQUID/sulfacytine: antibacterial

REPOISE/butaperizine: phenothiazine tranquilizer

RESCUDOSE/morphine: narcotic analgesic

RESERPAZIDE/reserpine, hydrochlorothiazide: antihypertensive, diuretic

reserpine/**RESERPOID, SERPASIL:** antihypertensive

reserpine, benzthiazide/**EXNA-R:** antihypertensive, diuretic

reserpine, chlorothiazide/**DIUPRES:** antihypertensive, diuretic

reserpine, chlorthalidone/**REGROTON:** antihypertensive, diuretic

reserpine, hydralazine/**SERPASIL-APRESOLINE:** antihypertensive, diuretic

reserpine, hydralazine, HCTZ/**SER-AP-ES, TRI-HYDRO-SERPINE:** antihypertensive, diuretic

reserpine, hydrochlorothiazide/**HYDROPRES, SERPASIL-ESIDRIX:** antihypertensive, diuretic

reserpine, hydroflumethiazide/**SALUTENSIN, SALUTENSIN-DEMI:** antihypertensive, diuretic

reserpine, methyclothiazide/**DIUTENSEN-R:** antihypertensive, diuretic

reserpine, polythiazide/**RENESE-R:** antihypertensive, diuretic

reserpine, quinethazone/**HYDROMOX-R:** antihypertensive, diuretic

reserpine, trichlormethiazide/**METATENSIN, NAQUIVAL:** antihypertensive

RESERPOID/reserpine: antihypertensive

RESPBID/theophylline: xanthine bronchodilator

RESTORIL/temazepam: benzodiazepine tranquilizer

RETET/tetracycline: antibiotic

RETIN-A/tretinoin: antiacne

RETROVIR/zidovudine: antiviral

RHINDECON/phenylpropanolamine: decongestant

RHYTHMOL/propafenone: ventricular antidysrhythmic

RIDAURA/auranofin: antiarthritic

rifabutin/**MYCOBUTIN:** antibiotic

RIFADIN/rifampin: antibiotic

RIFAMATE/rifampin, isoniazid: antibiotic

rifampin/**RIFADIN, RIMACTANE:** antibiotic

rifampin, isoniazid/**RIFAMATE:** antibiotic

RIMACTANE/rifampin: antibiotic

RITALIN/methylpenidate: antihyperactive, antinarcoleptic

ritodrine/**YUTOPAR:** decreases uterine activity

RMS/morphine: narcotic analgesic suppositories

ROBAMOL/methocarbamol: muscle relaxant

ROBAMOX/amoxicillin: antibiotic

ROBAXIN/methocarbamol: muscle relaxant

ROBIMYCIN/erythromycin: antibiotic

ROBITET/tetracycline: antibiotic

ROBITUSSIN/guaifenesin: expectorant

ROBITUSSIN A-C/guaifenesin, codeine: antitussive, expectorant

ROBITUSSIN DM/guaifenesin, dextromethorphan: antitussive, expectorant

ROCEPHIN/ceftriaxone: antibiotic

ROFERON-A/interferon: immune system stimulant

RONDOMYCIN/methacycline: antibiotic

ROXANOL 100/morphine: narcotic analgesic

ROXIDCET/oxycodone, APAP: narcotic analgesic

ROXIDCODONE/oxycodone: narcotic analgesic

RP-MYCIN/erythromycin: antibiotic

RUFEN/ibuprofen: analgesic, antiinflammatory

SALATIN with CODEINE/APC, codeine: narcotic analgesic

SALFLEX/salsalate: analgesic, antiinflammatory

salicylate, aminobenzoate/**PABALATE:** analgesic

salsalate/**DISALCID, SALFLEX:** analgesic, antiinflammatory

SALURON/hydroflumethiazide: antihypertensive, diuretic

SALUTENSIN/reserpine, hydroflumethiazide: antihypertensive, diuretic

SALUTENSIN-DEMI/reserpine, hydroflumethiazide: antihypertensive, diuretic

SANDIMMUNE/cyclosporine: immunosuppressant

SANDRIL/reserpine: antihypertensive

SANOREX/mazindol: appetite suppressant

SANSERT/methysergide: serotonin inhibitor (headaches)

SAS-500/sulfsalazine: antibacterial

secobarbital/**SECONAL:** barbiturate

secobarbital, amobarbital/**TUINAL:** barbiturate

SECONAL/secobarbital: barbiturate

SEDADROPS/phenobarbital: barbiturate

SEDAPAP/butalbital, APAP: analgesic

SEDAPAP #3/codeine, butalbital, APAP: narcotic analgesic

SELDANE/terfenadine: antihistamine

selegiline/**ELDEPRYL:** MAO inhibitor (Parkinson's disease)

senna/**SENOKOT, X-PREP:** laxative

SENOKOT/senna: laxative

SEPTRA/sulfamethoxazole, trimethoprim: antibacterial

SER-AP-ES/reserpine, hydralazine, HCTZ: antihypertensive, diuretic

SERAX/oxazepam: benzodiazepine tranquilizer

SERENTIL/mesoridazine: phenothiazine tranquilizer

SERPASIL/reserpine: antihypertensive

SERPASIL-APRESOLINE/reserpine, hydralazine: antihypertensive, diuretic

SERPASIL-ESIDRIX/reserpine, hydrochlorothiazide: antihypertensive, diuretic

SETAMINE/belladonna alkaloids, phenobarbital: antispasmodic

setraline/**ZOLOFT:** antidepressant

SILEXIN/guaifenesin, dextromethorphan: antitussive, expectorant

SINEMET/levodopa, carbidopa: antiparkinsonian

SINEQUAN/doxepin: tricyclic antidepressant

SINUBID/phenylpropanolamine, phenyltoloxamine, APAP: decongestant

SK-APAP/acetaminophen: analgesic, antiinflammatory

SK-APAP with CODEINE/acetaminophen, codeine: narcotic analgesic

SK-BAMATE/meprobamate: tranquilizer

SK-CHLOROTHIAZIDE/chlorothiazide: antihypertensive, diuretic

SK-DIPHENOXYLATE/diphenoxylate, atropine: narcotic antidiarrheal

SKELAXIN/metaxalone: muscle relaxant

SK-ERYTHROMYCIN/erythromycin stearate: antibiotic

SK-PHENOBARBITAL/phenobarbital: barbiturate

SK-PRAMINE/imipramine: tricyclic antidepressant

SK-65/propoxyphene: narcotic analgesic

SK-65-APAP/propoxyphene, acetaminophen: narcotic analgesic

SLO-BID/theophylline: xanthine bronchodilator

SLOPHYLLIN/theophylline: xanthine bronchodilator

SLOW FE/iron: iron supplement

SLOW-K/potassium: potassium supplement

SOFARIN/warfarin: anticoagulant

SOLFOTON/phenobarbital: barbiturate

SOLU-CORTEF/hydrocortisone: steroidal antiinflammatory

SOMA/carisoprodol: muscle relaxant

somatrem/**PROTROPIN:** hormone

SOMBULEX/hexobarbital: barbiturate

SOMOPHYLLIN/aminophylline: xanthine bronchodilator

SOMOPHYLLIN-T/theophylline: xanthine bronchodilator

SOPRODOL/carisoprodol: antispasmodic, sedative

SORATE/isosorbide dinitrate: antianginal, vasodilator

SORBIDE/isosorbide dinitrate: antianginal, vasodilator

SORBITRATE/isosorbide dinitrate: antianginal, vasodilator

SOSOL/sulfisoxazole: antibacterial

sotalol/**BETAPACE:** antidysrhythmic

SPALIX/belladonna alkaloids, phenobarbital: antispasmodic

SPANCAP/dextroamphetamine: stimulant

SPARINE/promazine: phenothiazine tranquilizer

SPASMOLIN/belladonna alkaloids, phenobarbital: antispasmodic

SPECTROBID/bacampicillin: antibiotic

SPINAXIN/methocarbamol: muscle relaxant

spironolactone/**ALDACTONE:** diuretic

spironolactone, hydrochlorothiazide/**ALDACTAZIDE:** diuretic

STADOL/butorphanol: narcotic analgesic

STAPHCILLIN/nafcillin: antibiotic

STELAZINE/trifluoperazine: phenothiazine tranquilizer

STEMETIL/prochlorperazine: phenothiazine tranquilizer

STERAPRED/prednisone: steroidal antiinflammatory

STERONE/prednisolone: steroidal antiinflammatory

STILPHOSTROL/diethylstilbestrol: hormone

STOXIL/idoxuridine: antiherpetic

STROPHANTHIN-G/ouabain: cardiac glycoside (CHF, SVT)

SUBLIMAZE/fentanyl: narcotic analgesic

SUB-QUIN/procainamide: antidysrhythmic

sucralfate/**CARAFATE:** antiulcer

SUFENTA/sufentanil: narcotic analgesic

sufentanil/**SUFENTA:** narcotic analgesic

SULDIAZO/sulfamethoxazole, phenazopyridine: antibacterial

sulfacytine/**RENOQUID:** antibacterial

SULFALAR/sulfisoxazole: antibacterial

sulfamethoxazole/**GANTANOL, METHOXAL:** antibacterial

sulfamethoxazole, phenazopyridine/**AZO GANTRISIN, AZO SOXAZOLE:** antibacterial

sulfamethoxazole, trimethoprim/**BACTRIM, SEPTRA:** antibacterial

sulfinpyrazone/**ANTURANE, ZYNOL:** uricosuric

sulfisoxazole/**GANTRISIN, SULFIZIN:** antibacterial

SULFIZIN/sulfisoxazole: antibacterial

sulfsalazine/**AZULFADINE, SAS-500:** antibacterial

sulindac/**CLINORIL:** analgesic, antiinflammatory

SUMOX/amoxicillin: antibiotic

SUMYCIN/tetracycline: antibiotic

SUPEN/ampicillin: antibiotic

SUPRAX/cefixime: antibiotic

SURFAK/docusate calcium: laxative

SURMONTIL/trimipramine: tricyclic antidepressant

SUSTAVERINE/papaverine: cerebral/peripheral vasodilator

SYMMETREL/amantadine: antiparkinsonian, antiviral

SYNALGOS-DC/APC, dihydrocodeine, promethazine: narcotic analgesic

SYNOPHYLATE-GG/theophylline, guaifenesin: bronchodilator, expectorant

SYNTHROID/levothyroxine: thyroid hormone

TACE/chlorotrianisene: hormone

TAGAMET/cimetidine: antiulcer

TALACEN/pentazocine, acetaminophen: narcotic analgesic

talbutal/**LOTUSATE:** barbiturate

TALWIN/pentazocine: narcotic analgesic

TALWIN COMPOUND/pentazocine, ASA: narcotic analgesic

TALWIN NX/pentazocine, naloxone: narcotic analgesic

TANDEARIL/oxyphenbutazone: analgesic, antiinflammatory

TARACTAN/chlorprothixene: tranquilizer

TAVIST/clemastine: antihistamine

TAVIST-D/clemastine, phenylpropanolamine: antihistamine

TEDFERN/theophylline, ephedrine, phenobarbital: bronchodilator, expectorant

TEDRAL/theophylline, ephedrine, phenobarbital: bronchodilator, expectorant

TEGA-FLEX/orphenadrine: analgesic, antiinflammatory

TEGOPEN/cloxacillin: antibiotic

TEGRETOL/carbamazipine: anticonvulsant

TELDRIN/chlorpheniramine: antihistamine

temazepam/**RESTORIL:** benzodiazepine tranquilizer

TEMPRA/acetaminophen: analgesic, antiinflammatory

TENUATE/diethylpropion: appetite suppressant

TEPANIL/diethylpropion: appetite suppressant

terazosin/**HYTRIN:** antihypertensive

terbutaline/**BRETHINE, BRICANYL:** bronchodilator

terfenadine/**SELDANE:** antihistamine

terpin hydrate, codeine/**CORTUSSIS:** narcotic antitussive, expectorant

TERRAMYCIN/oxytetracycline: antibiotic

tetracycline/**ACHROMYCIN, PANMYCIN:** antibiotic

TETRACYN/tetracycline: antibiotic

TETRAMINE/oxytetracycline: antibiotic

T-GESIC/hydrocodone, APAP: narcotic analgesic

THALFED/theophylline, ephedrine, phenobarbital: bronchodilator, expectorant

THEDRIZEM/theophylline, ephedrine, phenobarbital: bronchodilator, expectorant

THEELIN/estrone: hormone

THEOBID/theophylline: xanthine bronchodilator

THEOCLEAR/theophylline: xanthine bronchodilator

THEO-COL/theophylline, guaifenesin: bronchodilator, expectorant

THEODRINE/theophylline, ephedrine, phenobarbital: bronchodilator, expectorant

THEODUR/theophylline: xanthine bronchodilator

THEOFED/theophylline, ephedrine, phenobarbital: bronchodilator, expectorant

THEOFENAL/theophylline, ephedrine, phenobarbital: bronchodilator, expectorant

THEO-GUAIA/theophylline, guaifenesin: bronchodilator, expectorant

THEOLAIR/theophylline: xanthine bronchodilator

THEOLIXIR/theophylline: xanthine bronchodilator

THEOPHOZINE/theophylline, ephedrine, hydroxyzine: bronchodilator

THEOPHYL/theophylline: xanthine bronchodilator

theophylline/**SLOPHYLLIN, THEODUR:** xanthine bronchodilator

theophylline, ephedrine, hydroxyzine/**MARAX, THEOZINE:** bronchodilator, expectorant

theophylline, ephedrine, phenobarbital/**TEDRAL, THEOTABS:** bronchodilator, expectorant

theophylline, guaifenesin/**DIALIXIR, QUIBRON:** bronchodilator, expectorant

theophylline, guaifenesin, phenobarbital/**BRONKOLIXIR, MUDRANE GG:** bronchodilator, expectorant

THEORAL/theophylline, ephedrine, phenobarbital: bronchodilator, expectorant

THEODSPAN/theophylline: xanthine bronchodilator

THEOTABS/theophylline, ephedrine, phenobarbital: bronchodilator, expectorant

THEOZINE/theophylline, ephedrine, hydroxyzine: bronchodilator

thioridazine/**MELLARIL:** phenothiazine tranquilizer

thiothixene/**NAVANE:** tranquilizer

THORAZINE/chlorpromazine: phenothiazine tranquilizer

THYLOGEN/pyrilamine: antihistamine

THYRAR/thyroid: thyroid horomone

THYROCRINE/thyriod: thyroid horomone

thyroid/**THYRAR, THYROCRINE:** thyroid horomone

THYROLAR/liotrix: thyroid horomone

TICAR/ticarcillin: antibiotic

ticarcillin/**TICAR:** antibiotic

TIGAN/trimethobenzamide: antiemetic

TINACTIN/tolnaftate: antifungal

TINDAL/acetophenazine: phenothiazine tranquilizer

tobramycin/**NEBCIN:** antibiotic

TOFRANIL/imipramine: tricyclic antidepressant

tolazamide/**TOLINASE:** oral hypoglycemic

tolbutamide/**ORINASE:** oral hypoglycemic

TOLECTIN/tolmetin: analgesic, antiinflammatory

TOLINASE/tolazamide: oral hypoglycemic

tolmetin/**TOLECTIN:** analgesic, antiinflammatory

tolnaftate/**AFTATE, TINACTIN:** antifungal

TOLU-SED/guaifenesin, codeine: antitussive, expectorant

TOLU-SED DM/guaifenesin, dextromethorphan: antitussive, expectorant

TOTACILLIN/ampicillin: antibiotic

T-PHYL/theophylline: xanthine bronchodilator

TRAMACORT/triamcinolone: steroidal antiinflammatory

tramadol/**ULTRAM:** analgesic

TRANDATE/labetalol: antihypertensive

TRANDATE HCT/labetalol, HCTZ: antihypertensive

TRANMAP/meprobamate: tranquilizer

TRANSDERM NITRO/nitroglycerin: antianginal

TRANSDERM-SCOP/scopolamine: antiemetic

TRANXENE-SD/clorazepate: benzodiazepine tranquilizer

tranylcypromine/**PARNATE:** antidepressant

trazodone/**DESYREL:** tricyclic antidepressant

TRECATOR-SC/ethionamide: antibiotic (tuberculosis)

TREMIN/trihexyphenidyl: antiparkinsonian, antiextrapyramidal symptoms

TRENTAL/pentoxifylline: decreases blood viscosity

tretinoin/**RETIN-A:** antiacne

TREXAN/naltrexone: narcotic antagonist

triamcinolone/**ARISTOCORT, KENALOG:** steroidal antiinflammatory

triamterene/**DIRENIUM:** diuretic

triamterene, HCTZ/**DYAZIDE:** antihypertensive, diuretic

TRIAVIL/amitriptyline, perphenazine: tricyclic antidepressant, tranquilizer

triazolam/**HALCION:** benzodiazepine tranquilizer

trichlormethiazide/**METAHYDRIN, NAQUA:** antihypertensive, diuretic

TRIDIONE/trimethadione: anticonvulsant

trifluoperazine/**STELAZINE:** phenothiazine tranquilizer

triflupromazine/**VESPRIN:** phenothiazine tranquilizer

trihexyphenidyl/**ARTANE, TREMIN:** antiparkinsonian, antiextrapyramidal symptoms

TRI-HYDRO-SERPINE/reserpine, hydralazine, HCTZ: antihypertensive, diuretic

TRI-K/potassium: potassium supplement

TRIKATES/potassium: potassium supplement

TRILAFON/perphenazine: phenothiazine tranquilizer

trimethadione/**TRIDIONE:** anticonvulsant

trimethobenzamide/**TIGAN:** antiemetic

trimethoprim/**BACTRIM:** antibiotic

trimipramine/**SURMONTIL:** tricyclic antidepressant

TRIMOX/amoxicillin: antibiotic

tripelennamine/**PBZ, PYRIBENZAMINE:** antihistamine

triprolidine/**ACTIDIL:** antihistamine

TRI-SPAS/belladonna, phenobarbital: antispasmodic

TRITEN/dimethindene: antihistamine

TROCAL/guaifenesin, dextromethorphan: antitussive, expectorant

TUINAL/secobarbital, amobarbital: barbiturate

TUMOL/methocarbamol: muscle relaxant

TUSSEND/hydrocodone: narcotic antitussive

TUSSEND EXPECTORANT/hydrocodone, pseudoephedrine, guaifenesin: expectorant, narcotic antitussive

TUSSIONEX/hydrocodone, chlorpheniramine: narcotic antitussive

TUSS-ORNADE/phenylpropanolamine, caramiphen: antitussive, decongestant

TUZON/chlorzoxazone, acetaminophen: muscle relaxant, analgesic

TWIN-K/potassium: potassium supplement

TYLENOL/acetaminophen: analgesic, antiinflammatory

TYLENOL with CODEINE #2, #3, #4/acetaminophen with codeine: narcotic analgesic

TYLOX/oxycodone, acetaminophen: narcotic analgesic

U-GENCIN/gentamicin: antibiotic

ULTRACEF/cefadroxil: antibiotic

ULTRAM/tramadol: analgesic

UNIPEN/nafcillin: antibiotic

UNIPHYL/theophylline: xanthine bronchodilator

UNIPRES/reserpine, hydralazine, HCTZ: antihypertensive, diuretic

UNITENSEN/cryptenamine: antihypertensive

URECHOLINE/bethanechol: vagomimetic (urinary retention)

UREX/methenamine hippurate: antibacterial

URIDON/chlorothalidone: antihypertensive, diuretic

URISPAS/flavoxate: urinary antispasmodic

UTICILLIN VK/penicillin V: antibiotic

UTIMOX/amoxicillin: antibiotic

valacyclovir/**VALTREX**: antiviral

VALADOL/acetaminophen: analgesic, antiinflammatory

VALDRENE/diphenhydramine: antihistamine

VALISONE/betamethasone: steroidal antiinflammatory

VALIUM/diazepam: benzodiazepine tranquilizer

VALMID/ethinamate: tranquilizer

valproic acid/**DEPAKENE, DEPAKOTE**: anticonvulsant

VALRELEASE/diazepam: benzodiazepine tranquilizer

VALTREX/valacyclovir: antiviral

VANCERIL/beclomethasone: steroidal antiinflammatory

VAPONEFRIN/racepinephrine: bronchodilator

VASAL/papaverine: cerebral/peripheral vasodilator

VASCOR/bepridil: antianginal

VASERETIC/enalapril, HCTZ: antihypertensive, diuretic

VASODILAN/isoxsuprine: vasodilator

VASOSPAN/papaverine: cerebral/peripheral vasodilator

VASOTEC/enalapril: antihypertensive, diuretic

V-CILLIN/penicillin V: antibiotic

VEETIDS/penicillin V: antibiotic

VELOSEF/cephradine: antibiotic

venlafatine/**EFFEXOR**: antidepressant

VENTOLIN/albuterol: bronchodilator

VERACILLIN/hetacillin: antibiotic

verapamil/**CALAN, ISOPTIN**: antianginal, antihypertensive, antidysrhythmic

VERELAN/verapamil: antianginal, antihypertensive, antidysrhythmic

VEREQUAD/theophylline, guaifenesin, barbiturate: bronchodilator, expectorant

VERMOX/mebendazole: antihelminthic

VERSAPEN/hetacillin: antibiotic

VERSAPEN-K/methicillin: antibiotic

VERSTRAN/prazepam: benzodiazepine tranquilizer

VESPRIN/triflupromazine: phenothiazine tranquilizer

VIBRAMYCIN/doxycycline: antibiotic

VIBRA-TABS/doxycycline: antibiotic

VICODIN/hydrocodone, acetaminophen: narcotic analgesic

VISKEN/pindolol: antihypertensive

VISTARIL/hydroxyzine: antihistamine, tranquilizer

vitamin D/**CALCIFEROL**: vitamin (hypoparathyroidism)

VIVACTIL/protriptyline: tricyclic antidepressant

VOLMAX/albuterol: bronchodilator

VOLTAREN/diclofenac: analgesic, antiinflammatory

VONTROL/diphenidol: antiemetic

VORANIL/clortermine: appetite suppressant

WANS/pyrilamine, pentobarbital: antiemetic

warfarin/**COUMADIN, PANWARFIN**: anticoagulant

WIGRAINE/ergotamine, caffeine: antimigraine

WYAMYCIN/erythromycin: antibiotic

WYANOIDS HC/hydrocortisone, belladonna, ephedrine: antiinflammatory

WYCILLIN/penicillin G: antibiotic

WYGESIC/propoxyphene, acetaminophen: narcotic analgesic

WYMOX/amoxicillin: antibiotic

WYTENSIN/guanabenz: antihypertensive

XANAX/alprazolam: benzodiazepine tranquilizer

X-OTAG/orphenadrine: analgesic, antiinflammatory

X-PREP/senna: laxative

YODOXIN/iodoquinol: amebicide

YUTOPAR/ritodrine: decreases uterine activity

ZANTAC/ranitidine: antiulcer

ZARONTIN/ethosuximide: anticonvulsant (petit mal)

ZAROXOLYN/metolazone: antihypertensive, diuretic

ZESTORETIC/lisinopril, HCTZ: antihypertensive, diuretic

ZESTRIL/lisinopril: antihypertensive

zidovudine/**RETROVIR**: antiviral

ZOLOFT/setraline: antidepressant

ZOSTRIX/capsaicin: analgesic

ZOVIRAX/acyclovir: antiviral

ZYDONE/hydrocodone, APAP: narcotic analgesic

ZYLOPRIM/allopurinol: uricosuric

ZYNOL/sulfinpyrazone: uricosuric

3-6 Controlled Drug and Substance Categories

SCHEDULE I/CLASS I potential for abuse is so high as to be unacceptable, but may be used in research with appropriate limitations (e.g., heroin, LSD, peyote).

SCHEDULE II/CLASS II high potential for abuse with accepted medical usefulness; abuse can lead to severe psychological or physical dependence (e.g., amphetamines, narcotic analgesics, some barbiturates).

SCHEDULE III/CLASS III intermediate abuse potential (less than schedule II) with accepted medical usefulness; abuse can lead to moderate dependence. Prescriptions may be refilled up to five times in 6 months (e.g., anabolic steroids, codeine, or hydrocodone combined with nonnarcotic analgesics, some barbiturates, paregoric).

SCHEDULE IV/CLASS IV low abuse potential (less than schedule III) with accepted medical usefulness; limited dependence problem. Prescriptions may be refilled up to five times in 6 months (e.g., chloral hydrate, diazepam, phenobarbital).

SCHEDULE V low abuse potential with accepted medical usefulness; limited dependence problem. Prescriptions may be refilled at the discretion of the prescriber (e.g., cough syrups with codeine, Lomotil). Some Schedule V drugs may be sold by pharmacists to patients without a prescription.

(Modified from the United States Comprehensive Drug Abuse Prevention and Control Act of 1970; Section 202, Part 208 and revisions)

3-7 Drug Classification for Use During Pregnancy

CATEGORY A As demonstrated by studies that are adequate and well controlled, no risk to the fetus in the first trimester has been demonstrated. In addition, there does not appear to be risk in the second or third trimester.

CATEGORY B Studies in animals may or may not have shown risk. If risk has been shown in animals, no risk has been shown in human studies. If risk has not been seen in animals, there are insufficient data in pregnant women.

CATEGORY C Adverse effects have been demonstrated in animals, but there are insufficient data in pregnant women. In certain clinical situations, the benefits of using the medication could outweigh possible risks.

CATEGORY D Based on information collected in clinical investigations or postmarketing surveillance, human fetal risk has been demonstrated. In certain clinical situations, the benefits of using the medication could outweigh possible risks.

CATEGORY X Human fetal risk has been clearly documented in human studies, animal studies, clinical investigation, or postmarketing surveillance. Possible risks to the fetus outweigh potential benefits to pregnant women. Avoid use during pregnancy.

(U.S. Food and Drug Administration)

3-8 Cardiovascular Drug/Modality Intervention Recommendations

Class I A therapeutic option that is usually indicated, always acceptable, and considered useful and effective
(acceptable, definitely effective)

Class II A therapeutic option that is acceptable, is of uncertain efficacy, and may be controversial:

Class IIa A therapeutic option for which the weight of evidence is in favor of its usefulness and efficacy
(acceptable, probably effective)

Class IIb A therapeutic option that is not well established by evidence but may be helpful and is probably not harmful
(acceptable, possibly effective)

Class III A therapeutic option that is inappropriate, is without scientific supporting data, and may be harmful
(not indicated, may be harmful)

(Reproduced with permission, © *Textbook of Advanced Cardiac Life Support,* 1994, Copyright American Heart Association)

3-9 Antidysrhythmic Drug Classification

Group I   Sodium-channel blocking agents; causes slow depolarization and diminishes ectopics. Also known as **fast-channel blockers, membrane-stabilizing drugs.**

Type IA   Causes moderate slowing of conduction/depolarization; prolongs repolarization:
disopyramide
procainamide
quinidine

Type IB   Causes minimal slowing of conduction/depolarization; shortens repolarization:
lidocaine
phenytoin

Type IC   Causes profound slowing of conduction/depolarization; prolongs repolarization:
encainide
flecainide

Group II   Beta-adrenergic blocking agents:
acebutolol
esmolol
propranolol

Group III   Antiadrenergic agents causing increased contractility without suppressing automaticity; terminates re-entry dysrhythmias:
amiodarone
bretylium

Group IV   Calcium-channel blocking agents; decreases automaticity and myocardial muscle contraction. Also known as **slow-channel blocking agents:**
diltiazem
verapamil

Miscellaneous   Antidysrhythmics:
adenosine
digitalis
magnesium sulfate

Modified from Mosby-Year Book, Inc., *Emergency Medicine*, Rosen, et al.; Dysrhythmias, Yealy/Stapcynski, Vol. II, 3rd ed., p. 1207, St. Louis, 1992

3-10 Airway, Laryngoscope, Suction Catheter, and Tracheal Tube Sizing Guidelines

Age and Weight	Airway Oral / Nasal	Endotracheal Tube (inside diameter, mm)	Laryngoscope Blade	Suction Catheter (Fr)
Premature (1-5 lbs)	00 / 12	2.5-3.0 uncuffed	Miller 0	5-6
Term infant (>5-9 lbs)	0 / 12	3.0-3.5 uncuffed	Miller 0-1	6-8
Six months (>15-20 lbs)	1 / 14	3.5-4.0 uncuffed	Miller 1	8
One year (>20-25 lbs)	1 / 14	4.0-4.5 uncuffed	Miller 1-2	8
Two years (>25-32 lbs)	2 / 16	4.5-5.0 uncuffed	Miller 2	8
Four years (>32-41 lbs)	2 / 18	5.0-5.5 uncuffed	Miller 2	10
Six years (>41-51 lbs)	2 / 20	5.5 uncuffed	Miller 2	10
Eight years (>51-60 lbs)	2 / 22	6.0 either*	Miller 2 Macintosh 2	10
Ten years (>60-75 lbs)	3 / 24	6.5 either*	Miller 2 Macintosh 2	12
Twelve years (>75-85 lbs)	3 / 26	7.0 either*	Miller 2-3 Macintosh 3	12
Sixteen years (>85 lbs)	3 / 28	7.0-8.0 cuffed	Miller 3 Macintosh 3	12
Adult (>100 lbs)	4 / 30	7.5 cuffed	Miller 3 Macintosh 3	14-16
Adult (>150 lbs)	4 / 32	8.0 cuffed	Miller 3-4 Macintosh 3-4	16-18

*Uncuffed or cuffed

3-11 **Burn Calculation: Rule of Nines*—Adult and Child**

Adult

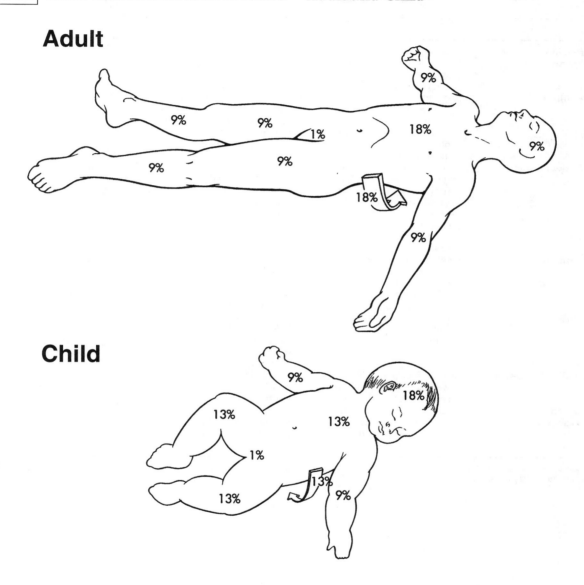

9%

9%   9%

1%

18%

9%

9%   9%

18%

9%

Child

9%

18%

13%

13%

1%

13%

13%   9%

*From Mosby-Year Book, Inc., *Wilderness Medicine: Management of Wilderness and Environmental Emergencies,* Auerbach; Emergency Care of the Burned Patient, Mann/Heimbach, 3rd ed., p. 247, St. Louis, 1995.

3-12 | Active Search Tactics Summary

Criterion	Type I	Type II	Type III
Objective	Speed Quickly search high-probability areas and gain information on search area	Efficiency Rapid search of large areas	Thoroughness Search with absolute highest probability of detection
Definition	Fast initial response of well trained, self-sufficient, mobile searchers, who check areas most likely to produce clues or the subject the soonest	Relatively fast, systematic search of high-probability segments of the search area that produce high results per searcher hour of effort	Slow, highly systematic search using the most thorough techniques to provide the highest probability of detection
Considerations	Works best with responsive subject; offers immediate show of effort; helps define search area; clue consciousness is critical; planning is crucial for effective use; often determines where not to search	Often employed after hasty searches, especially if clues were found; best suited to responsive subjects; often effective at finding clues; between-searcher spacing depends on terrain and visibility	Marking search segment is very important; should be used only as a last resort; very destructive of clues; used when other methods of searching are unsuccessful
Techniques	Investigation (personal physical effort); check last known position for clues; follow known route; run trails and ridges; check area perimeter, confine area; check hazards and attractions	Open grid line search with wide between-searcher spacing; compass bearings or specific guides are often used to control search; often applied in a defined area to follow up a discovered clue; no overlap in area coverage; critical separation; sound sweeps	Closed grid or sweep search with small between-searcher spacing; searched areas often overlap adjacent teams for better coverage
Usual team makeup	Two or three very mobile, well-trained self-sufficient searchers	May include three to seven skilled searchers, but usually just three	Four to seven searchers, including both trained and untrained personnel
Most effective resource	Investigators; trained hasty teams; human trackers; dogs; aircraft; any mobile trained resource	Clue-conscious search teams; human trackers; dogs; aircraft; trained grid search teams	Trained grid search teams

Modified from *Wilderness Medicine: Management of Wilderness and Environmental Emergencies,* 3rd edition, Auerbach: Search and Rescue, Cooper, Lavalla, Stoffel; Mosby, St. Louis, MO, 1995.

3-13 U.S. Navy Standard Air Decompression Table

DEPTH (FEET)	BOTTOM TIME (MIN)	TIME TO FIRST STOP (MIN:SEC)	DECOMPRESSION STOPS 50'	40'	30'	20'	10'	TOTAL ASCENT (MIN:SEC)	REPET-ITIVE GROUP
40	200	—					0	1:20	*
	210	1:00					2	3:20	N
	230	1:00					7	8:20	N
	250	1:00					11	12:20	O
	270	1:00					15	16:20	O
	300	1:00					19	20:20	Z
50	100	—					0	1:40	*
	110	1:20					3	4:40	L
	120	1:20					5	6:40	M
	140	1:20					10	11:40	M
	160	1:20					21	22:40	N
	180	1:20					29	30:40	O
	200	1:20					35	36:40	O
	220	1:20					40	41:40	Z
	240	1:20					47	48:40	Z
60	60	—					0	2:00	*
	70	1:40					2	4:00	K
	80	1:40					7	9:00	L
	100	1:40					14	16:00	M
	120	1:40					26	28:00	N
	140	1:40					39	41:00	O
	160	1:40					48	50:00	Z
	180	1:40					56	58:00	Z
	200	1:20				1	69	72:00	Z
70	50	—					0	2:20	*
	60	2:00					8	10:20	K
	70	2:00					14	16:20	L
	80	2:00					18	20:20	M
	90	2:00					23	25:20	N
	100	2:00					33	35:20	N
	110	1:40				2	41	45:20	O
	120	1:40				4	47	53:20	O
	130	1:40				6	52	60:20	O
	140	1:40				8	56	66:20	Z
	150	1:40				9	61	72:20	Z
	160	1:40				13	72	87:20	Z
	170	1:40				19	79	100:20	Z
80	40	—					0	2:40	*
	50	2:20					10	12:40	K
	60	2:20					17	19:40	L
	70	2:20					23	25:40	M
	80	2:00				2	31	35:40	N
	90	2:00				7	39	48:40	N
	100	2:00				11	46	59:40	O
	110	2:00				13	53	68:40	O
	120	2:00				17	56	75:40	Z
	130	2:00				19	63	84:40	Z
	140	2:00				26	69	97:40	Z
	150	2:00				32	77	111:40	Z
90	30	—					0	3:00	*
	40	2:40					7	10:00	J
	50	2:40					18	21:00	L
	60	2:40					25	28:00	M
	70	2:20				7	30	40:00	N
	80	2:20				13	40	56:00	N
	90	2:20				18	48	69:00	O
	100	2:20				21	54	78:00	Z
	110	2:20				24	61	88:00	Z
	120	2:20				32	68	103:00	Z
	130	2:00			5	36	74	118:00	Z

DEPTH (FEET)	BOTTOM TIME (MIN)	TIME TO FIRST STOP (MIN:SEC)	DECOMPRESSION STOPS 50'	40'	30'	20'	10'	TOTAL ASCENT (MIN:SEC)	REPET-ITIVE GROUP
100	25	—					0	3:20	*
	30	3:00					3	6:20	I
	40	3:00					15	18:20	K
	50	2:40				2	24	29:20	L
	60	2:40				9	28	40:20	N
	70	2:40				17	39	59:20	O
	80	2:40				23	48	74:20	O
	90	2:20			3	23	57	86:20	Z
	100	2:20			7	23	66	99:20	Z
	110	2:20			10	34	72	119:20	Z
	120	2:20			12	41	78	134:20	Z
110	20	—					0	3:40	*
	25	3:20					3	6:40	H
	30	3:20					7	10:40	J
	40	3:00				2	21	26:40	L
	50	3:00				8	26	37:40	M
	60	3:00				18	36	57:40	N
	70	2:40			1	23	48	75:40	O
	80	2:40			7	23	57	90:40	Z
	90	2:40			12	30	64	109:40	Z
	100	2:40			15	37	72	127:40	Z
120	15	—					0	4:00	*
	20	3:40					2	6:00	H
	25	3:40					6	10:00	I
	30	3:40					14	18:00	J
	40	3:20				5	25	34:00	L
	50	3:20				15	31	50:00	N
	60	3:00			2	22	45	73:00	O
	70	3:00			9	23	55	91:00	O
	80	3:00			15	27	63	109:00	Z
	90	3:00			19	37	74	134:00	Z
	100	3:00			23	45	80	152:00	Z
130	10	—					0	4:20	*
	15	4:00					1	5:20	F
	20	4:00					4	8:20	H
	25	4:00					10	14:20	J
	30	3:40				3	18	25:20	M
	40	3:40				10	25	39:20	N
	50	3:20			3	21	37	65:20	O
	60	3:20			9	23	52	88:20	Z
	70	3:20			16	24	61	105:20	Z
	80	3:00		3	19	35	72	133:20	Z
	90	3:00		8	19	45	80	156:20	Z
140	10	—					0	4:40	*
	15	4:20					2	6:40	G
	20	4:20					6	10:40	I
	25	4:00				2	14	20:40	J
	30	4:00				5	21	30:40	K
	40	3:40			2	16	26	48:40	N
	50	3:40			6	24	44	78:40	O
	60	3:40			16	23	56	99:40	Z
	70	3:20		4	19	32	68	127:40	Z
	80	3:20		10	23	41	79	157:40	Z

DEPTH (FEET)	BOTTOM TIME (MIN)	TIME TO FIRST STOP (MIN:SEC)	DECOMPRESSION STOPS 50'	40'	30'	20'	10'	TOTAL ASCENT (MIN:SEC)	REPET-ITIVE GROUP
150	5	—					0	5:00	C
	10	4:40					1	6:00	E
	15	4:40					3	8:00	G
	20	4:20				2	7	14:00	H
	25	4:20				4	17	26:00	K
	30	4:20				8	24	37:00	L
	40	4:00			5	19	33	62:00	N
	50	4:00			12	23	51	91:00	O
	60	3:40		3	19	26	62	115:00	Z
	70	3:40		11	19	39	75	149:00	Z
	80	3:20	1	17	19	50	84	176:00	Z
160	5	—					0	5:20	D
	10	5:00					1	6:20	F
	15	4:40				1	4	10:20	H
	20	4:40				3	11	19:20	J
	25	4:40				7	20	32:20	K
	30	4:20			2	11	25	43:20	M
	40	4:20			7	23	39	74:20	N
	50	4:00		2	16	23	55	101:20	Z
	60	4:00		9	19	33	69	135:20	Z
170	5	—					0	5:40	D
	10	5:20					2	7:40	F
	15	5:00				2	5	12:40	H
	20	5:00				4	15	24:40	J
	25	4:40			2	7	23	37:40	L
	30	4:40			4	13	26	48:40	M
	40	4:20		1	10	23	45	84:40	O
	50	4:20		5	18	23	61	112:40	Z
	60	4:00	2	15	22	37	74	155:40	Z
180	5	—					0	6:00	D
	10	5:40					3	9:00	F
	15	5:20				3	6	15:00	I
	20	5:00			1	5	17	29:00	K
	25	5:00			3	10	24	43:00	L
	30	5:00			6	17	27	56:00	N
	40	4:40		3	14	23	50	96:00	O
	50	4:20	2	9	19	30	65	131:00	Z
	60	4:20	5	16	19	44	81	171:00	Z
190	5	—					0	6:20	D
	10	5:40				1	3	10:20	G
	15	5:40				4	7	17:20	I
	20	5:20			2	6	20	34:20	K
	25	5:20			5	11	25	47:20	M
	30	5:00		1	8	19	32	66:20	N
	40	5:00		8	14	23	55	106.20	O

The time of decompression stops is in minutes. See next page for repetitive groups after no-decompression dives.

Instructions for use:

Enter table at the exact or next greater depth than the maximum depth attained during dive. Select the bottom time that is equal to or greater than the bottom time of the dive. The diver should maintain each decompression depth at chest level for the number of minutes listed. Rate of ascent **between** decompression stops is not critical for stops at 50 feet or less. Begin timing each stop on arrival at decompression depth. Resume ascent on completion of specified time.

From Naval Sea Systems Command, *U.S. Navy Diving Manual* 0994-LP-001-9111, Vol. 1, Revision 3/Change 1, July 1996.

No-Decompression Limits and Repetitive Group Designation Table

Table 3: Residual nitrogen times (minutes)

RESIDUAL NITROGEN TIMES BELOW (MINUTES) FOR REPETITIVE DIVE DEPTH ABOVE (FT)

	40'	50'	60'	70'	80'	90'	100'	110'	120'	130'	140'	150'	160'	170'	180'	190'
A	7	6	5	4	4	3	3	3	3	3	2	2	2	2	2	2
B	17	13	11	9	8	7	7	6	6	6	5	5	4	4	4	4
C	25	21	17	15	13	11	10	10	9	8	7	7	6	6	6	6
D	37	29	24	20	18	16	14	13	12	11	10	9	9	8	8	8
E	49	38	30	26	23	20	18	16	15	13	12	12	11	10	10	10
F	61	47	36	31	28	24	22	20	18	16	15	14	13	12	11	11
G	73	56	44	37	32	29	26	24	21	19	18	17	16	14	13	13
H	87	66	52	43	38	33	30	27	25	22	20	19	18	16	15	15
I	101	76	61	50	43	38	34	31	28	25	23	22	20	18	17	17
J	116	87	70	57	48	43	38	34	32	28	26	24	23	20	19	19
K	138	99	79	64	54	47	43	38	35	31	29	28	26	22	21	21
L	161	111	88	72	61	53	48	42	39	35	32	30	28	24	24	24
M	187	124	97	80	68	58	52	47	43	38	35	32	31	26	26	26
N	213	142	107	87	73	64	57	51	46	40	38	35	33	29	28	28
O	241	160	117	96	80	70	62	55	50	44	40	38	36	31	30	30
Z	257	169	122	100	84	73	64	57	52	46	42	40	37	32	31	31

REPETITIVE GROUP: A B C D E F G H I J K L M N O Z

Dives following surface intervals of more than 12 hours are not repetitive dives. Use the actual bottom times in the standard air decompression table (preceding page) to compute decompression for these dives.

Instructions For Use

These tables are used to calculate repetitive dive(s) following dives involving exposures up to and including no-decompression limits.

1 Enter Table 1 at the exact or next greater depth than that to which exposed. Select the exposure time that is exact or next greater than actual exposure time. Repetitive group designation is indicated by the letter at the head of the vertical column where the exposure time is listed.

2 Continue upward vertically along the lines joining Table 1 to Table 2. Enter Table 2 vertically and select the elapsed surface interval. The new repetitive group designation for the surface interval selected is to the right of the horizontal row where elapsed surface interval time is listed.

3 Enter Table 3 on the horizontal row to the right of the new repetitive group designation. Select the appropriate depth that will next be dived from the horizontal column at the top of the table. The intersection of that depth with the row of the new repetitive group designator is the appropriate residual nitrogen time. This time must be added to the anticipated bottom time of the following dive to determine safe exposure to that depth.

From Naval Sea Systems Command, *U.S. Navy Diving Manual* 0994-LP-001-9111, Vol. 1, Revision 3/Change 1, July 1996.

Table 2: Surface interval credit table (times in hr:min)

Triangular matrix of surface interval times joining repetitive group designations (A–Z). Each cell lists a time range in hr:min (e.g., 0:10–2:10 for group A, 2:11–10:06, etc.).

Table 1: "No-decompression" limits and repetitive group designation table for "no-decompression" air dives

BOTTOM TIME FOR "NO-D" DIVES (MINUTES)

DEPTH (FEET)	NO DECOMPRESSION LIMITS	A	B	C	D	E	F	G	H	I	J	K	L	M	N	O
10	–	60	120	210	300											
15	–	35	70	110	160	225	350									
20	–	25	50	75	100	135	180	240	325							
25	–	20	35	55	75	100	125	160	195	245	315					
30	–	15	30	45	60	75	95	120	145	170	205	250	310			
35	310	5	15	25	40	50	60	80	100	120	140	160	190	220	270	310
40	200	–	5	15	25	30	40	50	70	80	100	110	130	150	170	200
50	100	–	–	10	15	25	30	40	50	60	70	80	90	100		
60	60	–	–	10	15	20	25	30	40	50	55	60				
70	50	–	–	5	10	15	20	30	35	40	45	50				
80	40	–	–	5	10	15	20	25	30	35	40					
90	30	–	–	5	10	12	15	20	25	30						
100	25	–	–	5	7	10	15	20	22	25						
110	20	–	–	5	10	13	15	20								
120	15	–	–	5	10	12	15									
130	10	–	–	5	8	10										
140	10	–	–	5	7	10										
150	5	–	–	5												
160	5	–	–	5												
170	5	–	–	5												
180	5	–	–	5												
190	5	–	–													

Table 1: "No-decompression" limits and repetitive group designation table for "no-decompression" air dives

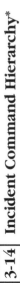

3-14 **Incident Command Hierarchy***

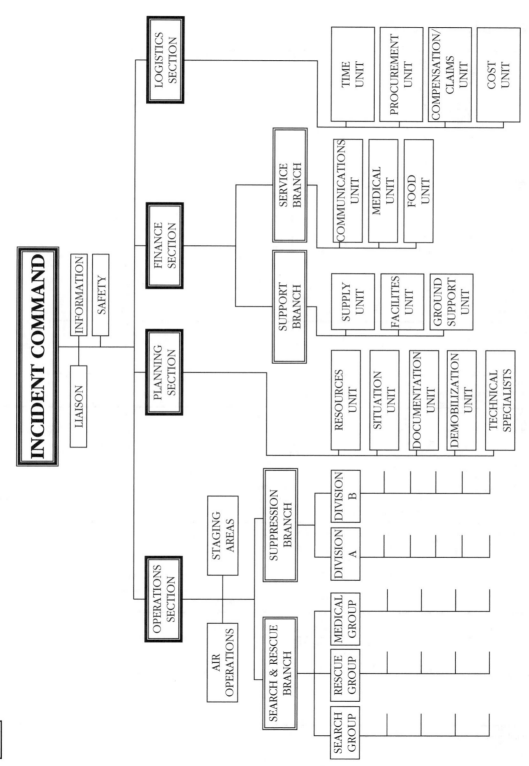

*Modified from National Interagency Incident Management System, Field Operations Guide-ICS 420-1, p. 1-2, 1982.

3-15   Compressed Gas Cylinders

Cylinder	A	AA	B	BB	D	DD	E	M	H
Diameter (inches)	3	2¾	3¼	2½	4¼	3¾	4¼	7	9
Height (inches)	10	11	18	19	20	23	26	47	55
Weight (pounds)	2½	3	5½	4	10½	8½	15	66	100

Contents	*Color*	*Outlet Connection/ Pin Index Number*
Carbon Dioxide	Gray	CGA-940
Compressed air	Yellow	CGA-400
Cyclopropane	Orange	CGA-920
Helium	Brown	CGA-930
Helium/Oxygen	Brown/Green	CGA-890
Oxygen	Green	CGA-870
Ethylene or Hydrogen	Red	CGA-400
Nitrous Oxide	Blue	CGA-910
Nitrogen	Black	CGA-580

(Color may cover the neck of the container, the entire container, or be indicated by a label/tag.)

Calculating Duration of Cylinder Flow

$$\frac{(\text{Gauge pressure in psi} - \text{Safe residual pressure}) \times \text{Cylinder factor}}{\text{Liter flow per minute}} = \text{Duration of flow (minutes)}$$

Example: For a D cylinder with gauge pressure of 1,800 psi and liter flow at 10 liters per minute:

$$\frac{(1,800 - 200) \times 0.16}{10} = \frac{256}{10} = 25.6 \text{ minutes of flow}$$

The safe residual pressure for all cylinder sizes is 200 psi. Common cylinder factors:
D - 0.16   M - 1.56
E - 0.28   H - 3.14

3-16 | Bite Patterns of Snakes

Nonpoisonous	Poisonous	Poisonous	Poisonous

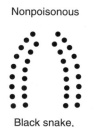 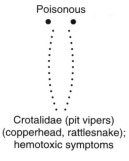 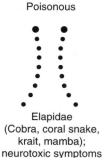 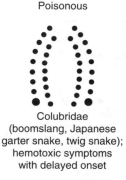

Black snake, garter snake

Crotalidae (pit vipers) (copperhead, rattlesnake); hemotoxic symptoms

Elapidae (Cobra, coral snake, krait, mamba); neurotoxic symptoms

Colubridae (boomslang, Japanese garter snake, twig snake); hemotoxic symptoms with delayed onset

Grades of Snake Envenomation*

Grade 0 Minimal pain; less than one inch of surrounding edema and/or erythema and no systemic symptoms in the first 12 hours (**no or minimal envenomation**)

Grade I Moderate pain or throbbing localized to fang wound, surrounded by 1 to 5 inches of edema and/or erythema with no systemic symptoms in the first 12 hours (**minimal envenomation**)

Grade II Widely distributed pain of increased severity; edema spreading toward trunk, ecchymosis and/or petechiae are limited to area of edema; nausea, vomiting, and/or giddiness usually present (**moderate envenomation**)

Grade III Rapidly progressive envenomation; hypoperfusion may develop within a few minutes of bite with tachycardia, pale/cool/moist skin and subnormal temperature; edema spreads up extremity and may involve part of the trunk within 12 hours; ecchymosis/petechiae may be generalized (**severe envenomation**)

Grade IV Sudden pain; rapidly progressive swelling that can reach/involve the trunk within a few hours; systemic symptoms, which begin soon after the bite, include nausea or vomiting, numbness or tingling around lips and face, vertigo, and weakness; ecchymosis, bleb forma-

tion, and necrosis may occur; other possible symptoms include coma, incontinence, muscle fasciculations, pale/cool/wet skin, seizures and tachycardia (**very severe envenomation**)

*Modified from Mosby-Year Book Inc., *Emergency Medicine,* Rosen et al; Venomous Animal Injuries, Otten, Edward J., Vol. I, 3rd ed., p. 881-882, St. Louis, 1992.

3-17 Wind Estimation Using the Beaufort Wind Scale

Observation on Land	Wind Category	MPH	Beaufort Number	Knots	Wind Category	Observation at Sea
Smoke rises vertically	calm	0-1	**0**	0-1	calm	Mirror smooth sea
Smoke drifts slowly	light air	1-3	**1**	1-3	light air	Small wavelets; no foam crests
Wind felt on face; leaves rustle; flags move slightly	slight breeze	4-7	**2**	4-6	slight breeze	Small wavelets; crests glassy
Leaves and twigs in motion; flags flap	gentle breeze	8-12	**3**	7-10	gentle breeze	Large wavelets (2 ft); breaking crests; scattered whitecaps
Small branches move; dust raised	moderate breeze	13-18	**4**	11-16	moderate breeze	Small waves (4 ft); numerous whitecaps
Small trees sway	fresh breeze	19-24	**5**	17-21	fresh breeze	Moderate waves (6 ft); many whitecaps; some spray
Large branches sway; whistling of small power lines; flags straight	strong breeze	25-31	**6**	22-27	strong breeze	Large waves (10 ft); extensive whitecaps; increased spray
Whole trees moving; difficulty walking;	near gale	32-38	**7**	28-33	near gale	Sea heaps up (14 ft) ; foam blown in streaks
Twigs break off	gale	39-46	**8**	34-40	gale	Moderately high waves (18 ft) ; foam blows in well-marked streaks
Branches break; possible minor building damage	strong gale	47-54	**9**	41-47	strong gale	High waves (23 ft) ; sea begins to roll; dense streaks of foam
Trees snapped and blown down; serious damage	whole gale	55-63	**10**	48-55	whole gale	Very high waves (29 ft) with overhanging crests; heavy rolling
Widespread damage	storm	64-75	**11**	56-65	storm	Exceptionally high waves (37 ft); sea covered with white foam
Extreme damage	hurricane	>75	**12**	>65	hurricane	Very deep troughs (45 ft); sea completely white; driving spray

3-18 | **Windchill Factors**

Windchill and state of comfort under varying conditions of temperature and wind velocity. The numbers along the left margin of the diagonal center block refer to windchill factor (the rate of cooling in kilogram-calories per square meter per hour of an unclad, inactive body exposed to specific temperatures and wind velocities). (Editor's note: Place a straightedge across the chart so that it connects the appropriate temperature to the appropriate wind velocity. The windchill factor (and danger) is read at the point that the straightedge crosses the center block. This procedure is most accurate at colder temperatures.) Windchill factors above 1400 are most hazardous.

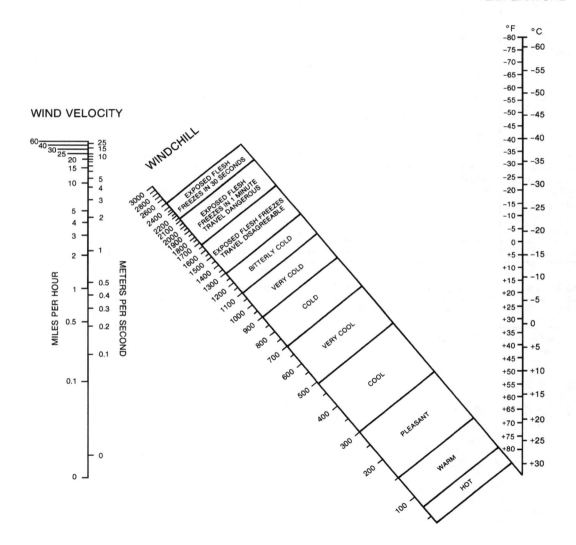

From Mosby-Year Book, Inc., *Wilderness Medicine: Management of Wilderness and Environmental Emergencies,* Auerbach; Wilderness Survival, Bowman, Warren D., 3rd ed., p. 367, St. Louis, 1995.

3-19 Windchill Index

Cooling power of wind on exposed flesh expressed as an equivalent temperature (under calm conditions)

Estimated wind speed (in mph)	Actual Thermometer Reading (°F)											
	50	40	30	20	10	0	−10	−20	−30	−40	−50	−60
	EQUIVALENT CHILL TEMPERATURE (°F)											
calm	50	40	30	20	10	0	−10	−20	−30	−40	−50	−60
5	48	37	27	16	6	−5	−15	−26	−36	−47	−57	−68
10	40	28	16	4	−9	−24	−33	−46	−58	−70	−83	−95
15	36	22	9	−5	−18	−32	−45	−58	−72	−85	−99	−112
20	32	18	4	−10	−25	−39	−53	−67	−82	−96	−110	−124
25	30	16	0	−15	−29	−44	−59	−74	−88	−104	−118	−133
30	28	13	−2	−18	−33	−48	−63	−79	−94	−109	−125	−140
35	27	11	−4	−21	−35	−51	−67	−82	−98	−113	−129	−145
40	26	10	−6	−21	−37	−53	−69	−85	−100	−116	−132	−148
Wind speeds greater than 40 mph have little additional effect.	Little danger in < $\frac{1}{2}$ hr with dry skin; maximum danger of a false sense of security.				Increasing danger; danger from freezing of exposed flesh within 1 minute.				GREAT DANGER Flesh may freeze within 30 seconds.			
	Trenchfoot and immersion foot may occur at any point on this chart.											

INSTRUCTIONS

Measure local temperature and wind speed if possible; if not, estimate. Enter table at closest 5°F interval along the top and with appropriate wind speed along left side. Intersection gives approximate equivalent chill temperature, that is, the temperature that would cause the same rate of cooling under calm conditions. Note that regardless of cooling rate, you do not cool below the actual air temperature unless wet.

From Sheehy: *Emergency Nursing*, ed. 3, St. Louis, 1992, Mosby.

3-20 | Modified Mercalli Earthquake Intensity Scale

I Not felt except by a very few under especially favorable circumstances.

II Felt only by a few persons at rest, especially on upper floors of buildings. Delicately suspended objects may swing.

III Felt quite noticeably indoors, especially on upper floors of buildings, but many people do not recognize it as an earthquake. Standing motorcars may rock slightly. Vibration like passing of truck. Duration estimated.

IV During the day felt indoors by many. Outdoors by few. At night some awakened. Dishes, windows, doors disturbed; walls make creaking sound. Sensation like heavy truck striking building. Standing motorcars rocked noticeably.

V Felt by nearly everyone; many awakened. Some dishes, windows, etc., broken. A few instances of cracked plaster. Unstable objects overturned. Disturbances of trees, poles, and other tall objects sometimes noticed. Pendulum clocks may stop.

VI Felt by all; many frightened and run outdoors. Some heavy furniture moved; a few instances of fallen plaster or damaged chimneys. Damage slight.

VII Everybody runs outdoors. Damage negligible in buildings of good design and construction, slight to moderate in well-built ordinary structures, considerable in poorly built or badly designed structures. Some chimneys broken. Noticed by persons driving motorcars.

VIII Damage slight in specially designed structures, considerable in ordinary substantial buildings with partial collapse, great in poorly built structures. Panel walls thrown out of frame structures. Fall of chimneys, factory stacks, columns, monuments, and walls. Heavy furniture overturned. Sand and mud ejected in small amounts. Changes in well water. Persons driving motorcars disturbed.

IX Damage considerable in specially designed structures. Well-designed structures thrown out of plumb, greatly in substantial buildings with partial collapse. Buildings shifted off foundations. Ground cracked conspicuously. Underground pipes broken.

X Some well-built wooden structures destroyed. Most masonry and frame structures with foundations destroyed; ground badly cracked. Rails bent. Landslides considerable from river banks and steep slopes. Shifted sand and mud. Water splashed (slopped) over banks.

XI Few, if any, (masonry) structures remain standing. Bridges destroyed. Broad fissures in ground. Underground pipelines completely out of service. Earth slumps and land slips in soft ground. Rails bent greatly.

XII Damage total. Practically all works of construction are damaged greatly or destroyed. Waves seen on ground surface. Lines of sight and level are distorted. Objects are thrown upward into the air.

From Mosby-Year Book, Inc., *Wilderness Medicine: Management of Wilderness and Environmental Emergencies,* Auerbach; Natural and Human-Made Hazards, Reed, Sheila B., 3rd ed., p. 587, St. Louis, 1995.

3-21 | Saffir/Simpson Hurricane Scale

Scale No. 1   Winds of 74 to 95 miles per hour. Damage primarily to shrubbery, trees, foliage, and unanchored mobile homes. No real damage to other structures. Some damage to poorly constructed signs. And/or: storm surge 4 to 5 feet above normal. Low-lying coastal roads inundated, minor pier damage, some small craft in exposed anchorage torn from moorings.

Scale No. 2   Winds of 96 to 110 miles per hour. Considerable damage to shrubbery and tree foliage; some trees blown down. Major damage to exposed mobile homes. Extensive damage to poorly constructed signs. Some damage to roofing materials of buildings; some window and door damage. No major damage to buildings. And/or: storm surge 6 to 8 feet above normal. Coastal roads and low-lying escape routes inland cut by rising water 2 to 4 hours before arrival of hurricane center. Considerable damage to piers. Marinas flooded. Small craft in unprotected anchorages torn from moorings. Evacuation of some shoreline residences and low-lying island areas required.

Scale No. 3   Winds of 111 to 130 miles per hour. Foliage torn from trees; large trees blown down. Practically all poorly constructed signs blown down. Some damage to roofing materials of buildings; some window and door damage. Some structural damage to small buildings. Mobile homes destroyed. And/or: storm surge of 9 to 12 feet above normal. Serious flooding at coast and many smaller structures near coast destroyed; larger structures near coast damaged by battering waves and floating debris. Low-lying escape routes inland cut by rising water 3 to 5 hours before hurricane center arrives. Flat terrain 5 feet or less above sea

level flooded inland 8 miles or more. Evacuation of low-lying residences within several blocks of shoreline possibly required.

Scale No. 4   Winds of 131 to 155 miles per hour. Shrubs and trees blown down; all signs down. Extensive damage to roofing materials, windows, and doors. Complete failure of roofs on many small residences. Complete destruction of mobile homes. And/or: storm surge 13 to 18 feet above normal. Flat terrain 10 feet or less above sea level flooded inland as far as 6 miles. Major damage to lower floors of structures near shore due to flooding and battering by waves and floating debris. Low-lying escape routes inland cut by rising water 3 to 5 hours before hurricane center arrives. Major erosion of beaches. Massive evacuation of all residences within 500 yards of shore possibly required, and of single-story residences on low ground within 2 miles of shore.

Scale No. 5   Winds greater than 155 miles per hour. Shrubs and trees blown down; considerable damage to roofs of buildings; all signs down. Very severe and extensive damage to windows and doors. Complete failure of roofs on many residences and industrial buildings. Extensive shattering of glass in windows and doors. Some complete building failures. Small buildings overturned or blown away. Complete destruction of mobile homes. And/or: storm surge greater than 18 feet above normal. Major damage to lower floors of all structures less than 15 feet above sea level within 500 yards of shore. Low-lying escape routes inland cut by rising water 3 to 5 hours before hurricane center arrives. Massive evacuation of all residential areas on low ground within 5 to 10 miles of shore possibly required.

Source: National Oceanic and Atmospheric Administration, *Tropical Cyclones of the North Atlantic Ocean, 1871-1977*, National Climatic Center, Asheville, North Carolina, 1978, p. 25.

3-22 | U. S. State and Territory EMS Office Directory

ALABAMA
Department of Public Health
Emergency Medical Services Division
434 Monroe Street
Montgomery, AL 36130-3017
334-613-5383
Fax 334-240-3061

ALASKA
Department of Health and Social Services
Emergency Medical Services Section
P. O. Box 110616
Juneau, AK 99811-0616
907-465-3027
Fax 907-465-4101

AMERICAN SAMOA
American Samoa Government
Emergency Medical Services
LBJ Tropical Medical Center
Pago Pago, AS 96799

ARIZONA
Arizona Department of Health Services
Office of Emergency Medical Services
1651 East Morten, Suite 120
Phoenix, AZ 85020
602-255-1170
Fax 602-255-1134

ARKANSAS
Arkansas Department of Health
Division of Emergency Medical Services
4815 West Markham Street, Slot 38
Little Rock, AR 72205-3867
501-661-2262
Fax 501-280-4901

CALIFORNIA
California Emergency Medical Services Authority
1930 9th Street, Suite 100
Sacramento, CA 95814
916-322-4336
Fax 916-324-2875

COLORADO
Colorado Department of Health
Emergency Medical Services Division
4300 Cherry Creek Drive
South Denver, CO 80222
303-692-2980
Fax 303-782-0904

CONNECTICUT
Connecticut Department of Public Health and Addiction
Services
Office of Emergency Medical Services
150 Washington Street
Hartford, CT 06106
203-566-7336
Fax 203-566-7172

DELAWARE
Delaware Department of Health and Social Services
Office of Emergency Medical Services
P.O. Box 637
Dover, DE 19903
302-739-4710
Fax 302-739-6617

DISTRICT OF COLUMBIA
District of Columbia Department of Human Services
Office of Emergency Health and Medical Services
613 G Street NW, Room 620
Washington, DC 20001
202-727-1622
Fax 202-727-0379

FLORIDA
Florida Department of Health and Rehabilitative Services
Office of Emergency Medical Services
2002-D Old St. Augustine Road
Tallahassee, FL 32301-4881
904-487-1911
Fax 904-488-2512

GEORGIA
Georgia Division of Public Health
Office of Emergency Medical Services
47 Trinity Avenue, Suite 104
Atlanta, GA 30334
404-657-6700
Fax 404-657-4255

GUAM
Guam Department of Health and Social Services
Office of Emergency Medical Services
P.O. Box 2816
Agana, GU 96910
671-472-8507
Fax 671-734-5910

HAWAII
Hawaii Department of Health
Emergency Medical Services System Branch
3627 Kilauea Avenue, Room 102
Honolulu, HI 96816
808-733-9210
Fax 808-733-8332

IDAHO
Idaho Emergency Medical Service System
3092 Elder Street
Boise, ID 83720
208-334-4000
Fax 208-334-4015

ILLINOIS
Illinois Department of Public Health
Div. of Emergency Medical Services and Highway Safety
525 West Jefferson Street, 3rd Floor
Springfield, IL 62761
217-785-2080
Fax 217-785-0253

INDIANA
State Emergency Management Agency
302 West Washington Street, Room 208E
Indianapolis, IN 46204
317-232-3980
Fax 317-232-3895

IOWA
Iowa Department of Public Health
Bureau of Emergency Medical Services
Lucas State Office Building
Des Moines, IA 50319
515-281-3741
Fax 515-281-4958

KANSAS
Kansas Board of Emergency Medical Services
109 SW Sixth Street
Topeka, KS 66603
913-296-7296
Fax 913-296-6212

KENTUCKY
Kentucky Department for Health Services
Emergency Medical Services Branch
275 East Main Street
Frankfort, KY 40621
502-564-8963
Fax 502-564-6533

LOUISIANA
Louisiana Department of Health and Hospitals
Bureau of Emergency Medical Services
1201 Capital Access Road, 5th Floor
Baton Rouge, LA 70804
504-342-4881
Fax 504-342-4876

MAINE
Maine Emergency Medical Services
16 Edison Drive
Augusta, ME 04330
207-287-3953
Fax 207-287-6251

MARYLAND
Maryland Institute for Emergency Medical Services Systems
636 West Lombard Street
Baltimore, MD 21201
410-706-5074
Fax 410-706-4768

MASSACHUSETTS
Massachusetts Department of Public Health
Office of Emergency Medical Services
150 Tremont Street
Boston, MA 02111
617-727-8338
Fax 617-727-3172

MICHIGAN
Michigan Department of Public Health
Division of Emergency Medical Services
P.O. Box 30195
Lansing, MI 48909
517-335-9502
Fax 517-335-8582

MINNESOTA
Minnesota Department of Health
Emergency Medical Services Regulatory Board
310 University Park Plaza
2829 University SE
Minneapolis, MN 55414-3222
612-627-6000
Fax 612-627-5442

MISSISSIPPI
Mississippi State Department of Health
Division of Emergency Medical Services
2423 North State Street
Jackson, MS 39215
601-987-3880
Fax 601-987-3993

MISSOURI
Missouri Bureau of Emergency Medical Services
1738 East Elm
Jefferson City, MO 65102
314-751-6356
Fax 314-526-4102

MONTANA
Montana Department of Public Health and Human Services
Emergency Medical Services Bureau
1400 Broadway
Helena, MT 59620
406-444-3895
Fax 406-444-1814

NEBRASKA
Nebraska State Department of Health
Emergency Medical Services Program
301 Centennial Mall South, 3rd Floor
Lincoln, NE 68509
402-471-2158
Fax 402-471-6446

NEVADA
Nevada State Health Division
EMS and Trauma Systems
1550 East College Parkway, Suite 158
Carson City, NV 89710
702-687-3065
Fax 702-687-6588

NEW HAMPSHIRE
New Hampshire Division of Public Health Services
Bureau of Emergency Medical Services
6 Hazen Drive
Concord, NH 03301
603-271-4568
Fax 603-271-4567

NEW JERSEY
Division of New Jersey Health Department Emergency Medical Services
300 Whitehead Road, CN 367
Trenton, NJ 08625-0367
609-588-7800
Fax 609-588-7698

NEW MEXICO
New Mexico Department of Health
Primary Care and Emergency Medical Services Bureau
900 West Alameda
Santa Fe, NM 87502
505-827-1400
Fax 505-827-1410

NEW YORK
New York State Department of Health
Emergency Medical Services Bureau
Commerce Plaza, Room 1126
Albany, NY 12260
518-474-2219
Fax 518-486-6216

NORTH CAROLINA
North Carolina Office of Emergency Medical Services
P.O. Box 29530
Raleigh, NC 27626
919-733-2285
Fax 919-733-7021

NORTH DAKOTA
North Dakota Department of Health
Division of Emergency Health Services
600 East Boulevard Avenue
Bismarck, ND 58505
701-328-2388
Fax 701-328-4727

OHIO
Ohio Department of Public Safety
Emergency Medical Services Division
P.O. Box 7167
240 Parsons Avenue
Columbus, OH 43205-0167
800-233-0785
614-466-9447
Fax 614-466-0433

OKLAHOMA
Oklahoma State Department of Health
Emergency Medical Services Division
1000 NE 10th Street
Oklahoma City, OK 73117
405-271-4027
Fax 405-271-3442

OREGON
Oregon Health Division
Emergency Medical Services and Systems
800 NE Oregon Street #607
Portland, OR 97232
503-731-4011
Fax 503-731-4077

PENNSYLVANIA
Pennsylvania Department of Health
Division of Emergency Medical Services Systems
P.O. Box 90
Harrisburg, PA 17108
717-787-8740
Fax 717-772-0910

PUERTO RICO
Bureau of Emergency Medical Services
Fire Department
P.O. Box 13325
San Juan, PR 00908
809-766-1733
Fax 809-765-5085

RHODE ISLAND
Rhode Island Department of Health
Division of Emergency Medical Services
3 Capitol Hill, Room 404
Providence, RI 02908
401-277-2401
Fax 401-277-1250

SOUTH CAROLINA
South Carolina Department of Health and Environmental Control
Division of Emergency Medical Services
2600 Bull Street
Columbia, SC 29201
803-737-7204
Fax 803-737-7212

SOUTH DAKOTA
South Dakota Department of Health
Emergency Medical Services
445 East Capitol Avenue
Pierre, SD 57501
605-773-4928
Fax 605-773-5683

TENNESSEE
Division of Emergency Medical Services
Tennessee Department of Health
Cordell Hull Building, 1st Floor
426 5th Avenue North
Nashville, TN 37247-0701
615-741-2584
Fax 615-741-4217

TEXAS
Texas Department of Health
Emergency Medical Services Division
1100 West 49th Street
Austin, TX 78756
512-834-6740
Fax 512-834-6736

UTAH
Utah Department of Health
Bureau of Emergency Medical Services
P.O. Box 142852
288 North 1460 West
Salt Lake City, UT 84114-2852
801-538-6435
Fax 801-538-6808

VERMONT
 Vermont Department of Health
 Emergency Medical Services Division
 108 Cherry Street
 Burlington, VT 05402
 802-863-7310
 Fax 802-863-7577

VIRGINIA
 Virginia Department of Health
 Office of Emergency Medical Services
 1538 East Parham Road
 Richmond, VA 23228
 800-523-6019
 804-371-3500
 Fax 804-371-3543

VIRGIN ISLANDS
 Virgin Islands Department of Health
 Division of Emergency Medical Services
 St. Thomas Hospital
 48 Sugar Estate
 Charlotte Amalie, VI 00802
 809-776-8311 ext. 2008
 Fax 809-777-4001

WASHINGTON
 Washington Department of Health
 Office of Emergency Medical Services and Trauma Systems
 P.O. Box 47853
 Olympia, WA 98504-7853
 360-705-6745
 Fax 360-705-6706

WEST VIRGINIA
 West Virginia Department of Health and Human Resources
 Office of Emergency Medical Services
 1411 Virginia Street East
 Charleston, WV 25301
 304-558-3956
 Fax 304-558-1437

WISCONSIN
 Wisconsin Department of Health and Social Services
 Emergency Medical Services Section
 P.O. Box 309
 Madison, WI 53701-0309
 608-266-1568
 Fax 608-267-4853

WYOMING
 Wyoming State Division of Health
 Office of Emergency Medical Services
 Hathaway Building, Room 527
 Cheyenne, WY 82002
 307-777-7955
 Fax 307-777-5639

3-23   EMS/Rescue Directory

Aerospace Medical Association
 320 South Henry Street
 Alexandria, VA 22314-3579
 703-739-2240
 Fax 703-739-9652

American Ambulance Association
 3800 Auburn Boulevard, Suite C
 Sacramento, CA 95821-2102
 916-483-3827
 Fax 916-482-5473

American College of Emergency Physicians
 P.O. Box 619911
 Dallas, TX 75261-9911
 214-550-0911
 Fax 214-580-2816

American Society For Testing and Materials
 Committee F30 on EMS
 100 Barr Harbor Drive
 West Conshohocken, PA 19428
 610-832-9726
 Fax 610-832-9666

Association of Air Medical Services
 35 South Raymond Avenue, Suite 205
 Pasadena, CA 91105
 818-793-1232
 Fax 818-793-1039

Association of Public-Safety Communications Officials International, Inc.
 2040 South Ridgewood Avenue
 South Daytona, FL 32119
 800-949-2726
 904-322-2500
 Fax 904-322-2501

Center for International Emergency Medical Services
 Humboldtstrasse 12A D-65189
 Wiesbaden, Germany
 49-611-307891
 Fax 49-611-370593

Congressional Fire Services Institute
 900 Second Street NE, Suite 303
 Washington, DC 20002
 202-371-1277
 Fax 202-682-FIRE

Emergency Care Information Center
P.O. Box 2789
Carlsbad, CA 92018
619-431-9797
Fax 619-431-8135
Emergency Nurses Association
216 Higgins Road
Park Ridge, IL 60068
708-698-9400
Fax 708-698-9407
Federal Emergency Management Agency
Emergency Management Institute
16825 South Seton Avenue
Emmitsburg, MD 21727
800-238-3358
301-447-1286
Fax 301-447-1598
Federal Emergency Management Agency
National Emergency Training Center
16825 South Seton Avenue
Emmitsburg, MD 21727
301-447-1186
Fax 301-447-1052
Federal Emergency Management Agency
Planning and Liaison Division
Response and Recovery Directorate
500 C Street SW, Room 602
Washington, DC 20472
202-646-4554
Fax 202-646-2901
Federal Emergency Management Agency
United States Fire Administration
16825 South Seton Avenue
Emmitsburg, MD 21727
301-447-1581
Fax 301-447-1102
Fire and Emergency Manufacturers and Services Association
808 17th Street NW, Suite 200
Washington, DC 20006
800-50-FEMSA
202-223-9669
Fax 202-223-9569
Helicopter Association International
1635 Prince Street
Alexandria, VA 22314-2818
800-435-4976
703-683-4646
Fax 703-683-4745
International Association of Dive Rescue Specialists
P.O. Box 5259
San Clemente, CA 92674-5259
800-423-7791
714-369-1660
Fax 714-369-1690
International Association of Fire Chiefs
4025 Fair Ridge Drive, Suite 300
Fairfax, VA 22033-2868
703-273-0911
Fax 703-273-9363

International Rescue and Emergency Care Association
9640 Guilford Road
Columbia, MD 21046
800-221-3435
Fax 800-221-3435
International Society of Fire Service Instructors
30 Main Street
Ashland, MA 01721
508-881-5800
Fax 508-881-6829
Medical Device and Laboratory Product Problem-Reporting Program
12601 Twin Brook Parkway
Rockville, MD 20852
800-638-6725
Fax 301-816-8247
National Association for Search and Rescue
4500 Southgate Place, #100
Chantilly, VA 22021
703-222-6277
Fax 703-222-6283
National Association of EMS Physicians
230 McKee Place, Suite 500
Pittsburgh, PA 15213
800-228-3677
412-578-3222
Fax 412-578-3241
National Center for Health Statistics
Office of Analysis and Epidemiology Programs
Presidential Building
6525 Belcrest Road, Suite 1064
Hyattsville, MD 20782
301-436-8500
Fax 301-436-4258
National EMS Pilots Association
35 South Raymond Avenue, Suite 205
Pasadena, CA 91105
818-405-9851
Fax 818-793-1039
National Fire Protection Association
1 Batterymarch Park
Quincy, MA 02269-9101
800-344-3555
617-770-3000
Fax 617-770-0200
National Flight Nurses Association
216 Higgins Road
Park Ridge, IL 60068
847-698-1733
Fax 847-698-9407
National Flight Paramedics Association
7136 South Yale, Suite 300
Tulsa, OK 74136
800-381-NFPA
Fax 918-496-1123

National Health Information Center
P.O. Box 1133
Washington, DC 20013-1133
800-336-4797
301-565-4167

National Highway Traffic Safety Administration
400 Seventh Street SW, NTS-42
Washington, DC 20590
202-366-5440
Fax 202-366-7721

National Institute for Occupational Safety and Health
Technical Information Branch
4676 Columbia Parkway
Cincinnati, OH 45226
800-356-4674

National Library of Medicine
8600 Rockville Pike
Bethesda, MD 20209
301-496-6193

National Native American EMS Association
P.O. Box 186
Park Hill, OK 74451
918-458-5403

National Registry of Emergency Medical Technicians
6610 Busch Boulevard (P.O. Box 29233)
Columbus, OH 43229
614-888-4484
Fax 614-888-8920

National Safety Council
1121 Spring Lake Drive
Itasca, IL 60143
708-285-1121
Fax 708-285-1315

National Speleological Society
National Cave Rescue Commission
2813 Cave Avenue
Huntsville, AL 35810-4431
205-852-1300
Fax 205-851-9241

National Tactical Officers Association
P.O. Box 529
Doylestown, PA 18901
800-279-9127
215-230-7616
Fax 215-230-7565

Office of the Assistant Secretary of Defense—Health Affairs
Pentagon, Room 1C545
Washington, DC 20301-1200
703-697-8233
Fax 703-693-1000

Undersea and Hyperbaric Medical Society
9650 Rockville Pike
Bethesda, MD 20814
301-571-1818
Fax 301-571-1815

Uniformed Services University of the Health Sciences
Military and Emergency Medicine—Casualty Care Research Center
4301 Jones Bridge Road
Bethesda, MD 20814-4799
301-295-6263

United States Department of the Interior
National Park Service
1849 C Street NW
Washington, DC 20242
202-208-6843

United States Department of Labor
Occupational Safety and Health Administration
200 Constitution Avenue NW, Room N3647
Washington, DC 20210
202-219-8151
Fax 202-219-5986

United States Food and Drug Administration
5600 Fishers Lane
Rockville, MD 20854
301-443-3170 (information line)

United States Public Health Service
Division of Trauma and Emergency Medical Systems
5600 Fishers Lane, Room 7-16
Rockville, MD 20857
310-443-3401
Fax 301-594-5999

United States Public Health Service
Office of Emergency Preparedness/National Disaster Medical Services
5600 Fishers Lane, Room 4-81
Rockville, MD 20857
800-872-6367
301-443-1167
Fax 301-443-5146/800-872-5945

Veterans Health Administration
Emergency Medical Preparedness Office
Training and Development
101 West Ohio Street, Suite 1510
Indianapolis, IN 46204-1997
317-226-5033
Fax 317-226-5135

Wilderness Medical Society
P.O. Box 2463
Indianapolis, IN 46206
317-631-1745
Fax 317-259-8150

COMMUNICATION AND TERMINOLOGY

4-1 Medical Root Words

acro extremity
adeno gland
aer air
alveol hollow cavity
angi vessel
arter artery
arth joint
asthen weakness
bar pressure
bio life
bili bile
brachi arm
brady slow
bronch air passage
bucc cheek
capn smoke
carcin, onco cancer
cardi heart
carp wrist
cephal head
cerebr brain
cerv, trachel neck (usually the cervix)
cheil, chil lip
chem chemical
chir hand
chol bile, gallbladder
chondr cartilage
colo large intestine
corp body
cortico the cortex
cost rib
crani skull
crypt hidden
cusp point
cutan skin
cyan blue
cyst bladder
cysto bladder, cyst, sac
cyt cell
dactyl finger, toes
dendr branched
dent tooth
derm skin
diastol relaxation
dips thirst
edem swelling
ejacul to throw out
electr electrical
emesis vomiting
encephal brain
enter intestine
eryth red
esthe sensation

febr fever
fibr fibers
gastr stomach
gingiv gums
glomer a ball, wound up
gloss tongue
gluc, glyc carbohydrate, glucose, sugar, sweet
glutin glue
gyn female
hem, hemat blood
hepat liver
hist tissue
hydra water
hydro water
hyster uterus
iatr treatment
ileo ileum, small intestine
ili flank, ilium
kal potassium
kary nucleus
kerat cornea
lact milk
lapar abdomen
leuk white
lig bind, tie
lip fat
lith stone
lys break up
mal bad
melan black
mening membrane
meningo meninges
men, mens month
muta change
my, myo muscle
myc fungus
myel marrow
nas nose
nat birth
natr sodium
nephr kidney, nephron
neur nerve
noct, nyct night
ocul eye
odont teeth
oo, ov egg
ophthalm eye
orchid testis
oss bone
osteo bone
oto ear
oxy oxygen
path disease

ped children
phag eat
phleb vein
photo light
physio function
plex twist, woven
pneumo air, breath, gas
pneumon lung
pod foot
poie create, produce
presby old
proct anus, rectum
pseud false
psych mind, soul
pyel renal pelvis
pyloro pylorus
pyo purulent material, pus
pyr fever
radi ray
ren kidney
rhino nose
rigor stiffness
salping tube (usually uterine)
sarco muscle
scler hard
semen, semin seed, sperm
sept contamination
sin cavity, recess
somat body
son sound
spire, spiro breathe
spondyl spinal column
stalsis wave-like contraction
stas, stat standing, stopping
sterno sternum
syn together
systol contraction
tachy fast, rapid
tact touch
therm heat
thorac thorax
thromb clot
tox poison
troph grow, nourish
tympan drum
tubercul tubercle (tuberculosis)
ureter kidney to bladder
urethra bladder to outside the body
uro urinary
varic enlarged vessel
vas duct, vessel
vesic bladder, blister
viscer viscera

4-2 Medical Prefixes and Suffixes

PREFIXES

a, an, ay no, not, without
a, ab away from
ab deviating from normal
ac pertaining to
acu a needle
af, ap, at toward
ambi, amph, amphi both
an, ana again, backward, excessive, up
anis unequal
ante, anter before, forward
anti against
apo upon
auto self
bi two
brady slow
brachy short
cac, caco bad, poor
cat, cata, cath down, downward
circum around
co, com, con, cor together, with
contra against, counter
de down, from, lack of
dec, deca ten
deci tenth
dext right
di double, two
di, dia across, complete, through
dipl double
dys bad, disordered, difficult, improper, poor
e, ec out, outside
ect, ecto outer, outside, without
ectop displaced
ef away from
em, en in, into
end inner, inside
endo within
ep, epi after, over, upon
eso inward
eu good
ex from, out of
ex, exo, extra beyond, in addition to, outside of
hapl single
hect one hundred
hem, hemat blood
hemi half
hen one
hept seven
heter, hetero different
hex six
holo all

homo, homeo equal, same
hyper extreme, more than normal
hypo below, less than normal, under
il, im, in, ir not
infra below, beneath, inferior
inter between
intra, intro within
iso equal
juxta close, near
kil, kilo one thousand
macro large
mal bad, poor
mega, megal great, large
mes, meso middle
meta after, beyond, change
micro small
mono one, single
multi many, much
neo new
non not
nulli none
ob, oc against, toward
oct eight
oligo few, scanty
ortho correct, straight, normal
par, para beside, near
pent five
per through
peri around, surrounding
poly excessive, many, much
post after, behind in place/time
pre, pro before, first, in front of
quad, quadr four
quinque five
re again, back
retro backward, behind
semi half, partly
sub, suf, sup below, under
supa, super, supra above, excessive, over, upper
sym, syn joined together
tachy fast
tetra four
trans across, over, through
tri three
ultra beyond
uni one, single

SUFFIXES

ac, al, ar, ary, ic, ior pertaining to
agogue introducing, leading
agra excessive pain
algesia oversensitivity to pain
algia pain

aps, apt fasten, fit
arche beginning
ase enzyme
asthenia weakness
blast embryonic, immature, make
capnia carbon dioxide
cele cyst, herniation, tumor
centesis piercing, puncture
chalasis relaxation
cidal killing
cide destruction, kill
cipient receiver
cise cut
clasis, clast break
clysis irrigation, washing
coccus berry-shaped
crescent grow
crine release, secrete, separate
crit separate
cusis hearing
cyesis pregnancy
cyte cell
cytosis condition of cells
desis binding together
drome run
dynia painful condition
dys bad, difficult, painful
eal pertaining to
ectasia dilation
ectomy surgical removal
emesis vomiting
emia condition of the blood
er one who
ferent, ferous bearing
form shape
flux flow
fugal, fuge driving away
fusion pour
gen creates, produced by
genesis creation
globin, globulin protein
grade go
gram a recording
graph draw, write
graphy recording procedure
hydrate containing water
ia, sia condition, process
iasis abnormal condition
in protein
ion, ism process
ism condition of
ist specialist
itis inflammation, irritation
ium structure, tissue
lemma covering, rind, sheath

lepsy seizure
lith rock, stone
logist one who studies
logy study
lunar moon
lysis destruction, killing
lytic destroy, reduce
malacia softening
mania obsessive preoccupation
megaly enlargement
meter measure
metric, metry length, measurement
mimetic copy, mimic
oid in the shape of, resembling
ole little, small
oma tumor
opia vision
opsy view
or one who
oscopy viewing
ose carbohydrate
osis abnormal condition or process
osmia smell
ous pertaining to
ostomy creation of a new opening
otomy cut
para births (viable)
paresis slight paralysis, weakness
partum birth, labor
pathy disease process
pellent drive
penia deficiency

pepsia digestion
pexy surgical fixation
phagia swallowing
pheresis removal
philia affinity for
phobia abnormal fear
phonia sound, voice
phoresis transmission
phoria feeling (mental state)
phragm dividing, partition
phylaxis prevention
physis grow, growth
phyte plant
plasia growth
plasm substance
plasty repair, shape
plegia paralysis
pnea breathing, respiration
poesis formation
porosis passage
prandial meal
praxia action
ptosis prolapse
ptysis spitting
rhage, rhagia breaking out, discharge, flow
rhaphy suture
rhea profuse flow (of fluid, not usually blood)
rrhexis rupture
salpinx fallopian tube
schisis split

sclerosis hardening
scope device for examining visually
scopy visual examination
sect cut
sis condition
some body
somnia sleep
spasm contraction of muscles
sphyxia pulse
stalsis contraction
stasis maintenance of a constant level
stenosis tightening, stricture
sthenia strength
stomy new opening
tensin, tension, tonic pressure
therapy treatment
thorax chest
thymia mind
tic pertaining to
tocia, tocin birth, labor
tome cutting instrument
tomy cutting process
tresia opening
tripsy crushing
trophia turn
trophy development, nourishment
tropin develop, nourish, stimulate
ule little, small
um structure, tissue
uresis urinary excretion
uria condition of urine
version turn

4-3 | Medical and Prehospital Abbreviations

⌒ semisitting

◦ sitting

◦ standing

◦⌐ supine

: ratio

– or (–) minus; negative

Ø no; none; not used

= equal

(L) left

(R) right

+ or (+) plus; positive

< less than

> greater than

pounds; number

& and

@ at

~ approximately

Δ change

↓ decrease

° degree

♀ female

♂ male

' foot; minute

≥ greater than or equal to

" inch; second

↑ increase; elevated

≤ less than or equal to

≠ not equal to

μ micron (same as micrometer)

μg microgram

μm micrometer

μqtt microdrop

1° first degree; primary

2° second degree; secondary

A assessment

a̅ ampere; anterior; artery

a̅ before

AA Alcoholics Anonymous

a̅a̅ one of each (ana, Greek)

AAA abdominal aortic aneurysm; American Ambulance Association

ab abortion

abd abdomen

ABG arterial blood gas

AC acromioclavicular

Ac actinium (89)

ac alternating current; antecubital; before meals (ante cibum, Latin)

ACEP American College of Emergency Physicians

ACh acetylcholine

ACH adrenal cortical hormone

AChE acetylcholinesterase

ACLS advanced cardiac life support

ACM air crew member

ACP American College of Physicians

ACS aeormedical communications specialist; American College of Surgeons

ACRV assured crew return vehicle

ACTH adrenocorticotropic hormone

ACV air cushion vehicle

AD right ear (auris dextra, Latin)

ad up to

ADF automatic direction finder

ADH antidiuretic hormone

ad lib as desired; freely (ad libitum, Latin)

AED automatic external defibrillator

AEIOU TIPS acidosis/alcohol, epilepsy, infection, overdose, uremia, trauma, insulin, psychosis, stroke

AF atrial fibrillation

AF 2:1 atrial flutter (with conduction ratio)

A Fib atrial fibrillation

AFFF aqueous film-forming foam

AFRCC Air Force Rescue Coordination Center

Ag silver (argentum, Latin) (47)

AGE arterial gas embolism

AI aortic insufficiency

AICD automatic implantable cardiac defibrillator

AIDS acquired immunodeficiency syndrome

AIS abbreviated injury scale

AIVR accelerated idioventricular rhythm

AJR accelerated junctional rhythm

aka also known as

Al aluminum (13)

ALS advanced life support

ALT alanine aminotransferase (formerly known as SGPT)

ALTE apparently life-threatening event

AM ante-meridian (morning)

Am americium (95)

ama against medical advice

AMA American Medical Association

amb ambulance; ambulatory

AMI acute myocardial infarction

amp ampere; ampule

AMPLE allergies, medications, past medical history, last oral intake (or menstrual period, etc., as appropriate), events before the emergency

AMS acute mountain sickness; atypical measles syndrome

amt amount

AMVER Automated Merchant Vessel Report

ANS autonomic nervous system

ANSI American National Standards Institute

Ant MI anterior myocardial infarction

AO area of operations

A/O x3 alert and oriented to person, place, and day

AOI apnea of infancy

AOP apnea of prematurity

AP anterior to posterior

ap apical; apical pulse

APAP acetaminophen

APR air-purifying respirator

Ar argon (18)

ARC AIDS-related complex

ARDS adult respiratory distress syndrome

ARRS Aerospace Rescue and Recovery Service

art arterial

AS aortic stenosis; left ear (auris sinistra, Latin)

As arsenic (33)

ASA acetylsalicylic acid (aspirin)

ASAP as soon as possible

ASD atrial septal defect

ASHD Arteriosclerotic Heart Disease

AST aspartate aminotransferase (formerly known as SGOT)

AT atrial tachycardia

At astatine (85)

ATA air traffic control area; atmosphere absolute

A-TACH atrial tachycardia

ATC air traffic control

ATF Bureau of Alcohol, Tobacco, and Firearms (U.S.)

ATLS advanced trauma life support

ATM atmosphere (of pressure)

ATP adenosine triphosphate

ATV all-terrain vehicle; automatic transport ventilator

AU both ears; each ear (auris uterque, Latin)

Au gold (79)

A-V atrioventricular (beat; block; bundle; conduction; dissociation; node)

AVB atrioventricular block

AVF augmented vector foot

AVL augmented vector left; automatic vehicle locator

AVPU alert, responds to verbal stimulus, responds to painful stimulus, unresponsive

AVR augmented vector right

Ax assessment

ax axis

B barometric (pressure); boron (5)

Ba barium (56)

BA blood alcohol; breathing apparatus

BBB bundle branch block

BCA bicycle accident

BCLS basic cardiac life support

BDR bedroom

Be beryllium (4)

BFB bifasicular block

Bi bismuth (83)

bid two times daily

bilat bilateral

Bk berkelium (97)

BLEVE boiling liquid expanding vapor explosion

BLS basic life support

bm bowel movement

BMR basal metabolic rate

BOW amniotic sac (bag of waters)

b/p blood pressure

B. P. Border Patrol (U.S.)

BR bathroom

Br bromine (35)

BRIM breathing, response to stimulus, eyes, movement

BS blood sugar; bowel sounds; breath sounds

BSA body surface area

BSH base station hospital

BTLS basic trauma life support

BTU British thermal unit

BUN blood urea nitrogen

BVM bag-valve mask

C calorie (large); carbon (6); Celsius; centigrade

c calorie (small); centi-

c̄ with

C 1 to 7 cervical (nerve, vertebra) (include appropriate number)

C-4 plastic explosive

C/A chest and abdomen

CA cancer; carcinoma; cardiac arrest; chronologic age

Ca calcium (20)

CABG coronary artery bypass graft

CAD coronary artery disease; computer-aided design; computer-aided dispatch

CAF centrifugal acceleratory force

CAGE cerebral arterial gas embolism

cap capsule; Civil Air Patrol (U.S.)

CAPD Continuous Ambulatory Peritoneal Dialysis

CAT clear air turbulence; coaxial tomography; computerized axial tomography (scan)

cath catheter; catheterize

CAVU ceiling and visibility unlimited

CBC complete blood count

CBF cerebral blood flow

CBR Chemical, Biological, Radiological

C/C chief complaint

cc cubic centimeter

CCP casualty collection point

CCT cardiac care technician

CCTV closed circuit television

CCU coronary care unit; critical care unit

Cd cadmium (48)

CDCP Centers for Disease Control and Prevention

Ce cerium (58)

CE continuing education

CEM Comprehensive Emergency Management

CEN Certified Emergency Nurse

CEU continuing education unit

Cf Californium (98)

CFR (aircraft) crash, fire, rescue (operations)

CGS centimeter-gram-second

cgs centimeter-gram-second

CHART chief complaint, history, assessment, treatment, transport

CHB complete heart block

CHEMTREC Chemical Transportation Emergency Center

CHF congestive heart failure

CHS classic (epidemic) heat stroke

CI comfort index

Ci curie

CID cervical immobilization device

CISD critical incident stress debriefing

CIVD cold induced vasodilatation

Cl chloride; chlorine (17)

Cm curium (96)

cm centimeter

CMV controlled mechanical ventilation

CN chloracetophenone (lacrimator)

CNG compressed natural gas

CNS central nervous system

CNT crisis negotiation team

CO carbon monoxide; cardiac output

CO₂ carbon dioxide

Co cobalt (27)

c/o complains of

COLD chronic obstructive lung disease

COPD chronic obstructive pulmonary disease

COSPAS satellite system for search of vessels in distress (Russian)

CP candle power; chest pain; cerebral palsy

CPAP continuous, or constant, positive airway pressure

CPK creatine phosphokinase

CPPV continuous, or constant, positive-pressure ventilation

CPR cardiopulmonary resuscitation

CPU central processing unit (computer)

C/R capillary refill

Cr chromium (24)

CRAMS circulation, respiration, abdomen/chest, motor, speech

CRT cardiac rescue technician

CS orthochlorobenzilidine malanonitrile (lacrimator)

Cs cesium (55)

C & S culture and sensitivity

CSAR combat search and rescue

C section cesarean section

CSF cerebrospinal fluid

CSM carotid sinus massage

CSR central supply room

CT computerized tomography (scan); counterterrorist

CTCSS continuous tone controlled subaudible squelch

CTS clear to send (signal)

Cu copper (29)

CUPS critical/CPR, unstable, potentially unstable, stable

CV cardiovascular

CVA cerebrovascular accident

CVP central venous pressure

CXR chest x-ray

D right (dexter, Latin)

d daily; day

DAN Divers Alert Network

dB decibel

db decibel

DC direct current

D/C discontinue

D & C dilatation and curettage

DCS decompression sickness

DEA Drug Enforcement Agency (U.S.)

D₅W dextrose 5% in water

D₅₀W dextrose 50% in water

DRG diagnosis-related group

DI diabetes insipidus

DIC disseminated intravascular coagulation

diff differential

dig digitalis

DIVP direct intravenous push (without an intravenous line)

DKA diabetic ketoacidosis

DM diabetes mellitus

DMAT Disaster Medical Assistance Team

DME distance measuring equipment

DMT dimethyltryptamine (hallucinogen)

DNA deoxyribonucleic acid

DNAR do not attempt resuscitation

DNIR do not initiate resuscitation

DNR do not resuscitate

DO doctor of osteopathic medicine

DOA dead on arrival

DOB date of birth

DOE Department of Energy (U.S.); dyspnea on exertion

DOM dimethoxymethylamphetamine (hallucinogen)

DOS dead on-scene

DOT Department of Transportation

DR dining room

DT delirium tremens

DTR deep tendon reflex

DUB dysfunctional uterine bleeding

DVT deep vein thrombosis

Dx diagnosis

Dy dysprosium (66)

E/B eastbound

EBL estimated blood loss

EBS emergency broadcast system

EBV Epstein-Barr virus

ECC external cardiac compression

ECF extracellular fluid

ECG electrocardiogram

ECMO extracorporeal-membrane oxygenation

ED effective dose; emergency department

EDC expected date of confinement (delivery date)

EEG electroencephalogram

EENT eye, ear, nose, throat

EGTA esophageal gastric tube airway

EHS exertional heat stroke

EJ external jugular

EKG electrocardiogram (Elektrokardiogramme, German)

elix elixir

ELT emergency locator transmitter

EMD electromechanical dissociation; emergency medical dispatcher

EMG electromyogram

EMS emergency medical services

EMT emergency medical technician

EMT-A emergency medical technician, ambulance

EMT-B emergency medical technician, basic

EMT-D emergency medical technician, defibrillation

EMT-I emergency medical technician, intermediate

EMT-IV emergency medical technician, intravenous (therapy)

EMT-NA emergency medical technician, nonambulance

EMT-P emergency medical technician, paramedic

EMT-R emergency medical technician, rescue

EMT-T emergency medical technician, tactical

EMT-W emergency medical technician, wilderness

ENT ear, nose, throat

EOA esophageal obturator airway

EOAG esophageal obturator airway with gastric tube

EOC emergency operations center

EOD explosive ordnance disposal

EOM extraocular movement

EPI electronic position indicator

EPIRB emergency position indicating radio beacon

EPT effective performance time

ER emergency room

Er erbium (68)

ERV expiratory reserve volume

Es einsteinium (99)

ESRD end-stage renal disease

ET elapsed time; endotracheal (intubation or route)

et and

ETA estimated time of arrival

ETD estimated time down

ETOH alcohol (ethyl)

ETT endotracheal tube

Eu europium (63)

EUD etiology undetermined

exp expiration; expire

F fahrenheit; fluorine (9)

FAA Federal Aviation Administration (U.S.)

fax facsimile

FB foreign body

FBI Federal Bureau of Investigation (U.S.)

FBS fasting blood sugar

FCC Federal Communications Commission (U.S.)

FD fetal dose; fire department; focal distance

FDA Food and Drug Administration (U.S.)

Fe iron (26)

FEF forced expiratory flow

FEMA Federal Emergency Management Agency (U.S.)

FET forced expiratory time

FEV forced expiratory volume

FFP fresh frozen plasma

FFW feet of fresh water

FHR fetal heart rate

FHT fetal heart tones

FiO$_2$ fractional inspired oxygen

FIRESCOPE Firefighting Resources of Southern California Organized for Potential Emergencies

fl fluid

FLIR forward looking infrared radar

Fm fermium (100)

FOD foreign object debris

fps foot-pound-second

Fr francium (87); French (scale)

FRC functional residual capacity

freq frequency; frequent

FSH follicle-stimulating hormone

FSW feet seawater

ft foot

FUO fever of undetermined origin

Fw F wave (fibrillatory wave; flutter wave)

Fx fracture

G gram, gravity

Ga gallium (31)

GB gallbladder

GC gonorrhea

GCA ground control approach

GCS Glasgow coma scale

Gd gadolinium (64)

GE gas embolism; gastroesophageal

Ge germanium (32)

GEM ground effect machine

gest gestation

GI gastrointestinal

gm gram

GOA gone on arrival

GPA gravida, para, abort

GPS global positioning system

gr grain

GSW gunshot wound

gtt drop

gtts drops

GU genitourinary

Gy gray (absorbed dose radiation measurement)

GYN gynecology

H hydrogen (1)

h hour

HA headache

HACE high-altitude cerebral edema

HAPE high-altitude pulmonary edema

HAV hepatitis A virus

HAZMAT hazardous materials (incident)

hbd has been drinking

HBV hepatitis B virus

HCl hydrochloric acid

H₂CO₃ carbonic acid

Hct hematocrit

HCTZ hydrochlorothiazide

HCV hepatitis C virus

HDV hepatitis D virus

He helium (2)

HEAR Hospital Emergency Administrative Radio (network)

HED high-energy defibrillation

HEENT head, eye, ear, nose, throat

HELP heat escape lessening posture (survival)

HEPA high-efficiency particulate mask

HEV hepatitis E virus

Hf hafnium (72)

HFJV high-frequency jet ventilation

Hg mercury (8)

Hgb hemoglobin

HHNC hyperglycemic hyperosmolar nonketotic coma

HHPPV high-frequency positive pressure ventilation

HIFR helicopter in-flight refueling

HIGE hover in ground effect

HIV human immunodeficiency virus

HMO Health Maintenance Organization

HNP herniated nucleus pulposus

H₂O water

H₂O₂ hydrogen peroxide

Ho holmium (67)

HOGE hover out of ground effect

hosp hospital

H & P history and physical

HPNS high-pressure nervous syndrome

hr hour

HRT hostage rescue team

hs bedtime; hour of sleep (hora somni, Latin)

HSV herpes simplex virus

H₂SO₄ sulfuric acid

ht height

HTLV human T cell lymphoma/leukemia virus

HTN hypertension

Hx history

I iodine (53)

IABC intraaortic balloon counterpulsation

IABP intraaortic balloon pump

IAFF International Association of Firefighters

IBL inflatable boat, large

IBS inflatable boat, small

IC incident commander; inspiratory capacity; intracardiac

ICC Interstate Commerce Commission (U.S.)

ICD implantable cardioverter defibrillator; International Classification of Diseases of the World Health Organization

ICDA International Classification of Diseases adapted for use in the United States

ICF intracellular fluid

ICP incident command post; intracranial pressure

ICS incident command system; intercostal space

ICU intensive care unit

ID identification; inside diameter; intradermal

I & D incision and drainage

IDDM insulin-dependent diabetes mellitus

IED improvised explosive device

IEM integrated emergency management

IEP isoelectric point

IFR instrument flight rules

IH infectious hepatitis

ILS instrument landing system

IM intramuscular

IMC instrument meteorological conditions

imp impression

IMS incident management system

IMV intermittent mandatory ventilation

In indium (49)

incis incision

Inf MI inferior myocardial infarction

insp inspiration

int internal

IOP intraocular pressure

IPAP inspiratory positive airway pressure

IPPB intermittent positive-pressure breathing

IPPV intermittent positive-pressure ventilation

IQ intelligence quotient

IR infrared

Ir iridium (77)

irreg irregular

irrig irrigation

IRV inspiratory reserve volume

IS intercostal space

ISA Industry Standards Architecture

ISO International Standards Organization

isol isolation

ISS injury severity scale

IU international unit

IUD intrauterine device

IV intravenous

IVP intravenous push; intravenous pyelogram

IVR idioventricular rhythm

J joule

JB junctional bradycardia

JR junctional rhythm

JT junctional tachycardia

JVD jugular venous distention

JVP jugular venous pressure

K Kelvin; potassium (19)

KCl potassium chloride

KED Kendrick extrication device

kg kilogram

km kilometer

KO keep open

Kr krypton (36)

KUB kidneys, ureter, bladder

KVO keep vein open (intravenous rate)

L liter

l liter

L 1 to 5 lumbar (nerve, vertebra) (with appropriate number)

La lanthanum (57)

lac laceration

LAD left axis deviation

LAF linear acceleratory force

LAHB left anterior hemiblock

LAP left atrial pressure

Lap laparotomy

LAST locate, access, stabilize, transport

lat lateral; latitude

lat MI lateral myocardial infarction

lb pound

LBBB left bundle branch block

LCM left costal margin

LD lethal dose

Ld II lead II (or appropriate number—I, II, III)

LDH lactic dehydrogenase

LEAN Lidocaine, Epinephrine, Atropine, Narcan (modified endotracheal medications)

LEC low energy cardioversion

LEL lower explosive limit

lg large

LH luteinizing hormone

Li lithium (3)

liq liquid

LLL left lower lobe

LLQ left lower quadrant

LMP last menstrual period

LOC level of consciousness; loss of consciousness

long longitude

LORAN long-range navigation system

LP lumbar puncture

LPG liquid propane gas

LPHB left posterior hemiblock

LPM liters per minute

LPN licensed practical nurse
LR lactated Ringer's (solution)
LS lumbosacral; lumbar spine
LSB left sternal border
LSD lysergic acid diethylamide (hallucinogen)
Lu lutecium (71)
LUL left upper lobe
LUQ left upper quadrant
LVAD left ventricular assist device
LVN licensed vocational nurse
LVR living room
Lw lawrencium (103)
LZ landing zone
m meter; milli-; minum
ma milliampere
MA mechanical advantage
MAC maximum allowable concentration
MACS multiagency coordination system
MAE moves all extremities
MAL midaxillary line
MAO monoamine oxidase
MAP mean arterial pressure
MAST medical antishock trousers; military antishock trousers; Military Assistance to Safety and Traffic
MCA motorcycle accident
mcg microgram
MCH mean cell hemoglobin
MCHC mean cell hemoglobin concentration
MCI multiple casualty incident
MCL midclavicular line; modified chest lead
MCV mean clinical value; mean cell volume
MD doctor of medicine
Md mendelevium (101)
MDA methylenedioxyamphetamine (stimulant)
MDI metered-dose inhaler
MDMA methylenedioxymethamphetamine (stimulant)
MED minimal effective dose; minimal erythema dose
med medication; medical
MEP maximal expiratory pressure
meq milliequivalent
mEq milliequivalent
Mg magnesium (12)
mg milligram
MI myocardial infarction
MICMD mobile intensive care physician
MICN mobile intensive care nurse
MICP mobile intensive care paramedic
MICU medical intensive care unit; mobile intensive care unit
min minimum; minute

MIP maximum inspiratory pressure
mks meter-kilogram-second
ml milliliter
mm millimeter
Mn manganese (25)
Mo molybdenum (42)
MOB man overboard
mod moderate
MRI magnetic resonance imaging
MS morphine sulfate; multiple sclerosis
MSDS material safety data sheet
MSE mental status exam
MSL midsternal line
MSO$_4$ morphine sulfate
MTV manual transport ventilator
MVA motor vehicle accident
MVP mitral valve prolapse
N nitrogen (7)
N/A no answer; not applicable
Na sodium (11)
NAD no acute/apparent distress; no appreciable disease
NaHCO$_3$ sodium bicarbonate
NALS Neonatal Advanced Life Support
NASAR National Association of Search and Rescue
NAT nonaccidental trauma
NAVEL Narcan, Atropine, Valium, Epinephrine, Lidocaine (endotracheal medications)
N/B northbound
Nb niobium (41)
NBC nuclear, biological, chemical
NC nasal cannula
Nd neodymium (60)
NDB nondirectional beacon
NDMS National Disaster Medical System
Ne neon (10)
NFPA National Fire Protection Association
NG nasogastric
NGT nasogastric tube
NGU nongonococcal arthritis
NH$_3$ ammonia
Ni nickel (28)
NIDDM non-insulin-dependent diabetes mellitus
NIH National Institutes of Health (U.S.)
NIIMS National Interagency Incident Management System (U.S.)
NIOSH National Institute for Occupational Safety and Health
nitro nitroglycerin(e)
NKA no known allergies
NKDA no known drug allergies
NKHC nonketotic hyperosmolar coma
NMR nuclear magnetic resonance (imaging)
No nobelium (102)

N$_2$O nitrous oxide
Np neptunium (93)
NPO nothing by mouth
npt normal pressure and temperature
NRC National Response Center
NRFM non-rebreather face mask
NS normal saline
NSAID nonsteroidal antiinflammatory drug
NSP National Ski Patrol
NSR normal sinus rhythm
NSU nonspecific urethritis
NTG nitroglycerin(e)
N/V nausea and vomiting
NVD neck vein distention
NWS National Weather Service
O oxygen (8); objective findings
O$_2$ oxygen
OA on arrival
OB obstetrics
OBA oxygen breathing apparatus
OBS organic brain syndrome
OC oleoresin capsicum (pepper gas) (lacrimator)
OCC occasional; operations coordination center
OD overdose (drug ingestion); right eye (oculus dexter, Latin)
OMS organic mental syndrome
ON every night (omni nocte, Latin)
OPP organophosphate poisoning
OR operating room
OS left eye (oculus sinister, Latin)
Os osmium (76)
OSHA Occupational Safety and Health Administration (U.S.)
OTC over the counter
OU both eyes (oculus uterque, Latin)
oz ounce
P plan; phosphorus (15); pressure; pulse; pupil
$\bar{p}$ after
P1 first pulmonic heart sound
P2 second pulmonic heart sound
P$_{50}$ oxygen tension at 50% hemoglobin saturation
PA posterior to anterior; Physician Assistant
Pa protactinium (91)
PAC premature atrial contraction
P$_a$CO$_2$ arterial carbon dioxide level (partial pressure)
P$_A$CO$_2$ alveolar carbon dioxide level (partial pressure)
PAL posterior axillary line
palp palpation
PALS Pediatric Advanced Life Support
P$_a$O$_2$ arterial oxygen level (partial pressure)

P_AO_2 alveolar oxygen level (partial pressure)

PAP pulmonary artery pressure

PASG pneumatic antishock garment

PAT paroxysmal atrial tachycardia

PB periodic breathing

Pb lead (82)

pc after meals (post cibum, Latin)

PCB polychlorinated biphenyl; printed circuit board

PCO_2 partial pressure carbon dioxide

PCP phencyclidine (stimulant/hallucinogen)

PCV packed cell volume

PCWP pulmonary capillary wedge pressure

PD police department

Pd palladium (46)

PDR *Physician's Desk Reference*

PE physical exam; pulmonary edema; pulmonary embolus

PEA pulseless electrical activity (formerly EMD)

pedi pediatric

PEL permissible exposure limit

PEEP positive end-expiratory pressure

PEFR peak expiratory flow rate

per according, by; through

PERL pupils equal and reactive to light

PERRLA pupils equal, round, reactive to light and accommodation

PFD personal flotation device

pH the hydrogen ion concentration of a liquid (gram equivalents/liter)

PHAD prehospital advanced directive

Pharm D doctor of pharmacy

PHI Prehospital Index (trauma scoring system)

PHTLS Prehospital Trauma Life Support

PID pelvic inflammatory disease

PJC premature junctional contraction

PKU phenylketonuria

PL private line tone

PLS point last seen; preloaded syringe; prolonged life support

PM paramedic; postmeridian (afternoon or evening)

Pm promethium (61)

PMH past medical history

PMI point of maximal impulse

PMS premenstrual syndrome; preventive maintenance

PND paroxysmal nocturnal dyspnea

Po polonium (84)

po by mouth; orally (per os)

PO_2 partial pressure oxygen

POA probability of area

POB persons onboard (aircraft)

POD probability of detection

POPS pulmonary overpressurization syndrome

POS probability of success

postop after surgery; post operative

POV privately owned vehicle

PPD purified protein derivative

PPE personal protective equipment

PPF plasma protein fraction

ppm parts per million

PPPPP pain, pallor, pulselessness, paresthesia, paralysis

PPV positive pressure ventilation

PQRST provokes, quality, region/radiation/recurrence, severity, time; cardiac electrical cycle

Pr praseodymium (59)

pr per rectum

preop before surgery; preoperative

PRH paramedic receiving hospital

prn as necessary

PSI pounds per square inch

PSIG pounds per square inch, gauge

PSV pressure supported ventilation

PSVT paroxysmal supraventricular tachycardia

PT patient; physical therapy; physical training; pint

Pt platinum (78)

PTA prior to arrival

PTCA percutaneous transluminal coronary angioplasty

PTLA pharyngeotracheal lumen airway

PTS pediatric trauma score

PTT partial thromboplastin time

PTV percutaneous transtracheal ventilation

P/U pickup (truck)

Pu plutonium (94)

PUD peptic ulcer disease

PVC polyvinyl chloride; premature ventricular contraction

$PvCO_2$ venous carbon dioxide (partial pressure)

PvO_2 venous oxygen (partial pressure)

PVR peripheral vascular resistance

Px physical exam

Q coulomb

q every

QA quality assurance

qd every day (quaque die, Latin)

qh every hour (quaque hora, Latin)

QI quality improvement

qid four times daily (quater in die, Latin)

ql as much as one pleases (quantum libet, Latin)

qm every morning (quaque matin, Latin)

qn every night (quaque nox, Latin)

qod every other day

qoh every other hour

qs as much as necessary; sufficient quantity (quantum sufficit, Latin)

qt quart

qtt drop

qv as much as you like (quantum vis, Latin)

R Rankine; respiration; roentgen

Ra radium (88)

RAD radiation absorbed dose; right axis deviation

RAM random access memory

Rb rubidium (37)

RBBB right bundle branch block

RBC red blood cell; red blood count

RBE relative biologic effectiveness

RCM right costal margin

RDF radio direction finder

Re rhenium (75)

REL recommended exposure limit

REM roentgen equivalent man; rapid eye movement

RES reticuloendothelial system

RESCAP rescue combat air patrol

resp respirations

Rh rhesus (factor); rhodium (45)

RHD rheumatic heart disease

RL Ringer's lactate

RLF retrolental fibroplasia

RLL right lower lobe

RLQ right lower quadrant

RML right middle lobe

RMP resting membrane potential

RN registered nurse

Rn radon (86)

RNA ribonucleic acid

RNAV area navigation

R/O rule out

ROM range of motion; read-only memory

ROS review of systems

ROSC return of spontaneous circulation

rpm revolutions per minute

RPM respiratory, pulse, motor (trauma scoring system)

RR respiratory rate

RSB right sternal border

RSM respiratory, systolic pressure, motor (trauma scoring system)

RSV respiratory syncytial virus

RTS request-to-send (signal); revised trauma score

Ru ruthenium (44)

RUL right upper lobe

RUQ right upper quadrant

RV recreational vehicle; residual volume

Rx prescription; to take (recipe, Latin); treatment

S̱ subjective findings, sulfur (16)

s̱ without (sine, Latin)

S 1 to 5 sacral (nerve, vertebra) (with appropriate number)

SA sinoatrial (node); sinus arrhythmia

SAMPLE signs/symptoms, allergies, medications, past medical history, last meal (or menstrual period, pain, etc. as appropriate), events before the emergency

SAP systemic arterial pressure

SAR search and rescue; supplied air respirator

SARSAT search and rescue satellite

SART search and rescue transponder

sat satisfactory, saturated

SB sinus bradycardia

S/B southbound

Sb antimony (51)

SC subcutaneous

Sc scandium (21)

SCBA self-contained breathing apparatus

SCF standard cubic foot

SCFM standard cubic foot per minute

SCM sternocleidomastoid

SCUBA self-contained underwater breathing apparatus

SD sheriff's department; standard deviation

Se selenium (34)

sec second

SGOT serum glutamic-oxyloacetic transaminase (now known as AST)

SGPT serum glutamic-pyruvic transaminase (now known as ALT)

SI International System of Units

Si silicon (14)

SICU surgical intensive care unit

SIDS sudden infant death syndrome

sig let it be labeled

SIMV spontaneous (synchronized) intermittent mandatory ventilation

SIPDE search, identify, predict, decide, execute (system, driving)

SK streptokinase

SL sublingual

SLE systemic lupus erythematosus

SLUDGE salivation, lacrimation, urination, diaphoresis, gastrointestinal symptoms, emesis

SM simple mask (oxygen)

Sm samarium (62)

Sn tin (50)

SO sheriff's office

SOAP subjective, objective, assessment, plan

SOB shortness of breath; souls on-board

SOFAR sound fixing and ranging

sol solution

SOLAS Safety of Life At Sea (agreements/conference)

soln solution

SOP standard operating procedure

SOS help; maritime distress call; if necessary (si opus sit, Latin)

sp gr specific gravity

SQ subcutaneous

SR sinus rhythm

Sr strontium (38)

SROM spontaneous rupture of membranes

SRS supplemental restraint system

S/S signs and symptoms

s̅s̅ half (semis, Latin)

SSB single side band (radio)

SSS sick sinus syndrome

ST sinus tachycardia

START simple triage and rapid treatment (system)

stat immediately (statim, Latin); now

STC supplemental type certificate

STCC Standard Transportation Commodity Code (number)

STD sexually transmitted disease

STEL short-term exposure limit

STP dimethoxymethylamphetamine (hallucinogen); standard temperature and pressure

STPD standard temperature and pressure, dry

sub q subcutaneous

supp suppository

SV sievert (radiation measurement)

SVR systemic vascular resistance

SVT supraventricular tachycardia

SWAT Special Weapons and Tactics (Team)

Sx seizure; symptoms

T temperature

T 1 to 12 thoracic (vertebrae) (include appropriate number)

Ta tantalum (73)

tab tablet

TACAN tactical air navigation

TB tuberculosis

Tb terbium (65)

tbsp tablespoon

TBV total blood volume

T & C type and crossmatch

Tc technetium (43)

TCA terminal control area; tricyclic antidepressant

TD therapeutic dose

Te tellurium (52)

temp temperature; temporary

TFB trifasicular block

Th thorium (90)

THC tetrahydrocannabinol (hallucinogen)

Ti titanium (22)

TIA transient ischemic attack

tid three times daily (ter in die, Latin)

TKO to keep open (intravenous rate)

Tl thallium (81)

TLC total lung capacity

TLJV translaryngeal jet ventilation

TLV threshold-limit value

TLV/C threshold-limit value/ceiling

TLV/STEL threshold-limit value/short term exposure limit

TLV/TWA threshold-limit value/time weighted average

Tm thulium (69)

TM tympanic membrane

TMJ temporomandibular joint

TOD time of death

TPA thermal protective aid; tissue plasminogen activator

TPR temperature, pulse, respiration

tr tincture; trail

TRISS Trauma Score/Injury Severity Score

TSH thyroid-stimulating hormone

tsp teaspoon

TSR terminate and stay resident (computer driver)

TSS toxic shock syndrome

TT transtracheal

TTP thrombotic thrombocytopenic purpura

TUC time of useful consciousness

TV tidal volume

TVI total volume infused

Tx transport; treatment

U unit; uranium (92)

UA urinalysis

UAO upper airway obstruction

UEL upper explosive limit

ug microgram (also µg, mcg)

UHF ultra-high frequency

um micrometer (also µm)

UPS uninterruptible power supply

uqtt microdrop (also µqtt)

URI upper respiratory infection

USAR urban search and rescue

USP United States Pharmacopeia

ut dict as dictated

UTI urinary tract infection

UTL unable to locate
UVA ultraviolet A radiation
UVB ultraviolet B radiation
UVC ultraviolet C radiation
UVR ultraviolet radiation
V vanadium (23)
v vein (vena, Latin); volt
VAD ventricular-assist device
VC vital capacity
VD venereal disease
vent ventilate; ventilator
V Fib ventricular fibrillation
V Tach ventricular tachycardia
VF ventricular fibrillation
VFR visual flight rules
VHF very high frequency
VHF omnirange very high frequency omnidirectional range

via by way of
VMC visual meteorological conditions
VNE velocity never exceeds
VOR very high frequency omnidirectional range
VORTAC very high frequency omnidirectional range/tactical air navigation
VR ventilation rate
V/S vital signs
vs versus (Latin)
VSD ventricular septal defect
VT tidal volume; ventricular tachycardia
VV volume ventilator
W tungsten (74)
w watt; week
W/B westbound

WAP wandering atrial pacemaker
WATS Wide Area Telephone Service
WBC white blood cell; white blood count
WCOE working capacity over an edge
WNL within normal limits
WPW Wolff-Parkinson-White (syndrome)
wt weight
x times
Xe xenon (54)
Y yttrium (39)
Yb ytterbium (70)
yd yard
y/o year(s) old
z zone
Zn zinc (30)
Zr zirconium (40)

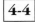 **4-4** **Anatomical Terminology**

abduction movement away from the midline
adduction movement toward the midline
anterior front
anterior to located in front of
caudad toward the tail; posterior
cephalad toward the head; superior
circumduction circular movement of a part, such as the eye
craniad toward the cranium
deep remote from the surface
depression lowering a body part
distal located away from the point of origin
dorsal back
dorsiflexion bending backward, as the foot
elevation raising a body part
erect standing
eversion turning outward, as the foot

extension moving parts away from one another; stretching
external outside
flexion moving parts closer to one another; bending
inferior below; toward the feet
internal inside
inversion turning inward, as the foot
lateral located toward the side; away from the midline
laterally recumbent lying horizontal on the right or left side
lateral rotation rotating outward away from the midline
medial located toward the midline
medial rotation rotating inward toward the midline
palmar the palm of the hand
peripheral away from the central area

plantar the sole of the foot
plantar flexion extending the foot
posterior back
posterior to located behind
pronation turning the hand (palm) downward or backward
prone lying face down
protraction pushing forward
proximal located toward the point of origin
recumbent lying generally horizontal
retraction pulling back
rotation turning around an axis
superficial near the surface
superior above; toward the head
supination turning the hand (palm) forward or upward
supine lying face up
ventral front

4-5 | Communication Prowords

These introductory and rudimentary words or phrases are used in special operations when communicating via radio or in any situation where absolute clarity of communication is a necessity. These words have an assigned meaning and are used because of their clarity when transmitted over the air.

affirmative Correct; yes.

all after Everything that follows.

all before Everything that precedes.

break Indicates a separation of the text just transmitted from other portions of the message.

clear Excellent quality transmission.

copy I have received your message, I understand it, and/or I will comply with it.

correct You are correct, or what you have transmitted is correct.

correction An error has been made in this transmission. The transmission will continue with the last word correctly sent. The correct version is. . . .

disregard this transmission This transmission is in error. Disregard it. [This is not used to cancel any message that has been completely transmitted and received.]

distorted Poor quality transmission.

figures Numerals follow.

from The originator of this message will be indicated by the address designation following.

good Transmission is good.

I read back I am repeating your instructions or message.

I say again I am repeating my transmission or portion indicated.

I spell I will spell the preceding word phonetically. [Use phonetic alphabet.]

leader The transmission following is for the group or team leader.

loud Transmission is strong.

message A message that requires recording is about to follow [immediately after this proword].

negative Incorrect; no.

out This is the end of my transmission to you, and no answer is required or expected.

over This is the end of my transmission to you and a response is necessary: Go ahead and transmit.

readable Good-quality transmission.

read back Repeat this entire transmission back to me exactly as received.

relay (to) Transmit this message to all involved or to the address designations immediately following.

roger I have received your transmission satisfactorily.

say again Repeat all of your last transmission.

silence [spoken three times] Cease transmission immediately. [Silence should be maintained until instructed to resume.]

silence lifted Resume normal transmissions. [Silence may be lifted only by the person or station imposing it or by a higher authority.]

speak slowly Reduce speed of transmission; it is too fast.

team The transmission following is for the entire group or team.

that is correct You are correct, or what you have transmitted is correct.

this is This transmission is from the person or station whose designation immediately follows.

time What follows is the time of the message.

to Those whose designations immediately follow are to be advised and/or take action on this message.

unknown station The identity of the person or station with whom I am attempting to establish communications is unknown.

very weak Transmission can be heard with great difficulty.

wait I must pause for a few seconds.

wait out I must pause longer than a few seconds.

weak Transmission can be heard with difficulty.

words twice Communications are difficult [high background noise, poor reception, or slow copying]. Transmit each phrase twice.

wrong Your last transmission was incorrect. The correct version is. . . .

(Modified from U.S. Coast Guard Institute, *Communications and Navigation*, p. 75-76, 1986.)

4-6 Phonetic Alphabet and Morse Code

Phonetic	Character	Morse code
ALPHA	A	· –
BRAVO	B	– · · ·
CHARLIE	C	– · – ·
DELTA	D	– · ·
ECHO	E	·
FOXTROT	F	· · – ·
GOLF	G	– – ·
HOTEL	H	· · · ·
INDIA	I	· ·
JULIET	J	· – – –
KILO	K	– · –
LIMA	L	· – · ·
MIKE	M	– –
NOVEMBER	N	– ·
OSCAR	O	– – –
PAPA	P	· – – ·
QUEBEC	Q	– – · –
ROMEO	R	· – ·
SIERRA	S	· · ·
TANGO	T	–
UNIFORM	U	· · –
VICTOR	V	· · · –
WHISKEY	W	· – –
XRAY	X	– · · –
YANKEE	Y	– · – –
ZULU	Z	– – · ·
ONE	1	· – – – –
TWO	2	· · – – –
THREE	3	· · · – –
FOUR	4	· · · · –
FIVE	5	· · · · ·
SIX	6	– · · · ·
SEVEN	7	– – · · ·
EIGHT	8	– – – · ·
NINE	9	– – – – ·
ZERO	0	– – – – –

4-7 **Sign Language (Manual) Alphabet**

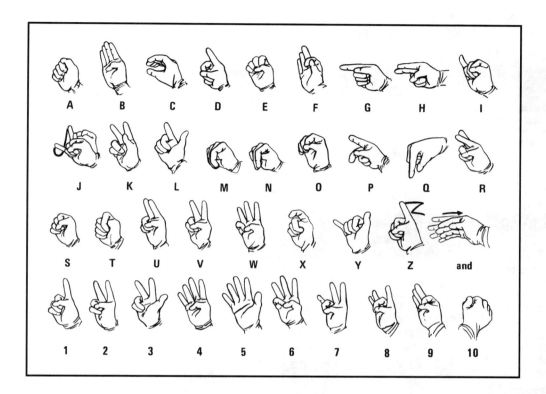

(From Mosby Year-Book Inc., *Advanced Sport Diver Manual*, Clinchy/Engstrom, 2nd Ed., p. 58, St. Louis, 1993)

4-8 Ground-to-Air Distress Signals I & II and Body Signals

I-PANEL SIGNALS

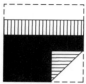

On Land: Walking
in this direction
At Sea: Drifting

Survivors use liferaft
sails to convey signals

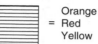 = Orange
Red
Yellow   side   = blue side

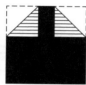

On Land: Need
quinine or atabrine
At Sea: Need
sun cover

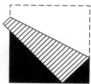

On Land: Need
warm clothing
At Sea: Need
exposure suit or
clothing indicated

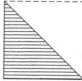

On Land & at Sea:
Plane is flyable,
need tools

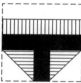

On Land & at Sea:
Need food
and water

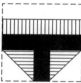

On Land: Need
gas and oil,
plane is flyable

On Land & at Sea:
Need medical
attention

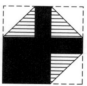

On Land & at Sea:
Need first aid
supplies

At Sea: Need
equipment as
indicated.
Signals follow

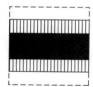

On land: Indicate
direction of
nearest civilization
At Sea: Indicate
direction of
rescue craft

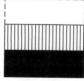

On land: should
we wait for
rescue plane?
At Sea: Notify
rescue agency
of my position

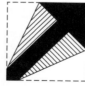

On land & at Sea:
O.K. to land,
arrow shows
landing direction

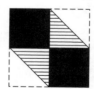

Land & Sea:
Do not
attempt landing

Continued

(Modified From U.S. Navy, Survival Training Guide, NAVWEPS 00-80T-56, p. 4-10, 1961)

Ground-to-Air Distress Signals I & II and Body Signals—cont'd

II-GROUND/AIR EMERGENCY CODE

I 1. Require doctor—serious injuries	**II** 2. Require medical supplies	**X** 3. Unable to proceed	**F** 4. Require food and water	**≋** 5. Require firearms and ammunition	**K** 6. Indicate direction to proceed
↑ 7. Am proceeding in this direction	**I)** 8. Will attempt to take off	**L7** 9. Aircraft badly damaged	**△** 10. Probably safe to land here	**LL** 11. All Well	**L** 12. Require fuel and oil
N 13. No—negative	**Y** 14. Yes—affirmative	**⅃L** 15. Not understood	**W** 16. Require engineer	**□** 17. Require compass and map	**⋮** 18. Require signal lamp

(Modified From U.S. Navy, *Survival Training Guide*, NAVWEPS 00-80T-56, p. 4-11 through 4-12, 1961)

Lay out these symbols using materials at hand, such as cloth strips, parachutes, stones, and wood. Provide as much color contrast as possible between the symbols and their background. These symbols should be at least 8 feet in height. Continue to use other means at hand to attract attention (fire, flares, mirror, radio). Fixed-wing rescue aircraft indicate understanding of message by rocking from side to side or flashing a green signal light. Confusion about message is indicated by the aircraft making a complete right-hand circuit or flashing a red signal light.

Ground-to-Air Distress Signals I & II and Body Signals—cont'd

BODY SIGNALS

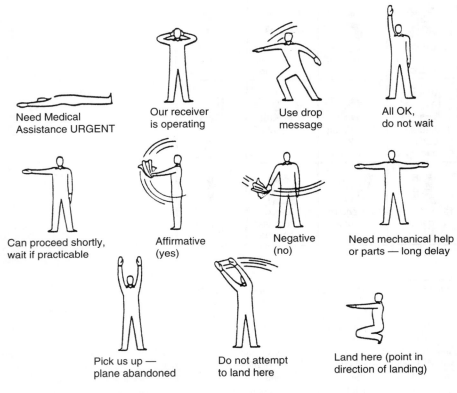

Need Medical
Assistance URGENT

Our receiver
is operating

Use drop
message

All OK,
do not wait

Can proceed shortly,
wait if practicable

Affirmative
(yes)

Negative
(no)

Need mechanical help
or parts — long delay

Pick us up —
plane abandoned

Do not attempt
to land here

Land here (point in
direction of landing)

(Modified From U.S. Navy, *Survival Training Guide*, NAVWEPS 00-80T-56, p. 4-11 through 4-12, 1961)

4-9   Maritime Distress Signals

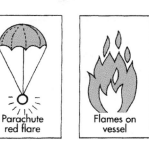

Flares and fire

Red flare

Parachute red flare

Flames on vessel

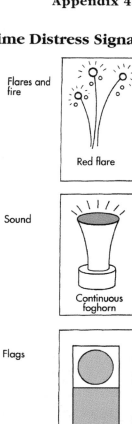

Sound

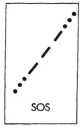

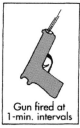

Continuous foghorn

Gun fired at 1-min. intervals

SOS

Flags

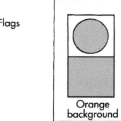

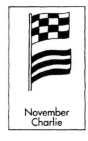

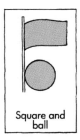

Orange background

November Charlie

Square and ball

Other

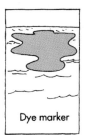

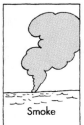

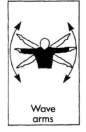

Dye marker

Smoke

Wave arms

Radio

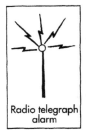

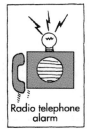

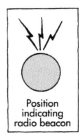

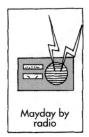

Radio telegraph alarm

Radio telephone alarm

Position indicating radio beacon

Mayday by radio

(From: Mosby Year-Book, Inc., *Wilderness Medicine: Management of Wilderness and Environmental Emergencies;* Auerbach; Survival at Sea, Oslund, Scott A. and Brooks, Christopher J., 3rd Ed., p. 1292, St. Louis, 1995. Courtesy U.S. Coast Guard.)

4-10 | Helicopter Landing/Takeoff Signals

Signal	From	To	Day	Night	Remarks
THUMBS DOWN	Landing Safety Officer	Pilot	Holds fist at shoulder level with thumb extended down.	Holds wand in "thumbs down" position.	Indicates that all is *not* OK.
READY TO ENGAGE ROTORS	Pilot	Landing Safety Officer	Moves hand in horizontal circle with index finger extended at eye level.	Same as day except hold red light in hand.	
ENGAGE ROTOR	Landing Safety Officer	Pilot	Facing pilot, holds left fist clenched above head. Moves right hand in horizontal circle with index finger at eye level.	Facing pilot, holds red wand in left hand above head. Moves right hand in horizontal circle with index finger at eye level.	Prior to giving signal, landing safety officer checks all rotor clearances and ensures that all unnecessary personnel and equipment are clear.
MOVE DOWNWARD	Landing Safety Officer	Pilot	Arms extended horizontally sideways beckoning downward, with palms turned down. Speed of movement indicates rate of descent.	Same as day except with wands.	
MOVE UPWARD	Landing Safety Officer	Pilot	Arms extended horizontally sideways beckoning upward, with palms turned up. Speed of movement indicates rate of ascent.	Same as day except with wands.	

Helicopter Landing/Takeoff Signals—cont'd

Signal	From	To	Day	Night	Remarks
MOVE TO LEFT	Landing Safety Officer	Pilot	Right arm extended horizontally sideways in direction of movement and other arm swung over the head in same direction, in a repeating movement.	Same as day except with wands.	
MOVE TO RIGHT	Landing Safety Officer	Pilot	Left arm extended horizontally sideways in direction of movement and other arm swung over the head in same direction, in a repeating movement.	Same as day except with wands.	
MOVE FORWARD	Landing Safety Officer	Pilot	With hands at head level and palms toward face, make closing motions toward head.	Same as day except with wands.	
MOVE BACK	Landing Safety Officer	Pilot	Arms by sides, palms facing forward, swept forward and upward repeatedly to shoulder height.	Same as day except with wands.	

Continued

Helicopter Landing/Takeoff Signals—cont'd

Signal	From	To	Day	Night	Remarks
TURN TO RIGHT OR LEFT	Landing Safety Officer	Pilot	Arm extended horizontally sideways in direction of movement and other arm swung over the head in the same direction, in a repeating movement.	Same as day except with wands.	
HOVER	Landing Safety Officer	Pilot	Arms extended horizontally sideways, palms downward.	Same as day except with wands.	

(Modified from U.S. Coast Guard Institute, *Aircraft Ground Handling and Firefighting*, p. 10-14, 1986.)